IADVL Atlas of DERMOSCOPY

Indian Association of Dermatologists, Venereologists and Leprologists

IADVL Atlas of DERMOSCOPY

Editor-in-Chief

Balachandra S Ankad MD
Professor and Head
Department of Dermatology
S Nijalingappa Medical College
Bagalkot, Karnataka, India

Associate Editor

Yasmeen J Bhat MD FACP
Associate Professor
Department of Dermatology, Venereology and Leprosy
Government Medical College
Srinagar, Jammu and Kashmir, India

Assistant Editor

Kinjal D Rambhia MD DNB
Fellowship in Diagnostic Dermatology (MUHS) Professional Diploma in Clinical Research
Assistant Professor
Department of Dermatology
HBT Medical College and Dr RN Cooper Hospital
Mumbai, Maharashtra, India

Foreword

Enzo Errichetti

Under the Aegis of IADVL Academy

JAYPEE BROTHERS MEDICAL PUBLISHERS
The Health Sciences Publisher
New Delhi | London

JAYPEE Jaypee Brothers Medical Publishers (P) Ltd

Headquarters
EMCA House
23/23-B, Ansari Road, Daryaganj
New Delhi 110 002, India
Landline: +91-11-23272143, +91-11-23272703
+91-11-23282021, +91-11-23245672
E-mail: jaypee@jaypeebrothers.com

Corporate Office
Jaypee Brothers Medical Publishers (P) Ltd.
4838/24, Ansari Road, Daryaganj
New Delhi 110 002, India
Phone: +91-11-43574357
Fax: +91-11-43574314
E-mail: jaypee@jaypeebrothers.com

Overseas Office
JP Medical Ltd.
83, Victoria Street, London
SW1H 0HW (UK)
Phone: +44-20 3170 8910
E-mail: info@jpmedpub.com

EU GPSR Authorised Representative
Logos Europe, 9 rue Nicolas Poussin
17000, La Rochelle, France
Phone: +33 (0) 6 67 93 73 78
E-mail: Contact@logoseurope.eu

Website: www.jaypeebrothers.com
Website: www.jaypeedigital.com

Inquiries for bulk sales may be solicited at: jaypee@jaypeebrothers.com

***IADVL Atlas of Dermoscopy* / Balachandra S Ankad**

First Edition: **2022**

Reprint: **2026**

ISBN: 978-93-90595-64-8

Printed at: Replika Press Pvt. Ltd.

CONTRIBUTORS

EDITOR-IN-CHIEF

Balachandra S Ankad MD
Professor and Head
Department of Dermatology
S Nijalingappa Medical College
Bagalkot, Karnataka, India

ASSOCIATE EDITOR

Yasmeen J Bhat MD FACP
Associate Professor
Department of Dermatology, Venereology and Leprosy
Government Medical College
Srinagar, Jammu and Kashmir, India

ASSISTANT EDITOR

Kinjal D Rambhia MD DNB Fellowship in Diagnostic Dermatology (MUHS) Professional Diploma in Clinical Research
Assistant Professor
Department of Dermatology
HBT Medical College and Dr RN Cooper Hospital
Mumbai, Maharashtra, India

CONTRIBUTING AUTHORS

Abhijeet Kumar Jha MD
Assistant Professor
Department of Dermatology
Patna Medical College
Patna, Bihar, India

Anuradha Bishnoi MD
Assistant Professor
Department of Dermatology
Venereology and Leprology
Postgraduate Institute of Medical
Education and Research
Chandigarh, India

Anuradha Jindal MD FRGUHS
Co-founder and Chief Dermatologist
Skin Win Clinics, Santhekatte and Udupi
Karnataka, India

Ashwini PK MD FRGUHS
Associate Professor
Department of Dermatology
JSS Medical College
JSS Academy of Higher Education and
Research
Mysuru, Karnataka, India

Aswath Rajan MD
Senior Resident
Goa Medical College
Bambolim, Goa, India

Atul Bothra MD FRGUHS
Chief Dermatologist
Skin Square Clinic
Guwahati, Assam, India

Balachandra S Ankad MD
Professor and Head
Department of Dermatology
S Nijalingappa Medical College
Bagalkot, Karnataka, India

Biswanath Behera MD DNB
Assistant Professor
Department of Dermatology and
Venereology
All India Institute of Medical Sciences
Bhubaneswar, Odisha, India

Chander Grover MD DNB MNAMS
Professor
Department of Dermatology and STD
University College of Medical Sciences
and GTB Hospital, New Delhi, India

Debjit Kar MD
Chief Consultant Dermatologist
DEBJIT DERMA 360
Department of Dermatology
JP Hospital
Rourkela, Odisha, India

Deepak Jakhar MD
Co-founder and Medical Director
Dermosphere Clinic
New Delhi, India

Devayani Pol MD
Assistant Professor
Department of Dermatology
Dr DY Patil Medical College, Hospital and Research Center, Pimpri
Pune, Maharashtra, India

Dilip Kumar NR MD DDVL
Assistant Professor
Department of Dermatology
Akash Institute of Medical Sciences and Research Center
Bengaluru, Karnataka, India

Dincy Peter CV MD
Professor
Department of Dermatology, Venereology and Leprosy
Christian Medical College
Vellore, Tamil Nadu, India

Dipali Rathod DNB DDVL
Assistant Professor
Department of Dermatology
Seth GS Medical College; KEM Hospital
Mumbai, Maharashtra, India

Faizan Younus Shah MD
Senior Resident
Department of Dermatology, Venereology and Leprosy
Government Medical College
Srinagar, Jammu and Kashmir, India

Harshit D Ranpara MD DVD
Diplomate of the American Board of Hair Restoration Surgery
Consultant Dermatologist
Rajkot, Gujarat, India

Ishmeet Kaur MD
Assistant Professor
Department of Dermatology
NDMC Medical College and Hindu Rao Hospital
New Delhi, India

Kinjal D Rambhia MD DNB Fellowship in Diagnostic Dermatology (MUHS) Professional Diploma in Clinical Research
Assistant Professor
Department of Dermatology
HBT Medical College and Dr RN Cooper Hospital
Mumbai, Maharashtra, India

Kumudhini Subramanian MD DVL FAGE DNB DVL FRGUHS
Chief Dermatologist
Deep Skin Dialogues
Chennai, Tamil Nadu, India

Malcom Noronha MD FRGUHS
Consultant Dermatologist
Skin Win Clinic
Udupi, Karnataka, India

Brig Dr Manas Chatterjee MD DNB
Brig Medical HQ 14 Corps
Consultant Dermatologist
153 General Hospital
C/O 56 APO

Mansi Kansal MD
Consultant Dermatologist
Kansal ENT and Skin Center
Patiala, Punjab, India

Muhammed Razmi T MD DNB MNAMS
Consultant Dermatologist and Clinical Head
IQRAA Aesthetics
IQRAA International Hospital
Kozhikode, Kerala, India

Nirmal B MD FRGUHS
Consultant Dermatologist and Head
Department of Dermatology
Meenakshi Mission Hospital and Dermal Square Skin Clinic
Madurai, Tamil Nadu, India

Niti Khunger MD DNB DDV
Consultant Dermatologist
Professor and Head
Department of Dermatology and STD
Vardhman Mahavir Medical College
Safdarjung Hospital
New Delhi, India

Priyanka Jaju MD FRGUHS
Consultant Aesthetic Dermatologist
Leelawanti Skin and Laser Center
New Delhi, India

Rachita Dhurat MD
Professor and Head
Department of Dermatology
LTM Medical College and LTMG Hospital Sion
Mumbai, Maharashtra, India

Samipa S Mukherjee MBBS DDV DDVL (CMC, Vellore) FRGUHS (Pediatric Dermatology)
Chief Dermatologist and Director
Dr Samipa's – The Skin Hair Nail Clinic
Consultant Pediatric Dermatologist
Cloudnine Hospitals
Bengaluru, Karnataka, India

Sanjeev Gupta MD DNB
Professor and Head
Department of Dermatology
MMIMSR, Mullana
Ambala, Haryana, India

Savitha L Beergouder MBBS DDVL
Consultant Dermatologist
Anagha Skin and Cosmetic Clinic
Bagalkot, Karnataka, India

Shagufta Rather MD
Associate Professor
Department of Dermatology, Venereology and Leprosy
Government Medical College
Srinagar, Jammu and Kashmir, India

Sharmila Patil MD DDV
Professor and Head
Department of Dermatology
Dr DY Patil Medical College, Nerul
Navi Mumbai, Maharashtra, India

Shazia Jeelani MD
Assistant Professor
Department of Dermatology, Venereology and Leprosy
Government Medical College
Srinagar, Jammu and Kashmir, India

Shekhar Neema MD
Associate Professor
Department of Dermatology
Armed Forces Medical College
Pune, Maharashtra, India

Shishira R Jartarkar MD DNB
Assistant Professor
Department of Dermatology
Vydehi Institute of Medical Sciences and Research Center
Bengaluru, Karnataka, India

Shital Poojary MD DNB FCPS
Professor and Head
Department of Dermatology
KJ Somaiya Medical College
Mumbai, Maharashtra, India

Smitha S Prabhu MD DVD
Additional Professor
Department of Dermatology and Venereology
Kasturba Medical College
Manipal
Manipal Academy of Higher Education
Mangalore, Karnataka, India

Soumil Khare MD
Assistant Professor
Department of Dermatology
BRLSABVM Government Medical College and Hospital
Rajnandgaon, Chhattisgarh, India

Suman Patra MD DNB MRCP SCE
Assistant Professor
Department of Dermatology, Venereology and Leprology
All India Institute of Medical Sciences
Jodhpur, Rajasthan, India

Sunanda Mahajan MD DVD
Additional Professor
Department of Dermatology
Seth GS Medical College and KEM Hospital
Mumbai, Maharashtra, India

Sushrut Nitin Save DNB MNAMS
Consultant Dermatologist
Dr Save's Clinic
Mumbai, Maharashtra, India

Tejas Vishwanath MD DNB MRCP SCE (UK) Fellow in Diagnostic Dermatology
Seth GS Medical College and KEM Hospital
Associate Consultant
Disha Skin and Laser Center
Thane, Maharashtra, India

Tejinder Kaur MD
Professor and Head
Department of Dermatology, Venereology and Leprology
Government Medical College
Amritsar, Punjab, India

Tishya Singh DNB MNAMS SCE (UK)
Consultant Dermatologist
Reviva Transplant Clinic
Apollo Clinic, Chandigarh
Chaudhary Hospital
Mohali, Punjab, India

Usha N Khemani MD
Associate Professor and Head
Department of Dermatology, Venereology and Leprology
Gokuldas Tejpal Hospital—Grant Medical College
Mumbai, Maharashtra, India

Vidya Kharkar MD DVD
Professor and Head
Department of Dermatology
Seth GS Medical College and KEM Hospital
Mumbai, Maharashtra, India

Vinay Keshavamurthy MD DNB FRCP (Lon)
Associate Professor
Postgraduate Institute of Medical Education and Research
Chandigarh, India

Vishal Gupta MD
Assistant Professor
All India Institute of Medical Sciences
New Delhi, India

Vrutika Hasmukh Shah MD DNB DVL
Consultant Dermatologist
Dr Vrutika's Dermanation
Thane, Maharashtra, India

Yasmeen J Bhat MD FACP
Associate Professor
Department of Dermatology, Venereology and Leprosy
Government Medical College
Srinagar, Jammu and Kashmir, India

MESSAGE FROM THE PRESIDENT IADVL

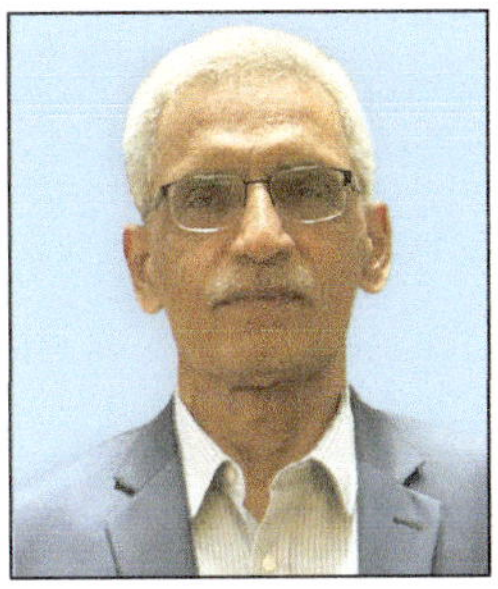

Jayadev Betkerur
President, IADVL 2021
Professor, Department of Dermatology
JSS Medical College
Mysuru, Karnataka, India

Examination of a lesion by naked eye or through a magnifying lens gives good information and we are able to diagnose. The finer details of the lesion will add to our diagnosis. Dermoscope is an instrument that gives us this information. The changes just below the epidermis can be delineated very well by a dermoscope. Various dermoscopic changes of different diseases have been described. The "Atlas of Dermoscopy" with details of these diseases and dermoscopic pictures will be of immense help to the dermatologist. This atlas in conjunction with histopathology will give us a correct diagnosis and help us in managing the disease better.

The chapters are well written and cover all dermatological diseases. The editors, Dr Balachandra S Ankad, Dr Yasmeen J Bhat and Dr Kinjal D Rambhia, are the pioneers of dermoscopy in India. I am sure their experience and valuable contributions by all the authors will make this atlas a most sought-after book by all of us.

I express my thanks to all those involved: The editors, authors, IADVL Academy headed by Chairperson Dr Deepika Pandhi and Convener Dr Dipankar De, and the publisher, in bringing out this "Atlas of Dermoscopy". As President of IADVL, I take pleasure in presenting you all this great work.

Long Live IADVL!

MESSAGE FROM THE HONORARY SECRETARY GENERAL IADVL

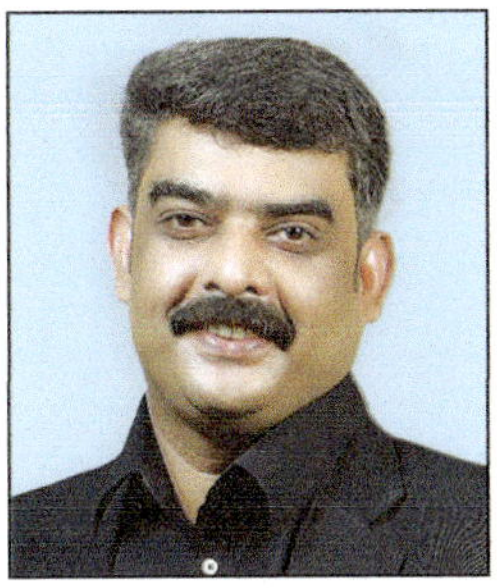

Feroz K
Honorary Secretary General, IADVL (2020–2022)
Dr Feroz's Skin Care Clinic
Kannur, Kerala, India

The Indian Association of Dermatologists, Venereologists and Leprologists (IADVL) is happy to present the first edition of the book "Atlas of Dermoscopy." This will serve as a ready reckoner for all dermatology residents and practitioners.

This book "Atlas of Dermoscopy" has been designed to address various dermatological conditions. The chapters have been contributed by dermatologists with experience, expertise, and interest in dermoscopy.

The editors have made sure to include details about basics, dermoscopic and histopathological correlation, clinical dermatology, cutaneous malignancies, infections, trichology, etc. The book will be a valuable addition for all residents as well as practitioners in dermatology, to sharpen their skills and to refresh their knowledge.

I sincerely congratulate the hard work and dedicated efforts of the editorial team—Drs Balachandra S Ankad, Yasmeen J Bhat, and Kinjal D Rambhia—and all the contributors. I also thank Dr Deepika Pandhi, Dr Dipanker De, and all the members of Academy for their support and help.

I wish this initiative all success!

MESSAGE FROM IADVL ACADEMY

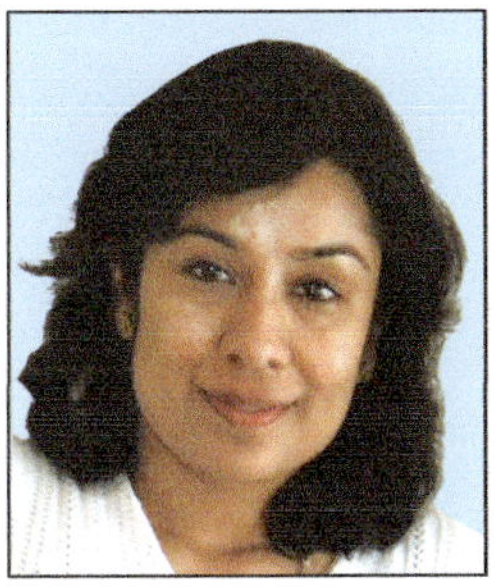

Deepika Pandhi
Chairperson, IADVL Academy

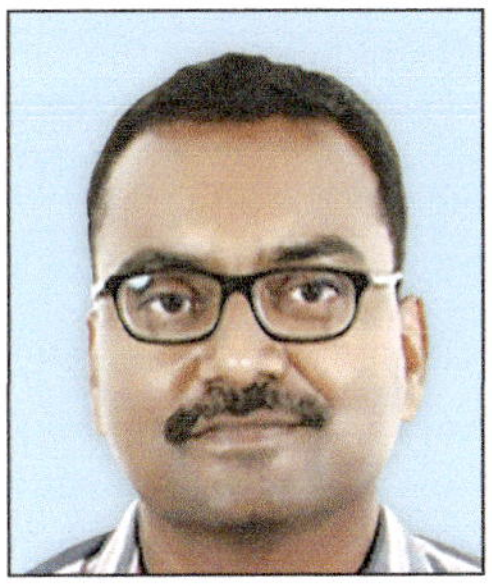

Dipankar De
Convener, IADVL Academy

Dermoscopy is an in vivo, noninvasive technique for examination of the skin by the use of a handheld device, which allows illumination and 10–14 times magnification of the lesion. While dermoscopy was initially used for the evaluation of melanocytic skin lesions, it has since been incorporated as a diagnostic modality for a wide variety of dermatoses. Due to its diagnostic accuracy and convenience, the interest in dermoscopy has increased in recent years with more dermatologists incorporating it in their diagnostic as well as interventional armamentarium. However, being a visual science, it has a learning curve and also the features may vary in skin of color. The specialty of dermoscopy has evolved tremendously over the years in India, with a steady rise in publications in Asian skin and reports of innovations in the technique of performing dermoscopy at various sites, which has paved the way for the growth of this specialty over the last decade. The Indian Association of Dermatologists, Venereologists and Leprologists (IADVL) is happy to present the first edition of the "Atlas of Dermoscopy."

The editorial team, comprising Drs Balachandra S Ankad, Yasmeen J Bhat, and Kinjal D Rambhia, has done a commendable job. They drafted an exhaustive table of content and selected eminent experts as authors from applications received from IADVL members. There are 19 chapters including details of "types of dermoscope and basic principles; dermoscopic and histopathological correlation; papulosquamous, pigmentary, and granulomatous disorders; infections; nevi; erythemas; cutaneous malignancies; mucoscopy, trichoscopy, and onychoscopy; and facial dermatoses." The chapters have been contributed by dermatologists with experience and expertise in dermoscopy and are well illustrated with more than 750 color images.

It has been a pleasure to be a part of the process of publication of this Atlas from conception to review and finally publication. Our thanks are due to members of the IADVL Academy 2021 for their critical inputs and to Dr Jayadev Betkerur, President, IADVL 2021, and Dr Feroz K, Honorary Secretary General, IADVL 2021, for their support for this endeavor.

We congratulate the dedicated efforts of the editors and all the contributors for achieving this mammoth task in a short while to bring out a book that will be a valuable reference material for all students and practitioners in dermatology.

We wish the "Atlas of Dermoscopy" great success!

FOREWORD

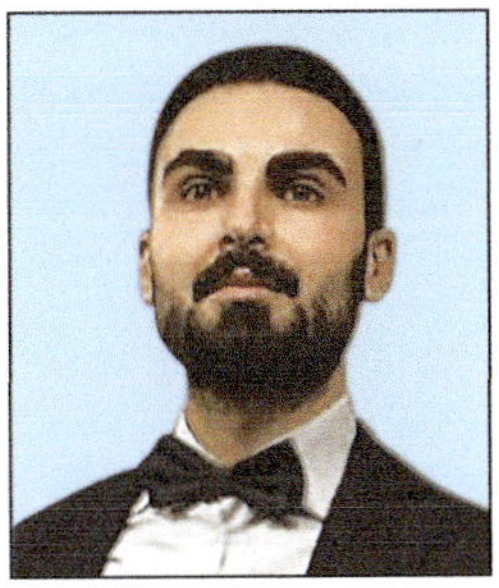

Enzo Errichetti MD MSc DVD
Senior Consultant Dermatologist and Venereologist
Institute of Dermatology
University Hospital "Santa Maria della Misericordia", Udine, Italy
General Secretary
Italian Association of Non-Invasive Diagnostics in Dermatology (AIDNID)
Executive Board Member
International Dermoscopy Society (IDS)

Diagnosis in dermatology mainly relies on the physician's ability to finely interpret the morphological changes of the skin, thus making such a discipline one of the most intriguing areas of clinical medicine. For a long time, naked-eye examination has been the only way to characterize skin lesions, with no consideration of all those subclinical dermoscopic details that are known nowadays.

The use of dermoscope has completely changed our daily practice and improved our diagnostic skills as it has let us better figure out microscopic structural changes of the lesions. Indeed, the dermoscopic assessment may be considered as a bridge between clinical and histological examination, with each dermoscopic feature corresponding to a specific histological finding. Besides, dermoscopy has also other invaluable properties, including being cheap, quick, and user-friendly, that have significantly contributed to its success.

The popularity of dermoscopy worldwide is also readily noticeable by the massive number of articles published on this topic in the literature. Indeed, by simply searching the word "dermoscopy" in the PubMed database, nearly 7,000 papers are found at time of this writing. However, it is of utmost importance to underline that dermoscopic assessment should not be regarded as a panacea for dermatologist but as a (relevant) piece in the puzzle of dermatological diagnostic process.

Albeit it has been classically used for the evaluation of both pigmented and nonpigmented skin tumors, dermoscopy has also been shown to be a helpful tool to assist the recognition of nonneoplastic dermatoses ("General Dermatology"), including inflammatory, infectious, and infiltrative disorders as well as nail and hair diseases. The enormous potential of such a technique may, however, be exploited to the full only by detailed knowledge on the topic.

The book you are holding has the virtue of representing a complete but at the same time concise guide for all those dermatologists who are seeking to improve their dermoscopic knowledge all-round. It also has the advantage of putting together information on both clinical and dermoscopic patterns of tumors and nonneoplastic dermatoses, thus letting the reader capture all the morphological dimensions of skin lesions.

I wish you a good reading!

PREFACE

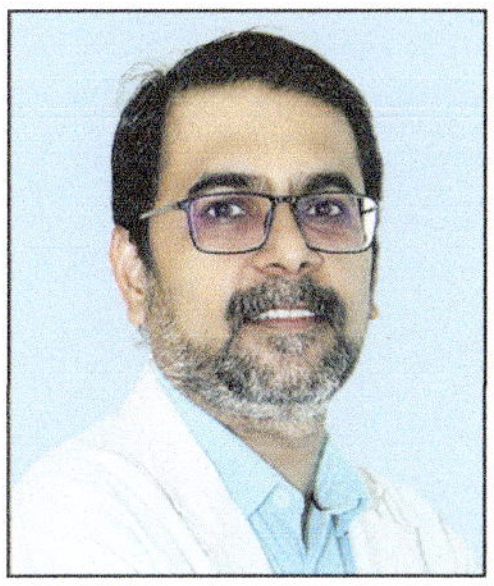

Balachandra S Ankad

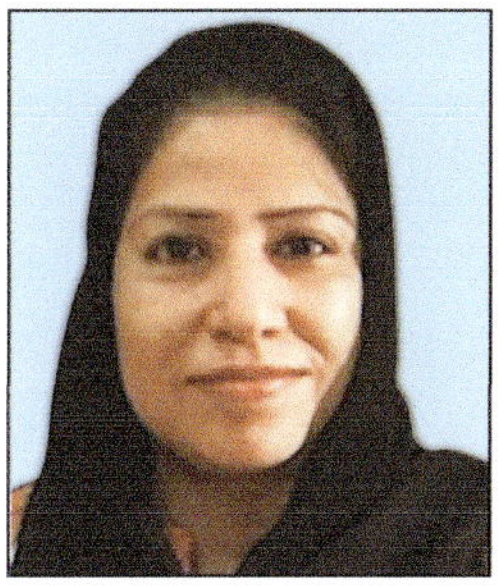

Yasmeen J Bhat

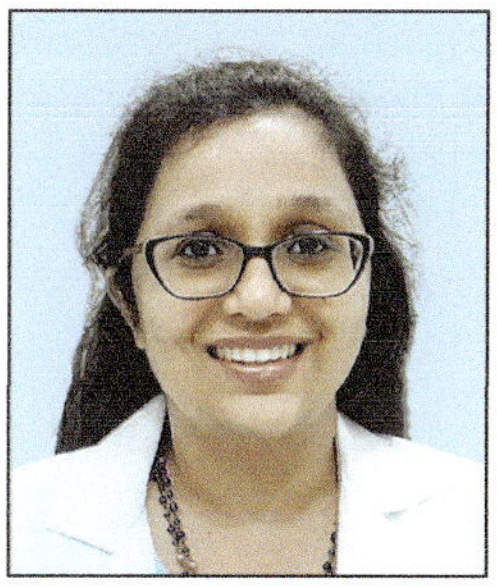

Kinjal D Rambhia

Dermoscopy, the visualization of surface and subsurface structures of the skin by a dermoscope, has been a prominent arena in the field of dermatology in the recent past. Factors attributable to its popularity are that it is a noninvasive method, quick and easy to perform. It is a known fact that dermatological conditions pose diagnostic challenges to dermatologists by virtue of varied and complex morphological features. Dermoscopy comes in handy to delineate similar clinical features by revealing definitive and specific patterns.

In view of a huge stride in the field of dermoscopy over the past few years, there is an increased zest among Indian dermatologists to learn dermoscopy. Keeping this in mind, the IADVL Atlas of Dermoscopy has been framed to encompass all the entities in the field of dermoscopy. We have tried to include all the topics which are relevant in the Indian scenario, to the academicians, practicing dermatologists as well as the dermatology residents. The high-quality dermoscopy images from the Indian skin will be of utmost help to the readers in understanding the dermoscopic patterns and structures. All the patterns of dermoscopy are labeled with accurate markings for the benefit of readers. Relevance is given to the histopathological correlation of dermoscopic findings, wherever necessary.

We, the editors, hope and wish that this atlas will be useful for practising the art of dermoscopy to the beginners and experienced dermoscopists as well. We would like to thank all the contributing authors for sharing their expertise and making this atlas possible. We render our heartfelt thanks to Dr Deepika Pandhi and Dr Dipankar De for their constant support and encouragement in bringing out this atlas. We are thankful to Dr Richa Saxena (Associate Director-Professional Publishing), Ms Nedup Denka Bhutia (Development Editor) and entire team of Jaypee Brothers Medical Publishers for their help and cooperation.

CONTENTS

1 CHAPTER

Introduction to Dermoscopy

Smitha Prabhu S, Sanjeev Gupta, Shishira R Jartarkar

INTRODUCTION

Dermoscopy or dermatoscopy is a noninvasive technique of mucocutaneous examination with an instrument known as the dermoscope or dermatoscope.[1] The dermoscope has a magnified lens with a polarized/nonpolarized or dual light source which can visualize superficial and deeper layers of skin yielding a better insight into the morphology and pathology of a condition.

A BRIEF HISTORY

Advent of dermoscopy started as early as 1655 when a French doctor, Pierre Borel pioneered the use of microscope to observe capillaries on the nail bed. Johan Kolhaus, Ernst Abbe, and Karl Heuter are the other pioneers in this field.[2] Johann Saphier, who is attributed with describing pigment globules, and using the term "dermatoscopy" in 1920s, is considered the father of dermoscopy,[3] and Leon Goldman is credited with the use of term "dermoscopy".[4] In 1970, Saitoh et al. initiated trichoscopy.[5]

In 1981, Fritsch and Pechlaner characterized the pigmented network.[6] Pehamberger et al. introduced pattern analysis in pigmented lesions in 1987.[7] In 1989, the first Consensus Conference on Skin Surface Microscopy (Hamburg, Germany) defined criteria for dermoscopy. Soyer et al. established a correlation between dermoscopic and histopathologic structures.[8]

In 1989, the first dermoscope consisting of halogen light with 10X magnification was marketed as DELTA 10. Application of immersion oil to skin surface aiding translucency was described in 1989 by Wilhelm Stolz et al.[9]

In 1994, the ABCD rule of dermoscopy was published by Wilhelm Stolz.[10] In the same year, Binder et al. used dermoscopic images to train an artificial neural network in differentiating melanomas from melanocytic nevi.[11] In 1997, MoleMax, the first dermoscopy system was released by Derma Medical Systems Company in cooperation with department of Dermatology of Medical University of Vienna.

In 2000, a virtual Consensus Net Meeting on Dermoscopy refined dermoscopic terminology and validity of various dermoscopic criteria and diagnostic algorithms.[12]

At the meeting of the American Academy of Dermatology in 2001 at Washington, DC, the World's first polarized pocket dermoscope—DermLite DL100 by 3Gen company was launched. HAM10000 (Human Against Machine with 10000 training images) dataset is a large collection of multi-source dermoscopic images of common pigmented skin lesions.[13]

CONCEPT OF DERMOSCOPY

Dermoscope works on the principle that transillumination of a lesion at higher magnification will reveal subtle variations in texture, color, and pattern of skin surface and subsurface lesions, thereby helping to delineate changes better as the light is absorbed and reflected by different skin surface components.[14]

The basic concepts of dermoscopy including pattern recognition, various algorithms, and steps and description of various terminologies will be covered in subsequent chapters.

STRUCTURES THAT CAN BE VISUALIZED

These include melanin, hemoglobin, keratin, collagen, follicular structures, eccrine gland openings, and vessels. Glandular concretions, pigment network and its variations, scar tissue, scaling, foreign particles, hair follicle and shaft, nail fold and its capillary network, and cuticle are also better delineated by dermoscopy.[15]

Normal skin is visualized as homogeneous pigment network which consists of darker reticulate lines with paler areas of pigmentation in between that make a grid pattern. The darker lines correspond to melanin in the vertical stem of rete ridges and paler hypopigmented areas are due to melanin in the horizontal stem of rete ridges.[16] Melanocytic pigmentation has characteristic appearance including: reticular pigment network, structureless pigment areas, dots, and globules. In addition, acral areas have parallel furrow, lattice, and fibrillary pattern.[17] The common morphological types of vascular structures include dotted, comma-like, linear, hairpin, glomerular, and arborizing vessels.[18]

Color variation: Though eumelanin is brown in color, Tyndall effect leads to color variegation depending upon the location and density of pigmentation which is of diagnostic significance.[19] The details of color variegation are depicted in **Table 1**.

Mucosa

Lesions located in accessible mucocutaneous areas like eyelids, lips, anogenital region, accessible part of oral mucosa are amenable to dermoscopy. Plastic food wraps or ice caps can be used to limit direct contact with the lens.[20] Pigment network is not seen in mucosae as rete ridges are absent. Mucosal pigmentation, benign and malignant tumors, inflammatory conditions can be identified.[20]

Hair

Trichoscopy is useful to visualize alopecia, scarring, variations in hair follicle, follicle unit, hair shaft anomalies, scalp pigmentation, scaling, vasculature, infections like piedra and pediculosis. Various descriptive terms are used which will be elaborated upon in coming chapters.

Nail

Normal nail fold capillary loops are placed at regular intervals and are thin, hairpin-like and of uniform diameter. Nail fold capillaroscopy is widely used in various connective tissue diseases.[21] Onychoscopy also assists in the visualization of the cuticle, lunula, nail plate, changes in the nail bed, free edge of nail plate, and hyponychium and onychomycotic changes.

USES IN DERMATOLOGICAL DIAGNOSIS[22,23]

Dermoscopy is a constantly upgrading diagnostic methodology based on algorithms and diagnostic criteria, which are frequently being put forth and refined.[24]

Common dermatological uses include:

- Differentiating melanocytic and nonmelanocytic lesions like nevi, seborrheic keratosis, lentigines, pigmented basal cell carcinoma, and dermatofibroma.
- Dermoscopy enhances diagnostic sensitivity of melanoma to 85% from the usual 65–80%.

TABLE 1: Color variegation in dermoscopy.

Color	Structures responsible	
Black to dark	Melanin in upper epidermis (stratum corneum and granulosum)	
Red black	Hemorrhagic crust on the skin	
Brown	Melanin in dermoepidermal junction, acanthosis	
Gray to slate blue	Melanin in papillary dermis	
Steel blue	Melanin in reticular dermis	
Red	Increase in number or dilation of blood vessels, angiogenesis and neovascularization, trauma	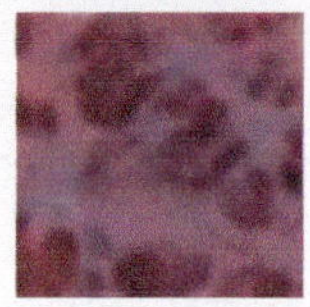
White	Increased collagen in scarring or fibrosis, absence of melanin, or due to calcium deposits	
Yellow	Compact keratin, sebaceous content, lipid, granuloma	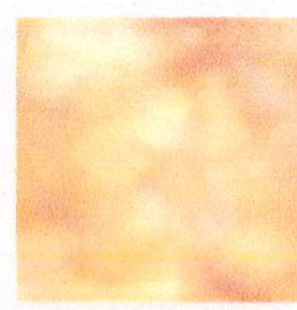
Orange	Dermal granuloma, keratin plus melanin	
Pink	Inflammation with vasodilation	
Purple	Nonoxygenated blood	

- Increasing diagnostic efficacy of inflammatory dermatoses like psoriasis, lichen planus, seborrhea, rosacea, granulomatous conditions, discoid lupus erythematosus, etc.
- Confirming diagnosis of ectoparasitic infestations like scabies, pediculosis, tungiasis, and Demodex folliculitis.
- Differentiating between various alopecias (cicatricial vs. noncicatricial).
- The diseases which can be diagnosed by dermoscopy are continually increasing in number and are shown in **Table 2**.

TABLE 2: Diagnostic dermoscopy in various skin conditions.

Condition	Well-defined criteria	Evolving criteria
Inflammatory conditions	• Psoriasis • Lichen planus • Urticaria • Urticarial vasculitis • Rosacea	• Nonscalp discoid lupus erythematosus • Pityriasis rosea • Eczematous dermatoses • Lichen sclerosus • Granuloma annulare • Cutaneous sarcoidosis • Necrobiosis lipoidica
Infections and infestations	• Scabies • Head and pubic lice • Tungiasis • Molluscum contagiosum • Human papillomavirus infections • Lupus vulgaris	• Tinea capitis • Tinea nigra
Lymphoproliferative disorders and tumors	• Clear cell acanthoma • Bowen's disease • Pyogenic granuloma • Sebaceous hyperplasia • Kaposi's sarcoma • Actinic porokeratosis • Xanthomatous neoplasms • Seborrheic keratosis • Melanoma • Basal cell carcinoma • Keratoacanthoma • Squamous cell carcinoma	• Primary cutaneous B cell lymphoma • Mycosis fungoides
Pigmentary disorders	• Pigmented purpuric dermatoses • Lichen planus pigmentosus • Cutaneous amyloidosis • Acanthosis nigricans • Melasma • Exogenous ochronosis	• Vitiligo • Idiopathic guttate hypomelanosis • Exogenous ochronosis
Miscellaneous dermatoses	• Port-wine stain • Aplasia cutis congenitalis	• Cutaneous mastocytosis • Aquagenic syringeal acrokeratoderma
Hair disorders	• Androgenetic alopecia • Alopecia areata • Lichen planopilaris • Discoid lupus erythematosus • Folliculitis decalvans • Trichostasis spinulosa • Trichotillomania • Hair shaft disorders	• Trichotillomania • Congenital triangular alopecia • Loose anagen hair syndrome • Frontal fibrosing alopecia • Erosive pustular dermatosis of scalp • Hair casts
Nail disorders	• Psoriasis • Onychomycosis • Lichen planus • Subungual hematoma	• Onychomycosis • Onychopapilloma • Onychomatricoma • Ectopic nails

Alternative Uses in Dermatological Practice

The nondiagnostic uses of dermoscopy include:[25,26]

- Disease activity evaluation: Alopecia areata, vitiligo, frontal fibrosing alopecia, skin tumors.
- For patient reassurance and follow-up of lesions at regular intervals.
- Wart mapping in areas like beard, face, even for genital warts to assess the extent of warts for treatment purpose.
- To detect intra- and subcutaneous foreign bodies like glass shards, suture bits, grit.
- For better and early visualization of adverse effects of topical corticosteroids.
- To define the exact surgical excision margin for skin tumors.
- Dermoscopy guided biopsy: For more accurate histopathological diagnosis.
- Dermoscopy is used in clinical studies as accurate measures of pre- and postinterventional changes.
- In evaluating efficacy of laser hair reduction.
- Dermoscopy in hair transplant: To assess the number and size of hair follicle units, and to diagnose early post-transplant folliculitis.
- Confirmation of imperceptible findings in skin tests like pathergy, patch test, and intradermal tests.

ADVANTAGES OF DERMOSCOPY

Dermoscopy aids in:[27]

- Diagnosis as well as assessment of border of tumoral pathologies likes basal cell.[28,29]
- Digital surveillance and monitoring of melanocytic lesions.
- Valuable in assessing pigmented and nonpigmented skin tumors and atypical and dysplastic nevi.[30]
- Monitoring the results of tumor treatment and is an assisting tool in tumor surgery.[31]
- Onychoscopy is helpful in evaluating nail disorders and in differentiating neoplastic and non-neoplastic diseases.[31]
- Entomodermoscopy is an effective and sensitive tool in diagnosis of viral, fungal, and parasitic diseases.[31]
- Trichoscopy is useful in detecting various alopecias and inflammatory scalp diseases and in monitoring and follow-up.

LIMITATIONS OF DERMOSCOPY[32]

- Adequate training and expertise is needed for dermoscopic analysis.
- Instruments are relatively expensive.
- The findings are subject to the light, type of dermoscope, and camera being used, also on application pressure and contact or noncontact method.[22]
- Dermoscopy has limited role in the diagnosis of very early and mainly featureless melanomas.[33]
- Anchoring bias: Diagnosis is based on a single dermoscopic finding.
- Search satisfaction: Tendency to fix the diagnosis based on partial information and not probing further.[27]
- In contact dermoscopy, faceplate of dermoscope needs to be disinfected before using in next patient.[25]
- Artifacts like colored powders, dust, dye, cosmetics can hinder proper visualization and cause confusion.
- Different dermoscopes yield different magnification and color grades, which lead to lack of uniformity.

FUTURE OF DERMOSCOPY

Dermoscopy is evolving into subcategories like pigmenteroscopy, inflammoscopy mucoscopy, and entodermoscopy.[26] The future trend is the use of artificial intelligence and teledermoscopy. Teledermoscopy and skin health self-inspection will become a new trend with the development of dermoscopic image analysis technology which will improve diagnostic accuracy.[34]

Artificial Intelligence

There is tremendous improvement in technology with periodic launch of newer and better handheld as well as videodermoscopy devices.

KEY POINTS

- First commercial dermoscope was manufactured in 1989.
- Various steps, algorithms, and pattern recognitions are set for diagnostic uniformity of conditions by dermoscopy.
- Dermoscopy now embraces various subcategories like trichoscopy, onychoscopy, mucoscopy, inflammoscopy, and entodermoscopy.
- It is used not only in diagnosis, but also in treatment monitoring, side effects of treatment, and for marking areas for biopsy and excision.
- Teledermoscopy is in the near future.

CONCLUSION

Dermoscopy, the method of noninvasive visualization of skin structures, is a helpful tool in the diagnosis and differentiation of many dermatoses. Trichoscopy is most evidence-based science of dermoscopy whereas onychoscopy is still evolving. Further research is recommended in the field of dermoscopy for validation of certain patterns.

REFERENCES

1. Ackerman AB. Dermatoscopy, not dermoscopy! J Am Acad Dermatol. 2006;55:728.
2. Domínguez-Espinosa AE. History of dermoscopy. Dermatol Rev Mex. 2014;58:165-72.
3. Berk-Krauss J, Laird ME. What's in a name-dermoscopy vs dermatoscopy. JAMA Dermatol. 2017;153:1235.
4. Goldman L. Some investigative studies of pigmented nevi with cutaneous microscopy. J Invest Dermatol. 1951;16:407-26.
5. Kharkar V. Overview of trichoscopy. In: Khopkar US (Ed). Dermoscopy and Trichoscopy in Diseases of the Brown Skin: Atlas and Short Text. New Delhi: Jaypee Brothers Medical Publishers (P) Ltd; 2012. pp. 167-81.
6. Fritsch P, Pechlaner R. Differentiation of benign from malignant melanocytic lesions using incident light microscopy. In: Ackerman AB, Mihara I (Eds). Pathology of Malignant Melanoma. New York: Masson; 1981. pp. 301-12.
7. Pehamberger H, Steiner A, Wolff K. In vivo epiluminescence microscopy of pigmented skin lesions. I. Pattern analysis of pigmented skin lesions. J Am Acad Dermatol. 1987;17:571-83.
8. Bahmer FA, Fritsch P, Kreusch J, Pehamberger H, Rohrer C, Schindera I, et al. Terminology in surface microscopy. Consensus meeting of the Committee on Analytical Morphology of the Arbeitsgemeinschaft Dermatologische Forschung, Hamburg, Federal Republic of Germany, Nov. 17, 1989. J Am Acad Dermatol. 1990;23:1159-62.
9. Stolz W, Bilek P, Landthaler M, Merkle T, Braun-Falco O. Skin surface microscopy. Lancet. 1989;2:864-5.
10. Stolz W, Riemann A, Cognetta AB. ABCD rule of dermatoscopy: a new practical method for early recognition of malignant melanoma. Eur J Dermatol. 1994;4:521-7.
11. Binder M, Steiner A, Schwarz M, Knollmayer S, Wolff K, Pehamberger H. Application of an artificial neural network in epiluminescence microscopy pattern analysis of pigmented skin lesions: a pilot study. Br J Dermatol. 1994;130:460-5.
12. Argenziano G, Soyer HP, Chimenti S, Talamini R, Corona R, Sera F, et al. Dermoscopy of pigmented skin lesions: results of a consensus meeting via the Internet. J Am Acad Dermatol. 2003;48:679-93.
13. Tschandl P, Rosendahl C, Kittler H. The HAM10000 dataset, a large collection of multi-source dermatoscopic images of common pigmented skin lesions. Sci Data. 2018;5:180161.
14. Nirmal B. Dermatoscopy: physics and principles. Indian J Dermatopathol Diagn Dermatol. 2017;4:27-30.
15. Witkowski A, Pellacani G, Gonzalez S, Longo C. Dermoscopy: basic knowledge of an innovative imaging tool. In: Humbert P, Fanian F, Maibach H, Agache P (Eds). Agache's Measuring the Skin. Cham: Springer Nature; 2017. pp. 211-28.
16. Nischal KC, Khopkar US. Principles and technique of dermoscopy and videodermoscopy. In: Khopkar US (Ed). Dermoscopy and Trichoscopy in Diseases of the Brown Skin: Atlas and Short Text. New Delhi: Jaypee Brothers Medical Publishers (P) Ltd; 2012. pp. 1-9.
17. Rosendahl C, Cameron A, McColl I, Wilkinson D. Dermatoscopy in routine practice—'chaos and clues'. Aust Fam Physician. 2012;41:482-7.
18. Ayhan E, Ucmak D, Akkurt Z. Vascular structures in dermoscopy. An Bras Dermatol. 2015;90:545-53.
19. Weismann K, Lorentzen HF. Dermoscopic color perspective. Arch Dermatol. 2006;142:1250.
20. Blum A, Simionescu O, Argenziano G. (2021). Dermoscopy of mucosal lesions. [online] Available from https://www.uptodate.com/contents/dermoscopy-of-mucosal-lesions [Last accessed October, 2021].
21. Jadhav P, Khopkar US. Nail fold capillaroscopy in connective tissue disorders. In: Dermoscopy and Trichoscopy in Diseases of the Brown Skin: Atlas and Short Text. Khopkar US (Ed). New Delhi: Jaypee Brothers Medical Publishers (P) Ltd; 2012. pp. 157-68.
22. Haldar SS, Nischal KC, Khopkar US. Dermoscopy: applications and patterns in diseases of the brown skin. In: Dermoscopy and Trichoscopy in Diseases of the Brown Skin: Atlas and Short Text. Khopkar US (Ed). New Delhi: Jaypee Brothers Medical Publishers (P) Ltd; 2012. pp. 10-37.
23. Kaliyadan F. The scope of the dermoscope. Indian Dermatol Online J. 2016;7:359-63.
24. Micali G, Verzì AE, Lacarrubba F. Alternative uses of dermoscopy in daily clinical practice: an update. J Am Acad Dermatol. 2018;79:1117-32.
25. Sonthalia S, Yumeen S, Kaliyadan F. Dermoscopy Overview and Extradiagnostic Applications. In: StatPearls [Internet]. Treasure Island (FL): Stat Pearls Publishing; 2021.
26. Sonthalia S, Pasquali P, Agrawal M, Sharma P, Jha AK, Errichetti E, et al. Dermoscopy update: review of its extradiagnostic and expanding indications and future prospects. Dermatol Pract Concept. 2019;9:253-64.
27. Marghoob AA, Usatine RP, Jaimes N. Dermoscopy for the family physician. Am Fam Physician. 2013;88:441-50.
28. Zalaudek I, Kreusch J, Giacomel J, Ferrara G, Catricalà C, Argenziano G. How to diagnose nonpigmented skin tumors: a review of vascular structures seen with dermoscopy: Part I. Melanocytic skin tumors. J Am Acad Dermatol. 2010;63:361-74.
29. Zalaudek I, Kreusch J, Giacomel J, Ferrara G, Catricala C, Argenziano G. How to diagnose nonpigmented skin tumors: Part II. Non-melanocytic skin tumors. J Am Acad Dermatol. 2010;63:377-86.
30. Venugopal SS, Soyer HP, Menzies SW. Results of a nationwide dermoscopy survey investigating the prevalence, advantages and disadvantages of dermoscopy use among Australian dermatologists. Australian J Dermatol. 2011;52:14-8.
31. Chappuis P, Duru G, Marchal O, Girier P, Dalle S, Thomas L. Dermoscopy, a useful tool for general practitioners in melanoma screening: a nationwide survey. Br J Dermatol. 2016;175:744-50.
32. Shen XW, Yu RX, Shen CB, Li CX, Jing Y, Zheng YJ, et al. Dermoscopy in China—current status and future prospective. Chin Med J. 2019;132:2096-104.
33. Skvara H, Teban L, Fiebiger M, Binder M. Limitation of dermoscopy in the recognition of melanoma. Arch Dermatol. 2005;14:155-60.
34. Uppal SK, Beer J, Hadeler E, Gitlow H, Nouri K. The clinical utility of teledermoscopy in the era of telemedicine. Dermatol Ther. 2021;34:e14766.

2 CHAPTER

Basic Principles of Dermoscopy

Shekhar Neema, Sharmila Patil, Devayani Pol

INTRODUCTION

Dermoscope is noninvasive diagnostic tool which helps in visualization of subsurface structures. It magnifies, illuminates, and helps in assessment of structures that are not usually visible to the naked eye. Dermoscopic structures have to be analyzed in the similar manner as we analyze histopathology for diagnosis. We will discuss basic principles and interpretation of visualized structures in this chapter. This chapter focuses on basics of dermoscopy which include principles of dermoscopy, melanocytic and vascular structures, and dermoscopy of normal skin. This chapter also deals with descriptive and metaphoric terminologies used in dermoscopy.

PRINCIPLES OF DERMOSCOPY

The visualization of any structure by human eye depends on the amount of light which reaches retina after getting reflected from the structure. When light falls on the skin, it undergoes reflection, refraction, diffraction, and absorption. The refractive index of the stratum corneum (1.55) is higher than that of air (1.00). Therefore, much of the incident light is reflected off the surface of the skin (stratum corneum) (**Fig. 1**).[1] This light overwhelms the retina and light that is reflected from the deeper layers of the skin cannot be visualized. Therefore, when one examines with naked eye or with magnifying glass, one can only see the morphologic structures that manifest on the surface layer of the skin (stratum corneum). The visualization of deeper structures requires less reflection from surface, so that more light gets reflected from deeper part of skin and reaches retina. Following features of dermoscope help in achieving this goal:

- *Contact plate or face plate*: When light travels in one medium to another of different refractive index, it changes path known as refraction. The change in path is more with higher difference in refractive index of two media. The interposition of glass contact plate having refractive index of 1.52 reduces refraction. The glass plate also has graduated scale. Smaller plates are available for difficult to access areas.
- *Linkage or interface fluid*: The skin surface has scales which traps air and creates multiple planes. To visualize

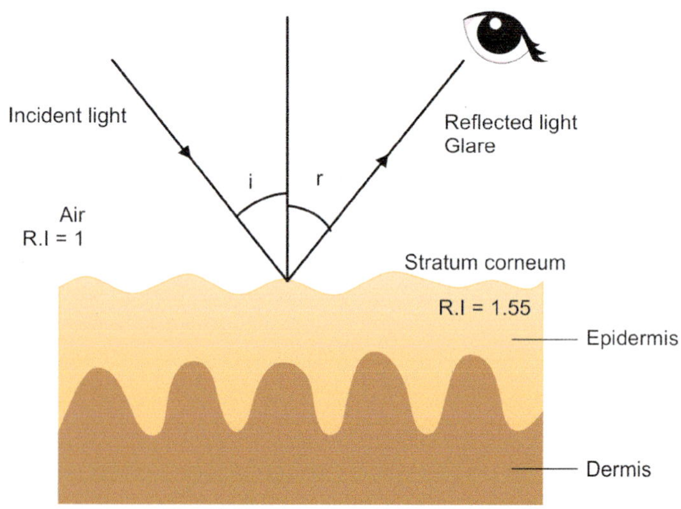

FIG. 1: As there is difference between refractive indices of air and skin surface, most of the incident light is getting reflected from skin surface, so deeper structures are not visible.

the deeper structures, the glare or reflection has to be reduced; for which the normal skin-air interface is replaced with skin-liquid interface, with the refractive index of fluid interface ideally equal to that of skin. Thereby stratum corneum becomes translucent and subsurface can be easily visualized (**Figs. 2** and **3**).[2] Various interface fluids like mineral oil, ultrasound gel or antibacterial gel, water, alcohol, liquid paraffin can be used. Immersion oil is not used as it is known to have teratogenic, fetotoxic, and carcinogenic effects.[3] The 70% alcohol appears to be the best immersion liquid as it yields fewer air bubbles, produces clearer images, and reduces cross-contamination.[1] For onychoscopy and dermoscopy of areas like periorbital region, ultrasound gel or antibacterial gels are useful, as gel fills up the curved areas because of its viscosity and also has less risk of dripping in the eyes.[1]

- *Polarized light*: Polarized lights are light waves in which vibration occurs in single plane. It is created by blocking one of the two planes of vibration using polarized filter. Polarized dermoscopy (PD) uses principle of cross-polarization. This technique utilizes two filters held perpendicular to each other. Polarized light incident on the stratum corneum is partly reflected from the surface and the rest enters the skin. The part that is reflected from the skin surface maintains its polarization while part that penetrates the skin scatters and loses its polarization. The second filter that is placed at 90°, blocks the reflected light while it allows light coming from deeper part to pass through. This technology is called as cross-polarization (**Fig. 4**).[4]

Nonpolarized dermoscopy (NPD) utilizes contact plate and interface fluids (**Figs. 5** and **6**). PD uses cross-polarization and does not need contact or interface fluid.

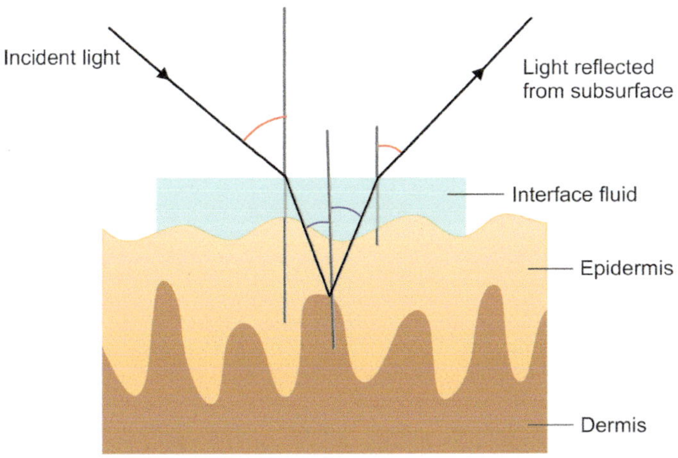

FIG. 2: Application of linkage fluid creates liquid-skin interface and allows light to reach deeper structures.

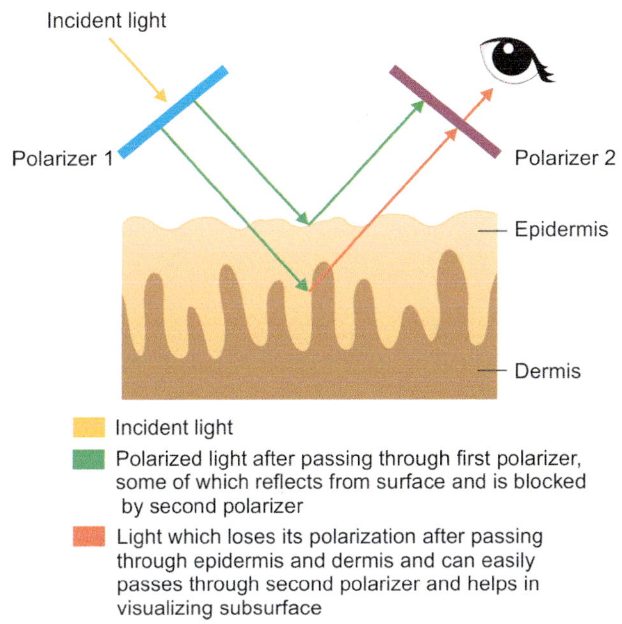

FIG. 4: Principle of cross-polarization: Reflected light from surface is blocked by second polarizer, while light which reaches deeper structures loses its polarization and deeper structures are visible.

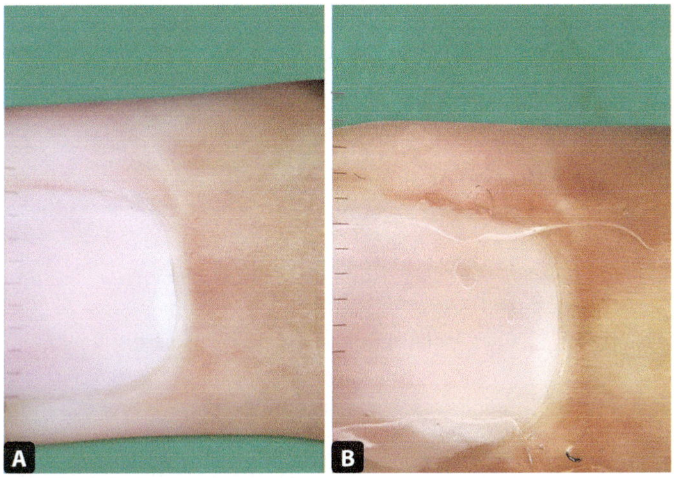

FIGS. 3A AND B: (A) Polarized dermoscopy shows nail unit with glare from nail plate; (B) Application of ultrasound jelly as linkage fluid improves visualization of nail unit structure including proximal nail fold capillaries (polarized, DermLite DL4, 10×).

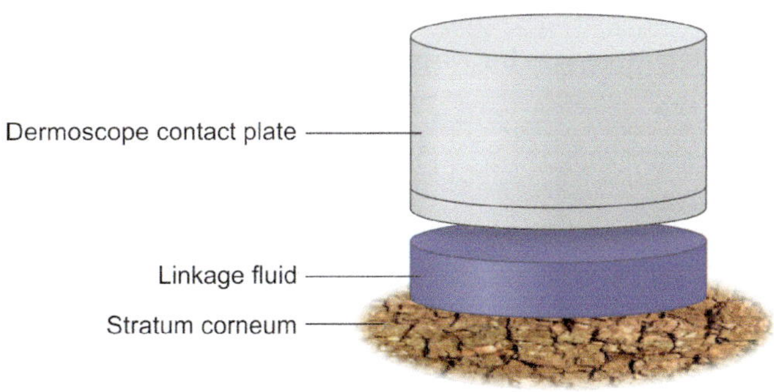

FIG. 5: Relationship between contact plate and interface fluids in nonpolarized dermoscopy.

It prevents blanching of vascular structures and cross-contamination. NPD is better for visualizing superficial structures while PD is better for deeper structures (**Figs. 7A** and **B**). To evaluate a lesion completely both NPD and PD should be performed. Hybrid dermoscope is a device which has both polarized and nonpolarized mode. The difference between NPD and PD is tabulated in **Table 1**.

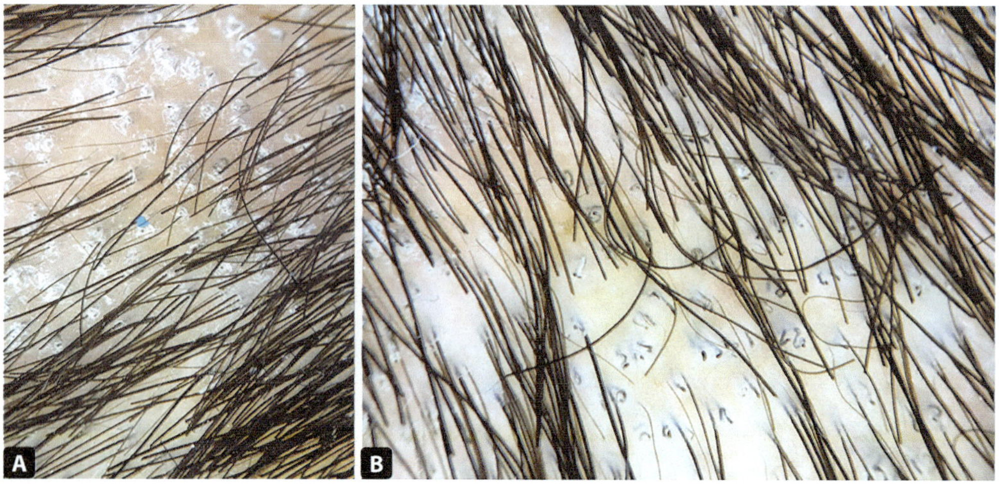

FIGS. 6A AND B: (A) Polarized dermoscopy without application of linkage fluid shows scales on trichoscopy; (B) Application of 70% alcohol as linkage fluid allows visualization of underlying structures and helps in rapid diagnosis (polarized, DermLite DL4, 10×).

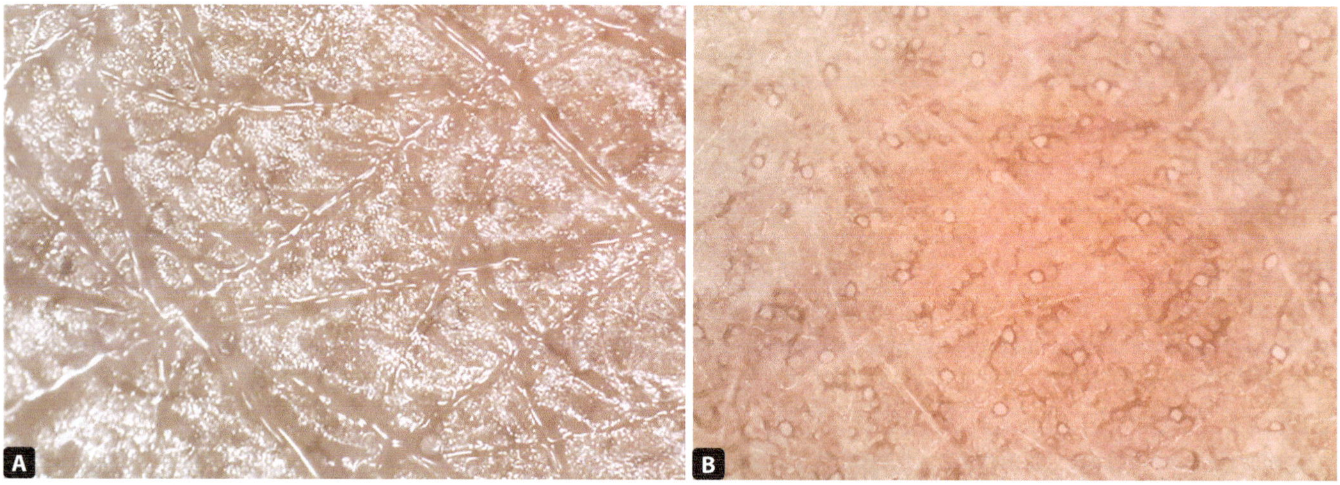

FIGS. 7A AND B: (A) Nonpolarized dermoscopy shows surface structures; (B) Polarized dermoscopy of same area shows pigment network (Dino-Lite Edge, 20×).

TABLE 1: Differences between polarized and nonpolarized modes and application of differences.

	Nonpolarized dermoscopy	Polarized dermoscopy
Direct contact with skin	Required	Not required
Interface fluid	Required	Not required
Principle used	Glass plate-interface fluid-skin surface set up to decrease the glare	Cross-polarization to decrease the glare
Structures more conspicuous	Milia-like cysts, comedo-like openings, and scales (**Fig. 7A**)	Blood vessels, vascular blush, chrysalis strands, white scar-like area, pigment (**Fig. 7B**)
Colors enhanced	Blue-white veil	Pink-red

EVALUATION OF DERMOSCOPIC PARAMETERS

The evaluation of a lesion by dermoscopy should be systematic and should include assessment of:

1. Color and morphology of structures
2. Pigment and vascular pattern
3. Follicular structures

- *Color*: The color seen in dermoscopy depends on the chromophore and its location.[5] Melanin in epidermis absorbs all the incident light resulting in black color (**Fig. 8**). Melanin in dermoepidermal junction, some light gets reflected from superficial layer, prevents black color and it appears brown (**Fig. 9**). Melanin in superficial dermis, light gets reflected in epidermis and scattering occurs in collagen leading to Tyndall effect, thus causing blue shift of color and the resultant color is gray (**Fig. 10**). When melanin is present in deep dermis, majority of light gets scattered by collagen leading blue color (**Fig. 10**). Different colors seen are orange (**Fig. 11**), yellow (**Fig. 12**), white (**Figs. 13** and **14**), and red (**Fig. 15**).[5]
- *Pigment and vascular pattern*: Structures and patterns seen in dermoscopy are akin to alphabets to a language. Structures can be described in metaphoric or descriptive form. In this chapter, authors have focused on descriptive terminologies as described by Professor Harald Kittler. The metaphoric terminologies will be described in respective chapters. The descriptive pigmentary and vascular terminologies are described in **Tables 2** and **3**.[6,7] When structures are present in particular manner, they are called patterns and summation of these patterns suggests diagnosis. It should be noted that these patterns must be repetitive and reproducible. It is also important to know normal before one can identify abnormal. The normal findings on dermoscopy of skin and mucosa are described in **Table 4**.[8]

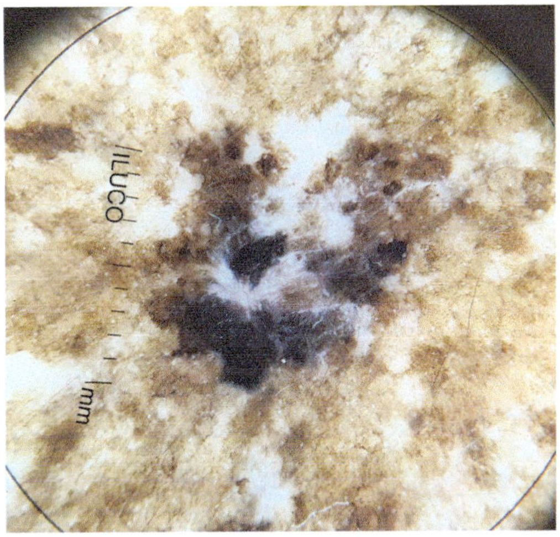

FIG. 8: Polarized dermoscopy shows black, brown, and blue color depicting melanin in epidermis, dermoepidermal junction and papillary dermis, respectively (polarized, Illuco, 10×).

Courtesy: Dr Rohit Kothari , Senior Resident, Department of Dermatology, Command Hospital, Airforce Bengaluru, Karnataka, India.

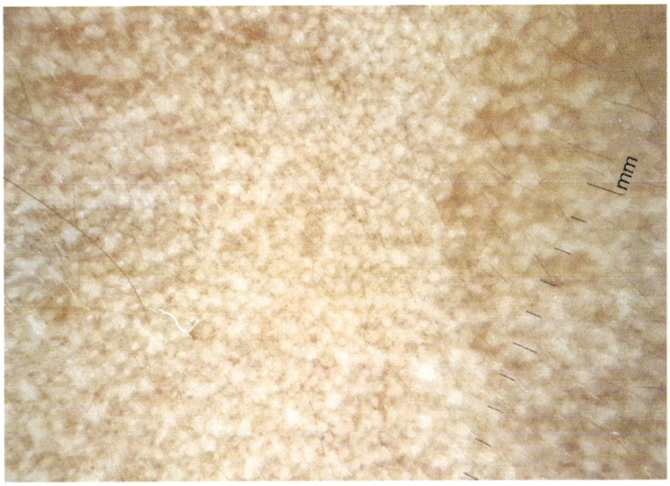

FIG. 9: Polarized dermoscopy shows brown reticular pigment network with few scattered brown blotches depicting melanin in epidermis or at dermoepidermal junction (polarized, DermLite DL4, 10×).

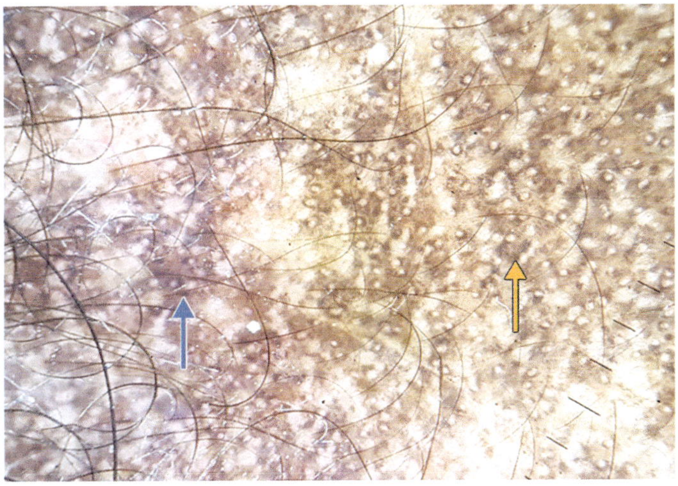

FIG. 10: Polarized dermoscopy shows dots and clods of gray color (orange arrow) and of blue color (blue arrow) depicting melanin in upper and lower papillary dermis, respectively (polarized, DermLite DL4, 10×).

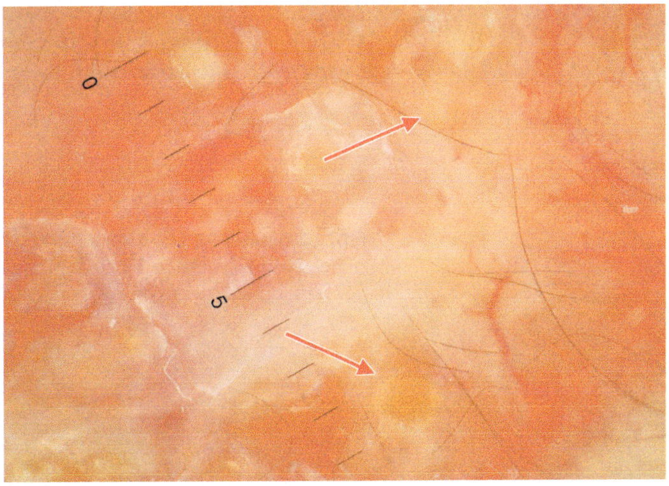

FIG. 11: Polarized dermoscopy shows orange-yellow color (red arrows) depicting granuloma in a case of cutaneous tuberculosis (polarized, DermLite DL4, 10×).

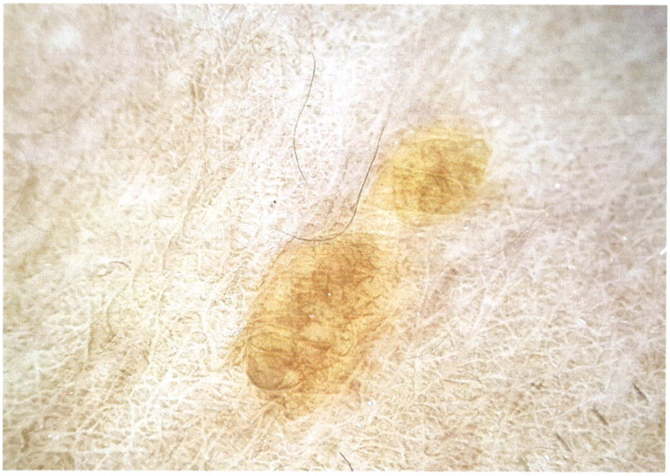

FIG. 12: Dermoscopy shows predominantly brownish-yellow (in skin of color) color in a xanthoma depicting lipid deposits (polarized, DermLite DL4, 10×).

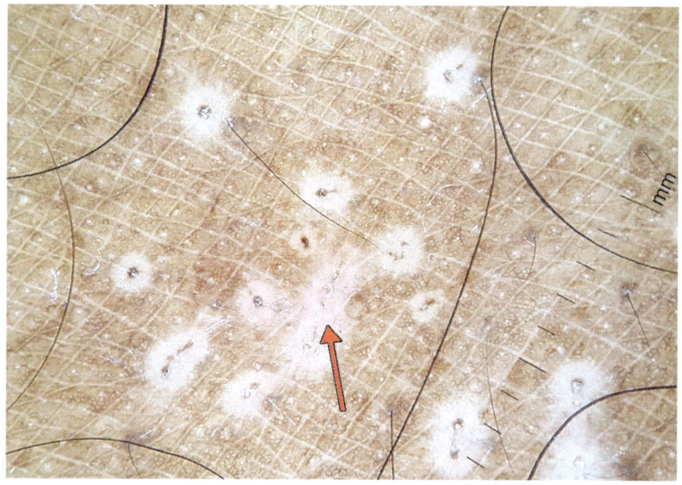

FIG. 13: Dermoscopy shows white color (red arrow) due to collagen in a case of lichen sclerosus et atrophicus (polarized, DermLite DL4, 10×).

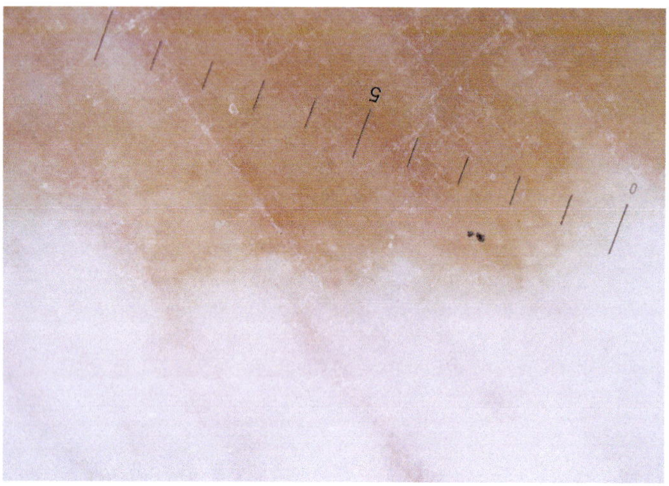

FIG. 14: Dermoscopy shows white color resulting from absence of melanin in a case of vitiligo (polarized, DermLite DL4, 10×).

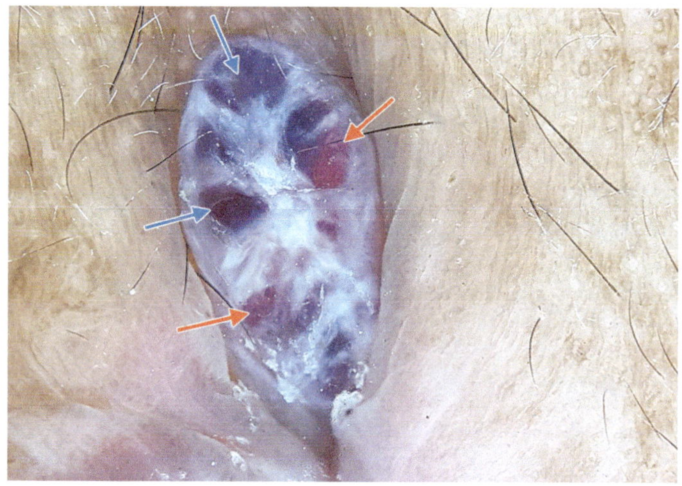

FIG. 15: Dermoscopy shows red and purple color depicting oxygenated blood (red arrows) and deoxygenated blood (blue arrows), respectively (polarized, DermLite DL4, 10×).

TABLE 2: Descriptive terminologies for pigmented structures.[6]

Descriptive terminology	Definition	Schematic image
Lines	Straight or curved structure with parallel edges having length more than width	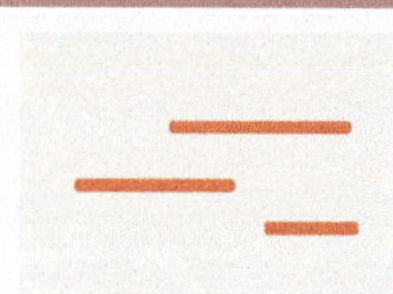
	The patterns which can be seen are parallel lines, reticular lines, branched lines, curved lines, and radial lines (**Figs. 16** to **18**)	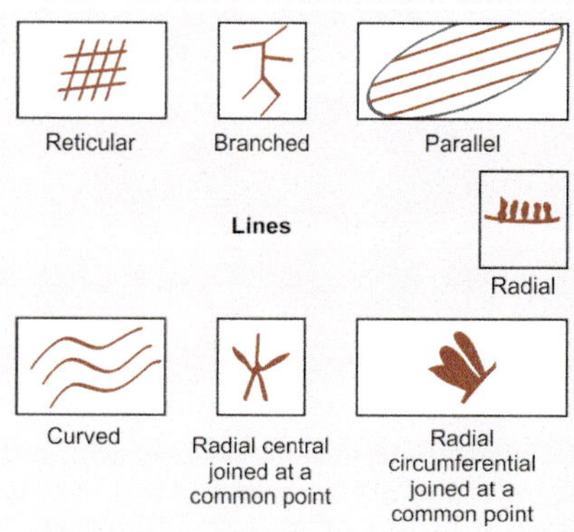

Continued

Continued

Descriptive terminology	Definition	Schematic image
	These patterns can be further subclassified on the basis of colors or thickness as white lines, delicate or thick lines. Radial lines can be connected to a common base or converging to a central dot or clod	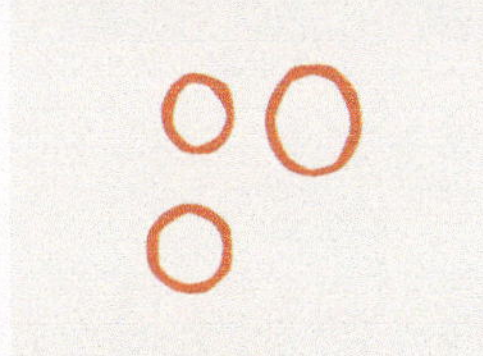
Pseudopod	It is a line with a bulbous end	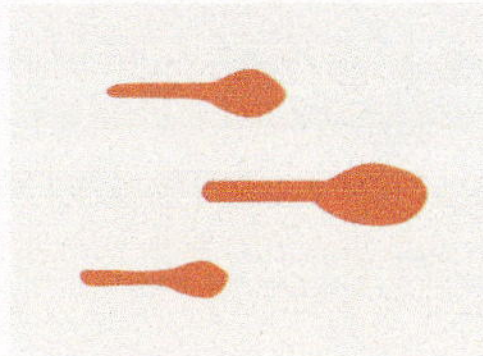
Dots	• Small solid pigmented spot (**Fig. 19**) • Dots can be further described depending on color as gray, brown, etc. and arrangement as linear, central, and so on	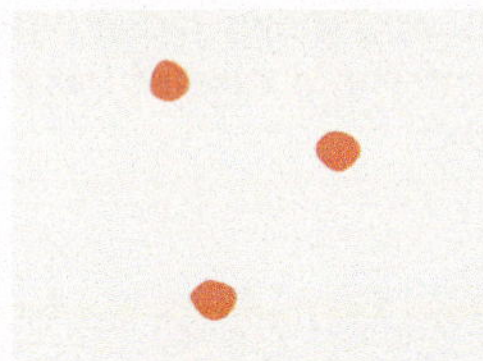
Clod	Circumscribed solid, pigmented spot larger than a dot (**Fig. 20**). Shape and color can vary and it can be described as large or small; red, blue, pink, purple, white, and so on	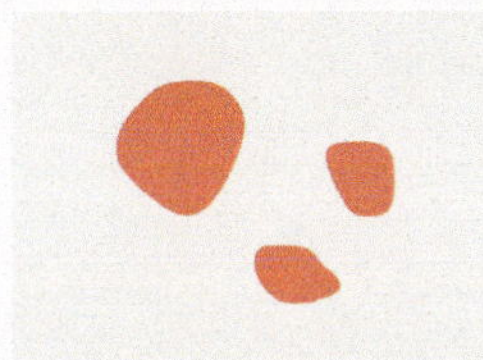
Circle	It is a curved line equidistant from central point	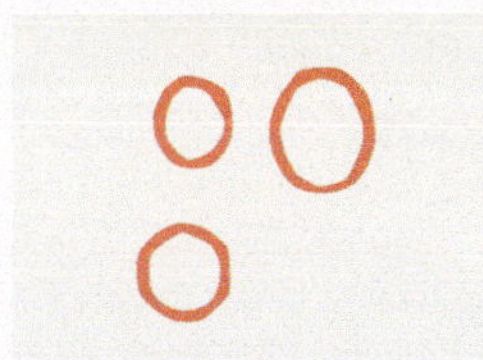
Structureless area	An area with absence of basic structures	

FIG. 16: Dermoscopy shows reticular brown lines in case of pigmented purpuric dermatoses (polarized, DermLite DL4, 10×).

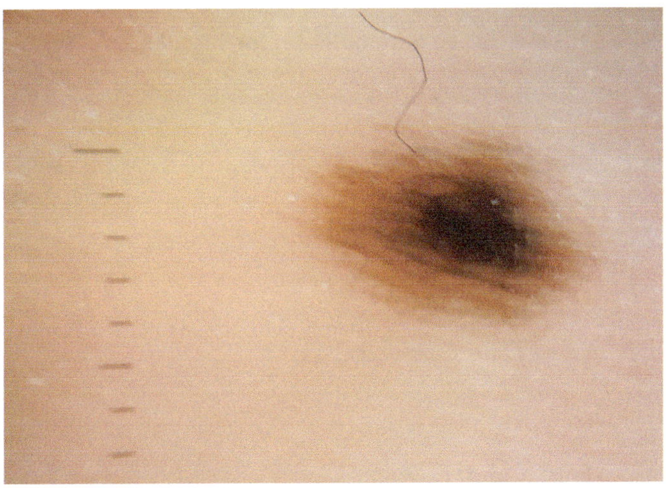

FIG. 17: Dermoscopy shows parallel pigmented lines in case of acral nevi (polarized, DermLite DL4, 10×).

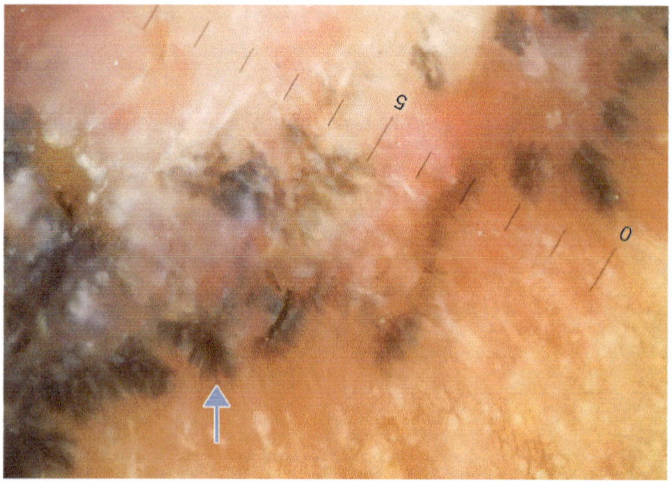

FIG. 18: Dermoscopy shows radial lines (blue arrow) connecting to a common center in a case of basal cell carcinoma (polarized, DermLite DL4, 10×).

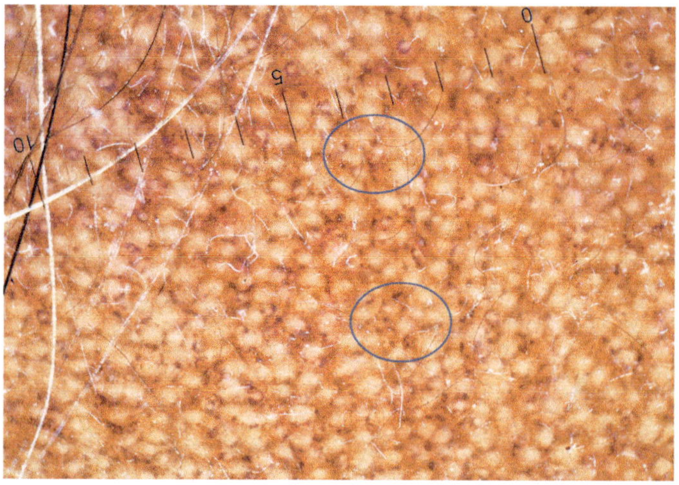

FIG. 19: Dermoscopy shows brown-gray dots/clods (blue circles) in a case of lichen planus pigmentosus (polarized, DermLite DL4, 10×).

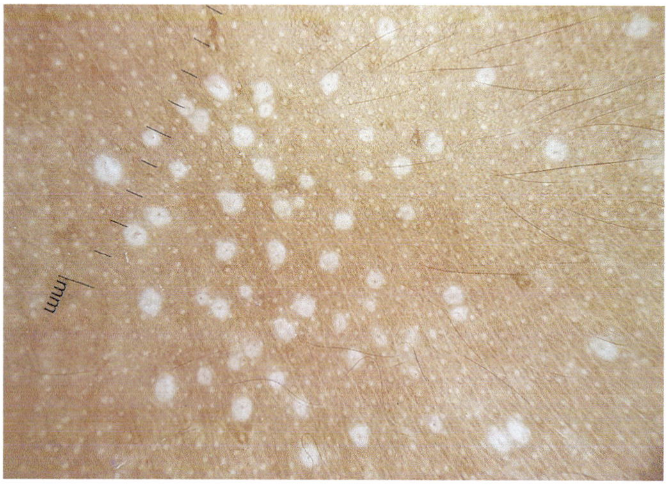

FIG. 20: Dermoscopy shows white clods in a case of lichen nitidus (polarized, DermLite DL4, 10×).

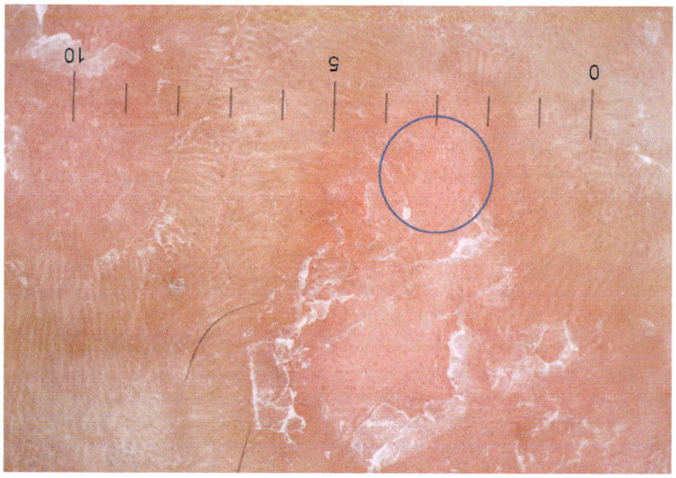

FIG. 21: Dermoscopy shows regular, red-dotted vessels (blue circle) in a case of psoriasis (polarized, DermLite DL4, 10×).

TABLE 3: Descriptive terminologies for vascular structures and arrangement.[7]

Descriptive terminology	Definition	Schematic image
Dots	Tiny pinpoint vessels (**Fig. 21**)	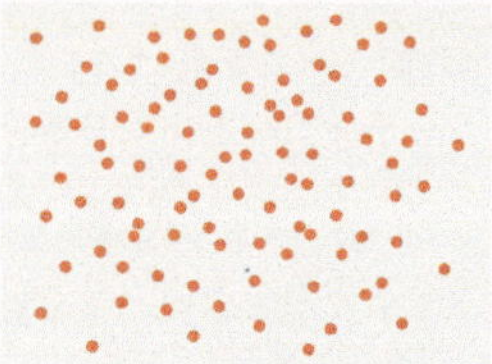
Clods	Sharply demarcated round to oval areas bigger than dots (**Fig. 22**)	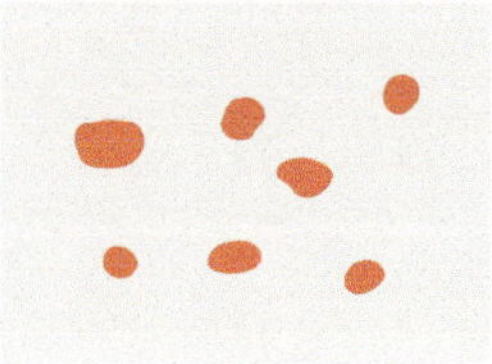

Continued

Continued

Descriptive terminology	Definition	Schematic image

Linear	• Linear vessels (**Fig. 23**)
	• *Subtypes:*
	  ○ Straight
	  ○ Coiled—tightly coiled vessels resembling glomerular apparatus of the kidney
	  ○ Looped—two parallel linear vessels forming a hairpin-like structure (**Fig. 24**)
	  ○ Curved—linear curved short vessels
	  ○ Serpentine—linear vessels with multiple bends
	  ○ Helical—twisted looped vessels with bends twisted along a central axis
		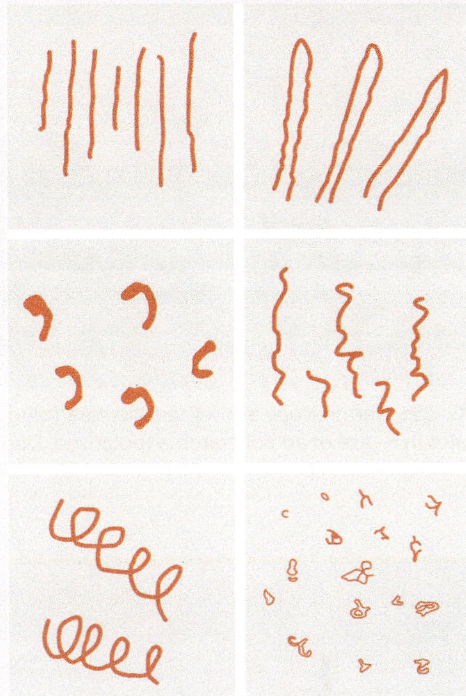

Terminologies for arrangement of vascular structures		
Radial	Radial serpentine or arborizing vessels at the periphery of the lesion that radiate toward the center (**Fig. 25**)	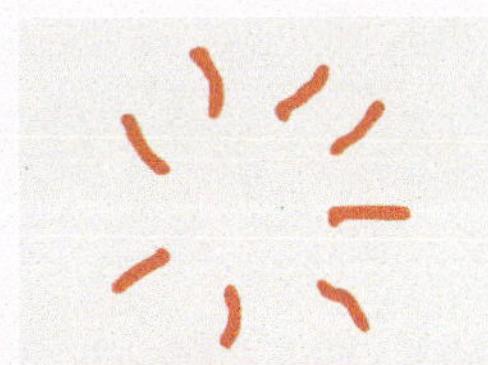
Serpiginous	Coiled or dotted vessels arranged in lines	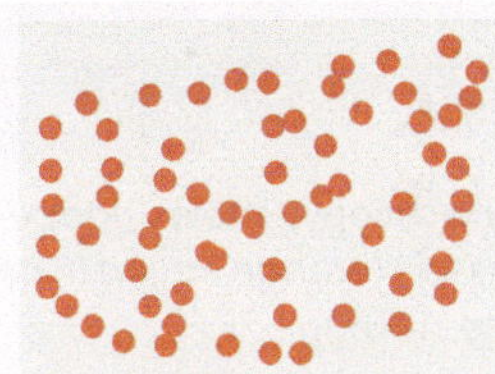
Branched	Bright red sharply in focus large or thick diameter vessels (**Fig. 26**)	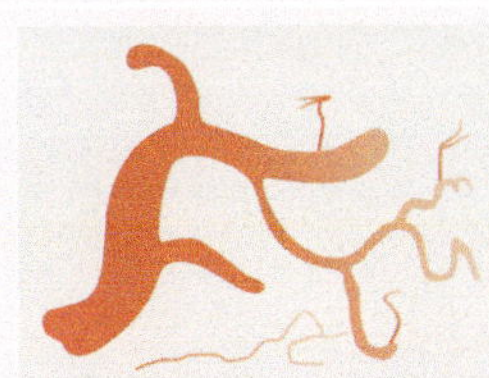
Clustered	Coiled vessels arranged in groups (**Fig. 27**)	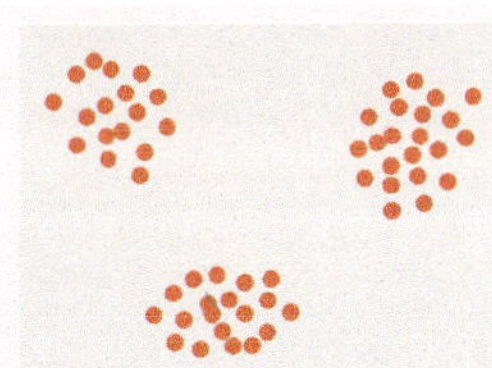

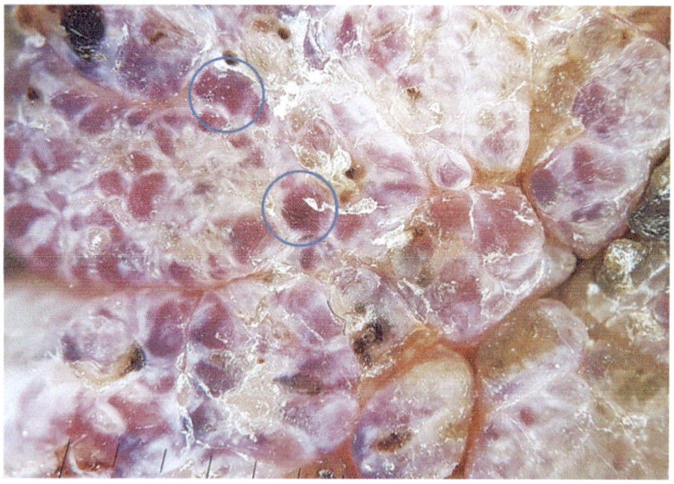

FIG. 22: Dermoscopy shows red lacunae (blue circles) and white scales in a case of angiokeratoma (polarized, DermLite DL4, 10×).

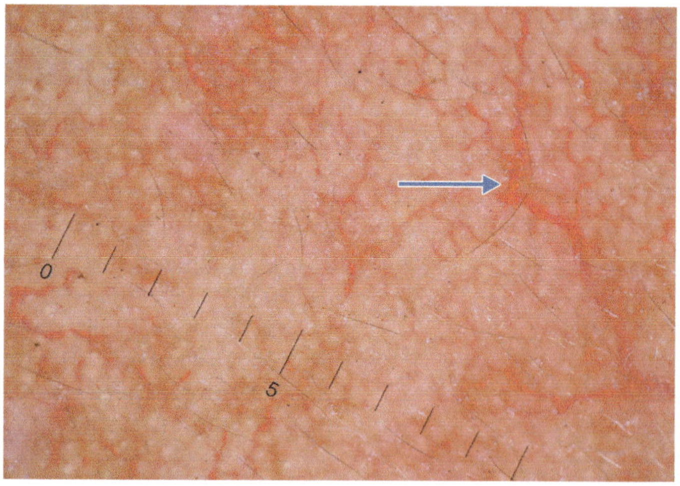

FIG. 23: Dermoscopy shows linear vessels (blue arrow) in a case of steroid damaged face (polarized, DermLite DL4, 10×).

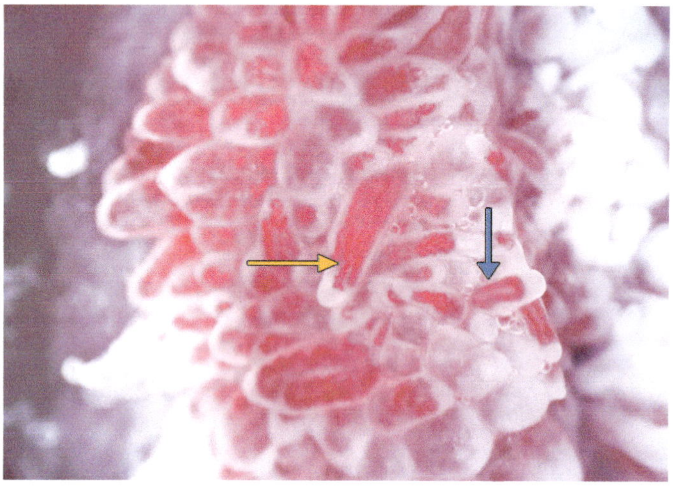

FIG. 24: Dermoscopy shows looped vessels (blue arrow) and serpentine vessels (orange arrow) in case of oral verrucae (polarized, Dino-Lite Edge, 100×).

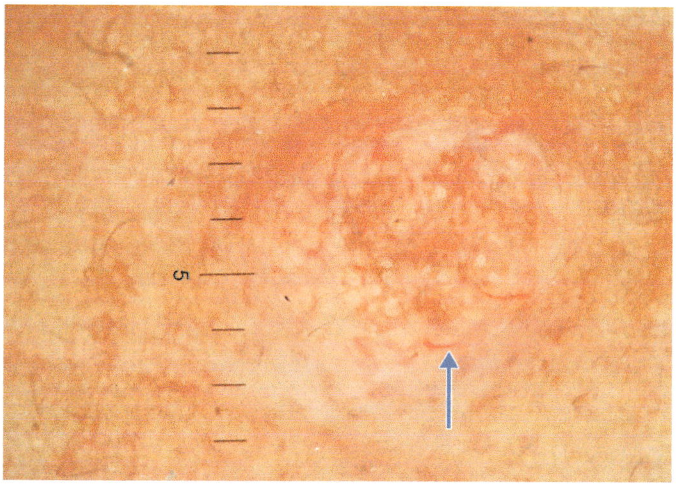

FIG. 25: Dermoscopy shows radial arrangement of crown vessels (blue arrow) in a case of sebaceous hyperplasia (polarized, DermLite DL4, 10×).

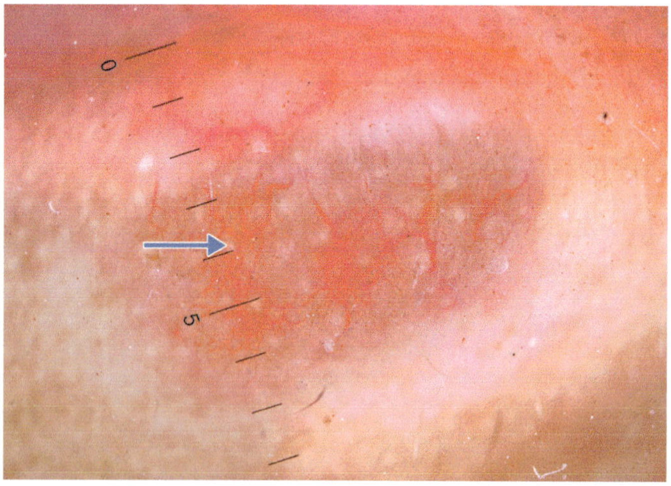

FIG. 26: Dermoscopy shows branching vessels (blue arrow) in a case of granulomatous lesion (polarized, DermLite DL4, 10×).

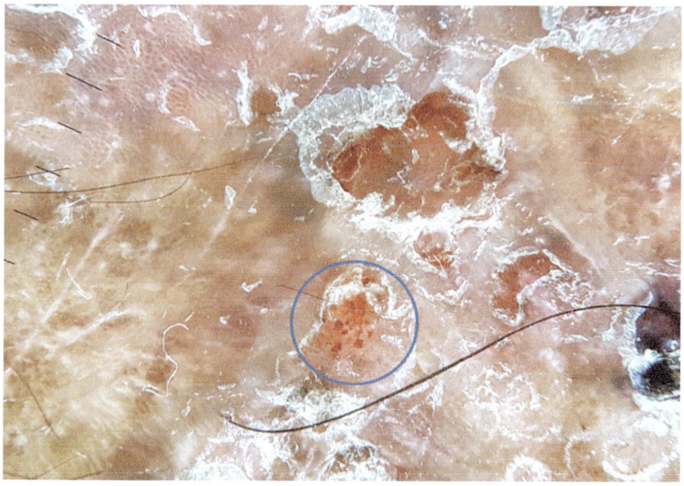

FIG. 27: Dermoscopy shows clustered glomerular vessels (blue circle) and white scales in a case of Bowen's disease (polarized, DermLite DL4, 10×).

TABLE 4: Dermoscopy of normal skin over various body parts.[8]

Body part	Dermoscopy pattern	Description
Trunk and extremities	Reticular pigment network (**Fig. 28**)	Homogeneous brown-colored network forming uniform and regular mesh with white circles in-between representing eccrine duct opening
Face	Pseudonetwork (**Fig. 29**)	Pigment network interrupted by multiple light brown circles and yellow clods, this appearance is due to relatively flat rete ridges and abundant pilosebaceous units
Acral skin	Ridges and furrows (**Fig. 30**)	Alternate banding of light brown furrows and dark brown ridges with tiny white dots of eccrine gland openings present on ridges
Mucosa	Pigment network is not present, nonspecific patterns which can be seen are parallel pattern and ring-like pattern. Looped, dotted or linear vessels can be seen (**Fig. 31**)	
Nail (**Fig. 32**)	• Nail plate • Nail bed • Proximal nail fold (PNF) • Cuticle • Hyponychium	• Smooth translucent structure • Pink structure directly visible through nail plate with linearly arranged vessels at distal end of plate • Looped vessels having convexity distally and density of nearly 30 linear vessels per 5 mm. Absence of dropouts and hemorrhage • Transverse transparent band attaching PNF to nail plate • Dotted vessels
Hair and scalp (**Fig. 33**)	• Hair shaft • Follicular units • Perifollicular and interfollicular skin • Blood vessels	• Presence of both terminal hair and vellus hair. Vellus hair density < 20% of total hair • 2–3 hairs emerge from single ostia • Honeycomb reticular network with small regular white dots corresponding to eccrine glands • Looped vessel around follicular unit usually on frontal scalp, thin arborizing vessels usually on temporal or occipital scalp

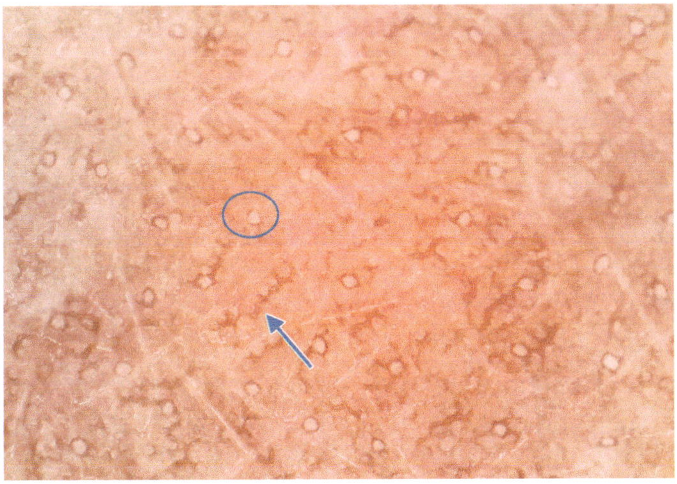

FIG. 28: Dermoscopy of extremities shows reticular pattern of pigment (blue arrow) and regular white dots (blue circle) representing eccrine ducts opening (polarized, Dino-Lite Edge, 20×).

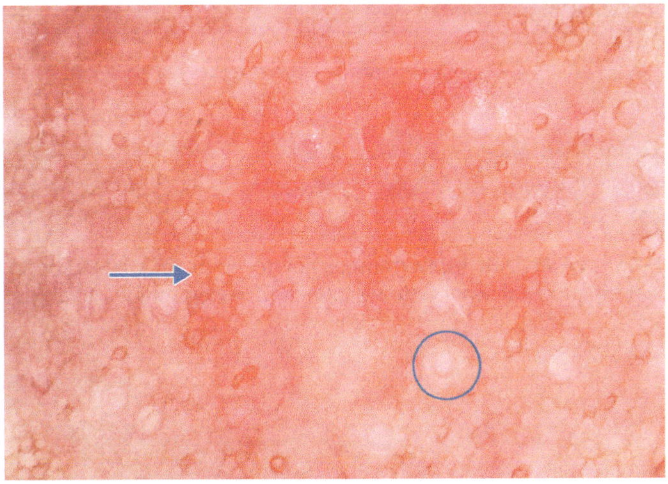

FIG. 29: Dermoscopy of facial skin shows pseudoreticular pattern of pigment (blue arrow) and yellow clods (blue circle) representing patulous follicular opening (polarized, Dino-Lite Edge, 20×).

- *Characteristic dermoscopic features*: These features are specific to certain disease and suggest a diagnosis. For example, presence of regular red dots on an erythematous background suggests psoriasis (**Fig. 21**). Specific features are in metaphoric term like maple leaf area in basal cell carcinoma (**Fig. 34**).
- *Dermoscopic criteria*: The collection of dermoscopic features with reasonable positive or negative predictive value for diagnosis forms a criterion. There are well-documented criteria for melanoma, basal cell carcinoma, and seborrheic keratosis.[9]

METAPHORIC AND DESCRIPTIVE TERMINOLOGIES

Metaphor is a word representative or symbolic of something else. It helps learner to connect commonly seen or used object with new or unfamiliar description. The advantage of metaphor is that it is easier to remember and recall. There are many problems associated with use of metaphors:

- Metaphors depend on imagination and largely described in the form of commonly seen objects locally.
- Metaphoric descriptions are ambiguous and may mean different to different individuals.

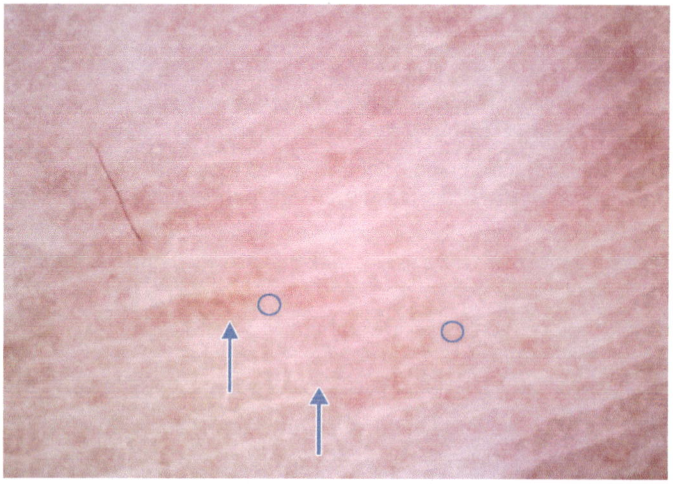

FIG. 30: Dermoscopy of palmar skin shows light brown furrows and dark brown ridges (blue arrows). Ridges show regular white dots (blue circles) representing eccrine ducts opening (polarized, Dino-Lite Edge, 20×).

- Similar metaphoric structures may be present in many diseases.
- The search for metaphoric structures prevents complete analysis of dermoscopic findings and may result in misdiagnosis.
- The number of metaphors is increasing exponentially and it is not possible to remember all.

Because of these disadvantages, descriptive terminologies as discussed above, are now preferred. The use of descriptive terminologies is not without problems. Pigment network which is a simple term understood by all is described as "grid-like pattern consisting of interconnecting pigmented lines surrounding hypopigmented holes". These descriptions are complex, verbose, and difficult to reproduce. The use of descriptive terminologies in many instances is more effective and intuitive like the term "peppering" is more difficult to imagine than "fine dots with blue-gray color". In our opinion, a mix of metaphoric

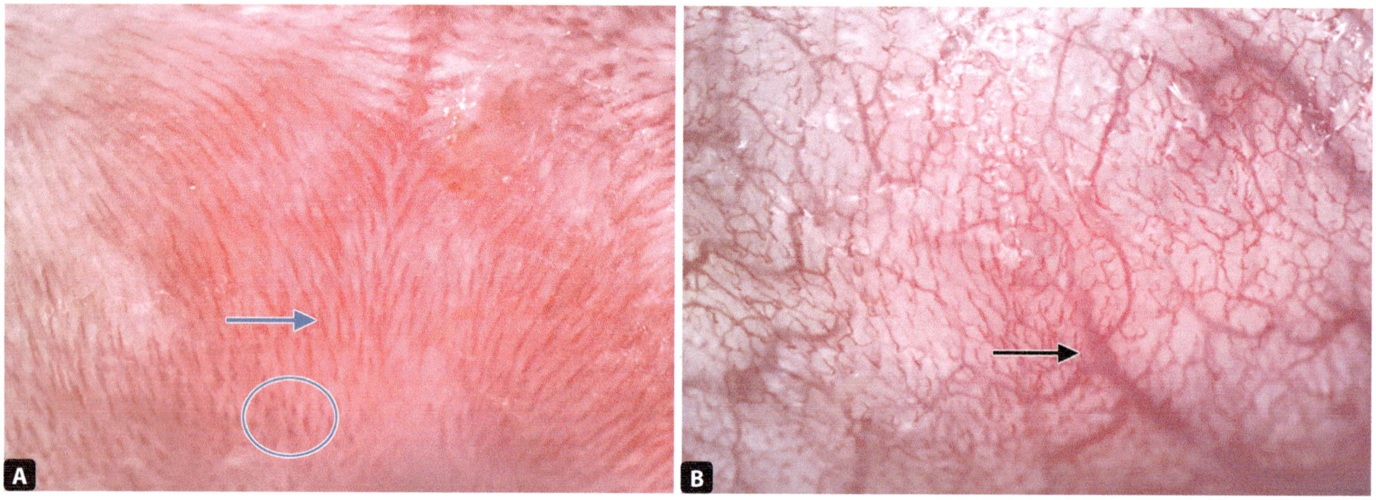

FIGS. 31A AND B: (A) Dermoscopy of dry lip (outer aspect) shows parallel (blue arrow) and dotted vessels (blue circle); (B) Dermoscopy of wet lip (mucosal aspect) shows branched vessels (black arrow) (polarized, Dino-Lite Edge, 20×).

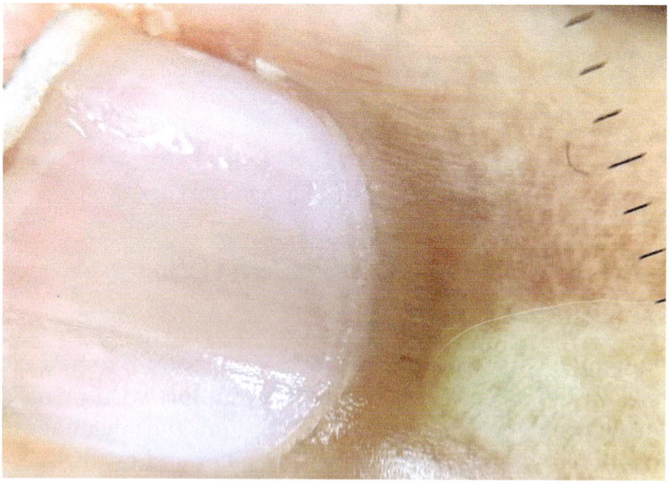

FIG. 32: Polarized dermoscopy of nail unit shows translucent nail plate, nail bed, cuticle, and nail fold capillaries (polarized, Illuco, 10×).

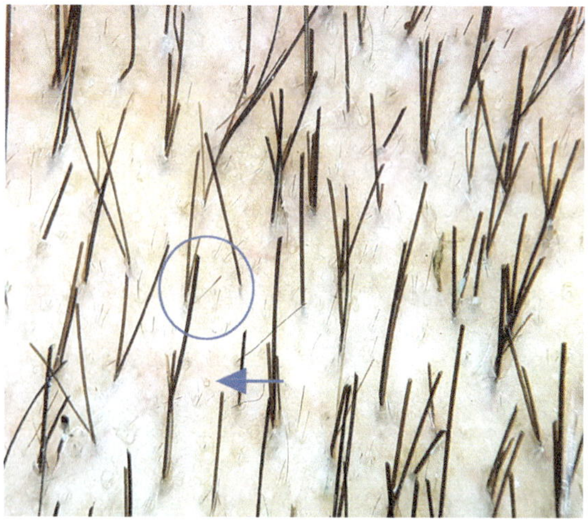

FIG. 33: Dermoscopy of scalp shows honeycomb pigment pattern (blue circle), white dots (blue arrow), and terminal hairs (polarized, DermLite DL4, 10×).

and descriptive terminologies is best for better dermoscopic description. The commonly used metaphoric terminologies and their descriptive counterparts are tabulated in **Table 5**.[10]

TIPS WHILE USING DERMOSCOPE

Capturing good dermoscopic image is an art and essential to perform dermoscopy effectively:

- Keep dermoscope fully charged.
- Use adapter which fits the dermoscope properly.
- Clean the lesion to remove artifact.
- Application of linkage fluid like 70% alcohol improves picture quality even in polarized dermoscope.
- Nonpolarized dermoscopy, noncontact polarized and contact PD should be performed in all cases.
- Apply ultrasound gel for dermoscopy of nail unit.
- Lesser pressure, removal of contact plate, use of linkage fluid, and use of videodermoscope prevent blanching of vessels and result in better visualization of vascular structures.
- Toggling

TABLE 5: Common metaphors and their description.[10]

Metaphor	Description	Condition
Spoke-wheel area	Brown, gray, tan-colored radial projection from central clod of same color	Basal cell carcinoma (BCC)
Starburst pattern	Peripheral pseudopods around the perimeter of the lesion	Spitz nevus
Maple leaf like pigmentation (**Fig. 34**)	Discrete, brown to gray-blue, bulbous extensions resembling a maple leaf	BCC
Cerebriform pattern (**Fig. 35**)	Brain-like appearance created due to gyri and keratin-filled sulci	Seborrheic keratoses
Cobblestone	Polygonal globules, symmetrically distributed	Congenital nevus
Strawberry pattern	Reddish pseudonetwork (erythema and wavy vessels) around hair follicle openings which are accentuated with white halo appearance	Actinic keratoses
Fingerprint pattern	Light brown thin-curved lines that do not interconnect to form a network	Seborrheic keratoses
Milia-like cyst	White to yellow round opalescent structures corresponding to intraepidermal cysts	Seborrheic keratoses
Comedo-like openings	Round-oval keratin-filled clefts	Seborrheic keratoses
Blue-whitish veil (**Fig. 36**)	An irregular-shaped blotch of blue hue with an overlying whitish ground glass haze	Melanoma
Crypts (**Fig. 37**)	Keratin-filled invaginations that are larger than comedo-like openings	Seborrheic keratoses
Typical pigment network	• Network with minimal variability of color, thickness, and spacing • Symmetrically distributed	• Nevi • Delicate pigment network in dermatofibroma
Atypical pigment network	• Network with increased variability of color, thickness, and spacing • Asymmetrically distributed	Melanoma, dysplastic nevi
Hub and spoke pattern (**Fig. 38**)	Dark-colored radial lines with central dot or clod	Cutaneous amyloidosis

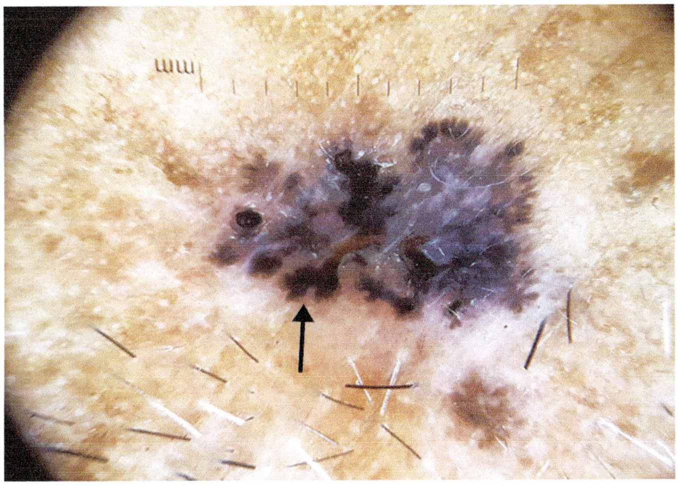

FIG. 34: Dermoscopy shows maple leaf-like areas (black arrow) in a case of basal cell carcinoma (polarized, DermLite DL4, 10×).

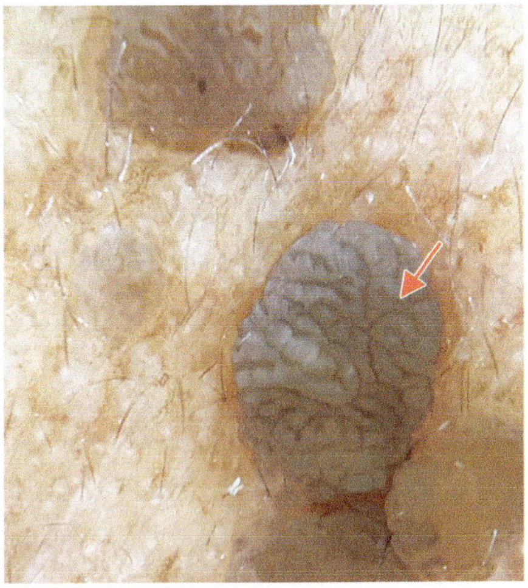

FIG. 35: Dermoscopy shows cerebriform appearance (red arrow) in a case of seborrheic keratosis (polarized, DermLite DL4, 10×).

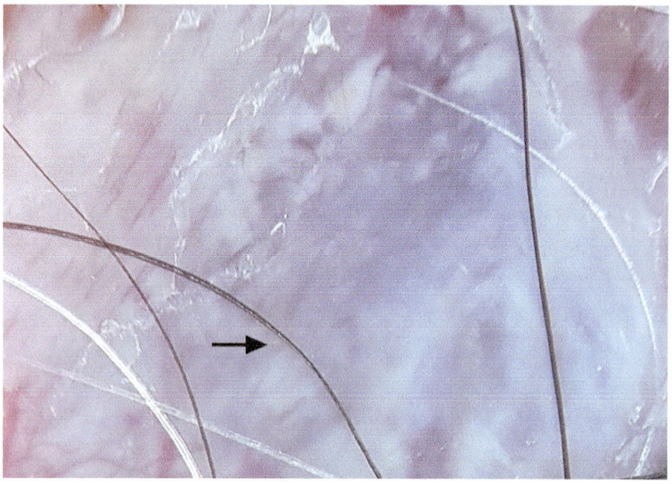

FIG. 36: Dermoscopy shows blue-white veil (blue arrow) in a case of melanoma (polarized, DermLite DL4, 10×).

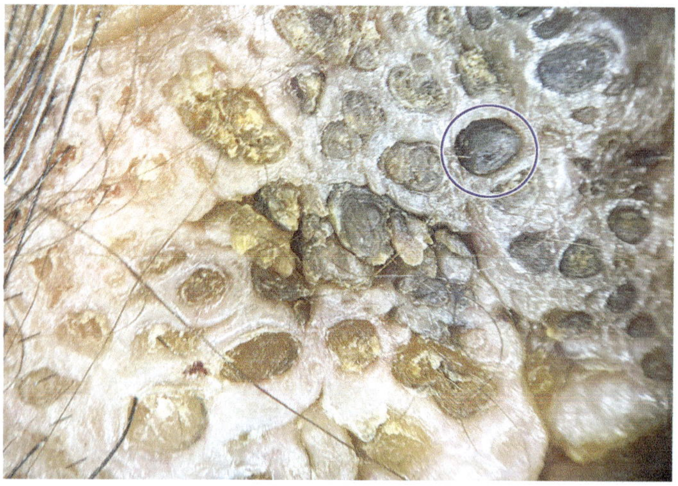

FIG. 37: Dermoscopy shows crypts (blue circle) in a case of seborrheic keratoses (polarized, Dino-Lite Edge, 20×).

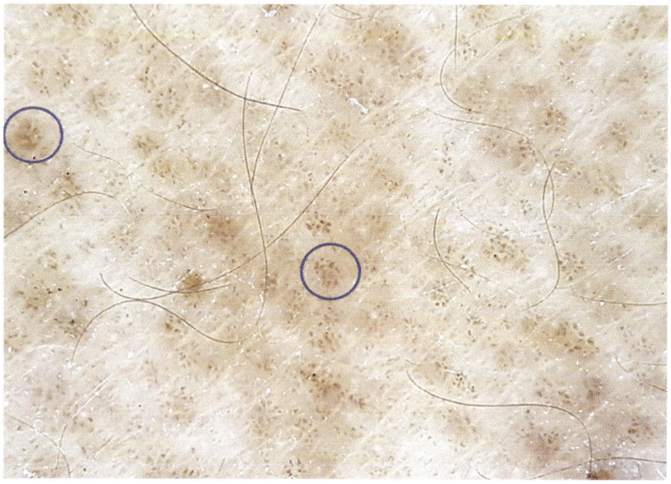

FIG. 38: Dermoscopy of macular amyloidosis shows hub and spoke pattern (blue circles) (polarized, DermLite DL4, 10×).

KEY POINTS

- The contact plate, interface fluid, and polarizing light are essential components of dermoscopy.
- There are two main types of dermoscopy: PD and NPD.
- Descriptive and metaphoric terminologies are used to describe the patterns.
- Dermoscopy of normal skin differs according to different parts of the body.

CONCLUSION

Dermoscopy is rapid and noninvasive tool for diagnosis of many skin disorders. Understanding basic principles of dermoscopy and knowledge of structures and patterns seen on dermoscopy are essential to use dermoscope as a diagnostic tool effectively.

REFERENCES

1. Wang SQ, Dusza SW, Scope A, Braun RP, Kopf AW, Marghoob AA. Principles of dermoscopy and dermoscopic equipment. In: Marghoob AA, Malvehy J, Braun RP (Eds). Atlas of Dermoscopy, 2nd edition. New York: CRC Press; 2012. pp. 3-10.
2. Wang SQ, Dusza SW, Scope A, Braun RP, Kopf AW, Marghoob AA. Difference in dermoscopic images from nonpolarized dermoscope and polarized dermoscope influence the diagnostic accuracy and confidence level: a pilot study. Dermatol Surg. 2008;34:1389-95.
3. Binder M, Kittler H, Pehamberger H, Wolff K. Possible hazard to patients from immersion oil used for epiluminescence microscopy. J Am Acad Dermatol. 1999;40:499.
4. Anderson RR. Polarized light examination and photography of the skin. Arch Dermatol. 1991;127:1000-5.
5. Kittler H, Rosendahl C, Cameron A, Tschandl P. Principal pigmented skin lesions relevant to dermatoscopy. In: Dermatoscopy-Pattern Analysis. Kittler H, Rosendahl C, Cameron A, Tschandl P (Eds), Vienna: facultas.wuv, 2011. pp. 25-48.
6. Kittler H. Dermatoscopy: Introduction of a new algorithmic method based on pattern analysis for diagnosis of pigmented skin lesions. Dermatopathology: Practical and Conceptual. 2007;13(1):3.
7. Kittler H, Riedl E, Rosendahl C, Cameron A. Dermatoscopy of unpigmented lesions of the skin: a new classification of vessel morphology based on pattern analysis. Dermatopathology: Practical and Conceptual. 2008;14(4):4.
8. Nirmal B. Dermoscopy of normal skin and appendages. In: Khopkar US (Ed). Dermoscopy and Trichoscopy in Diseases of the Brown Skin: Atlas and Short Text. New Delhi: Jaypee Brothers Medical Publishers (P) Ltd; 2012. pp. 47-59.
9. Puig S, Cecilia N, Malvehy J. Dermoscopic criteria and basal cell carcinoma. G Ital Dermatol Venereol. 2012;147(2):135-40.
10. Kittler H, Marghoob AA, Argenziano G, Carrera C, Curiel-Lewandrowski C, Hofmann-Wellenhof R, et al. Standardization of terminology in dermoscopy/dermatoscopy: results of the third consensus conference of the International Society of Dermoscopy. J Am Acad Dermatol. 2016;74:1093-106.

3

CHAPTER

Parts and Types of Dermoscopes

Shital Poojary, Atul Bothra

INTRODUCTION

The dermoscope assists to visualize the subsurface features of the skin which are otherwise not visible to the naked eye. It helps us to see the intricate details of the epidermis and superficial dermis including pigment patterns, vascular patterns, and appendageal structures.

Light incident on the skin undergoes reflection, refraction, diffraction, and absorption. Normal dry skin reflects most of the light incident on it and, smooth, oily skin allows most of the light to pass through and reach the deeper dermis. Application of appropriate linkage fluids over the cutaneous lesions prevents reflection and scattering of light and increases the transparency of the stratum corneum.

In polarized dermoscopes, the polarization prevents scattering of light and allows visualization of subsurface structures even without usage of linkage fluid.

PARTS OF A DERMOSCOPE (FIG. 1)[1-4]

- *Achromatic lens*: The lens in standard dermoscopes gives 10–20x magnification. Lenses in FotoFinder can provide magnification up to180x.
- *Illumination system*: Light-emitting diodes (LEDs) provide high intensity white light. Number of LEDs may differ in different dermoscopes (from 4 to 40). The light can be adjusted by switching on only specific set of LEDs. Dermoscopes can also be designed to emit different colored light based on requirement: yellow, red, blue LEDs (multispectral dermoscope).[5,6] Level of penetration of light into the skin depends on the wavelength of light. LED lamps provide much better illumination than the halogen lamps which were used previously. Also, since halogen lamps give a yellowish light, the actual color of the lesion may be masked.
- *Power supply*:
  - Handheld dermoscopes are powered by batteries. Types of batteries:
    - Lithium ion battery
    - Rechargeable lithium battery
    - Alkaline battery.
  - Some dermoscopes are provided with a compatible charging dock.
  - Videodermoscope—via USB cable.
- *Contact plate*: For contact dermoscopy, a glass plate with a refractive index similar to that of the stratum corneum is used. Hence, the amount of light reflected is considerably reduced. If contact fluid is additionally applied to the skin lesion, the light can better penetrate depths of the skin, and the epidermis becomes almost transparent.

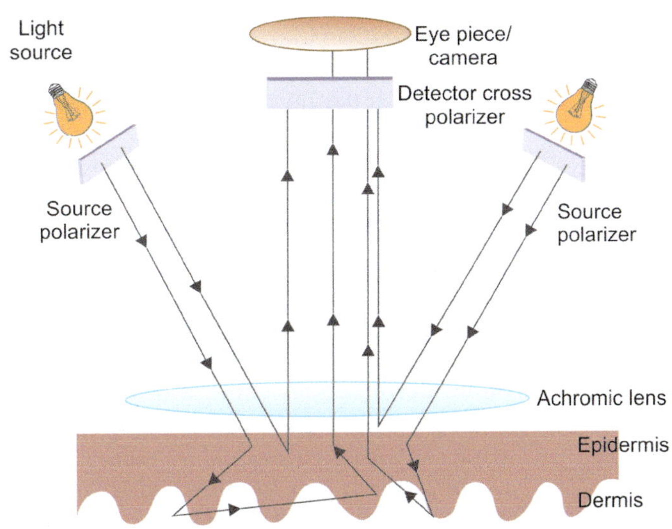

FIG. 1: Schematic diagram of cross-polarization and parts of dermoscope.

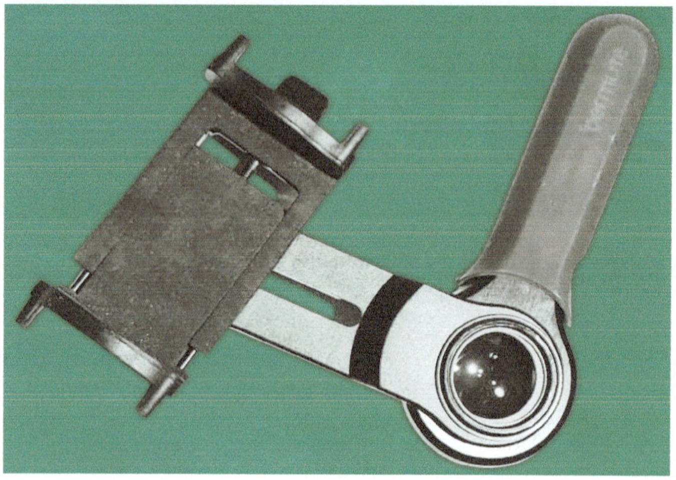

FIG. 2: Universal adapter attached to DermLite DL4.

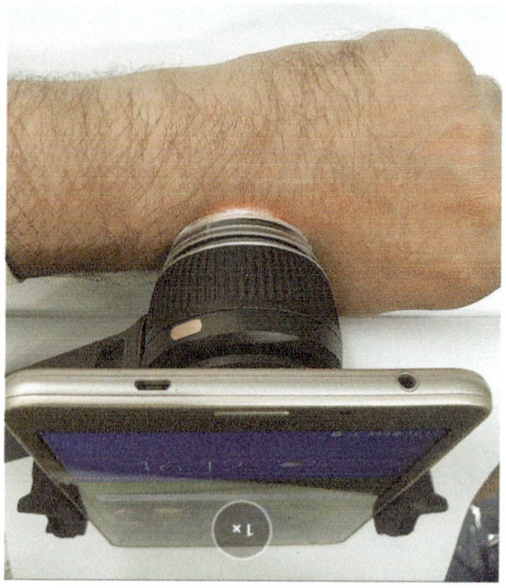

FIG. 3: Dermoscope attached to a cell phone using universal adapter.
Courtesy: Dr Saurabh Jaiswal.

Autoclavable contact plates are available in different sizes for difficult to access contact areas. Small disks measuring 8 mm in diameter can be used by simply clicking them onto the head of the dermoscope. Contact plates are composed of multicoated silicone glass and either graduated or nongraduated. Graduated plates have a scale inscribed to measure the size of the lesion examined.

Disposable contact plate caps, known as ice caps which snap over the faceplate of dermoscope are available and can be used to prevent cross-contamination while using the dermoscope.

Retractable contact plates are available to switch between contact and noncontact modes during dermoscopy.

- *Dermoscopy photography system*:
  - Inbuilt camera, e.g., in videodermoscope
  - Attached digital camera: Camera can be attached with an adapter
  - USB cable to transfer photographs to laptop/desktop Attachments for cameras:[7]
    - Lenses: They are attached to digital cameras—commonly DSLRs (Canon or Nikon) that can be used to store images with high quality. They are available for dermoscopes such as DermLite (3Gen) and Heine Delta 20T.
    - Adapters: They are used for attaching to mobile phones for taking images:
      - Special cases contoured for the mobile phone or tablet device either slide over or snap to the phone or tablet. They have a built-in magnet which is compatible with a specific dermoscope.
      - Some dermoscopes come with a universal smartphone adapter which is compatible with any smartphone. It comes with clamps which can be attached to various smartphones (**Figs. 2** and **3**).
      - Magnetic rings are available that attach to smartphone case which can be attached by a simple magnetic adapter to the dermoscope.
      - Three-dimensional (3D) printing can also be used to prepare adapters for attaching dermoscopes wherever facilities are available for the same. These are low cost compared to commercially available ones and are customisable.[8]
- *Software*:
  - Mobile apps are available to digitally store images.
  - Inbuilt software for measuring area and disease severity scoring.

TYPES OF DERMOSCOPES

A. Depending on presence/absence of polarization filters, there are two types of dermoscopes:
   1. *Nonpolarized dermoscopes*: In nonpolarized dermoscopes, linkage fluid requires to be used to provide an interface between the skin surface and the optical plate of the dermoscope.
      Linkage fluids which can be used are ultrasonography gel, mineral oil, alcoholic disinfectant, glycerine, and water. Immersion oil is generally avoided as it contains chlorinated paraffin and dibutyl phthalate which have teratogenic, fetotoxic, and carcinogenic effects. Water and alcohol antiseptic solutions are also not preferred as they evaporate quickly and hence are less preferred than oils.
   2. *Polarized dermoscopes*: Polarized dermoscopes have cross-polarization filters. Placement of filters is depicted in **Figure 1**.
      The cross-polarization allows the scattered light to be absorbed allowing light to pass through in a single plane. This allows the structures to be better visualized. In polarized dermoscopes, contact fluid

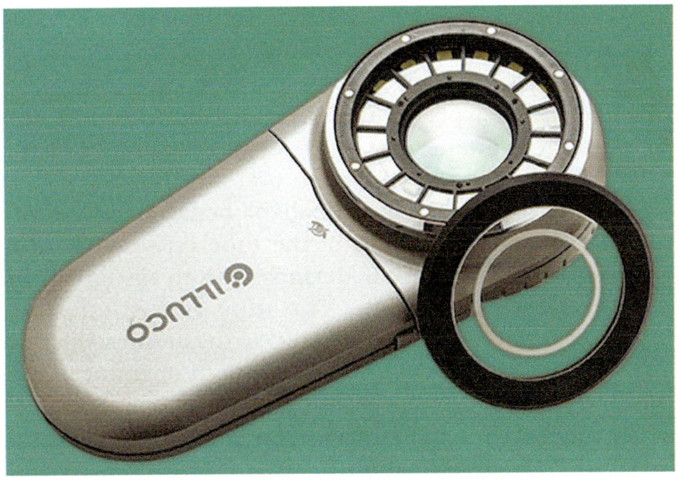

FIG. 4: Illuco IDS-1100.

Source: https://dermoscan.de/en/products/illuco-1-1/.

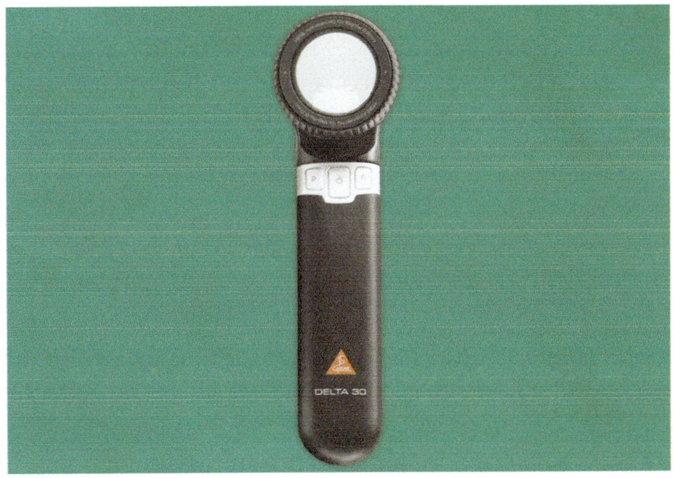

FIG. 5: Heine Delta 30 dermatoscope.

Source: https://www.heine.com/en/products/dermatoscopes-and-digital-documentation/dermatoscopes/detail/100034-heine-delta-30-dermatoscope.

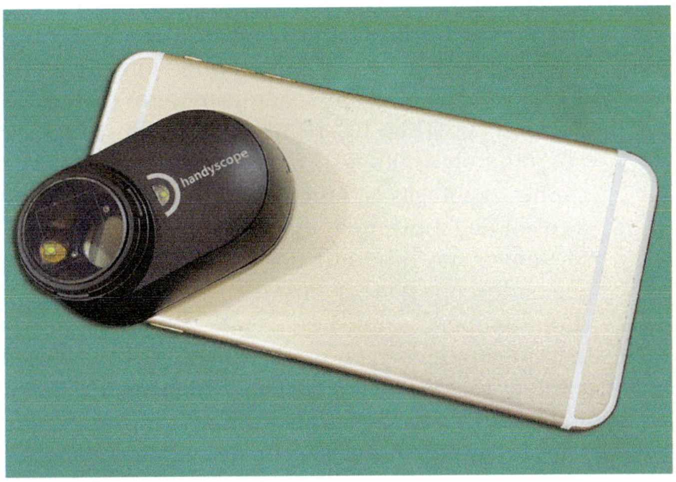

FIG. 6: Handyscope by FotoFinder.

Courtesy: Dr Balachandra Ankad, SN Medical College, Bagalkot, Karnataka, India.

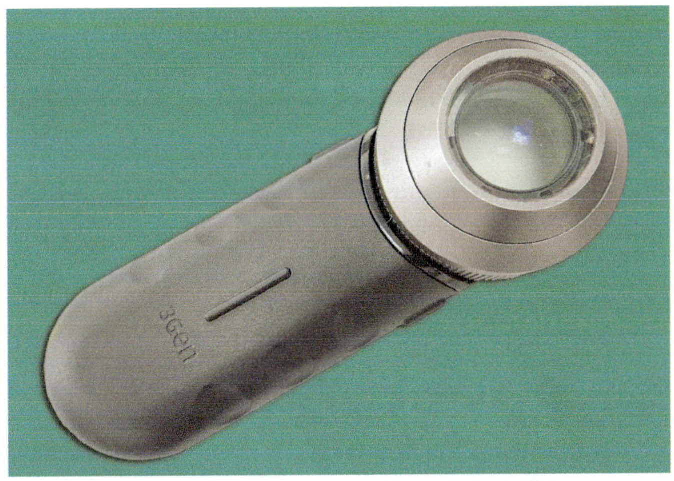

FIG. 7: Handheld hybrid dermoscope—DermLite (3Gen) DL3.

is not required. Polarized dermoscopes allow noncontact dermoscopy.

Hybrid dermoscopes: These devices allow switching between polarized and nonpolarized mode. These help in better diagnosis as the nonpolarized mode assists in identifying structures on the surface while the polarized mode helps in visualizing pigmentary and vascular changes. Examples are Illuco IDS-1100, Heine Delta 30, and Handyscope FotoFinder (**Figs. 4** to **6**).

B. Dermoscopes can also be classified as follows:
   1. *Handheld dermoscope*: This needs to be attached to a camera or a phone to obtain images (**Figs. 6** and **7**).
   2. *USB dermoscope*: This dermoscope is attached via USB cable to a laptop/desktop which enables to see and interpret images (**Fig. 8**).

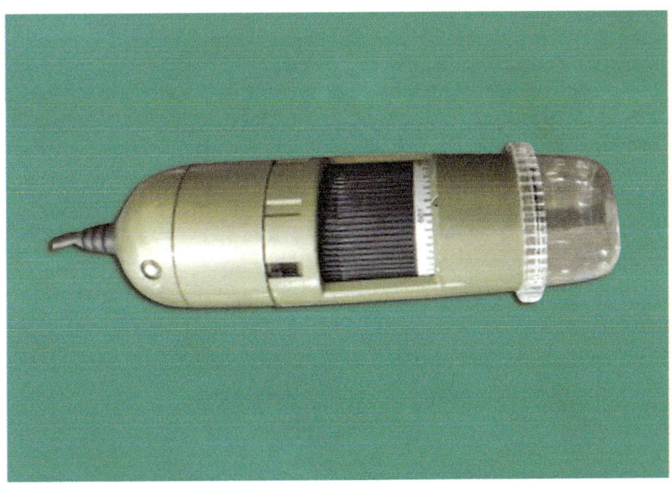

FIG. 8: USB dermoscope.

SYSTEMS FOR DIGITAL DERMOSCOPY

Some sophisticated systems are available especially abroad which enable full body images in 2D or 3D. They are either integrated into digital dermoscopic systems, work with smartphone, or have a separate rigging system. Examples include:

- DermEngine (MetaOptima)
- FotoFinder (**Fig. 9**)
- MoleMax HD (Derma Medical Systems)
- Vectra 3D (Canfield)

PARAMETERS OF THE LENSES

Magnification and resolution: Magnification of the lenses varies between 10× and 20× with occasional dermoscopes having 40× magnifications. Higher magnification may not always mean a better image as the patterns may not be visible.

Optical resolution describes the ability of the dermoscope lens to resolve detail in the lesion that is being imaged. Optical resolution depends on the quality of the lens. Sharpness and details of the image are affected by the resolution.

Size of the lenses: Size of the lenses should be optimum. Large lenses are useful to cover large areas but these cannot be used in smaller specific areas, e.g., between the toes. Hence, optimal size of the lenses is essential or a smaller contact plate can be used to adapt to smaller areas.

MODIFICATIONS OF DERMOSCOPE

- *For inaccessible areas*: Dermoscopy of sites like mucosa and body folds is a challenge due to the inherent shape of the dermoscope. Endoscopes and oral mucoscopes have been tried previously, but are unsuitable for use in routine practice. The following are the modifications described to ease dermoscopy of inaccessible areas:
    - Modification of a USB dermoscope: Sterilized disposable plastic tubes that form core of leukoplast adhesive tapes are used as an attachment of the dermoscope to access the oral mucosa. The plastic tube is clenched by the patient, between the incisors leaving a small part of the tube outside which is attached to a USB dermoscope to visualize the mucosal structures. The tube is cost-effective, disposable, provides stability to the dermoscope and allows patient to hold their mouth open for longer durations. Moreover, as the dermoscope itself does not come in contact with the mucosa, it avoids the risk of contamination.[9]
    - Use of otoendoscope: Contact dermoscopy using rigid handheld otoendoscope attached to a smartphone has been described for less accessible sites such as mucosal surface and interdigital spaces. The advantage of using an otoendoscope is the long shape which allows to access difficult areas and attachment to the smartphone allows image capture and storage without any separate monitor (as for USB dermoscope) (**Fig. 10**). However, otoendoscopes are not routinely available in a dermatological setup and capturing images is difficult with the otoendoscope as even fine movement leads to significant blurring. Moreover, no inherent magnification property of the endoscope goes against the basic principles of a dermoscope.[10]
- *For dermoscopy guided biopsy*: Dermoscope can be used intraoperatively to identify the site of biopsies. However, stabilization of dermoscopes mid-air during guided biopsies is difficult. Agrawal et al. described the use of a syringe barrel cut circumferentially approximately 1 cm from the base with a rectangle window on one side of the barrel as an adapter for handheld dermoscopes to

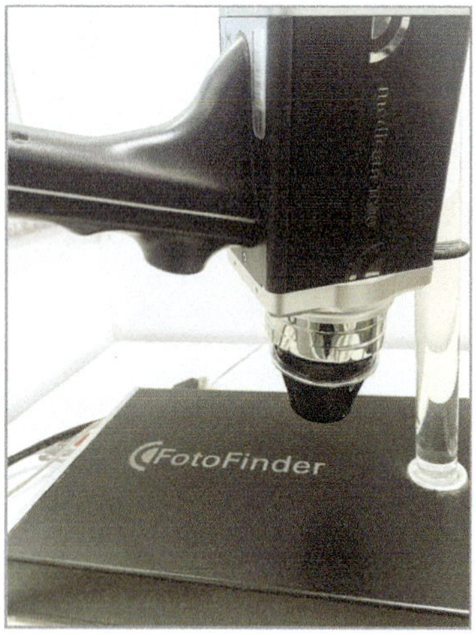

FIG. 9: FotoFinder videodermoscope.

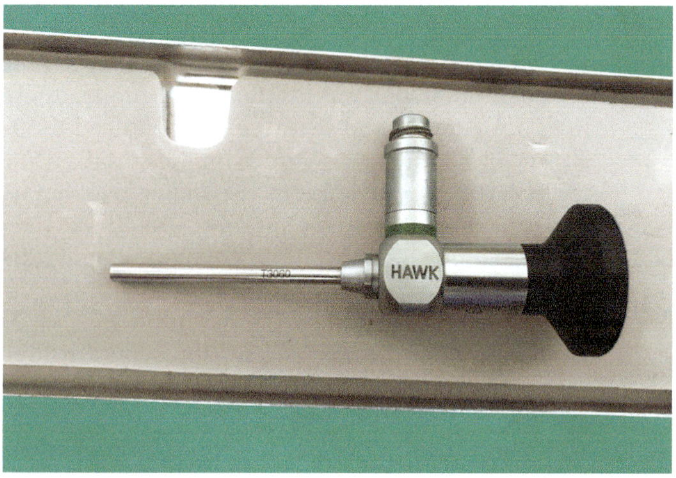

FIG. 10: Otoendoscope.

be used intraoperatively to ease dermoscopic guided biopsies.[11]

- *Dermoscopes for resource-limited settings*: One of the limitations of dermoscope is the high cost of the device which limits its widespread use, especially in developing countries. The following have been described as low-cost alternatives:
    - Tape dermoscopy: After applying immersion fluid, the lesion is covered with transparent adhesive tape with lateral tension.[12] Under ambient indoor or outdoor lighting, the image is captured using a mobile phone or digital camera placed 25–30 cm from the lesion and held at approximately 45° to avoid light reflection. Limitations of tape dermoscopy are unfocused images, blanching of the vessels while applying the tape and absence of polarized light. Moreover, exophytic tumors and lesions on certain difficult locations (e.g., convex surfaces of the nose, ears, and nails) may not be recorded with adequate image quality.
    - Eyepiece lens of a microscope: After application of Echogel on the lesion, a glass slide is mounted over it followed by illumination of the lesion using a torch, and lastly examining the lesion using the eyepiece lens of a microscope.[13]
    - Jeweler's loupe: A jeweler's loupe with 10x magnification and an inbuilt LED light can be used as a low-cost alternative to a dermoscope (**Fig. 11**) after applying linkage gel.[14] The loupe can be taped to the back of a cell phone to collect and store images. However, the clarity is not as good as a dermoscope, although essential skin features are easily discernable.
    - Clip-on lens: A clip-on lens can be used as an alternative to dermoscope in resource-limited settings.[13] The magnification of the device is 30–60x and it is compatible with all smartphones. However, it lacks polarized light and the structures are not as clear as with a dermoscope but being economical it can be used as an alternative handy device.

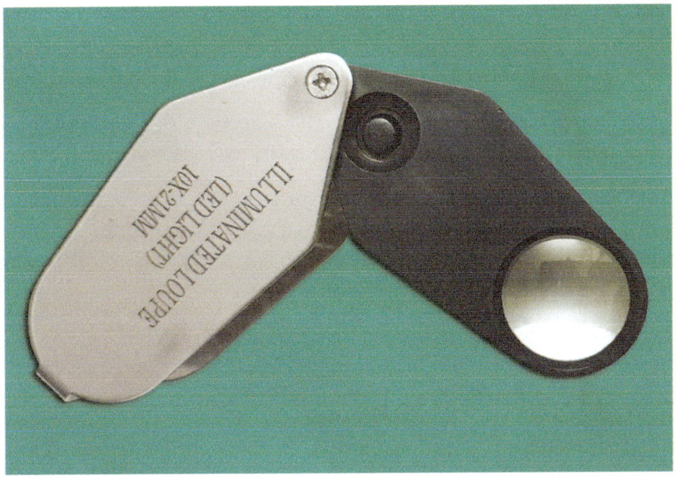

FIG. 11: Jeweler's loupe.

A low-cost 3D-printed clip-on polarizing dermoscope compatible with all smartphone has been described by Sahoo et al.[8] The clip-on was designed by AutoCAD modeling and printed on a 3D printer. It contains a magnifying lens of focal length 10 mm along with two polarizing sheets. This clip-on dermoscope can be attached to any smartphone and images can be stored. The light emitted from the flash of the camera passes through the polarizing sheet aligned to the flash of the camera and gets polarized to view the skin structures. This clip-on dermoscope does not require its own light source as it utilizes the flash of the Smartphone camera. It does not require any power source/battery or any accessories, thus making it a very affordable polarized dermoscope (**Figs. 12A** and **B**).[15]

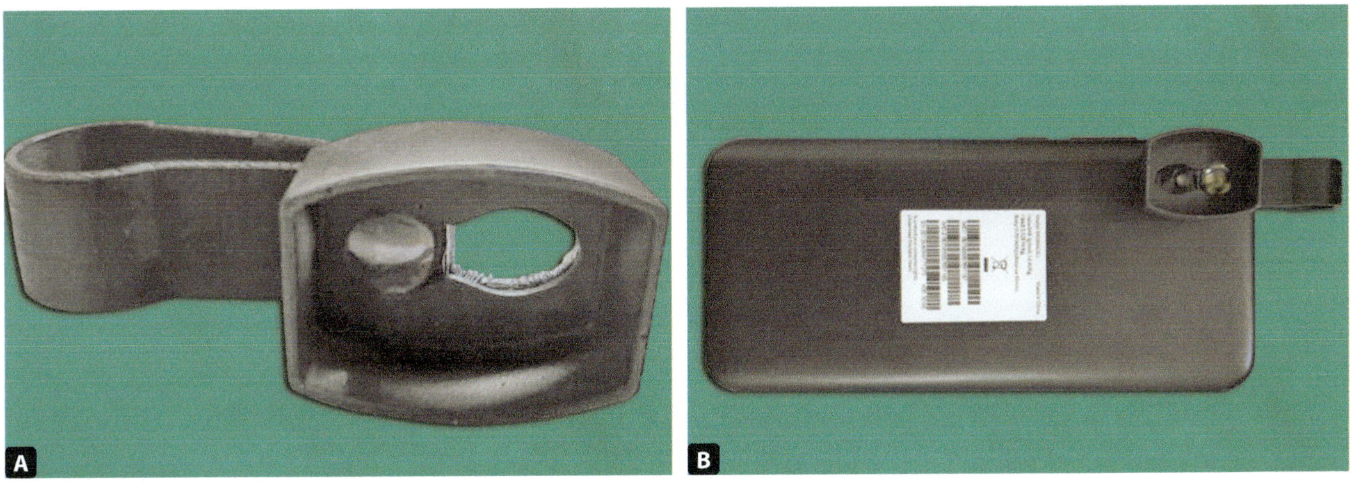

FIGS. 12A AND B: (A) 3D-printed clip-on polarizing dermoscope; (B) Attachment of clip-on polarizing dermoscope to mobile phone.
Source: REDX Innovation Lab, Welingkar Institute of Management Development and Research, Mumbai in collaboration with KJ Somaiya Medical College, Mumbai, Maharashtra, India.

KEY POINTS

- Polarized and nonpolarized modes of the dermoscope are useful to visualize the subsurface and surface structures, respectively.
- Recent modifications in dermoscopic techniques have eased mucosal and intraoperative dermoscopy.
- Potential low-cost dermoscopes, e.g., 3D-printed dermoscopes will be helpful in resource-restricted settings.

CONCLUSION

Dermoscopy, the examination of skin lesions in a noninvasive fashion, is being adored by many dermatologists across the world. Hence, we find many types of dermoscopes in the market. User should choose a scope based on the budget, workload, type of clinical material, and need for the documentation. It should be noted that polarized and nonpolarized modes are complementary to each other and should be practiced in examining a given skin lesion.

REFERENCES

1. Ankad BS, Smitha SV, Koti VR. Basic science of dermoscopy. Clin Dermatol Rev. 2020;4:69-73.
2. Nirmal B. Dermatoscopy: physics and principles. Indian J Dermatopathol Diagn Dermatol. 2017;4:27-30.
3. Nischal KC, Khopkar US. Principles and technique of dermoscopy and videodermoscopy. In: Khopkar US (Ed). Dermoscopy and trichoscopy in diseases of the brown skin: Atlas and Short Text. New Delhi, India: Jaypee Brothers Medical Publishers (P) Ltd; 2012. pp. 1-9.
4. Mukherjee S. The dermoscope. In: Malakar S (Ed). Dermoscopy: Text and Atlas. New Delhi, India: Jaypee Brothers Medical Publishers (P) Ltd; 2019. pp. 4-10.
5. Nirmal B. Yellow light in dermatoscopy and its utility in dermatological disorders. Indian Dermatol Online J. 2017;8:384-5.
6. Weekenstroo HH, Cornelissen BM, Bernelot Moens HJ. Green light may improve diagnostic accuracy of nailfold capillaroscopy with a simple digital videomicroscope. Rheumatol Int. 2015;35:1069-71.
7. DermLite. [online] Available from https://dermlite.com/collections [Last accessed October, 2021].
8. Sahoo A, Wahi A, Patel S, Poojary S, Jaiswal S, Das A. A novel clip-on for smartphone dermoscopy in India. Bethesda, MD: Healthcare Innovations and Point of Care Technologies (HI-POCT), 2017 IEEE; 2017. pp. 101-4.
9. Jakhar D, Grover C. Innovative modification of the USB dermatoscope for mucoscopy. J Am Acad Dermatol. 2018;78(1):e3-4.
10. Kaliyadan F, Mohammed AW. Modification of dermoscopes for difficult to access sites. Indian Dermatol Online J. 2019;10(3):346.
11. Agrawal S, Dhurat R, Daruwalla S, Sharma A. A simple modification of a syringe barrel as an adapter for dermoscopic guided biopsy. J Am Acad Dermatol. 2020;83(1):e5-6.
12. Blum A, Giacomel J. Tape dermatoscopy: constructing a low-cost dermatoscope using a mobile phone, immersion fluid and transparent adhesive tape. Dermatol Pract Concept. 2015;5(2):87-93.
13. Sawada M, Tanaka M. Self-assembly of a simple low-cost dermoscope for examination of skin lesions. Dermatol Pract Concept. 2013;3(4):35.
14. Kaliyadan F. Using a simple jeweler's loupe as a dermoscopic instrument. Indian J Dermatol Venereol Leprol. 2011;77(5):617-20.
15. Gupta S, Aggarwal K, Yadav A, Gujrathi A. Low-cost video dermatoscope using an inexpensive clip-on lens. JAAD International. 2020;1(1):9-10.

4 CHAPTER

Dermoscopic-Histopathological Correlation

Biswanath Behera, Kinjal D Rambhia, Tejas Vishwanath

INTRODUCTION

Dermoscopic features are the direct reflection of pathological changes of a particular lesion. The various colors observed are due to the chromophores present in epidermis, dermis, or both. The colors observed are white, red, black, brown, gray, blue, and yellow. In addition, the above colors can have different shades.

Different chromophores such as melanin, blood (oxygenated and deoxygenated), keratin, collagen, xanthomatous histiocytes (lipids), and sebocytes (lipids) produce different colors (**Figs. 1A** to **F**). Out of various chromophores, melanin plays a significant role in orchestrating various pigment structures. So, the skin color of the patient is very important while analyzing the dermoscopic features. For the same dermatosis, dermoscopic differences can be observed between fair-skinned and dark-skinned individuals.

The appreciation of different colors or their shades depends upon the distance of the chromophore from the skin surface. Another factor that affects the appreciation of color is the presence and location of melanin, which can hinder the visibility of other chromophores based upon their concentration and location.[1] For example, pigment structure masks the visibility of vascular structures in basal cell carcinoma (BCC).[1]

The perception of various dermoscopic features or patterns depends upon the epidermal and/or dermal components and their proliferative or reaction patterns. Besides, all the patterns/features will have a background color. For example, a cerebriform pattern in seborrheic keratosis in the skin of color will have a brown to gray-brown background color.

DERMOSCOPIC PATTERNS AND STRUCTURES

- *Melanocytic lesions*:
  - Pigment network (lines, reticular): It is due to the interconnecting pigmented lines surrounding the hypopigmented hole arranged in a grid-like pattern. The pigmented lines correspond to melanin in vertical arms of rete ridges and holes correspond to the hypopigmented horizontal width between the adjacent rete ridges:
    - Typical network: It is typified by the presence of symmetrically distributed lines and holes with minimal variability in the color, thickness, and gap between the lines and commonly seen in a melanocytic nevus and Becker's nevus (**Figs. 2A** and **B**).[2]
    - Atypical network: It is characterized by asymmetrical distribution of pigmented lines of variable thickness, color, and arrangement and the holes are of different sizes. It is seen in dysplastic nevus and superficial spreading melanoma.[2]
  - Pseudonetwork (structureless brown area, interrupted by follicular openings): It consists of a structureless brown area interrupted by adnexal openings (**Fig. 2C**) on face. The holes correspond to follicular, eccrine, or sebaceous gland openings and the structureless brown area to the melanin in the basal layer.[2]
  - Negative network (lines, reticular, hypopigmented, around brown clods): It is seen in Spitz nevus and melanoma. The broad hypopigmented serpiginous

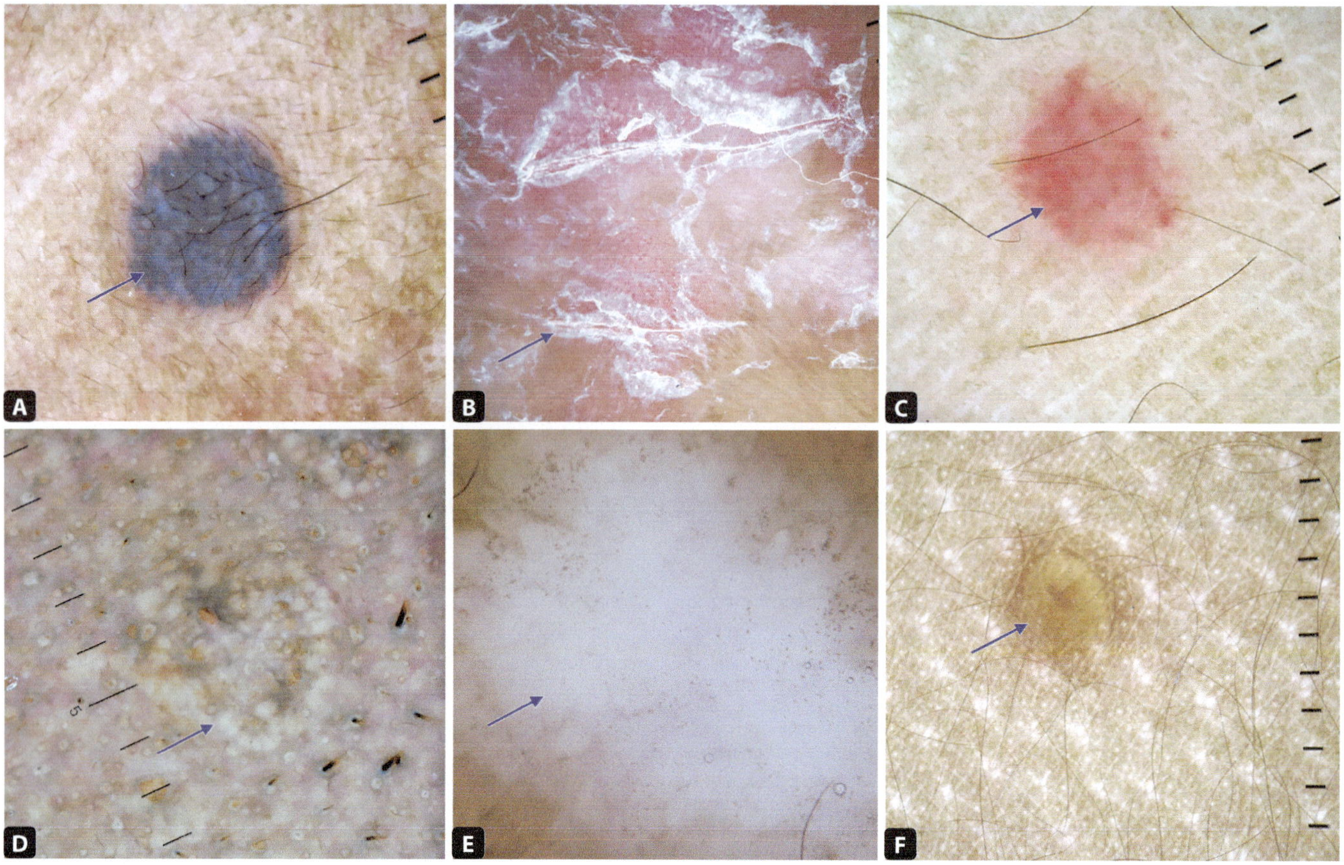

FIGS. 1A TO F: (A) Dermoscopy showing blue-gray homogeneous area (arrow) in a case of melanocytic nevus (chromophore-melanin) (polarized, DermLite DL4, 10×); (B) Diffuse white scales (arrow) in the case of psoriasis (chromophore-keratin) (polarized, DermLite, DL4, 10×); (C) Homogeneous pink area (arrow) in the case of small vessel vasculitis (chromophore-erythrocytes) (polarized, DermLite DL4, 10×); (D) Dermoscopy showing homogeneous yellow area (arrow) in a case of sebaceous hyperplasia (chromophore-lipid-containing sebocytes) (nonpolarized, Heine Delta, 10×); (E) Homogeneous white area (arrow) in the case of extragenital lichen sclerosus (chromophore-collagen) (polarized, DermLiteDL4, 10×); (F) Dermoscopy showing homogeneous yellow area (arrow) in a case of xanthogranuloma (chromophore-lipid inside xanthomized histiocytes) (polarized, DermLite DL4, 10×).

Source: AIIMS, Bhubaneswar, Odisha and JIPMER, Puducherry, India.

interconnecting lines surround the elongated and curvilinear globules. The lines correspond to the elongated hypopigmented rete ridges and globules to the large nests of melanocytes within the dermal papillae.[2,3]

- Structureless area: It is defined as the area without discernible basic elements and covers at least 10% of the whole lesion. It can be hyperpigmented, hypopigmented, and normal pigmented structureless area:[2]
  - White structureless area: BCC, squamous cell carcinoma (SCC) (**Fig. 2D**), idiopathic guttate hypomelanosis, and vitiligo (**Figs. 3A** to **C**)
  - Skin-colored structureless area: Neurofibroma, trichoepithelioma
  - Blotch (hyperpigmented structureless area): It is observed in melanoma and melanocytic nevus (**Figs. 3D** to **F**) and corresponds to the melanin in the stratum corneum, epidermis, and dermis.
- Homogeneous area: An area with a single color involving most of the lesion. It can be of various colors:
  - Homogeneous blue area: It corresponds to densely pigmented dermal melanocytes as in blue nevus and melanoma.
  - Homogeneous white area: It corresponds to depigmented epidermis in vitiligo
  - Homogeneous yellow area: Steatocystoma, xanthoma owing to lipids (**Figs. 4A** to **C**)
  - Homogeneous red or pink area: Small vessel vasculitis (**Figs. 4D** to **F**)
- Starburst pattern (pseudopods, circumferential, radial, lines): A central pigmented clod with radiating pigmented lines with bulbous ends, seen in Reed nevus.[2]
- Streaks [lines, radial (always at periphery)]: It comprises both radial streaming and pseudopods. It corresponds to the melanocytes' confluent nests at the periphery and is seen in the radial growth phase of malignant melanoma and Reed nevus:[2]
  - Radial streaming (lines, radial, and segmental): Linear radial extensions at the edge of a lesion
  - Pseudopods (lines, radial, and segmental with knobs at their tips): Bulbous and often kinked projections

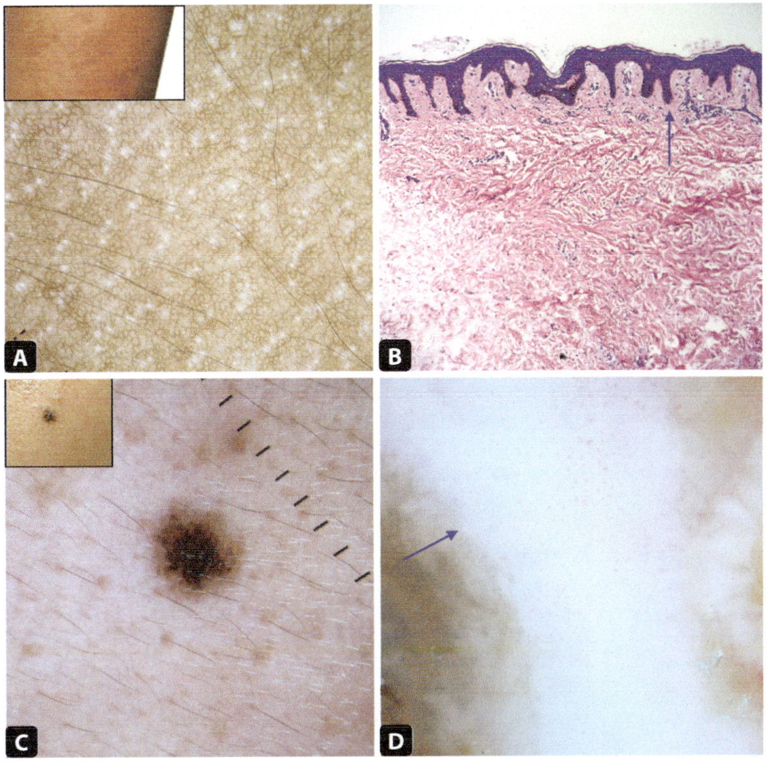

FIGS. 2A TO D: (A) Dermoscopy showing pigment network in a case of Becker's nevus (inset) (polarized, DermLite DL4, 10×); (B) The pigmented keratinocytes over the rete ridges (arrow) correspond to the brown lines and the dermal papillae with suprapapillary plate to the hypopigmented holes [hematoxylin and eosin (H&E), 100×]; (C) Pseudonetwork in a case of melanocytic nevus (inset) over the face (polarized, DermLite DL4, 10×); (D) Dermoscopy showing a homogeneous white area in a case of squamous cell carcinoma (nonpolarized, Heine Delta, 10×).

Source: AIIMS, Bhubaneswar, Odisha and JIPMER, Puducherry, India.

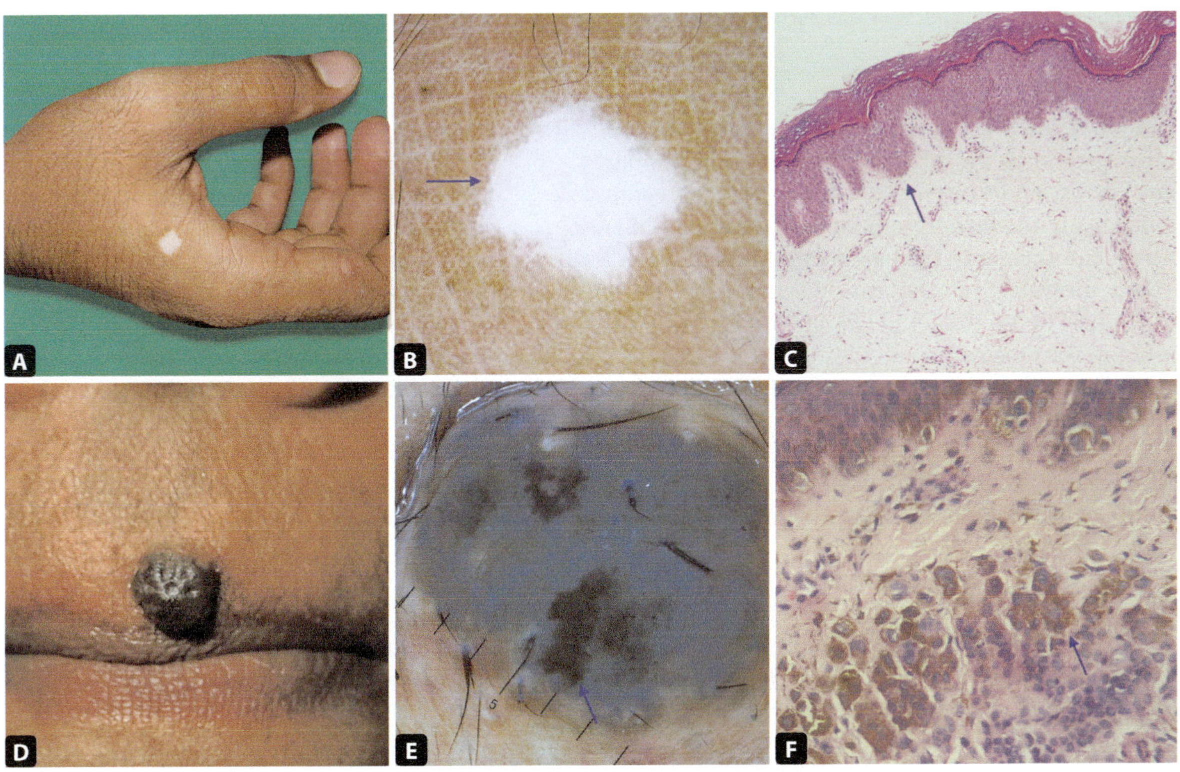

FIGS. 3A TO F: (A) Solitary depigmented macule in a case of vitiligo; (B) Dermoscopy showing white structureless area (arrow) (polarized, DermLite DL4, 10×); (C) Histology showing complete loss of melanin (arrow) (H&E, 100×); (D) Intradermal nevus; (E) Dermoscopy showing brown blotch (arrow) (nonpolarized, Heine Delta, 10×); (F) Histology showing pigmented nevocyte nests (arrow) and increased epidermal pigmentation (H&E, 400×).

Source: AIIMS, Bhubaneswar, Odisha and JIPMER, Puducherry, India.

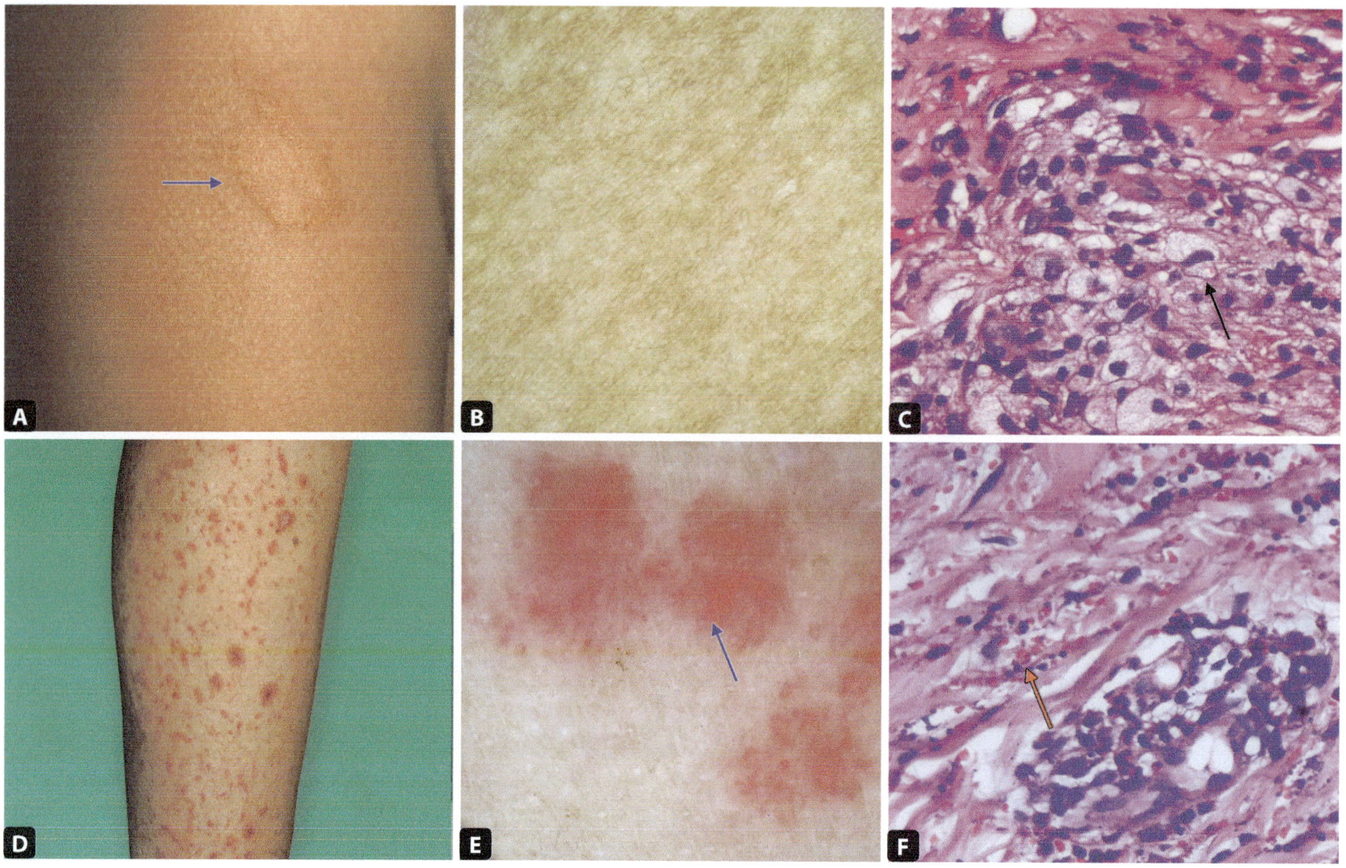

FIGS. 4A TO F: (A) Solitary yellow plaque in a case of a xanthoma; (B) Dermoscopy shows yellow homogeneous area (polarized, Dermlite DL4, 10×); (C) Histology shows upper dermal xanthomized histiocytes that correspond to yellow color (arrow) (H&E, 400×); (D) Multiple purpura and petechiae in a case of small vessel vasculitis; (E) Dermoscopy shows red homogeneous area (arrow) (polarized, DermLite DL4, 10×); (F) Histology shows erythrocyte extravasation that corresponds to red color (arrow) (H&E, 400×).
Source: AIIMS, Bhubaneswar, Odisha and JIPMER, Puducherry, India.

- Angulated lines (lines, angulated, or polygonal): These structures are observed in lentigo maligna. They correspond to atypical melanocytes' aggregate along an attenuated dermoepidermal junction (DEJ) and melanophages in the papillary dermis.[2]
- Brown globules (clods, round, or oval): They correspond to the clustered nevomelanocytes at the DEJ or in the dermis:[2]
  - Regular: Minimal variation in the size, shape, and color of the globules
  - Cobblestones: Symmetrically distributed polygonal globules
  - Rim of brown globules: Globules at the periphery of the lesion
  - Irregular: Asymmetrically distributed globules with varying size, shape, and color
- Dots: These are small, round, and well-circumscribed structures smaller than globules (<0.1 mm).[1] The color can vary from black, brown, or blue-gray, depending upon the level of pigmentation.[2]
- Parallel furrow pattern (lines, parallel, thin, in the furrows): It is seen in acral nevus and corresponds to the pigmented melanocytes and keratinocytes in the furrow.[2,3]
- Parallel ridge pattern (lines, parallel, thick, on the ridges): It is commonly noted in acral lentiginous melanoma and corresponds to the pigmented melanocytes in the rete ridges associated with acrosyringia.[2,3]

- *Epithelial tumors*:[2,3]
  - Comedo-like openings [clods, brown, yellow, or orange (rarely black)]: These are round to oval keratin-filled clefts, commonly seen in seborrheic keratosis. They correspond to the concave, keratin-filled invaginations of the epidermis or dilated follicular infundibulum (**Figs. 5A** and **B**).
  - Milia-like cyst (dots or clods, white or yellow, clustered or disseminated): It corresponds to the keratin-filled cystic structure and is seen in seborrheic keratosis, trichoepithelioma, and melanoma (**Figs. 5A** and **C**).
  - Moth-eaten border (sharply demarcated, scalloped border): A feature observed in seborrheic keratosis and solar lentigo.
  - Fissures and ridges or cerebriform pattern (lines, curved, and thick): The thick curved lines, formed by the gyri and the keratin-filled sulci impart a brain-like appearance. This pattern is seen in seborrheic

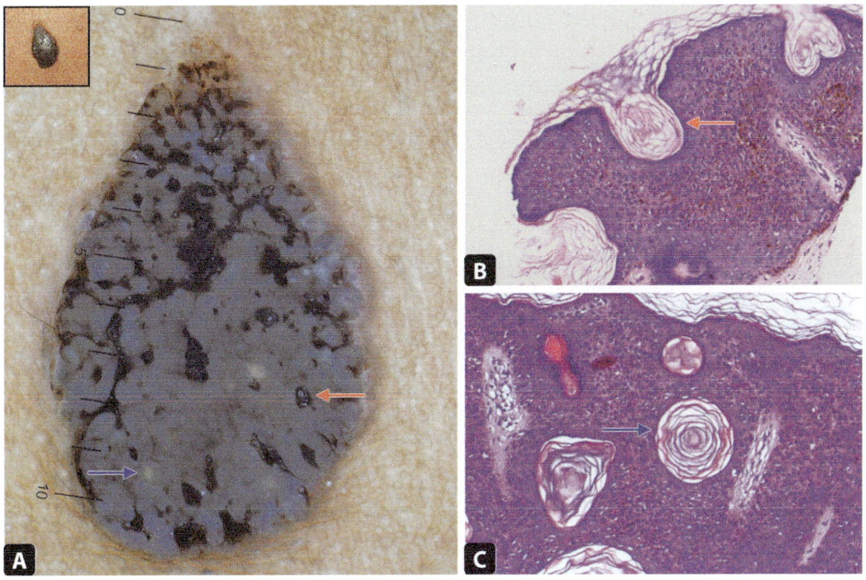

FIGS. 5A TO C: (A) Dermoscopy shows comedo-like openings (red arrow) and milia-like cysts (blue arrow) in a case of seborrheic keratosis (inset) (nonpolarized, Heine Delta, 10×); (B) Keratin-filled epithelial invagination (arrow) corresponds to the comedo-like opening (H&E, 100×); (C) Horn cyst (arrow) corresponds to milia-like cyst (H&E, 100×).

Source: AIIMS, Bhubaneswar, Odisha and JIPMER, Puducherry, India.

keratosis, nevus sebaceous, verrucous epidermal nevus, and dermatofibroma (**Figs. 6A** and **B**). Fissures correspond to wedge-shaped, keratin-filled invaginations of the epidermis, and ridge to the exophytic proliferation of the epidermis (**Fig. 6C**).

- Fingerprint pattern (lines, brown, curved, parallel, thin): Thin, light brown curved lines arranged in a linear or curvilinear fashion (**Fig. 7A**). They correspond to the thin and small gyri.
- Strawberry pattern (structureless, red, interrupted by follicular openings): This pattern is characteristically seen in nonpigmented actinic keratosis and consists of erythematous pseudonetwork interrupted by keratin-filled follicular openings. The increased vasculature leads to erythematous pseudonetwork and the follicular hyperkeratosis responsible for keratin-filled follicular opening.
- Annular granular pattern (gray dots, gray circles): It results from the perifollicular distribution of dots and structureless areas and involves adnexal opening. It is observed in pigmented actinic keratosis, lichen planus pigmentosus (**Figs. 7B** to **D**), and lichen planus-like keratosis.
- Linear dark dots/globules (dots, clods, peripheral, arranged in lines): Linearly arranged brown to gray dots or globules seen in pigmented Bowen's disease. They represent pigmented atypical keratinocytes.
- White circles: Bright white circles surrounding the yellow or orange keratin plug are commonly seen in SCC and keratoacanthoma. They correspond to infundibular acanthosis and hypergranulosis.
- Blue-gray ovoid nests (clods, blue, large, clustered): These are well-circumscribed ovoid structures with confluent or near confluent blue-gray pigmentation (**Fig. 8A**) and correspond to heavily pigmented large nests of tumor cells in the dermis (**Fig. 8B**).
- Multiple blue-gray globules and dots (clods, dots, blue/gray, not aggregated): They correspond to the basaloid nodule or nest in the dermis or at DEJ.

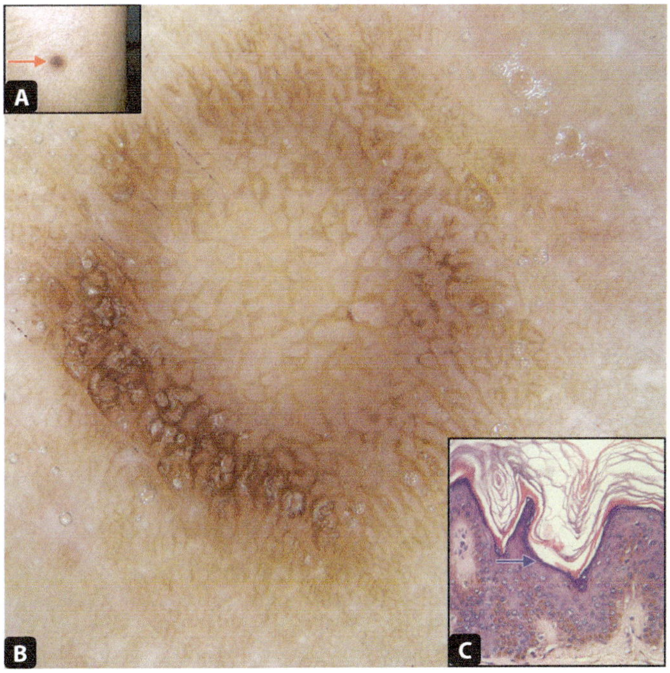

FIGS. 6A TO C: (A) Solitary pigmented papule of a dermatofibroma; (B) Dermoscopy shows a cerebriform pattern in a case of dermatofibroma (nonpolarized, Heine Delta, 10×); (C) The wedge-shaped, keratin-filled invaginations (arrow) correspond to fissure and the acanthotic and papillomatous epidermis to the ridge (H&E, 400×).

Source: AIIMS, Bhubaneswar, Odisha and JIPMER, Puducherry, India.

- Leaf-like areas (lines, radial, connected to a common base): Brown to gray/blue discrete linear or bulbous structures coalescing at a common off-center base creating structures that resemble a leaf-like pattern (**Fig. 8C**). They correspond to the large pigmented nests connected at DEJ (**Fig. 8D**).

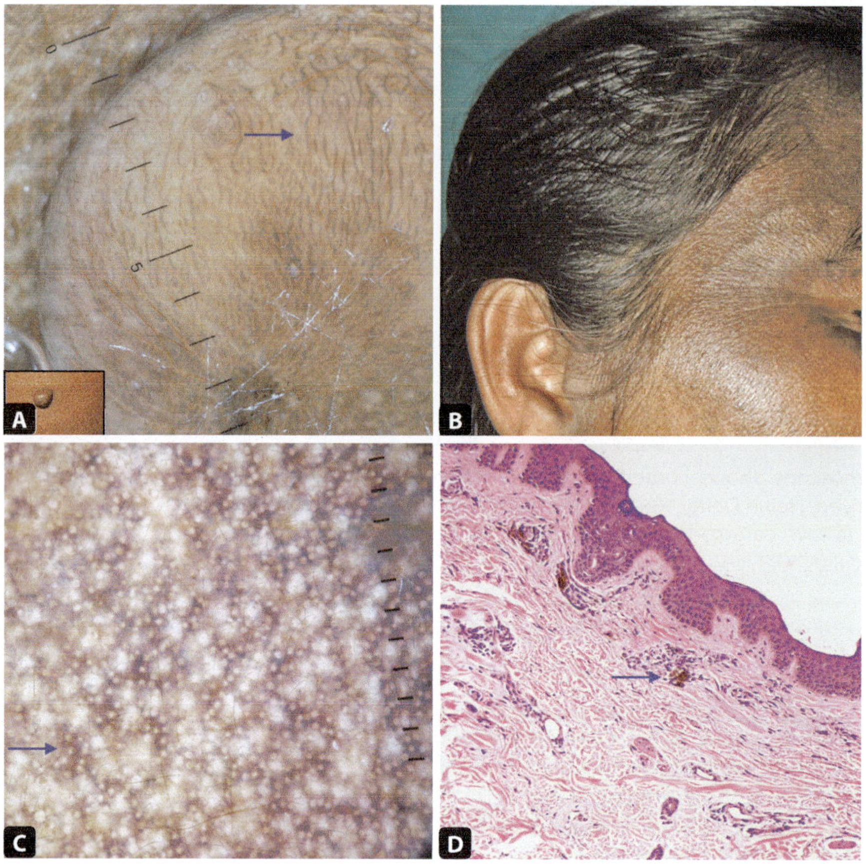

FIGS. 7A TO D: (A) Dermoscopy shows fingerprint-like structures in a case of neurofibroma (inset) (nonpolarized, Heine Delta, 10×); (B) Brown-gray macules in a case of lichen planus pigmentosus; (C) Dermoscopy shows a annular granular pattern (arrow) (polarized, DermLite DL4, 10×); (D) Dermal pigment incontinence (arrow) and increased basal pigmentation that correspond to the gray-brown color (H&E, 100×).

Source: AIIMS, Bhubaneswar, Odisha and JIPMER, Puducherry, India.

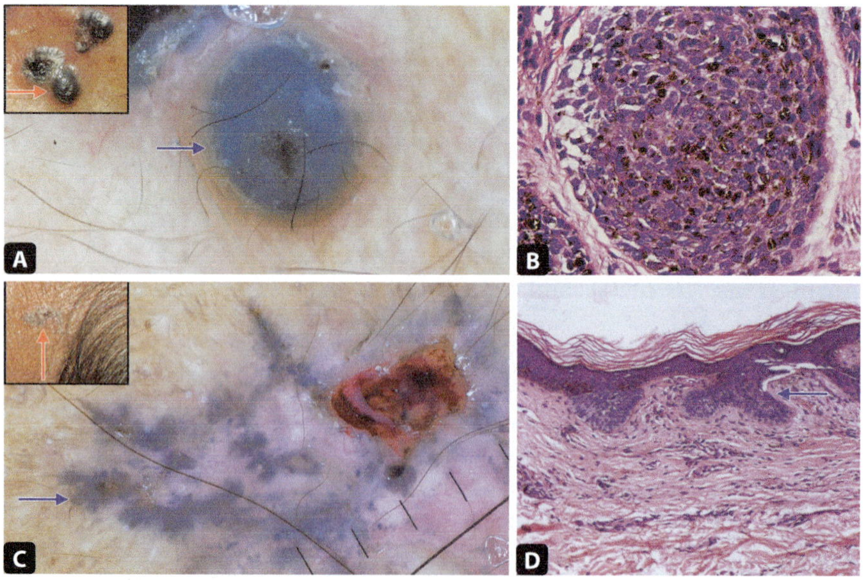

FIGS. 8A TO D: (A) Dermoscopy shows blue-gray ovoid nest (arrow) in a case of basal cell carcinoma (inset) (nonpolarized, Heine Delta, 10×); (B) The large pigmented nest of tumor cells in the dermis corresponds to the blue-gray ovoid nest (H&E, 400×); (C) Dermoscopy shows leaf-like area (arrow) in a case of superficial basal cell carcinoma (inset) (nonpolarized, Heine Delta, 10×); (D) The pigmented tumor nests connected at the dermoepidermal junction correspond to the leaf-like area (H&E, 100×).

Source: AIIMS, Bhubaneswar, Odisha and JIPMER, Puducherry, India.

- Spoke wheel areas (lines, radial, converging to a central dot or clod): The presence of a darker central clod (dark brown, black, or blue color) and radially projecting lines (light brown, blue, or gray in color) that are well-circumscribed and equidistant from the center imparts a spoke wheel pattern. They correspond to large pigmented nests connected to each other at DEJ.
- Concentric structures (clod within a clod): It is considered a precursor of spoke wheel areas.
- Blue-white veil (structureless zone, blue): An irregular-shaped blotch of blue hue with an overlying whitish ground-glass haze (**Fig. 9A**). It corresponds to compact orthokeratosis and aggregation of heavily pigmented cells (melanocytes and/or melanophages) or melanin in the dermis (**Fig. 9B**). It is noted in BCC and melanoma.

- *Fibrohistiocytic tumors*:
  - Scar-like area (structureless zone, white): It corresponds to dermal fibrosis/sclerosis and is a notable feature in dermatofibroma.
  - Crypts: These structures, seen in dermatofibroma and seborrheic keratosis, are keratin-filled epithelial invaginations (**Figs. 10A** and **B**) larger than comedo-like openings (**Figs. 10C** and **D**).
- *Non-Langerhans cell histiocytosis*:
  - Yellow globules, yellow structureless area: They correspond to xanthomized histiocytes and are seen in xanthogranuloma (**Fig. 1F**).

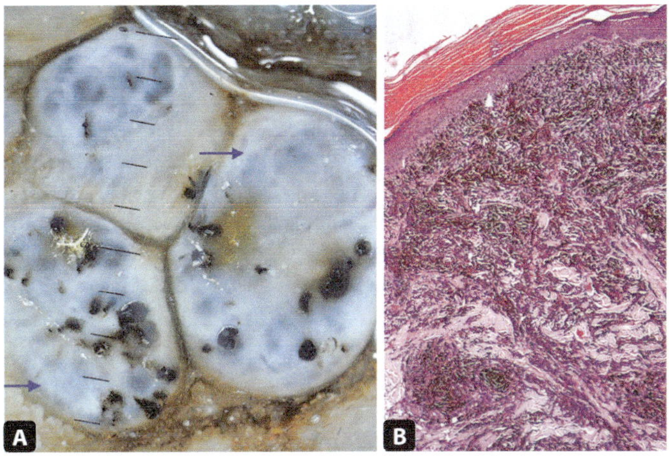

FIGS. 9A AND B: (A) Dermoscopy shows blue-white veil (arrows) in a case of metastatic melanoma (nonpolarized, Heine Delta, 10×); (B) The blue-white veil corresponds to the heavily pigmented melanocytes and overlying orthokeratosis (H&E, 100×).

Source: AIIMS, Bhubaneswar, Odisha and JIPMER, Puducherry, India.

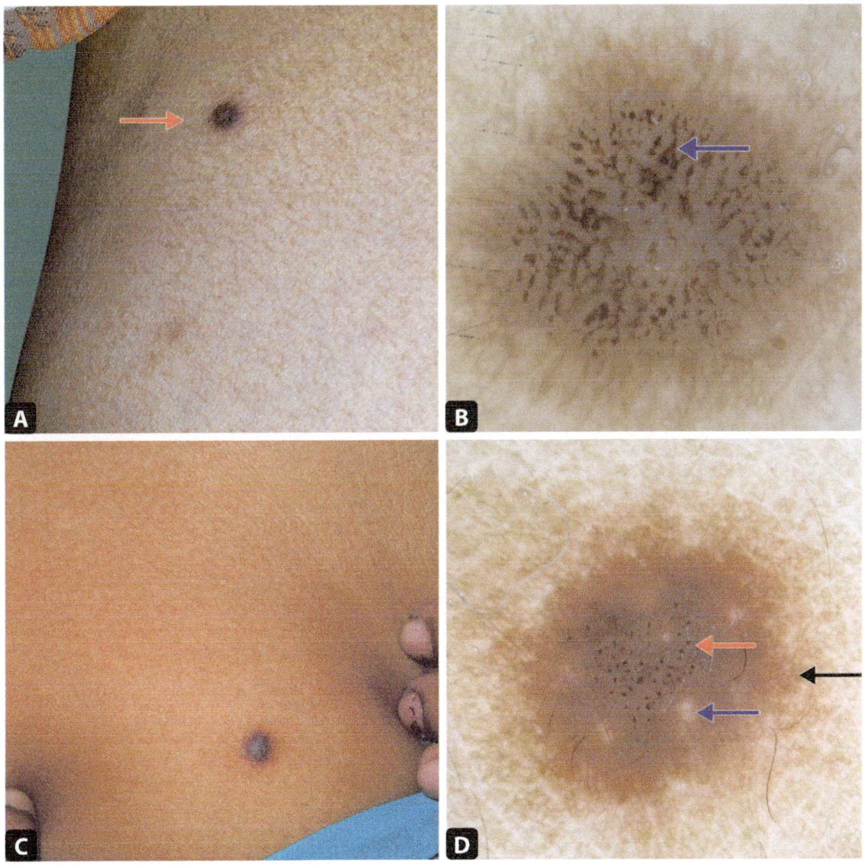

FIGS. 10A TO D: (A) Solitary pigmented papule of dermatofibroma (arrow); (B) Dermoscopy shows linear-irregular crypts (arrow) (nonpolarized, Heine Delta, 10×); (C) Solitary pigmented papule of dermatofibroma; (D) Dermoscopy shows multiple comedo-like openings with keratotic plugging (red arrow), focal white structureless area (blue arrow), and peripheral delicate pigment network (black arrow) (nonpolarized, Heine Delta, 10×).

Source: AIIMS, Bhubaneswar, Odisha and JIPMER, Puducherry, India.

- Setting sun sign/pattern: Orange-yellow background and globules with a subtle erythematous border.

- *Lymphoproliferative disorders*:
  - Salmon or orange color: It is seen both in cutaneous B-cell lymphoma and cutaneous pseudolymphoma. It is due to dense dermal lymphocytic infiltrate.
- *Lymphovascular tumors*:
  - Lacunae (red): It corresponds to the thin-walled dilated blood vessels in the papillary dermis and is a feature of angioma, angiokeratoma, and lymphangioma circumscriptum (**Figs. 11A** and **B**).
- *Papulosquamous disorders*:
  - Wickham's striae: It corresponds to compact hyperkeratosis overlying wedge-shaped or beaded hypergranulosis with acanthosis in lichen planus (**Figs. 11C** and **D**).
  - White starburst pattern: It corresponds to the fibrosis in the papillary dermis in prurigo nodularis (**Figs. 12A** to **C**).
  - Collarette sign: It is due to the peripheral scales in pityriasis rosea (**Figs. 12D** and **E**).
- *Granulomatous disorders*:
  - *Orange or yellowish-orange structureless area*: It is due to the mass effect of dense and compact dermal granulomatous infiltrate in many granulomatous conditions like sarcoidosis, lupus vulgaris, leprosy (**Figs. 13A** to **C**).
- *Vasculitic disorders*:
  - Red or pink homogeneous area: It is due to extravasated red blood cells.
- *Infections and infestations*:
  - Molluscum contagiosum: White clod corresponds to the endophytic lobule of acanthotic squamous epithelium and crown vessels to the peripherally displaced dilated vessels (**Figs. 14A** and **B**).
- *White shiny structures*:[4] These are seen only under polarized light. Their pathological correlation is unclear (**Figs. 14C** and **D**):
  - Rosette (4 white dots arranged in a square): Actinic keratosis, SCC
  - White shiny lines (lines, white, perpendicular): Melanoma, Spitz nevus
  - White shiny structureless area (clods, white, shiny): BCC
- *Multi-colored rainbow pattern (structureless zone, polychromatic)*:[5] The pattern was initially described in Kaposi's sarcoma, and the exact pathological correlate is debatable.

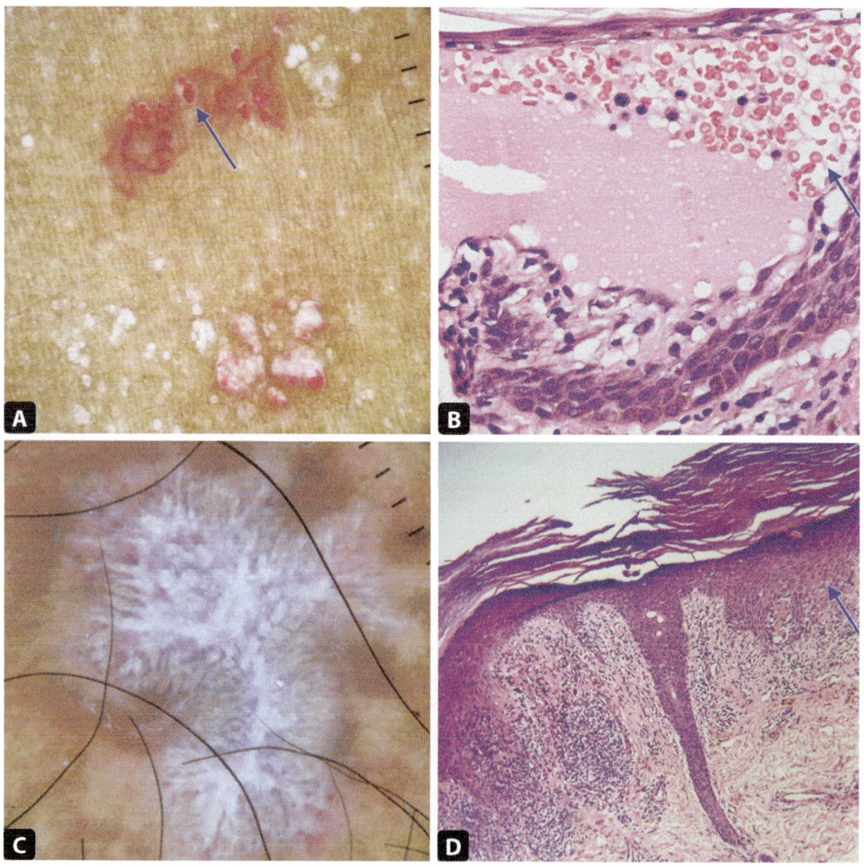

FIGS. 11A TO D: (A) Dermoscopy shows red lacunae (arrow) in a case of lymphangioma circumscriptum (polarized, DermLiteDL4, 10×); (B) The red blood cells inside the dilated lymphatic space correspond to the red lacuna (H&E, 400×); (C) Wickham's striae in the case of lichen planus (polarized, DermLite DL4, 10×); (D) The acanthotic epidermis and the wedge-shaped hypergranulosis (arrow) correspond to Wickham's striae (H&E, 100×).

Source: AIIMS, Bhubaneswar, Odisha and JIPMER, Puducherry, India.

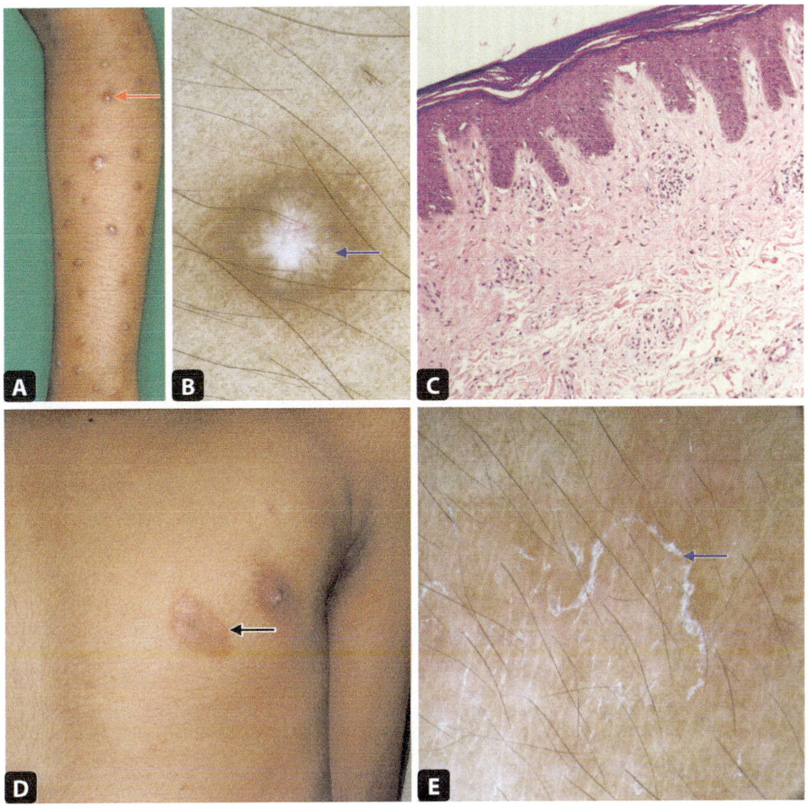

FIGS. 12A TO E: (A) Multiple pigmented papules in case of prurigo nodularis (arrow); (B) Dermoscopy shows a white starburst pattern (arrow) and peripheral brown structureless area (polarized, DermLite DL4, 10×); (C) Histology showing acanthotic epidermis and increased dermal collagen (H&E, 100×); (D) Herald patch in the case of pityriasis rosea (arrow); (E) Dermoscopy shows collarette of white scales (arrow) (polarized, DermLite DL4, 10×).

Source: AIIMS, Bhubaneswar, Odisha and JIPMER, Puducherry, India.

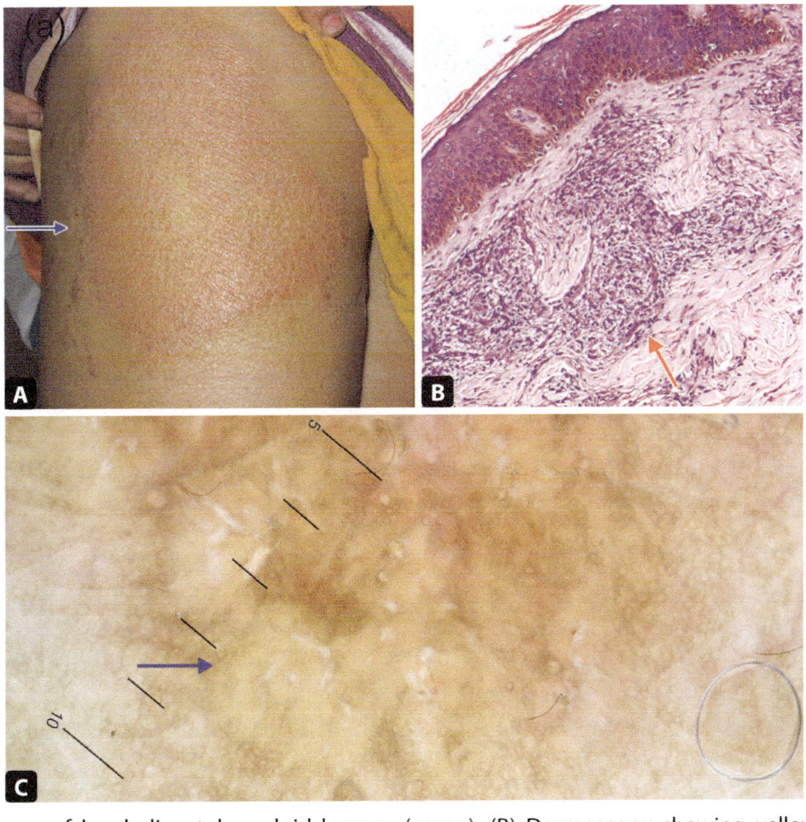

FIGS. 13A TO C: (A) A plaque of borderline tuberculoid leprosy (arrow); (B) Dermoscopy showing yellow structureless area (arrow) (polarized, Heine Delta, 10×); (C) Histology shows upper dermal epithelioid granulomas responsible for the mass effect (H&E, 100×).

Source: AIIMS, Bhubaneswar, Odisha and JIPMER, Puducherry, India.

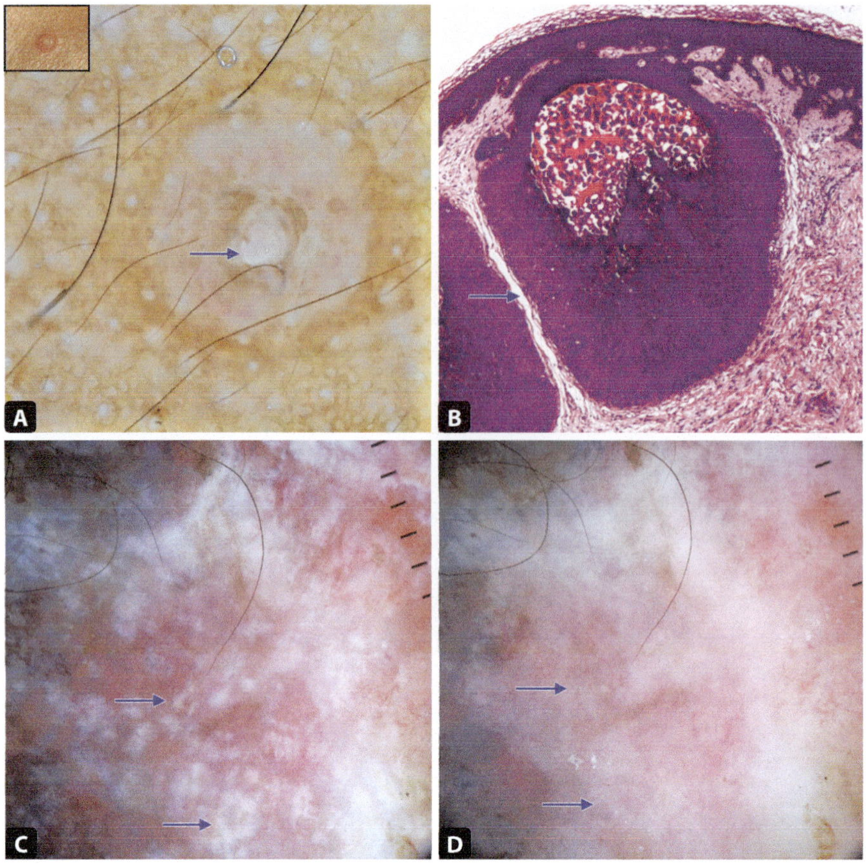

FIGS. 14A TO D: (A) Dermoscopy shows a central white clod in a case of molluscum contagiosum (inset) (nonpolarized, Heine Delta, 10×); (B) The endophytic lobule (arrow) corresponds to the white clod (H&E, 100×); (C) Dermoscopy shows white shiny structure (arrows) (polarized, DermLite DL4, 10×); (D) The disappearance of white shiny structures under nonpolarized mode (arrows) (nonpolarized, DermLite DL4, 10×).

Source: AIIMS, Bhubaneswar, Odisha and JIPMER, Puducherry, India.

- *Trichoscopic-pathologic correlation*:[6]
  - Yellow dots correspond to follicular infundibular orifices with inspissated keratin and sebum. They are noted in alopecia areata, patterned alopecia, and active discoid lupus erythematosus.
  - White dots correspond to acrosyringeal openings or acrotrichia with fibrosis.
  - Red dots, glomerular vessels, signet ring vessels, twisted red loops—correspond to dilated blood vessels in various orientations and are seen in discoid lupus erythematosus, scalp psoriasis, and seborrheic dermatitis.
  - Follicular microhemorrhages: Juxta-acrosyringeal red dots due to hemorrhage caused by traumatic plucking of hair.
  - Black dots are hair shafts that are ruptured at the scalp level and are seen in alopecia areata, tinea capitis, and chemotherapy-induced alopecia.
  - Peripilar sign in active patterned (hormone-dependent) alopecia is a brown halo around the hair follicle on polarized dermoscopy. It is due to perifollicular inflammation and signifies active disease.
  - Target sign: Blue pigmentation around hair follicles in lichen planopilaris and is a diagnostic hallmark. Folliculocentric lichenoid inflammation in lichen planopilaris causes melanin incontinence in the adjacent adventitial dermis, which, due to the Tyndall effect, appears blue (**Figs. 15A** and **B**).
  - Large irregular white dot: It corresponds to dermal fibrous tract and seen in lichen planopilaris (**Figs. 15C** and **D**).
  - Honeycomb pigmentation: Accentuated normal pigment network on photo exposed scalp as a consequence of alopecia.
  - Follicular plug and milky-red areas: These correspond respectively to infundibular hyperkeratosis (**Figs. 16A** and **B**) and recent onset fibrosis with increased vascularity (**Figs. 16C** and **D**) in cicatricial alopecia.
  - Peripilar tubular casts: Scales along the hair shaft for a few millimeters seen classically in lichen planopilaris.[7]
  - Ivory-white background: It corresponds to the fibrotic dermis with complete absence of hair follicles. It is seen in frontal fibrosing alopecia and pseudopelade of Brocq.

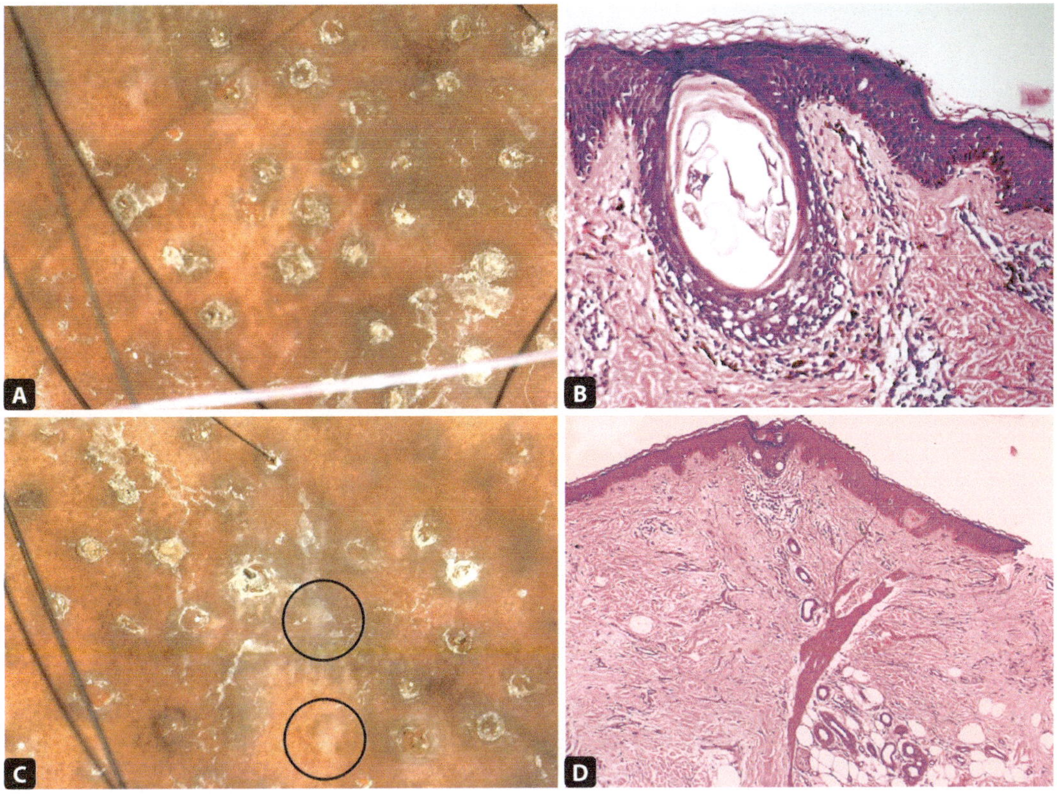

FIGS. 15A TO D: (A) Follicular plugging and peripilar target sign comprising blue-gray pigmentation around hair follicular openings (polarized Dino-Lite videodermoscope); (B) Peripilar target sign corresponds to adventitial dermal melanin incontinence due to lichenoid inflammatory infiltrate of the follicular infundibulum. Note also the follicular plug (H&E, 100×); (C) Large irregular white dots (black circles) (polarized Dino-Lite videodermoscope); (D) Histology shows follicular fibrous tracts that correspond to large irregular white dots (H&E, 100×).

Source: Seth GS Medical College and KEM Hospital, Mumbai, Maharashtra, India.

- *Advantages of dermoscopic-histopathological correlation*: Comprehensive knowledge regarding dermoscopic-histopathological correlation will benefit the clinicians in the following ways:[8]
  - It can serve as a tool to guide the dermatologists in choosing the most representative area for biopsy preoperatively and sectioning postoperatively.
  - *Ex vivo* dermoscopy can be extremely useful in evaluating large and complex pigmented lesions:
    - Dermoscopy can detect the different histopathological subtypes of skin cancers such as BCC.
  - The dermoscopic examination can provide the following prognostic information: Atypical pigment network and brown color may indicate thin melanoma without mitosis while black color and peripheral streaks may indicate the presence of mitosis; invasive melanomas can be significantly associated with three or more colors, atypical pigment network or streaks, white shiny streaks, milky-red color, and blue-white veil, while in-situ melanomas commonly have up to two colors, and absence of white shiny streaks, milky-red color, and blue-white veil. The absence of pigment network and the presence of ulceration and blotch may predict lymph node metastsis.[9-12]
  - Dermoscopy can aid in deciding the therapy.

KEY POINTS

- Dermoscopy reveals what is happening in the skin layers.
- Most of patterns correlate well with the histopathological changes. However, discrepancy is expected due to epidermal hyperplasia and hyperkeratosis.
- Vascular structures are not seen as they appear under dermoscopy.

CONCLUSION

Dermoscopy is quick and noninvasive tool which gives information about the happenings in the different skin layers. It demonstrates specific patterns which correspond to histopathological findings. It is recommended that one should always correlate the dermoscopic features with corresponding histopathological changes.

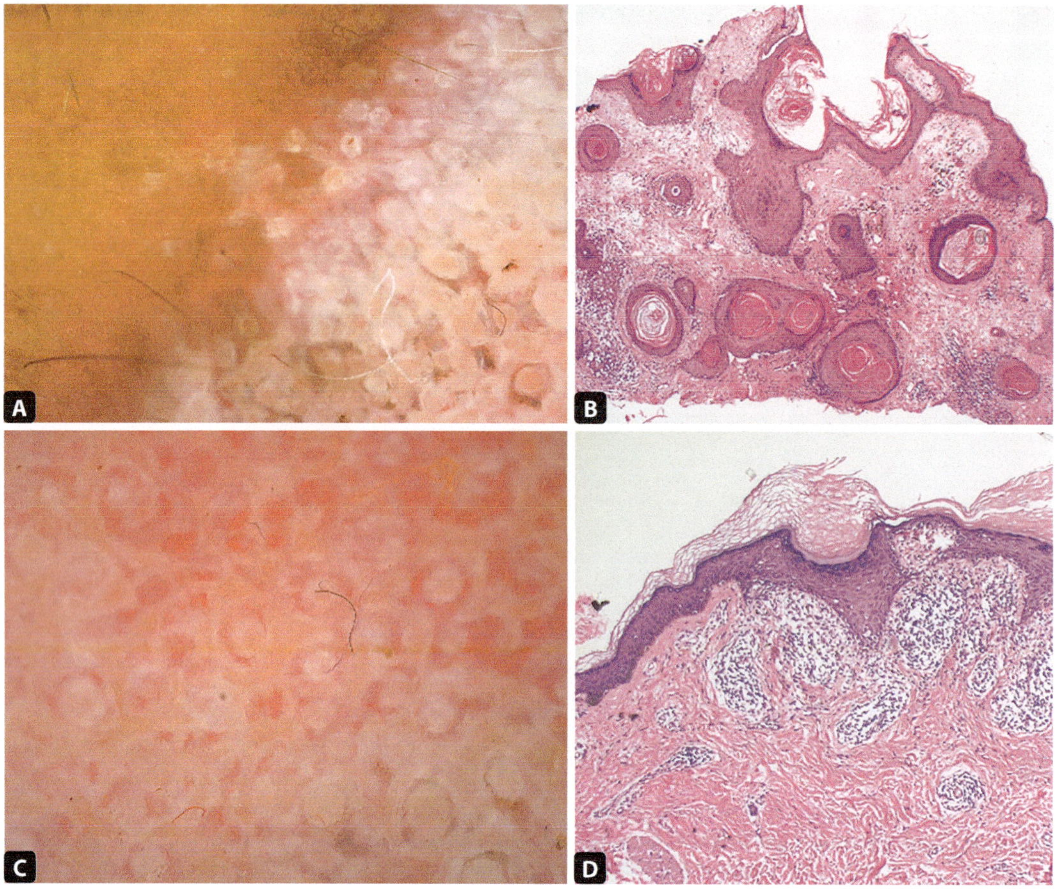

FIGS. 16A TO D: (A) Follicular plugs in discoid lupus erythematosus (Dino-Lite polarized videodermoscope); (B) Infundibular hyperkeratosis in the dilated follicular ostia corresponds to the keratotic plug (H&E, 100×); (C) Milky-white areas around follicular plugs (Dino-Lite polarized videodermoscope); (D) Active inflammation with increased vascularity corresponds to milky-white area (H&E, 100×).

Source: Seth GS Medical College and KEM Hospital, Mumbai, Maharashtra, India.

REFERENCES

1. Suppa M, Micantonio T, Di Stefani A, Soyer HP, Chimenti S, Fargnoli MC, et al. Dermoscopic variability of basal cell carcinoma according to clinical type and anatomic location. J Eur Acad Dermatol Venereol. 2015;29:1732-41.
2. Kittler H, Marghoob AA, Argenziano G, Carrera C, Curiel-Lewandrowski C, Hofmann-Wellenhof R, et al. Standardization of terminology in dermoscopy/dermatoscopy: results of the third consensus conference of the International Society of Dermoscopy. J Am Acad Dermatol. 2016;74:1093-106.
3. Yélamos O, Braun RP, Liopyris K, Wolner ZJ, Kerl K, Gerami P, et al. Dermoscopy and dermatopathology correlates of cutaneous neoplasms. J Am Acad Dermatol. 2019;8:341-63.
4. Liebman TN, Rabinovitz HS, Dusza SW, Marghoob AA. White shiny structures: dermoscopic features revealed under polarized light. J Eur Acad Dermatol Venereol. 2012;262:1493-7.
5. Draghici C, Vajaitu C, Solomon I, Voiculescu VM, Popa MI, Lupu M. The dermoscopic rainbow pattern—a review of the literature. Acta Dermatovenerol Croat. 2019;27:111-5.
6. Khopkar U, Bharti A. Trichoscopy. In: Khopkar US (Ed). Dermoscopy and Trichoscopy in Diseases of the Brown Skin: Atlas and Short Text. New Delhi: Jaypee Brothers Medical Publishers (P) Ltd; 2012. pp. 332-85.
7. d'Ovidio R, Sgarra C, Conserva A, Angelotti UF, Erriquez R, Foti C. Alterated integrin expression in lichen planopilaris. Head Face Med. 2007;3:11.
8. Yélamos O, Braun R, Morgado D, Mc Loughlin CR. Importance of dermoscopy and histopathology correlates. Dermoscopedia. 2019;16:25. [online] Available from https://dermoscopedia.org/w/index.php?title=Importance_of_dermoscopy_and_histopathology_correlates&oldid=16700 [Last accessed October, 2021].
9. Ribero S, Argenziano G, Lallas A, Moscarella E, Benati E, Raucci M, et al. Dermoscopic features predicting the presence of mitoses in thin melanoma. J Dermatol Sci. 2017;86:158-61.
10. Silva VP, Ikino JK, Sens MM, Nunes DH, Di Giunta G. Dermoscopic features of thin melanomas: a comparative study of melanoma in situ and invasive melanomas smaller than or equal to 1 mm. An Bras Dermatol. 2013;88:712-7.
11. Balagula Y, Braun RP, Rabinovitz HS, Dusza SW, Scope A, Liebman TN, et al. The significance of crystalline/chrysalis structures in the diagnosis of melanocytic and nonmelanocytic lesions. J Am Acad Dermatol. 2012;67:194.e1-8.
12. González-Álvarez T, Carrera C, Bennassar A, Vilalta A, Rull R, Alos L, et al. Dermoscopy structures as predictors of sentinel lymph node positivity in cutaneous melanoma. Br J Dermatol. 2015;172:1269-77.

5 CHAPTER

Papulosquamous Disorders

Sunanda Mahajan, Vidya Kharkar, Sushrut Save, Muhammed Razmi T, Tishya Singh

INTRODUCTION

Papulosquamous disorders are a heterogeneous group of inflammatory conditions of the skin characterized by eruptions that exhibit erythema and squamous components. These disorders account for a large number of patients in day-to-day practice. Dermoscopy can be an effective noninvasive tool, helpful in differentiating these conditions further and not only minimize the need for invasive skin biopsies but also helpful in determining the treatment outcomes.

PSORIASIS AND ITS TYPES

Clinical Features

Psoriasis is a chronic papulosquamous disorder involving the skin, nails, and joints and is characterized clinically by erythematous papules and plaques covered with silvery white scales, particularly over extensor surfaces, and scalp (**Fig. 1**).[1]

Dermoscopic Features

- Characteristic dermoscopic features in a chronic plaque psoriasis include uniformly distributed red dots on a light red/pink background and diffuse bright white scales (**Fig. 2**)[2-5] which are characteristics of psoriasis (**Fig. 3**).[1-3,6,7]
- On higher magnifications (50–200 fold), the lesions predominantly demonstrate "bushy" glomerular vessels that are coiled capillaries believed to be due to the presence of tortuous loops of vertically arranged vessels within the elongated and thinned-out dermal papillae (**Fig. 4**).[1]
- In hyperkeratotic lesions, scales impede the visualization of the vasculature, which can be better appreciated by mechanically scraping the scales or by using an interface fluid.[2,6]
- Palmoplantar psoriasis lesion shows a dull red background and the scales are dull white. Dotted vessels are arranged along the skin markings of the acral areas (**Fig. 5**).[2,6]
- Dermoscopy can also be used for treatment response monitoring. After use of topical steroids, the number of glomerular vessels decreases and linear vessels (linear telangiectasias) become apparent on dermoscopy (**Fig. 6**).[8-10]
- Scalp psoriasis reveals red dots, glomerular vessels, and twisted red loops (**Fig. 7**).[8,11]

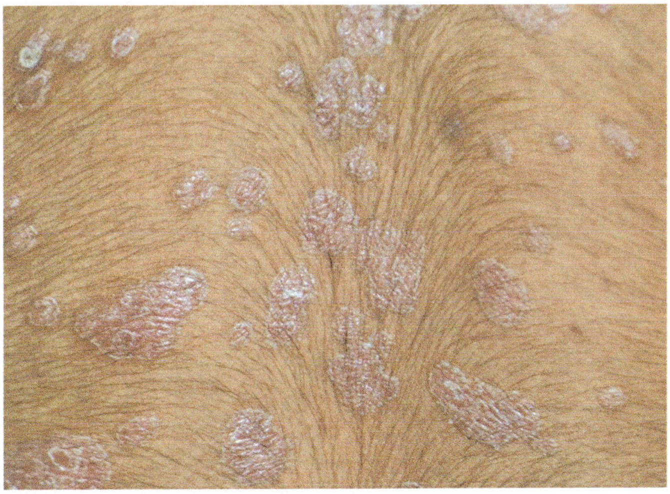

FIG. 1: Clinical image of chronic plaque psoriasis showing erythematous papules and plaques covered with silvery white scales on back.

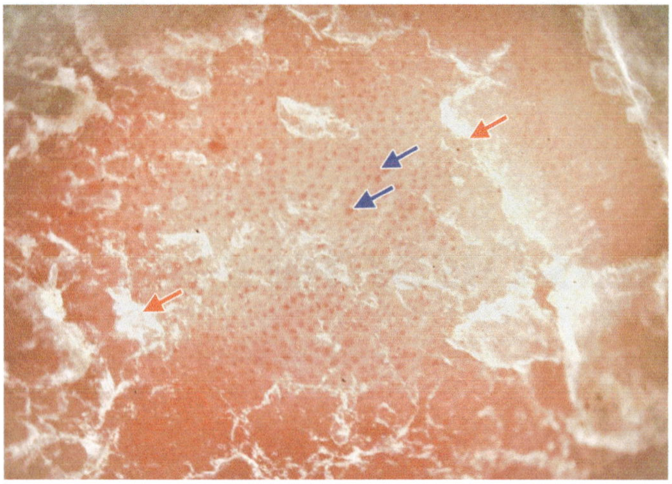

FIG. 2: Dermoscopy of plaque psoriasis demonstrating bright white diffuse scale (red arrows) uniformly distributed dotted and glomerular vessels (blue arrows) over a light red background (polarized, Oitez dermoscope, 20×).

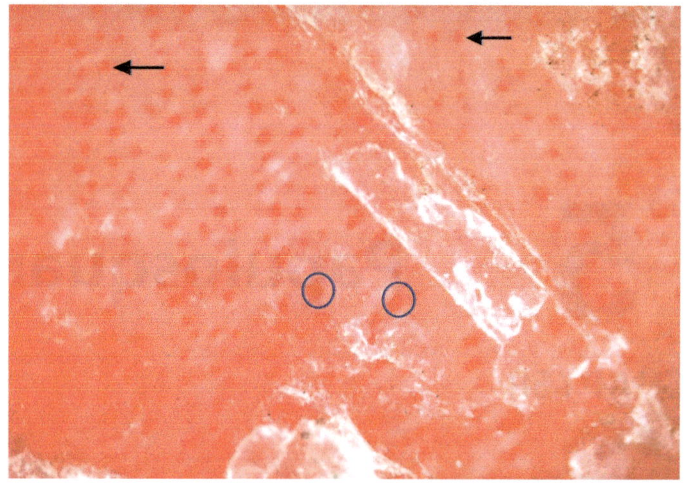

FIG. 3: Dermoscopy of psoriasis demonstrating uniform distribution of dotted (black arrows) and glomerular vessels (blue circles) (polarized, Oitez dermoscope, 20×).

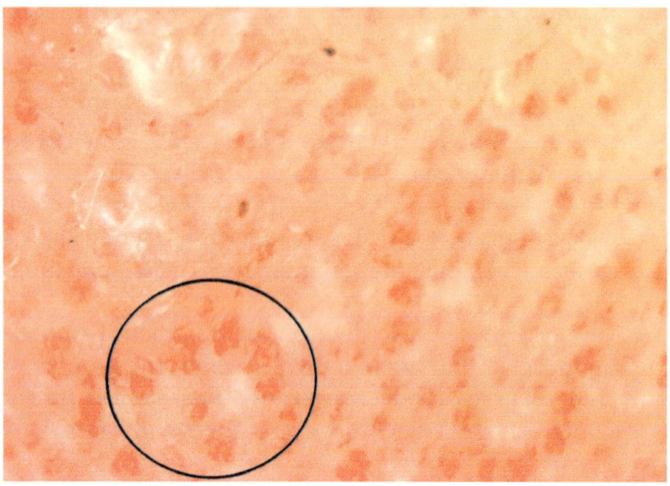

FIG. 4: Dermoscopy of psoriasis on higher magnification shows the "bushy" glomerular vessels (black circle) (polarized, Oitez dermoscope, 200×).

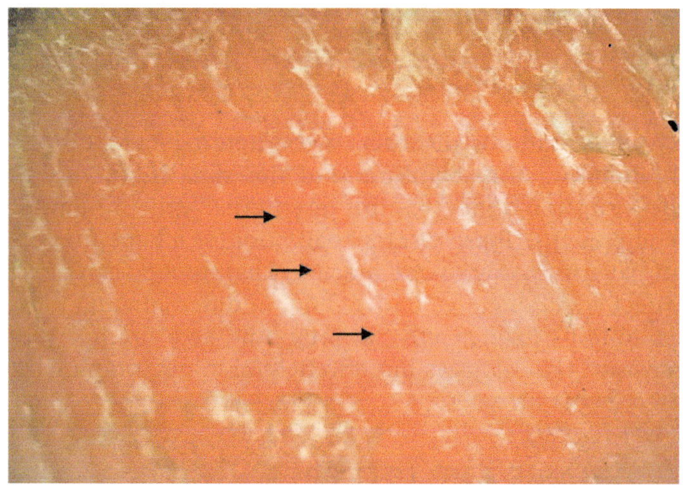

FIG. 5: Dermoscopy of palmoplantar lesions of psoriasis showing dull white scales and regular dotted vessels arranged along the dermatoglyphics (black arrows) (polarized, Oitez dermoscope, 200×).

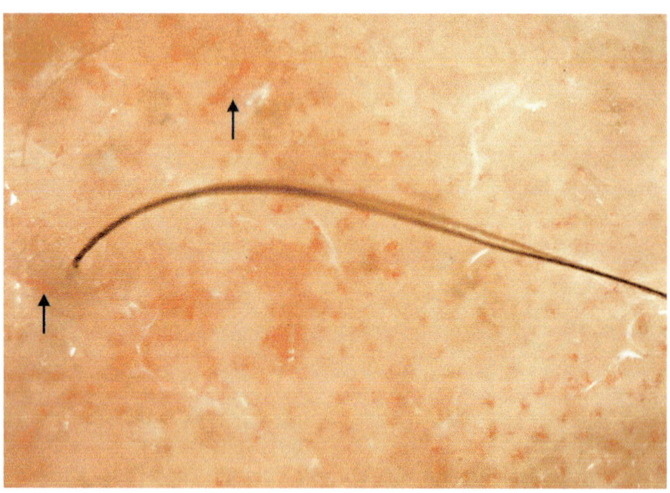

FIG. 6: Dermoscopy of psoriasis lesion treated with topical 0.1% mometasone furoate cream for 3 weeks demonstrating a smaller number of bushy capillaries and few linear vessels (black arrows) (polarized, Oitez dermoscope, 20×).

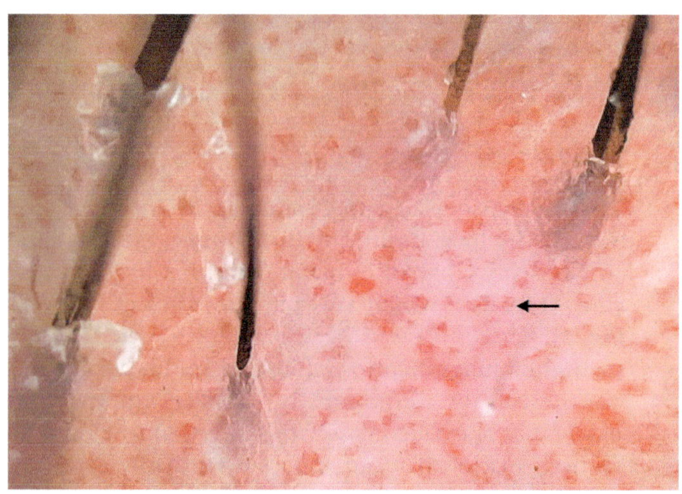

FIG. 7: Dermoscopy of scalp psoriasis lesion showing multiple red dots, globules, and twisted vessels (black arrow) on light red background (polarized, Oitez dermoscope, 20×).

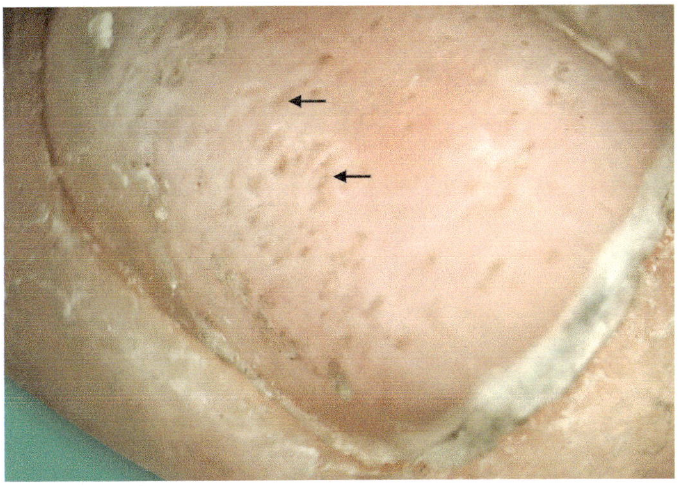

FIG. 8: Dermoscopy of nail psoriasis showing multiple coarse pits as tiny depressed areas with surrounding scale (black arrows) (polarized, Oitez dermoscope, 20×).

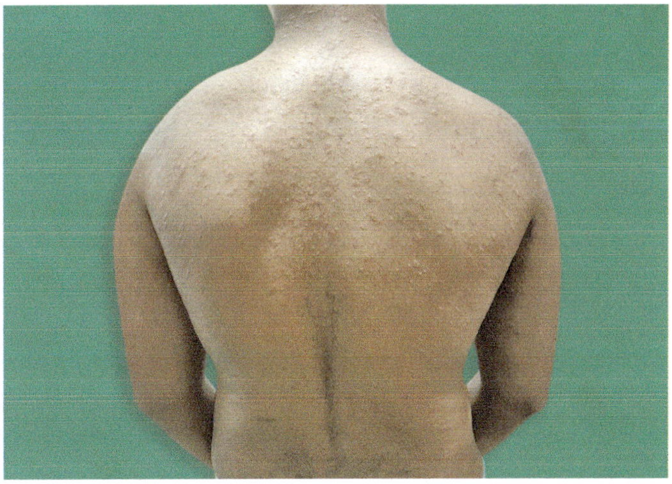

FIG. 9: Clinical photograph of pityriasis rosea showing Christmas tree pattern of multiple erythematous macules and papules with overlying scaling.

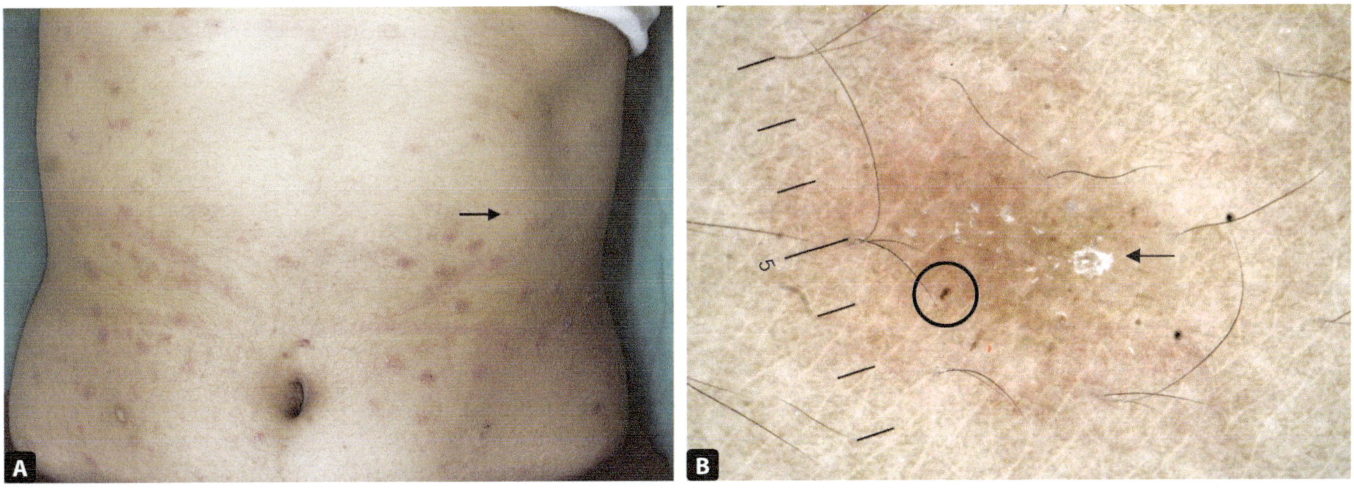

FIGS. 10A AND B: (A) Clinical picture of lesions of pityriasis rosea present on the abdomen demonstrating multiple erythematous macules and papules. Lesion for which dermoscopy was done is marked (black arrow); (B) Dermoscopy of early lesion of pityriasis rosea shows centrally placed scale (black arrow) denoting the beginning of scaling with brown globule (black circle) (polarized, Heine Delta 20, 20×).

- Nail psoriasis demonstrates coarse pits (most common finding), onycholysis, splinter hemorrhages, oil drop sign, leukonychia, and subungual hyperkeratosis (**Fig. 8**).[12,13]

Key Points

- Light red background
- Homogeneous uniform distribution of red dots
- Palmoplantar psoriasis lesion—dotted vessels are arranged along the skin markings of the acral areas
- Topical steroid treated psoriasis lesion—number of glomerular vessels decrease with appearance of linear vessels
- Scalp psoriasis—twisted red loops

PITYRIASIS ROSEA

Clinical Features

Pityriasis rosea (PR) is characterized clinically by erythematous scaly plaques which are called as herald patches that appear usually on the trunk or neck. These are followed by an eruption of multiple secondary small erythematous scaly lesions located predominantly on the trunk. These are termed as daughter patches and these lines of cleavage on the back give a Christmas tree or inverted fir tree appearance (**Figs. 9, 10A** and **11A**). Peripheral scale referred to as collarette scaling is seen typically (**Figs. 12A** and **13A**).

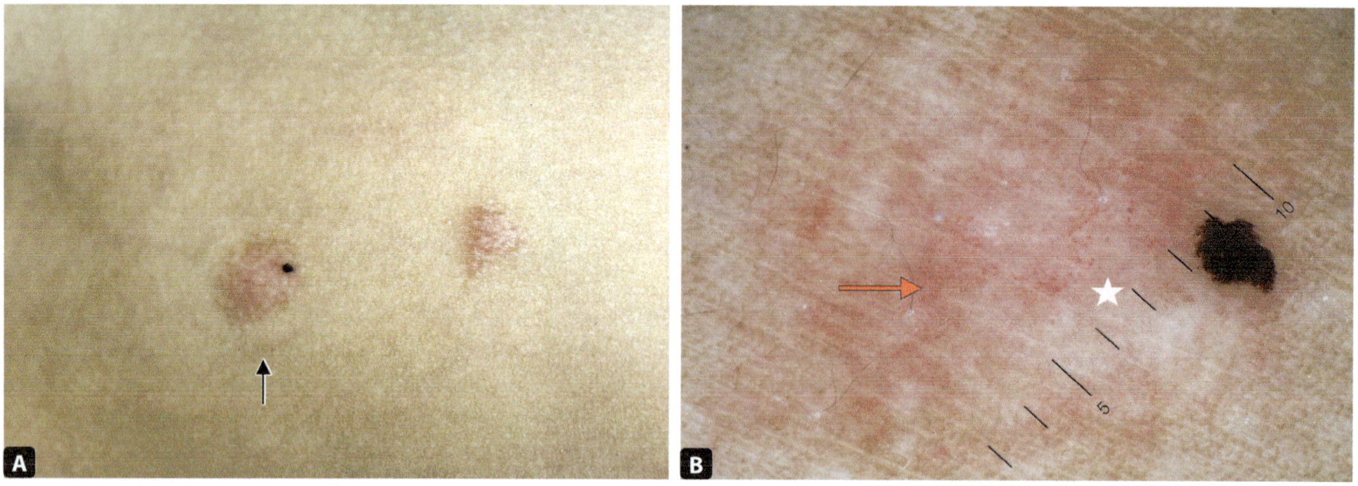

FIGS. 11A AND B: (A) Clinical image of pityriasis rosea on the abdomen demonstrating two discrete erythematous papules. Lesion for which dermoscopy was done is marked (black arrow); (B) Dermoscopy of early lesion of pityriasis rosea shows white areas (white star) with irregular distribution of red dots (red arrow) (polarized, Heine Delta 20, 20×).

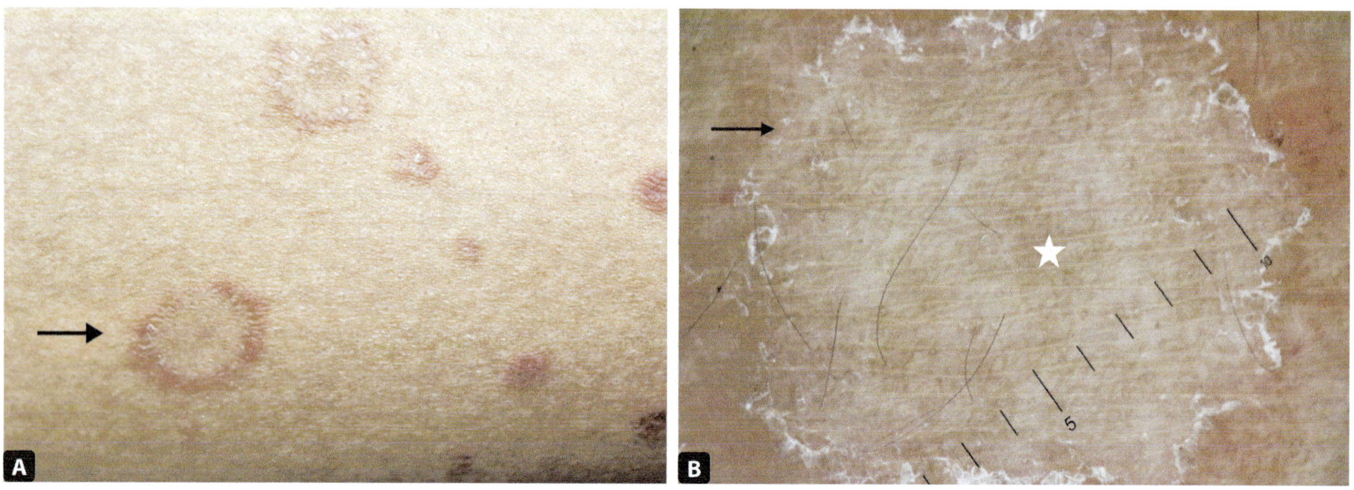

FIGS. 12A AND B: (A) Clinical images of pityriasis rosea showing multiple discrete erythematous plaques with a collarette of scales on the thigh. Lesion for which dermoscopy was done is marked (black arrow); (B) Dermoscopy of late lesion of pityriasis rosea shows a peripheral white scaling (black arrow) with a brownish background (white star) (polarized, Heine Delta 20, 20×).

Dermoscopic Features

Dermoscopy of both herald patch and secondary lesions of PR displays similar findings of fine scales present at the periphery (collarette sign) with dotted blood vessels present in an irregular pattern over a red or brown background.[14] Red dots are due to dilatation of vessels and scaling is due to parakeratosis and hyperkeratosis.[15] Early lesions demonstrate milky-red globules indicating extravasated red blood cells (RBCs) in dermis with more centrally placed scales with occasional white areas. Brown globules may be seen (**Figs. 10B** and **11B**).[3] Lesions in later stages present with brown dots, a yellowish-brown background, and collarette scales (**Figs. 12B** and **13B**). The brown dots are due to the spongiotic tissue reaction and hemosiderin deposits from extravasated RBCs.[3] In Indian skin, a brownish hue in the background is more conspicuous.[16]

Key Points

- An irregular distribution of blood vessels over a reddish/brownish background
- Collarette of scale

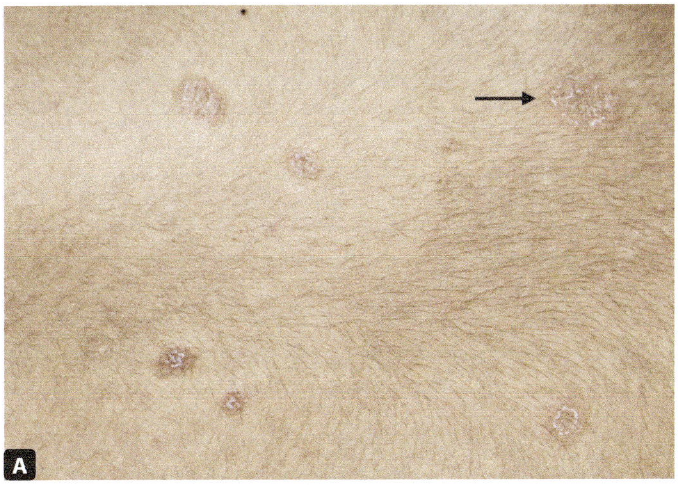

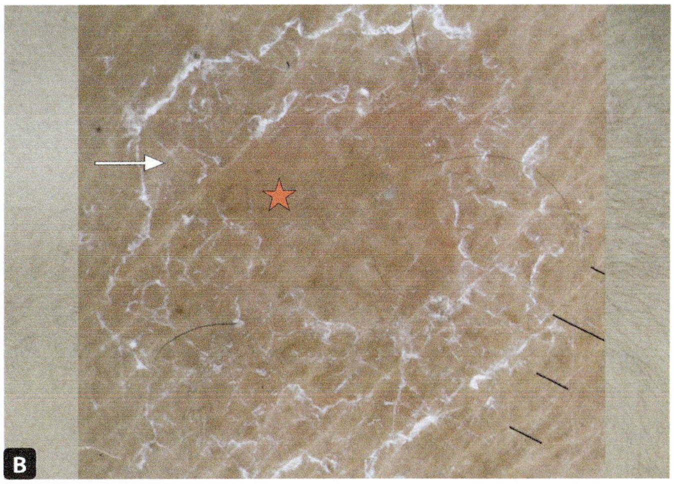

FIGS. 13A AND B: (A) Clinical image of pityriasis rosea demonstrating multiple scaly plaques on the back. Lesion for which dermoscopy was done is marked (black arrow); (B) Dermoscopy of late lesions of pityriasis rosea shows peripheral collarette of white scales (white arrow) with multiple brown dots (red star) with a brownish background (polarized, Heine Delta 20, 20×).

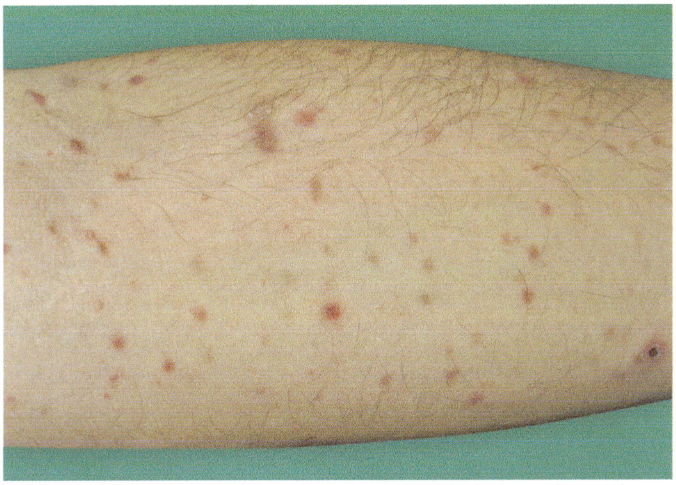

FIG. 14: Clinical image of pityriasis lichenoides et varioliformis acuta showing multiple, small, red papules with hemorrhagic crusts and scarring on arm.

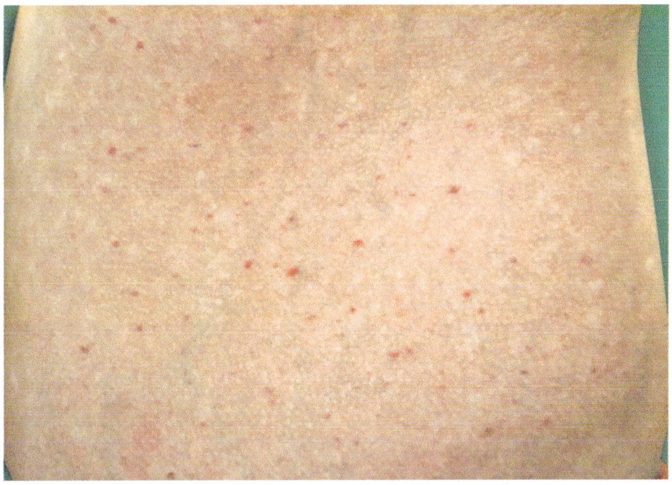

FIG. 15: Clinical image of pityriasis lichenoides chronica showing multiple erythematous and purpuric macules, and papules, with postinflammatory hypopigmentation on back.

PITYRIASIS LICHENOIDES ET VARIOLIFORMIS ACUTA AND PITYRIASIS LICHENOIDES CHRONICA

Clinical Features

Pityriasis lichenoides is a group of inflammatory skin disorders that include pityriasis lichenoides et varioliformis acuta (PLEVA), febrile ulceronecrotic Mucha-Habermann disease (a subtype of PLEVA), and pityriasis lichenoides chronica (PLC).[17] PLEVA presents as acute multiple, small, red papules that develop into polymorphic lesions and heal with residual varioliform scars (**Fig. 14**). PLC presents as small, erythematous papules that develop a reddish-brown hue with centrally adherent micaceous scales and resolve leaving hypopigmentation (**Fig. 15**).

Dermoscopic Features

Pityriasis Lichenoides et Varioliformis Acuta

- Features observed in early lesions of PLEVA include amorphous brownish area and central crust around the hair follicles within a rim of white scale and dotted vessels at the periphery (**Fig. 16**).[18-20]
- Red dots and globules are seen at the periphery. These correspond to microhemorrhages and extravasations of RBCs in the papillary dermis (**Fig. 17**).[18]
- Late-phase lesions show white structureless areas and central white crust and white scales, focal blue gray areas and few dotted and linear vessels at periphery (**Fig. 18**).[18,19]

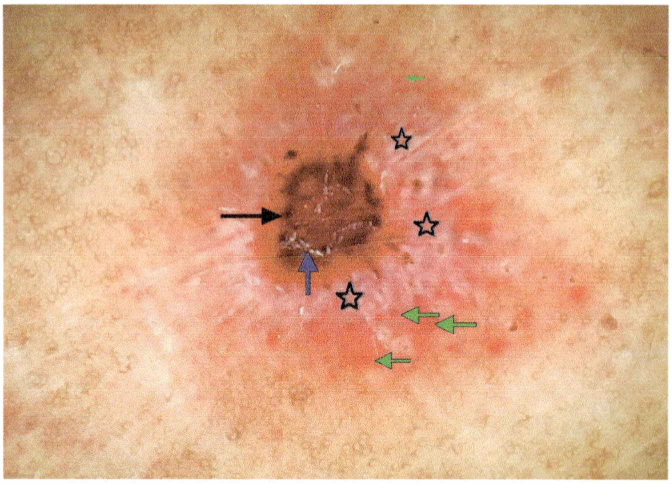

FIG. 16: Dermoscopy of early lesion of pityriasis lichenoides et varioliformis acuta demonstrating central amorphous brown area with crust (black arrow), rim of white scales (blue arrow), white structureless areas (black stars), dotted vessels at periphery (green arrows) (polarized, Oitez dermoscope, 20×).

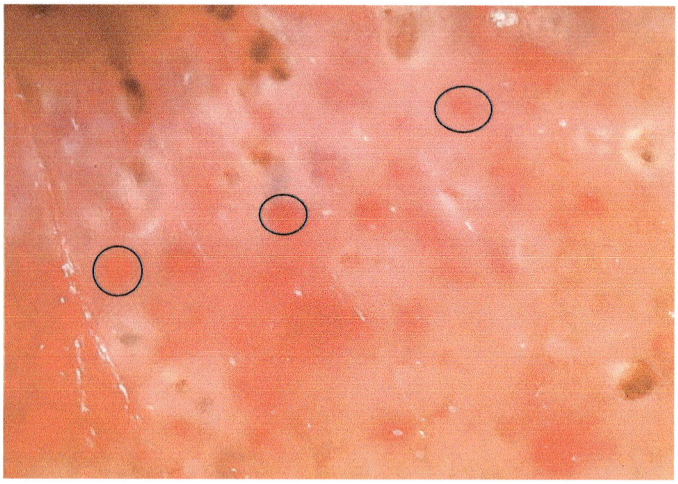

FIG. 17: Dermoscopy of early lesion of pityriasis lichenoides et varioliformis acuta showing globular vessels at periphery (black circles) (polarized, Oitez dermoscope, 200×).

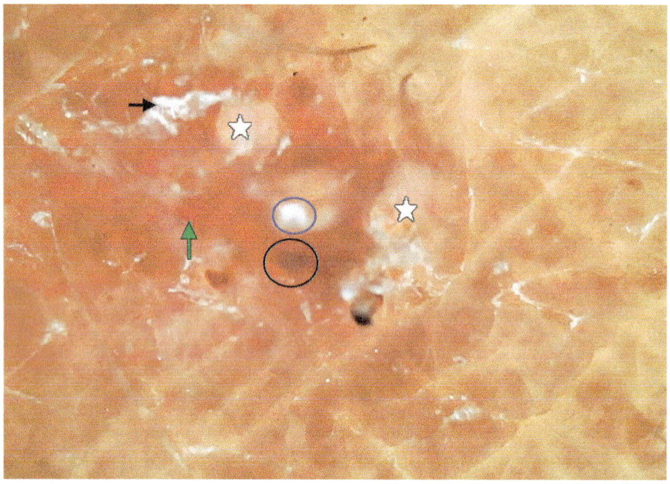

FIG. 18: Dermoscopy of late lesion of pityriasis lichenoides et varioliformis acuta demonstrating white areas (white stars) and central white crust (blue circle) and white scales (black arrow) with focal blue-gray areas (black circle) and few dotted vessels at periphery (green arrow) (polarized, Oitez dermoscope, 20×).

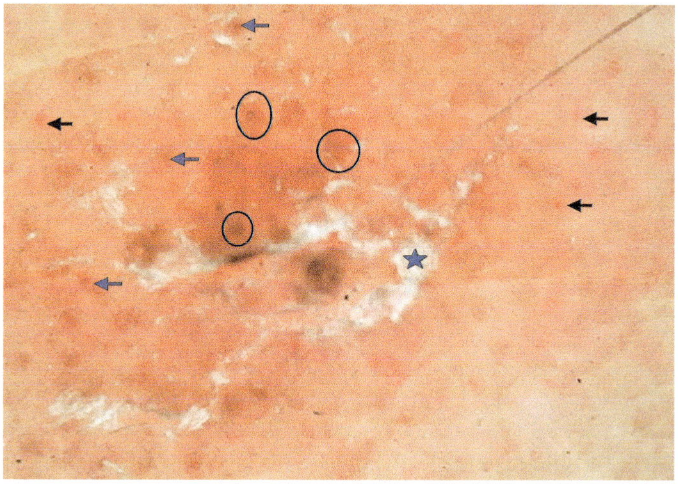

FIG. 19: Dermoscopy of late lesion of pityriasis lichenoides chronica demonstrating brownish red background color, brown dots (blue arrows), brownish areas (black circles) with focal dotted vessels (black arrows) and white diffuse scales (blue star) (polarized, Oitez dermoscope, 20×).

Pityriasis Lichenoides Chronica

- Dermoscopic features include brownish-red background color, brown dots, brownish structureless areas, focal dotted and linear vessels and white diffuse scale (**Fig. 19**).[3,21]
- A brownish background is likely due to hemosiderin deposition (due to extravasated RBCs) and melanophages.[3]
- Dispersed brown and black colored clods on a brownish-red background are observed characteristically in PLC (**Fig. 20**).[21] These are believed to be due to the postinflammatory hyperpigmentation in darker skin types.[21]

Key Points

Pityriasis Lichenoides et Varioliformis Acuta

- Early lesion—amorphous brown area, rim of white scale and dotted vessels at periphery
- Late lesion—white areas, central white crust, focal blue-gray areas, and few dotted and linear vessels at periphery

Pityriasis Lichenoides Chronica

- Brownish-red background color
- Brown dots and brownish areas

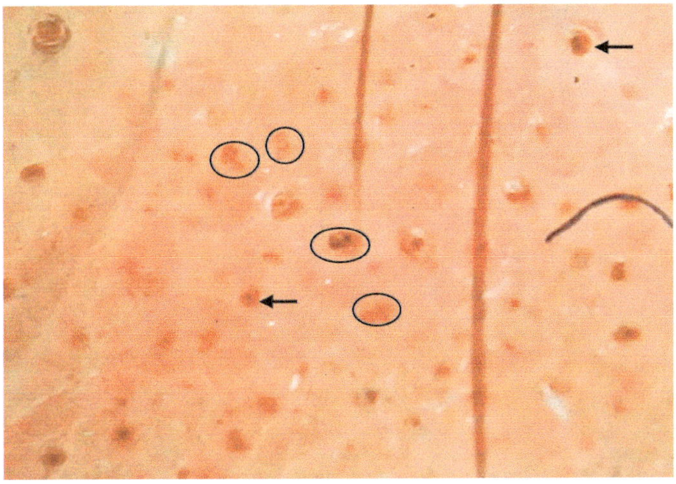

FIG. 20: Dermoscopy of late lesion of pityriasis lichenoides chronica showing multiple brown black-colored granules, dots (black arrows) and brownish structure less areas (black circles) (polarized, Oitez dermoscope, 200×).

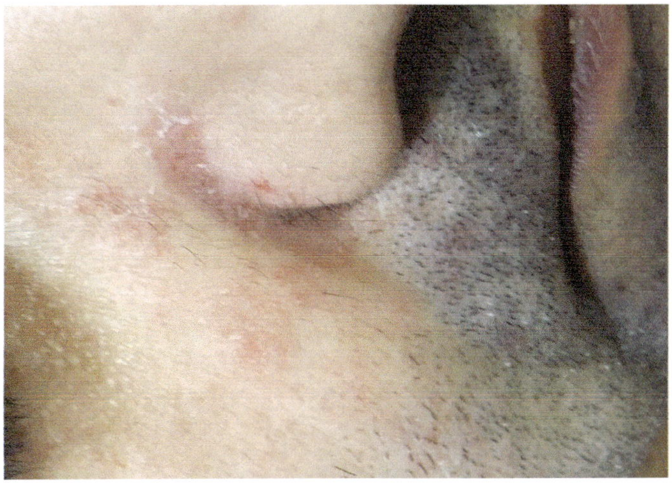

FIG. 21: Clinical photograph of seborrheic dermatitis over face showing fine whitish-yellow greasy scales and erythema over nasolabial region of face and nose.

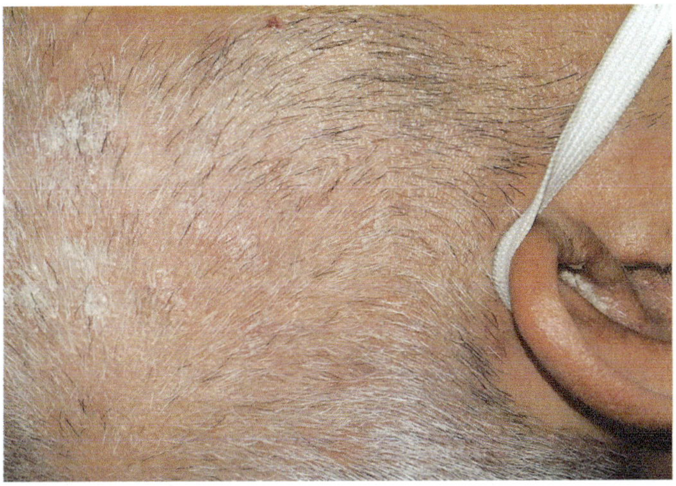

FIG. 22: Clinical photograph of seborrheic dermatitis of scalp showing scaly plaque.

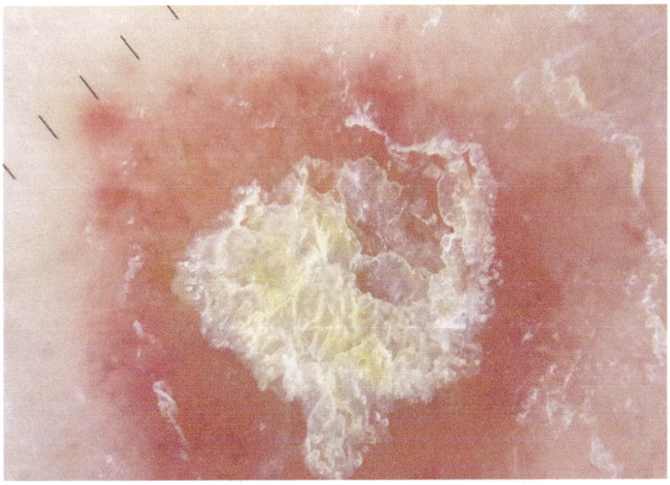

FIG. 23: Dermoscopic image of seborrheic dermatitis on the face shows prominent yellowish-white scales with an erythematous background. Note the few dotted vessels at the periphery (polarized, DermLite 3N, 10×).

- Focal dotted and linear vessels
- Diffuse white scale

SEBORRHEIC DERMATITIS

Clinical Features

Seborrheic dermatitis is a chronic relapsing erythematosquamous dermatosis that can affect the scalp.[22] It is characterized by erythematous skin covered with yellowish-greasy scales and is observed over areas rich in sebaceous glands namely, scalp, nasolabial folds, ears, eyebrows, chest, back and flexural areas (**Figs. 21** and **22**).[22]

Dermoscopic Features

The characteristic dermoscopic features of seborrheic dermatitis over face include the presence of yellowish greasy scales present in a patchy distribution over a pinkish red background (**Fig. 23**).[14,23] The dotted or comma vessels correspond to the dilated blood vessels within the dermal papillae with overlying psoriasiform epidermal hyperplasia.[14,23] Few lesions also demonstrate the tail of *Demodex* mite (**Fig. 24**). Seborrheic dermatitis of the scalp is characterized by the presence of arborizing vessels and atypical vessels in the absence of red dots and globules (**Fig. 25**).[24] Yellow, greasy scales are usually observed, mostly presenting as peripilar cluster of scales. Orange-yellow or white structureless areas may also be seen.[25,26]

Key Points

Body area:
- Yellowish, patchy scales
- Pinkish-red background
- Comma and dotted vessels

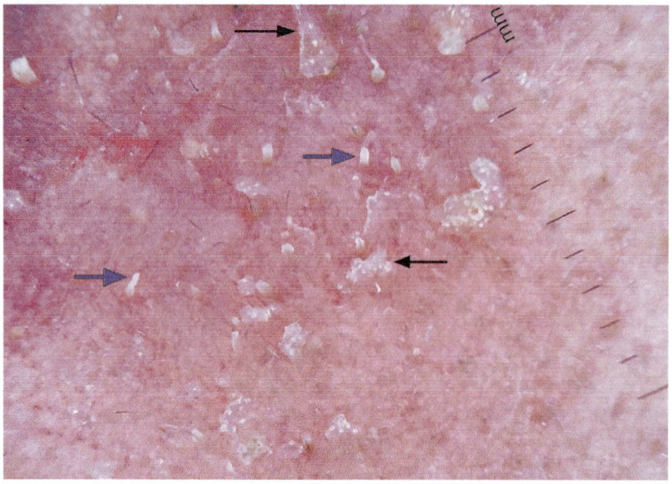

FIG. 24: Dermoscopic image of seborrheic dermatitis on the face shows yellowish-white scales (black arrows) along with presence of *Demodex* tails (blue arrows). Note the dotted and linear vessels in the background (polarized, DermLite 3N, 10×).

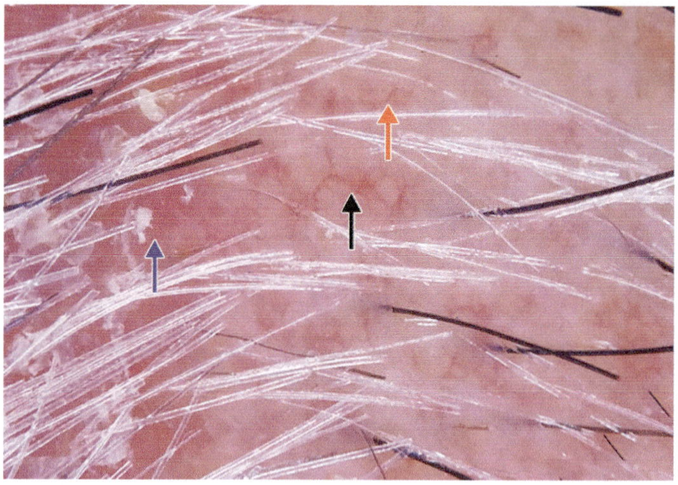

FIG. 25: Dermoscopic image of seborrheic dermatitis of scalp demonstrating arborizing red vessels (black arrow), atypical red vessels (red arrow), and yellowish scales (blue arrow) (polarized, DermLite 3N, 10×).

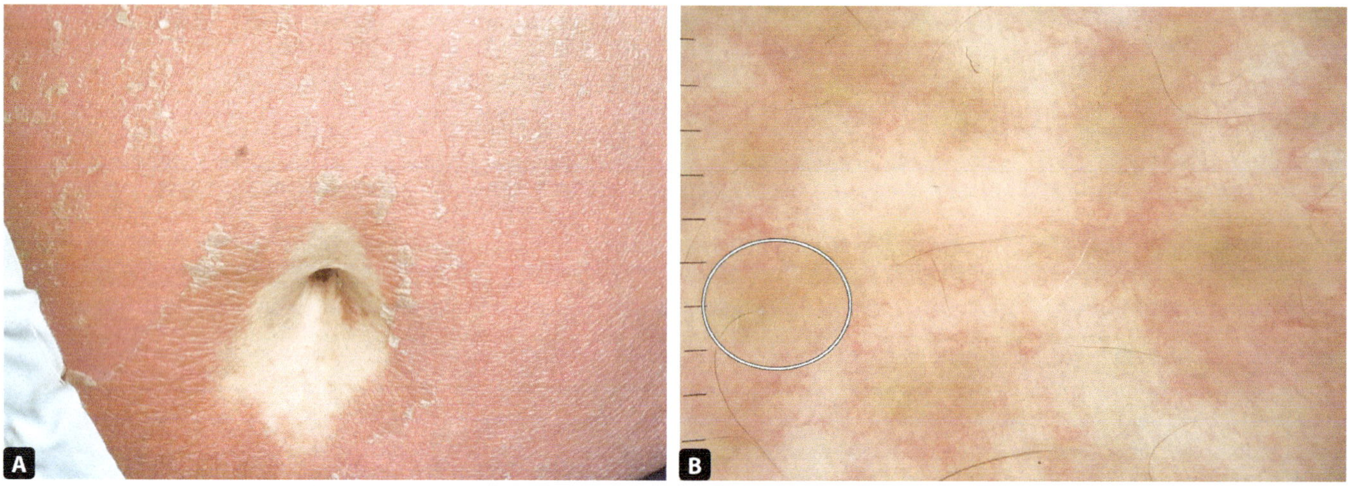

FIGS. 26A AND B: (A) Clinical image of pityriasis rubra pilaris showing diffuse salmon erythema with branny scaling of abdomen with areas of sparing around umbilicus; (B) Dermoscopy of pityriasis rubra pilaris showing whitish keratotic plugs with central hairs with perifollicular yellowish areas (circle) and surrounding erythema. Linear and dotted vessels can also be noted (polarized, DermLite DL4, 10×).
Courtesy: Dr Vinay Keshavamurthy, Chandigarh, India.

Scalp:

- Arborizing vessels and atypical vessels
- The absence of red dots and globules, albeit twisted red loops may be seen.
- Structureless areas devoid of any particular vascular patterns.
- Yellowish scales
- Mostly single scales over slightly yellowish background. Scales may also be present over the hair shaft.

PITYRIASIS RUBRA PILARIS

Clinical Features

Pityriasis rubra pilaris (PRP) is characterized by reddish-orange scaly plaques with well-defined borders, involving some parts of body like elbows/knees or entire body (**Fig. 26A**). Cephalocaudal progression with areas of sparing palmoplantar keratoderma, and follicular hyperkeratosis are characteristic clinical features.

Dermoscopic Features

Characteristic dermoscopic findings of PRP include whitish keratotic plugs with hair shaft in the center surrounded by perifollicular yellowish rings, and peripheral erythema. Few authors have reported presence of linear vessels with or without dotted vessels as a feature of classical PRP, while others have not.[27,28] However, erythrodermic PRP typically shows linear and dotted vessels[29] along with the classical dermoscopic features (**Fig. 26B**).

Key Points

- Whitish keratotic plugs with central hairs surrounded by yellowish and erythematous ring.
- Linear vessels, with or without dotted vessels can also be seen.

ECZEMA

Clinical Features

Eczema or eczematous dermatitis encompasses a wide spectrum of distinct clinical conditions that demonstrate epidermal spongiosis on histopathology. These include conditions such as atopic dermatitis, nummular eczema, allergic contact dermatitis, and asteatotic eczema.[23] Eczemas usually present as erythematous to hyperpigmented plaques, generally distributed over the extremities. Clinically, they may demonstrate oozing, serocrusts in the acute stage (**Figs. 27** and **28**) and patchy white scales or lichenification in chronic stage (**Figs. 29** to **31**).

Dermoscopic Features

The characteristic dermoscopic features of eczematous dermatitis include the presence of dotted vessels in a patchy distribution or in an unspecified arrangement, along with the presence of yellow scales and serocrusts, referred to as "yellow clod" sign (**Fig. 32**).[14] The dermoscopic feature may vary depending upon the stage of the eczema. The yellow serocrusts or the "yellow clod" sign is considered as a distinct feature of acute exudative eczema and it represents the spongiosis and hyperkeratosis and the serous discharge.[14,30] It is commonly observed in nummular dermatitis.[14,23] Subacute eczema may also present with similar dermoscopic findings (**Fig. 33**). The dotted vessels appearing in clusters correspond to the dilated capillaries within the irregularly elongated dermal papillae.[14] Under higher magnification, the red dots appear

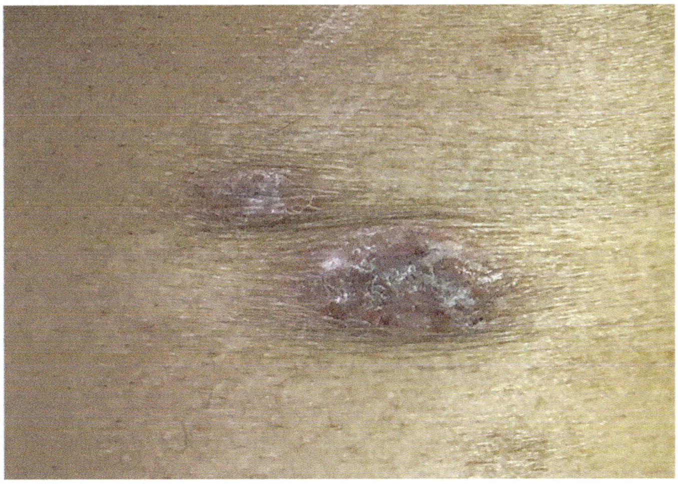

FIG. 27: Clinical photograph of acute eczema over the thigh showing a circular erythematous plaque with scaling and crusting.

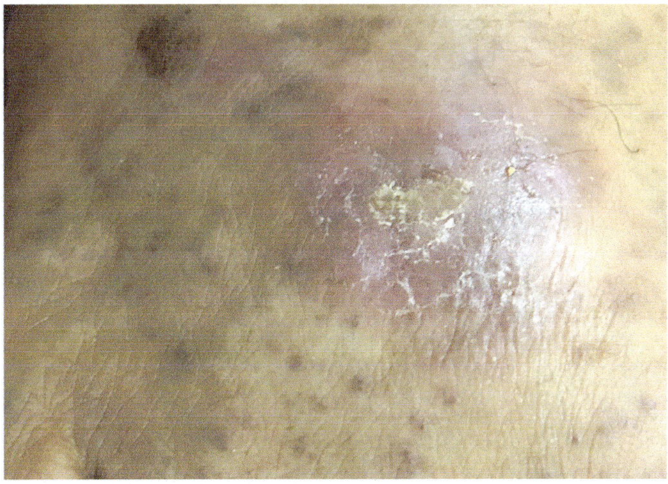

FIG. 28: Clinical photograph of subacute eczema over the right foot showing an erythematous plaque with scaling.

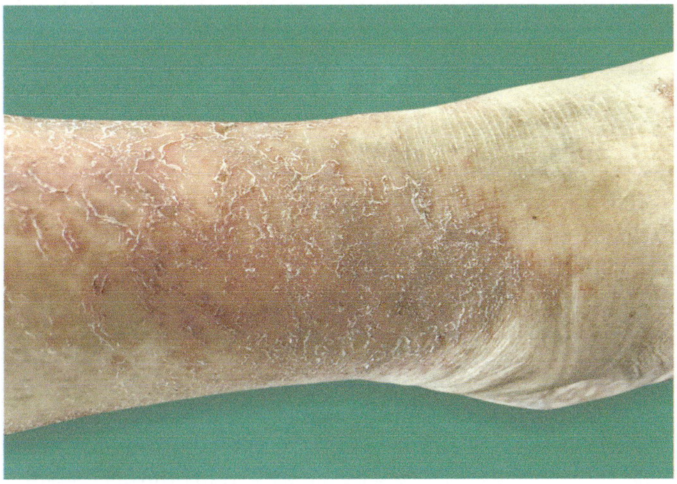

FIG. 29: Clinical image of asteatotic eczema showing dry patch with chapped skin and scaling on the surface.

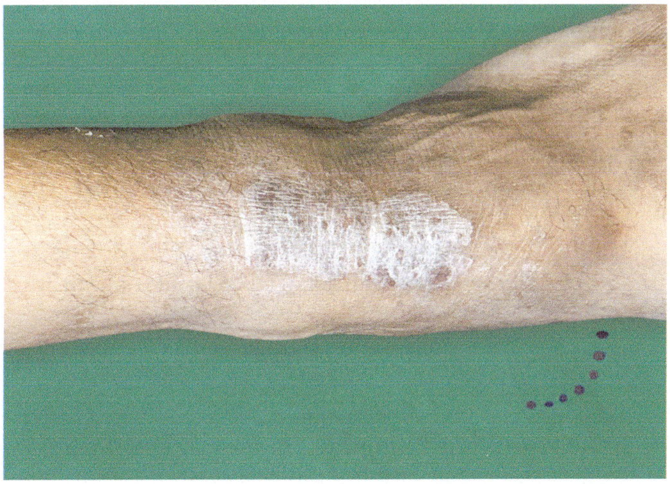

FIG. 30: Clinical photograph of chronic eczema over the foot showing hyperpigmented lichenified plaque with scaling.

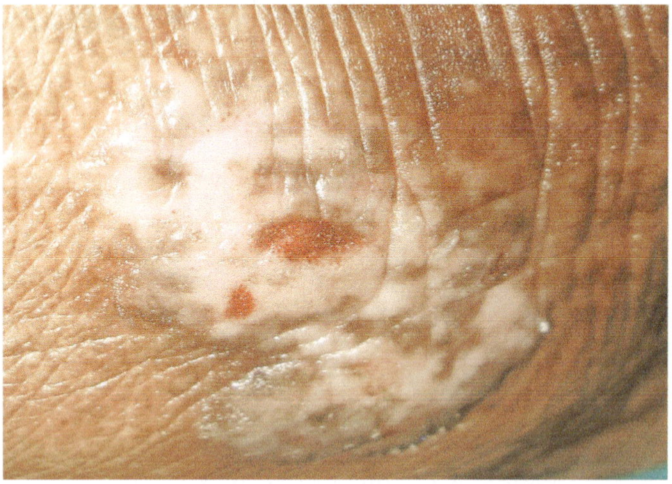

FIG. 31: Clinical image of lichen simplex chronicus showing depigmented plaque with lichenification and thickening.

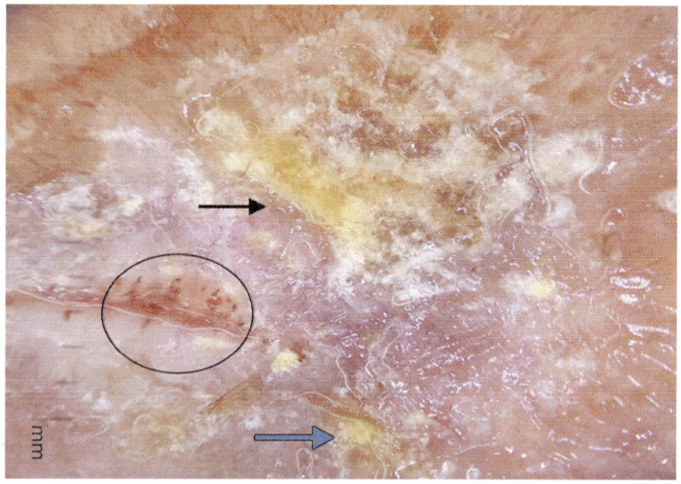

FIG. 32: Dermoscopic image of acute eczema showing dotted vessels in a patchy distribution (black circle) and the presence of yellowish serocrusts (black arrow)/yellow clods (blue arrow) (polarized, DermLite 3N, 10×).

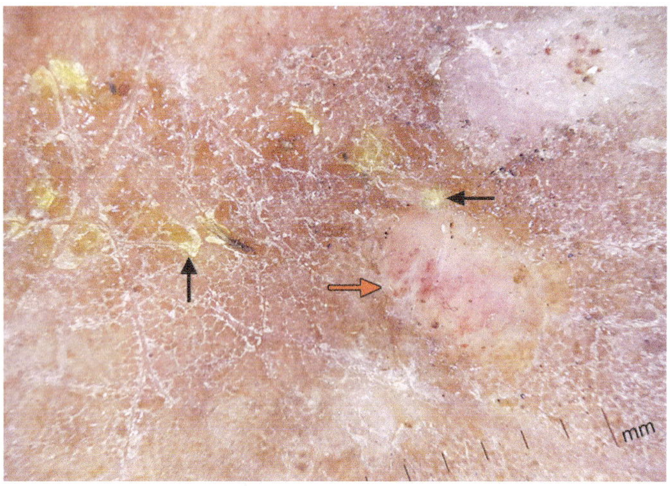

FIG. 33: Dermoscopic image of subacute eczema showing dotted vessels in a patchy distribution (red arrow) and yellowish serocrusts (black arrows) (polarized, DermLite 3N,10×).

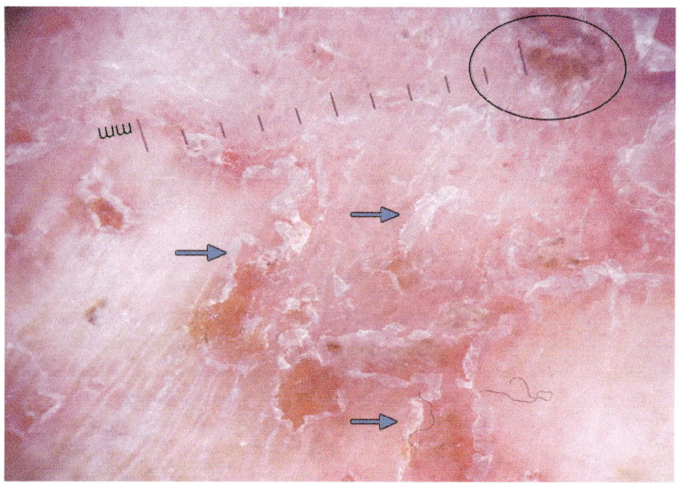

FIG. 34: Dermoscopic image of asteatotic eczema demonstrating white scales with everted edges (blue arrows) along with patchy red dots and globules (black circle) (polarized, DermLite 3N,10×).

as dots and globules, especially in subacute eczema and asteatotic eczema, in contrast to the regular red dots seen in psoriasis. Focal white scales resulting from hyperkeratosis are also observed in the acute stage.[14] In case of asteatotic eczema, the scales may appear whitish with everted edges (**Fig. 34**).[14]

In chronic eczema, patchy dotted vessels and white scales are predominantly seen. In the lichenified stages, intermittent white areas are also observed (**Figs. 35** and **36**). The dotted vessels may demonstrate a white halo around them on account of lichenification.[14]

Key Points

- Dotted vessels in clusters or patchy distribution
- Yellow serocrusts ("yellow clod" sign)

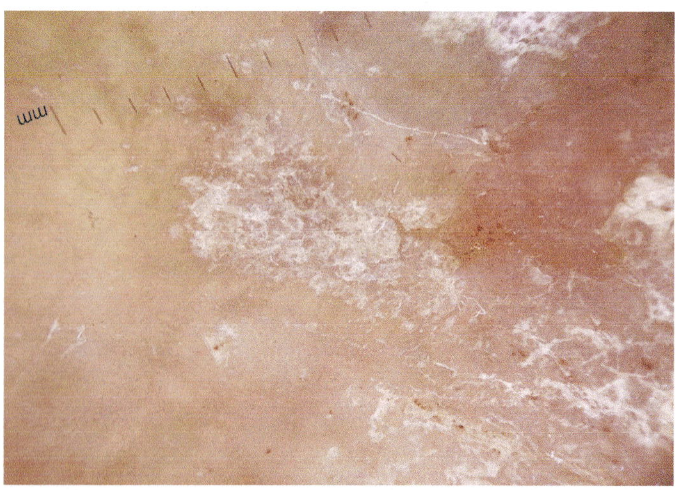

FIG. 35: Dermoscopic image of chronic eczema showing red dots in patchy distribution along with white scales (polarized, DermLite 3N, 10×).

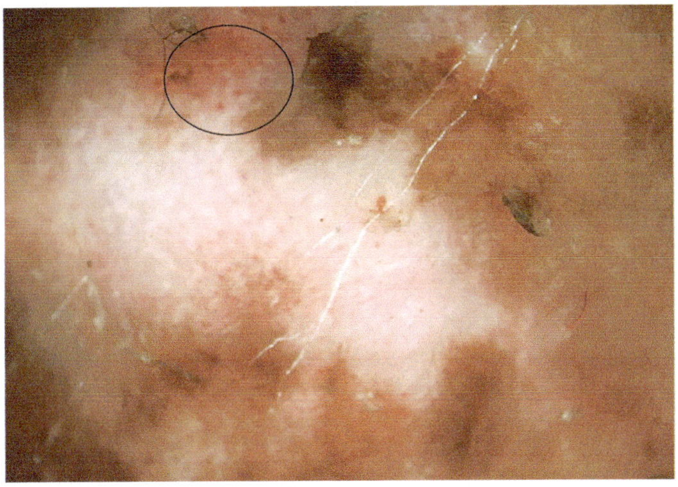

FIG. 36: Dermoscopic image of lichen simplex chronicus showing white areas along with patchy red dots and globules (black circle) (polarized, Otiez dermoscope, 20×).

LICHEN PLANUS

Clinical Features

Lichen planus (LP) typically presents as pruritic, violaceous, flat-topped, polygonal papules predominantly over the flexors of extremities but can affect trunk, mucous membranes, scalp, palms, soles, and nails. The scales are adherent and not usually visible. It runs a very chronic course and pigmentation tends to persist for a long time.

Dermoscopic Features

- *Wickham's striae (WS)*: Pearly whitish and sometimes yellowish or blue-white opaque structures seen in various patterns or configurations (**Figs. 37A to D**)[1,4,31-33] and are considered pathognomonic of LP and an activity marker.[31]
- *Vascular structures*: Seen as red dots, globules or linear vessels are more prominent in active lesions and become inconspicuous in late lesions (**Fig. 37E**).[4,34]

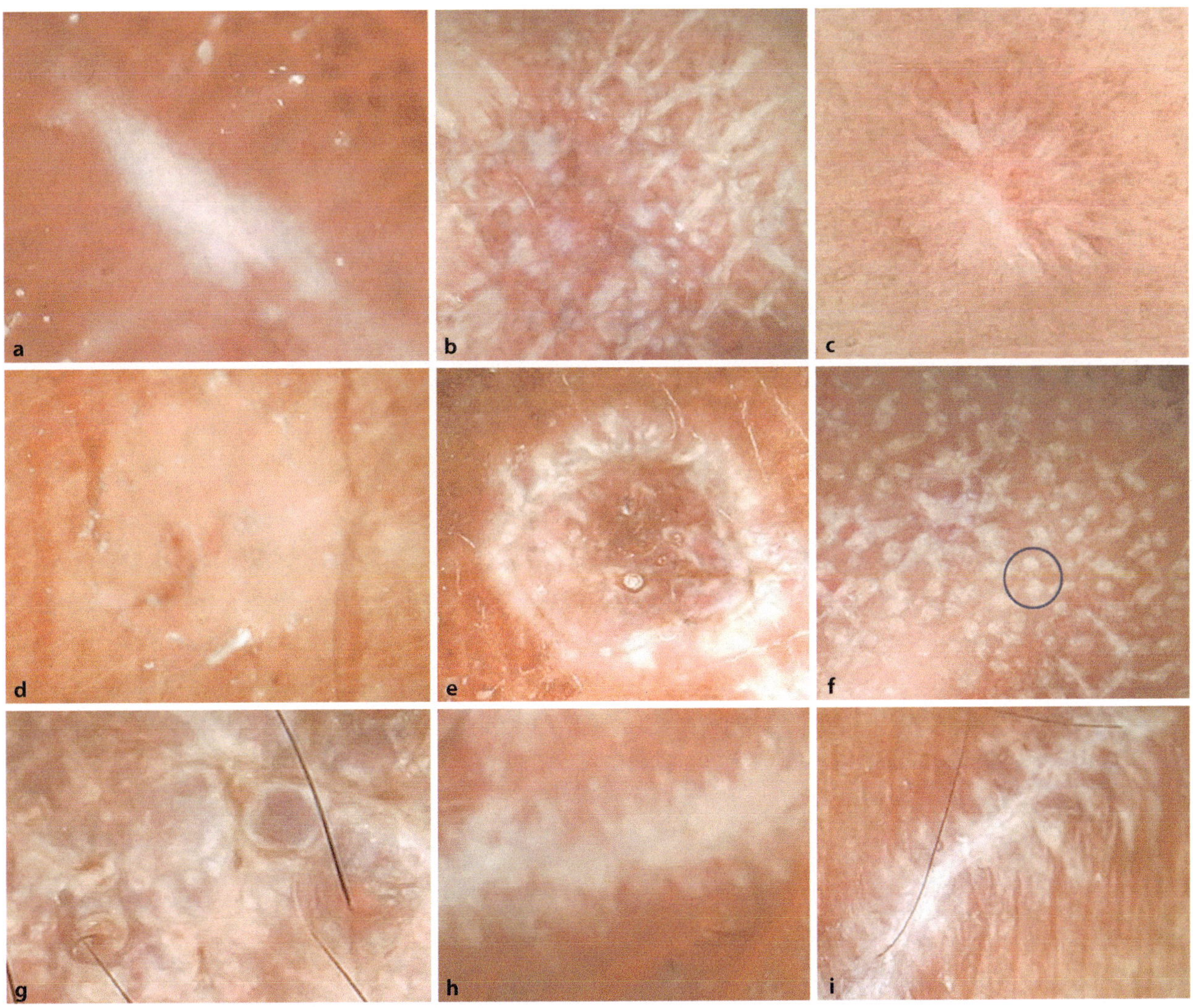

FIG. 37A: Wickham's striae in various morphological patterns: a—linear, b—reticular, c—radially arranged or starburst, d—structureless or veil-like, e—annular, f—globular (circle), g—circular, h—fern leaf-like pattern, i—leaf venation pattern.

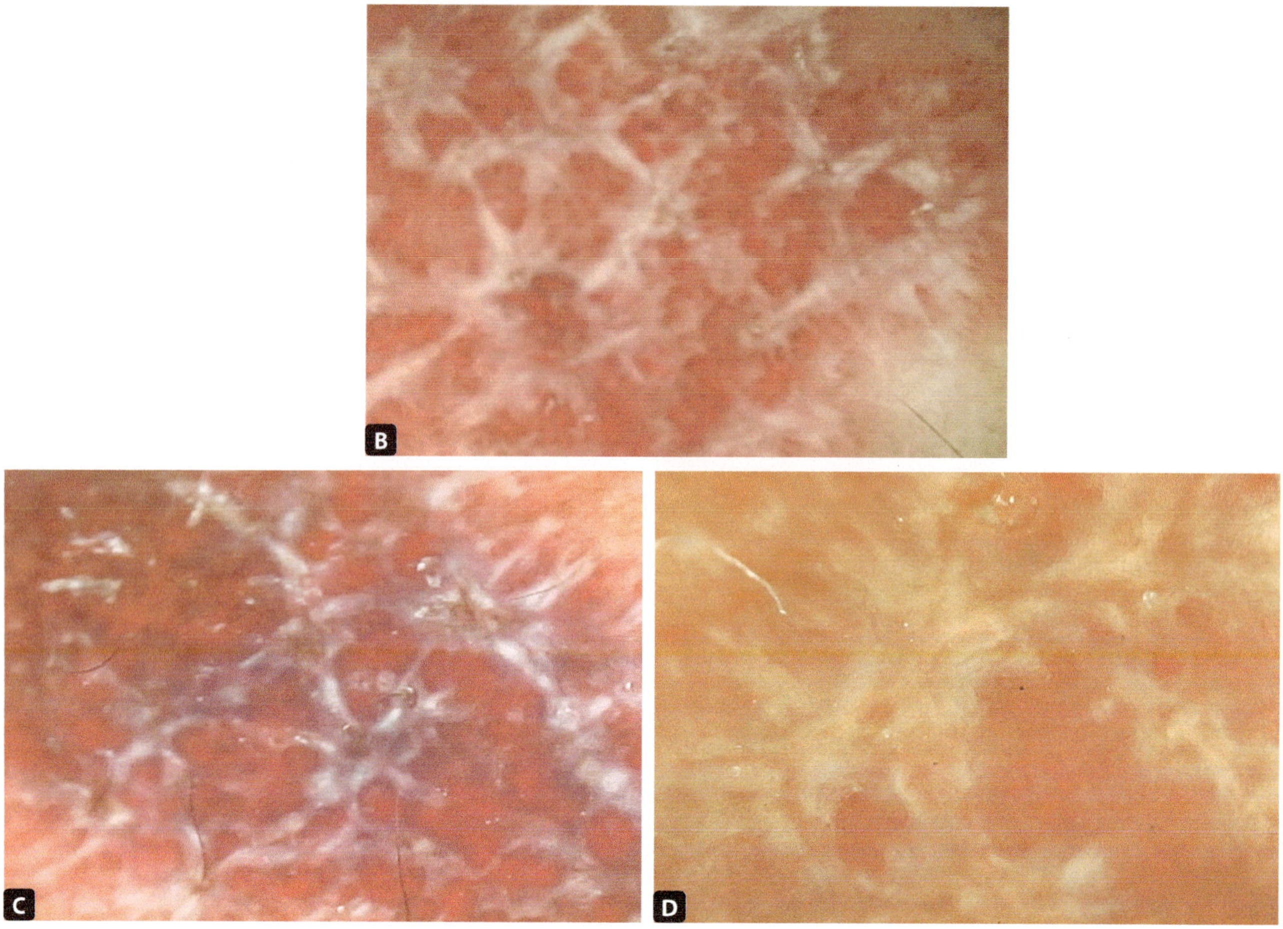

FIGS. 37B TO D: (B) White-colored Wickham's striae; (C) Violaceous-colored Wickham's striae; (D) Yellowish-colored Wickham's striae.

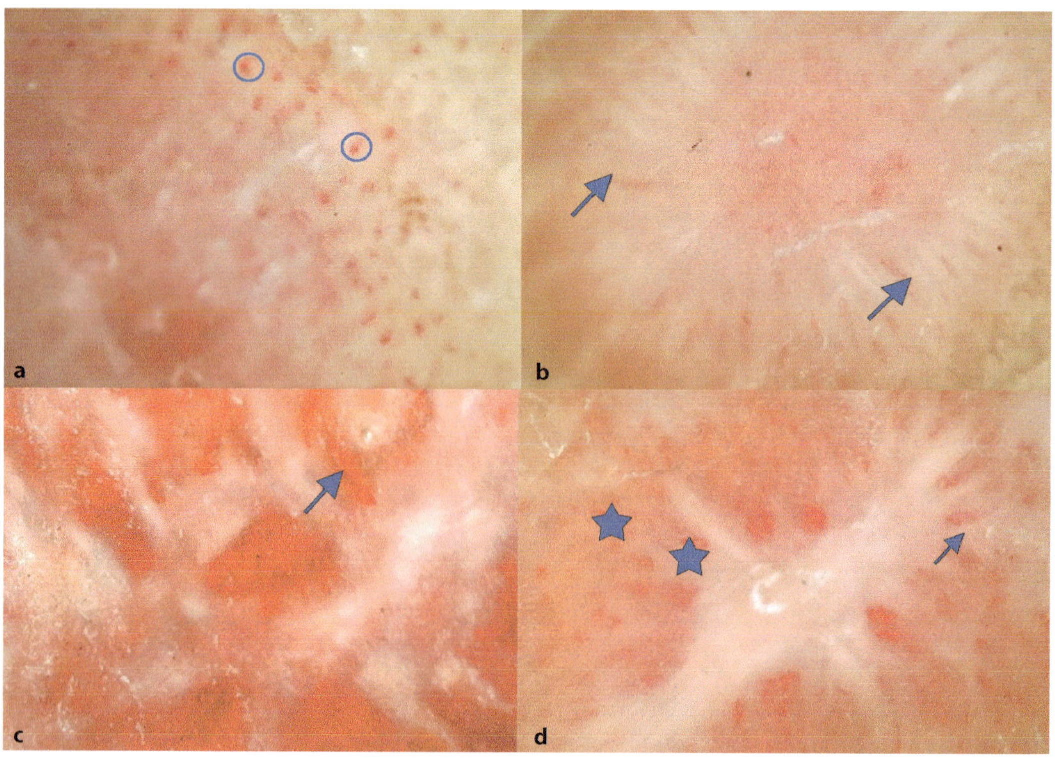

FIG. 37E: Vascular structures seen in lichen planus: a—red globules (circles), b—linear vessels (arrows), c—linear vessels (arrow) in higher magnification with few twisted vessels, d—red globules (stars) and linear vessels (arrow) (polarized, Oitez dermoscope, 200×).

- *Pigmentation*: Diffuse structureless brownish areas, coarse gray-blue/brown dots or globules and mixed pattern showing both diffuse brownish areas with dotted structures.[35] Pigmentation increases gradually as the lesions evolve and is predominant feature in the resolved lesions.[4]
- Complete evolution and regression of LP lesion could be followed with dermoscope, and also it aids in determining the prognosis in residual pigmentation.[4,36]
- There are many clinical types depending upon the morphology, configuration, and the sites involved.
- Classical dermoscopic features, dermoscopy in evolving and resolving lesions, and dermoscopic features in various morphological variants of LP are depicted in **Tables 1** to **3**, respectively. Dermoscopic and histopathological correlation is shown in **Table 4**.

Key Points

- Pearly white polymorphic Wickham's striae often showing projections at the periphery
- Dotted or linear vessels in the periphery
- Brown and gray pigmented dots and globules
- Brownish area

TABLE 1: Classical dermoscopic features of lichen planus.

Wickham's striae	• Various patterns • Color of Wickham's striae—white, blue-white (in dark skinned) or yellowish
Vascular structures	• Red dots and globules • Red lines
Pigmentation patterns	• Diffuse brown pigmentation • Granular—blue-gray dots and globules • Mixed pattern—diffuse and globular • Background color—red, violaceous, brown

TABLE 2: Dermoscopy findings in evolving and resolving lesions of lichen planus.[4,31,36]

Evolution stage of lichen planus	Dermoscopic features		
	Wickham's striae	**Vascular structures**	**Pigmentation**
Very early lesion—skin colored or pink tiny papule (**Fig. 38A**)	Structureless veil-like or rounded, small Wickham's striae (**Figs. 38B** and **C**)	May or may not be visible	A central yellow-brown dot
Early papule—tiny violaceous papule (**Fig. 39A**)	Irregularly rounded Wickham's striae, with projections of the border giving radial or starburst appearance (**Figs. 39B** and **C**)	Peripheral vasculature in form of red lines or red globules	With or without central yellow brown area
Classical evolved lesion—violaceous papules and plaques (**Figs. 40A** and **C**)	Dense Wickham's striae (rounded, arboriform or annular) with border showing comb-like projections (**Figs. 40B** and **D**)	Prominent linear vessels and globules in between these projections (**Figs. 40B** and **D**)	Violaceous or reddish or brownish background
Koebner's phenomenon—elongated papules or violaceous papules arranged in linear fashion at sites of trauma (**Figs. 41A, 42A,** and **42C**)	Central linear white Wickham's striae with comb-like projections (**Figs. 41B, 42B,** and **42D**)	Linear and globular vascular structures in between the projections	Areas of blotchy violaceous pigmentation
Long-standing lesion—hyperpigmented papule (**Figs. 43A** and **43D**)	Reticulate dense Wickham's striae showing projections at periphery and few keratin-filled plugs (**Figs. 43B, C,** and **E**)	Few scattered red globules (**Figs. 43B** and **C**)	Center with bluish globules on a diffuse brownish pigmentation (**Figs. 43B, C,** and **E**)
Resolving lesion (**Fig. 44A**)	Thin sparse reticulate Wickham's striae at periphery (**Fig. 44B**)	Usually not seen	Pigmentation (multiple brown and grayish-blue globules) in the center (**Fig. 44B**)
Resolved lesions (**Fig. 45A**)	Absent	Absent	Diffuse structure less brownish areas with gray-blue or brown dots or globules (**Figs. 45B** to **D**)

TABLE 3: Clinical and dermoscopic features in various types of lichen planus.

Clinical type	Clinical features	Dermoscopic features
Classical	Violaceous flat-topped polygonal papules	Wickham's striae in variable configurations with vascular structures (red dots, globules, and lines) and gray blue pigmentation[34]
Hypertrophic (**Figs. 46A** to **F**)	Thick lichenified plaques or verrucous lesions (**Figs. 46A** and **C**)	Keratin-filled craters or comedo-like structures with sparse Wickham's striae and pigmentation. Corneal structures or corn pearls seen over the surface of some comedo-like structures[4,31] (**Figs. 46B, D,** and **E**)
Annular (**Figs. 47A** to **C**)	Ring-shaped lesions with central flattening (**Fig. 47A**)	Peripheral ring-shaped Wickham's striae with radially arranged projections and linear red vessels in between the projections and pigmentation in the center[4,31] (**Figs. 47B** and **C**)
Linear	Lesions arranged along Blaschko's lines or dermatomal distribution	Similar to classical lichen planus
Follicular lichen planus (**Figs. 48A** to **E**)	• Scalp—follicular scaly papules with scarring and pigmentation (**Fig. 48A**) • Body—violaceous follicular papules with keratotic plugs (**Fig. 48C**)	• Early—perifollicular erythema, peripilar casts, whitish veil-like Wickham's striae • Fibrotic stage—absence of follicular openings, scarring seen as structureless white areas, gray-brown dots in targetoid pattern around follicular ostia[31,33,37,38] (**Figs. 48B, D,** and **E**)
Vesicular and bullous (**Figs. 49A** and **B**)	Vesicles/bullae on lichen planus lesion (**Fig. 49A**)	Clear fluid-filled vesicle with base showing grayish-blue pigmented blotches and structureless or whitish veil like Wickham's striae against an erythematous background[26] (**Fig. 49B**)
Palmoplantar (**Figs. 50A** to **G**)	Keratotic plaques, punctate keratosis, and pitted plaques (**Figs. 50A** and **D**)	• Absence of classical Wickham's striae • Keratotic lesions—yellowish or brownish areas with or without peripheral projections giving a star-like appearance (**Figs. 50B** and **C**)[23,39] • Punctate keratoses—keratin-filled irregular craters with scales in lacy reticular or polycyclic pattern (**Figs. 50E** to **G**)[39,40]
Mucosal LP-Lip (**Figs. 51A** to **E**)	Reticular, annular, papular, plaque-like (**Figs. 51A** and **D**)	Linear, annular, or reticulate Wickham's striae with dotted, linear, or curvilinear vessels and bluish-black pigmentation (**Figs. 51B, C,** and **E**)[39,41,42]
Atrophic lichen planus (**Figs. 52A** and **B**)	Multiple violaceous lesions with slight depression in the center and perilesional hypopigmentation (**Fig. 52A**)	Diffuse brownish pigmentation with multiple blue-gray dots and perilesional white halo. Classical Wickham's striae absent (**Fig. 52B**)

TABLE 4: Dermoscopic and histopathological correlation of lichen planus with their significance.[4]

Dermoscopy finding	Definition	Histopathology correlation	Clinical significance
Wickham's striae	Pearly white opaque structures in various patterns	Compact orthokeratosis with wedge-shaped hypergranulosis	Diagnostic of lichen planus, marker of activity
Red globules	Rounded dilated red structures	Tortuous and dilated capillaries in the dermal papilla	Commonly seen in active lesions of lichen planus
Red dots	Punctate red dots	Tips of normal capillaries in the papillary dermis	Commonly seen in active lesions of lichen planus
Linear vessels	Linear red structures	Horizontally placed dilated capillaries in the papillary dermis	Commonly seen in active lichen planus, subside in regressing lesions
Brown pigmentation	Diffuse brown pigmentation	Pigmentation in the epidermis	Good prognosis
Gray-blue globules and dots	Rounded grayish-blue structures	Dermal melanophages	Long-lasting, resistant to treatment
Comedo-like openings	Crateriform depressions filled with keratin	Hyperplastic, dilated, infundibula with orthokeratosis and hypergranulosis	Commonly seen in hypertrophic lichen planus
Corn pearls	Round corneal structures	Transepidermal elimination	Common in hypertrophic lichen planus
Central yellow-brown area	Yellowish brown blotch	Basal keratinocytes vacuolization and spongiosis in the spinous zone	Seen in early lesions of lichen planus

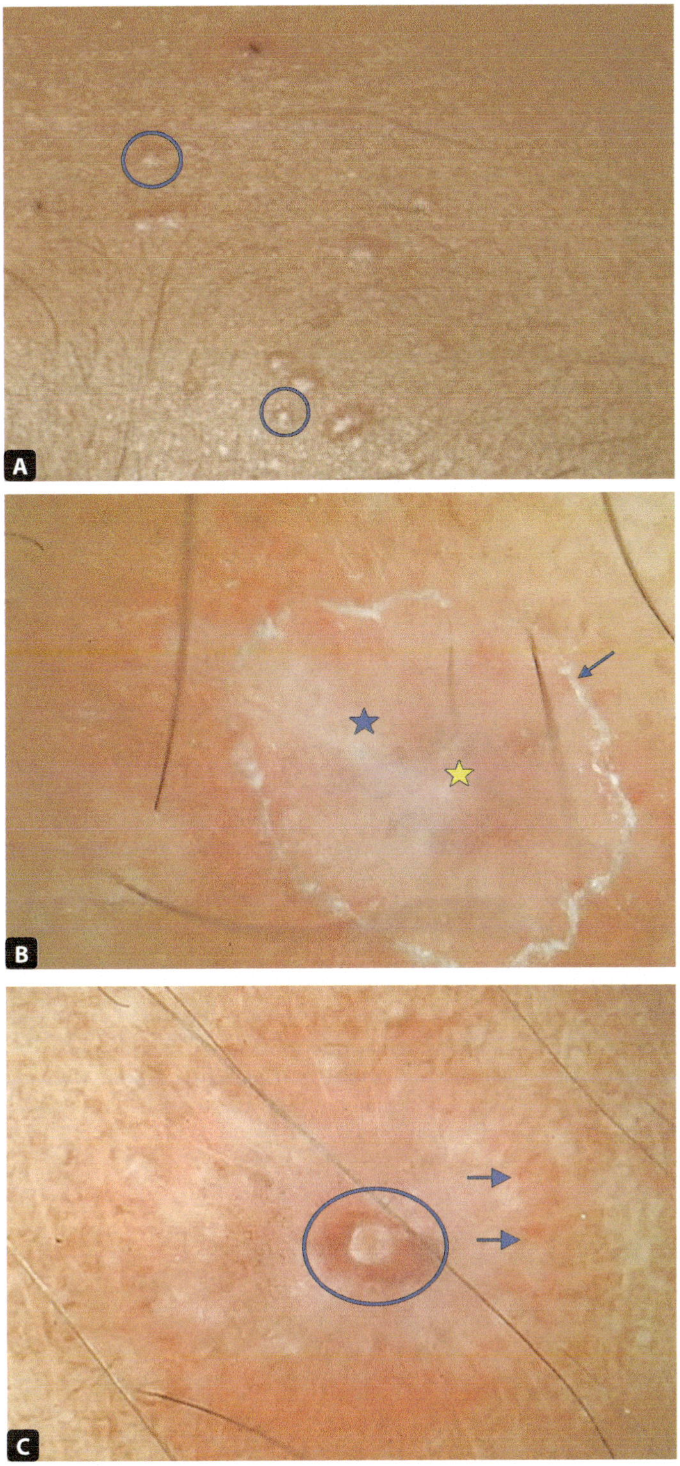

FIGS. 38A TO C: (A) Clinical image of very early lesion of lichen planus showing tiny pinhead-sized pink papules (circles); (B) Dermoscopy of very early lesion of lichen planus showing whitish structureless veil-like Wickham's striae (blue star) with pale pink background (yellow star) and collarette of scale in the periphery (blue arrow) (polarized, Oitez dermoscope, 20×); (C) Dermoscopy of lichen planus showing whitish structureless veil-like Wickham's striae with yellowish area in the center (circle) and multiple linear vessels at the periphery (arrows). Few scattered brown dots are noted (polarized, Oitez dermoscope, 20×).

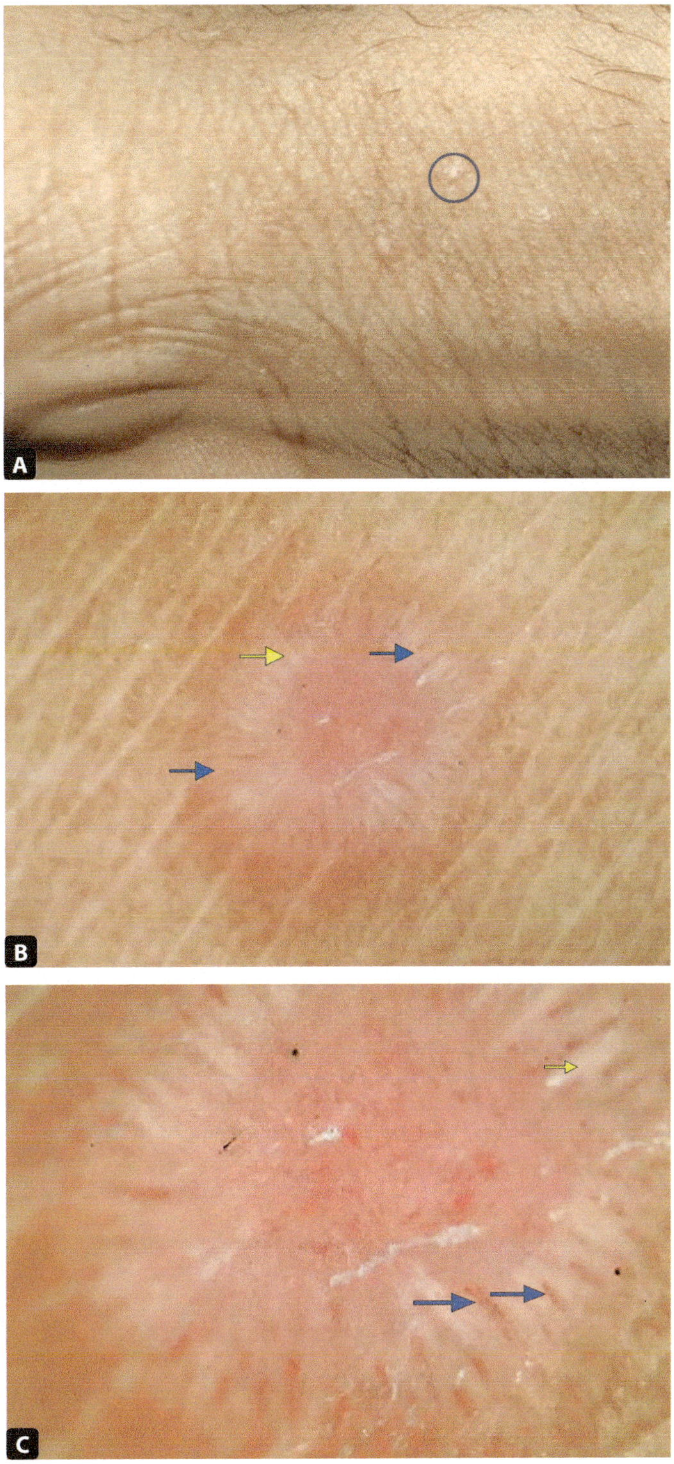

FIGS. 39A TO C: (A) Clinical image of early lesion of lichen planus showing tiny violaceous papules on the wrist (blue circle); (B) Dermoscopy of early lesion of lichen planus showing ill-defined and linear Wickham's striae (yellow arrow) in radial or starburst pattern, with linear vessels (blue arrows) in between the projections (polarized, Oitez dermoscope, 20×); (C) Better visualization of radially arranged Wickham's striae (yellow arrow) and linear vessels (blue arrows) (polarized, Oitez dermoscope, 200×).

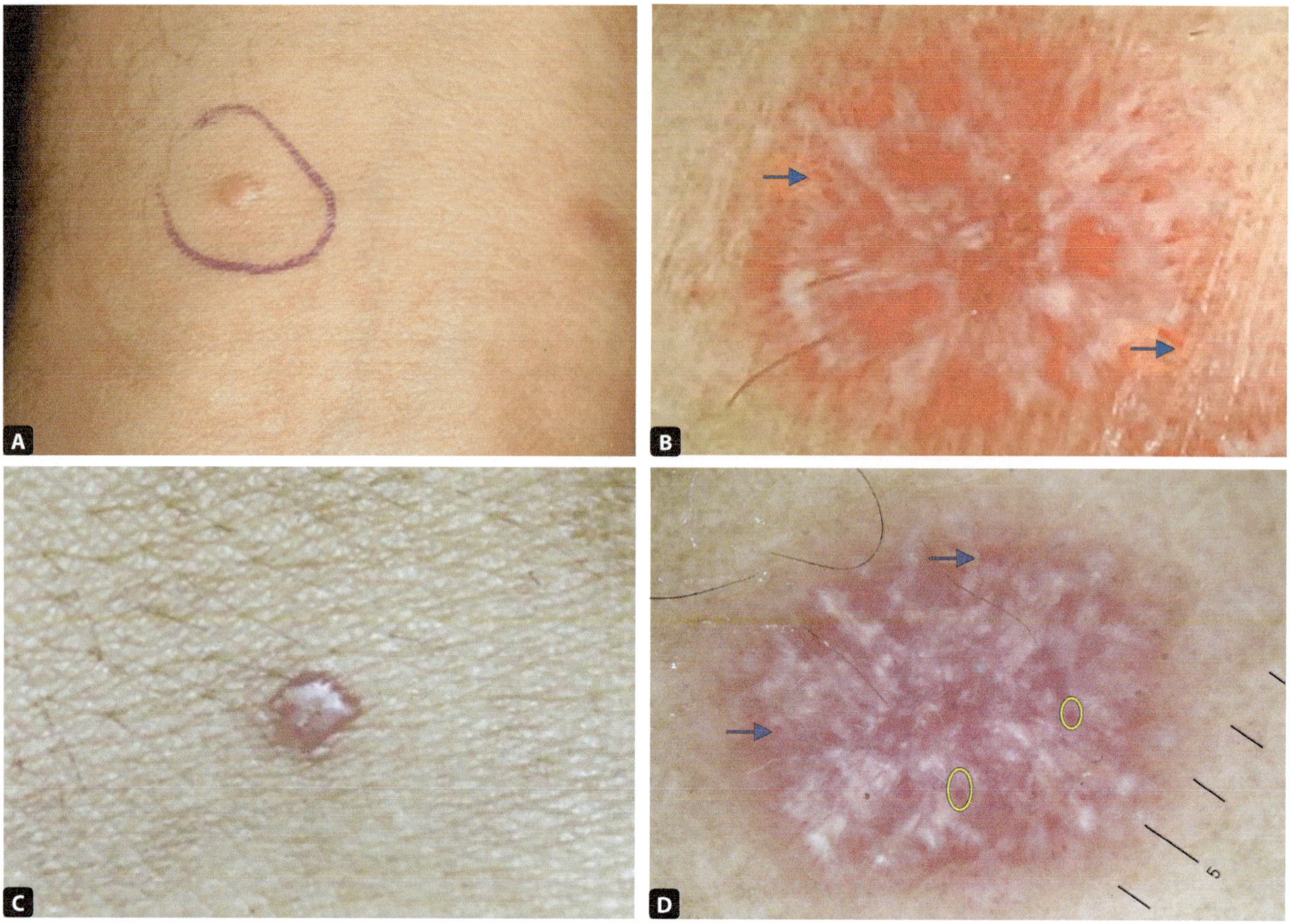

FIGS. 40A TO D: (A) Clinical image of classical evolved lesion of lichen planus showing violaceous flat-topped polygonal papules; (B) Dermoscopy of lichen planus showing arboriform or reticular Wickham's striae with border showing comb-like projections and prominent linear vessels (arrows) and red globules in between these projections against a reddish background (polarized, Oitez dermoscope, 20×); (C) Clinical image of classical lichen planus showing violaceous polygonal papule; (D) Dermoscopy of lichen planus showing arboriform Wickham's striae and prominent linear vessels (blue arrows) and globules (yellow circles) in between these projections against a violaceous background (polarized, Heine Delta 20, 10×).

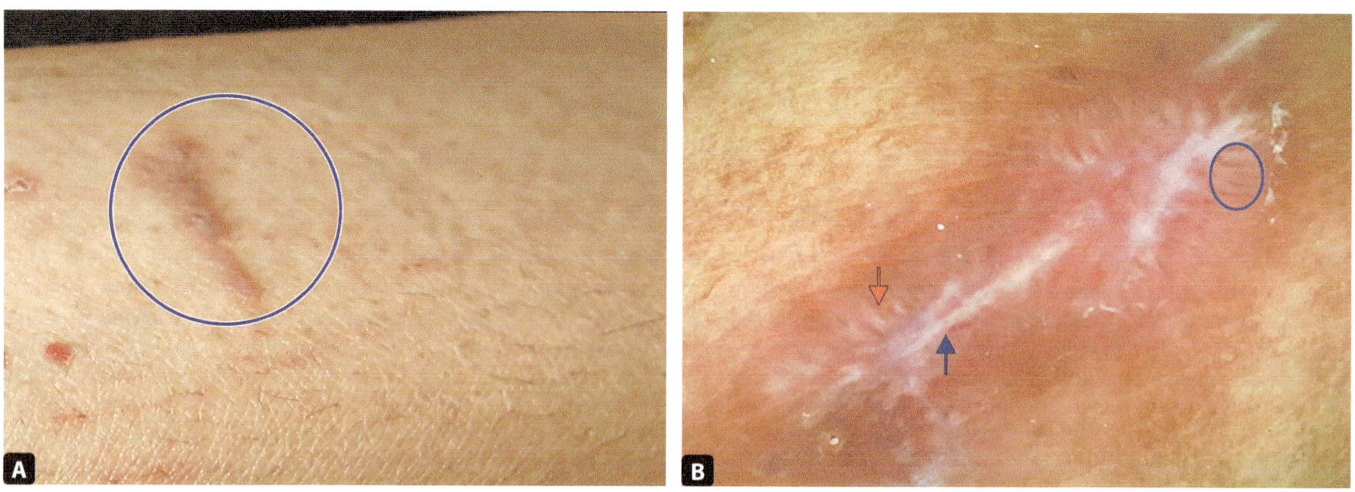

FIGS. 41A AND B: (A) Clinical image of lichen planus showing violaceous papules in Koebner's phenomenon; (B) Dermoscopy of lesions in Koebner's phenomenon shows central linear white Wickham's striae (blue arrow) with comb-like projections (red arrow) and linear and globular vascular structures (blue circle) (polarized, Oitez dermoscope, 20×).

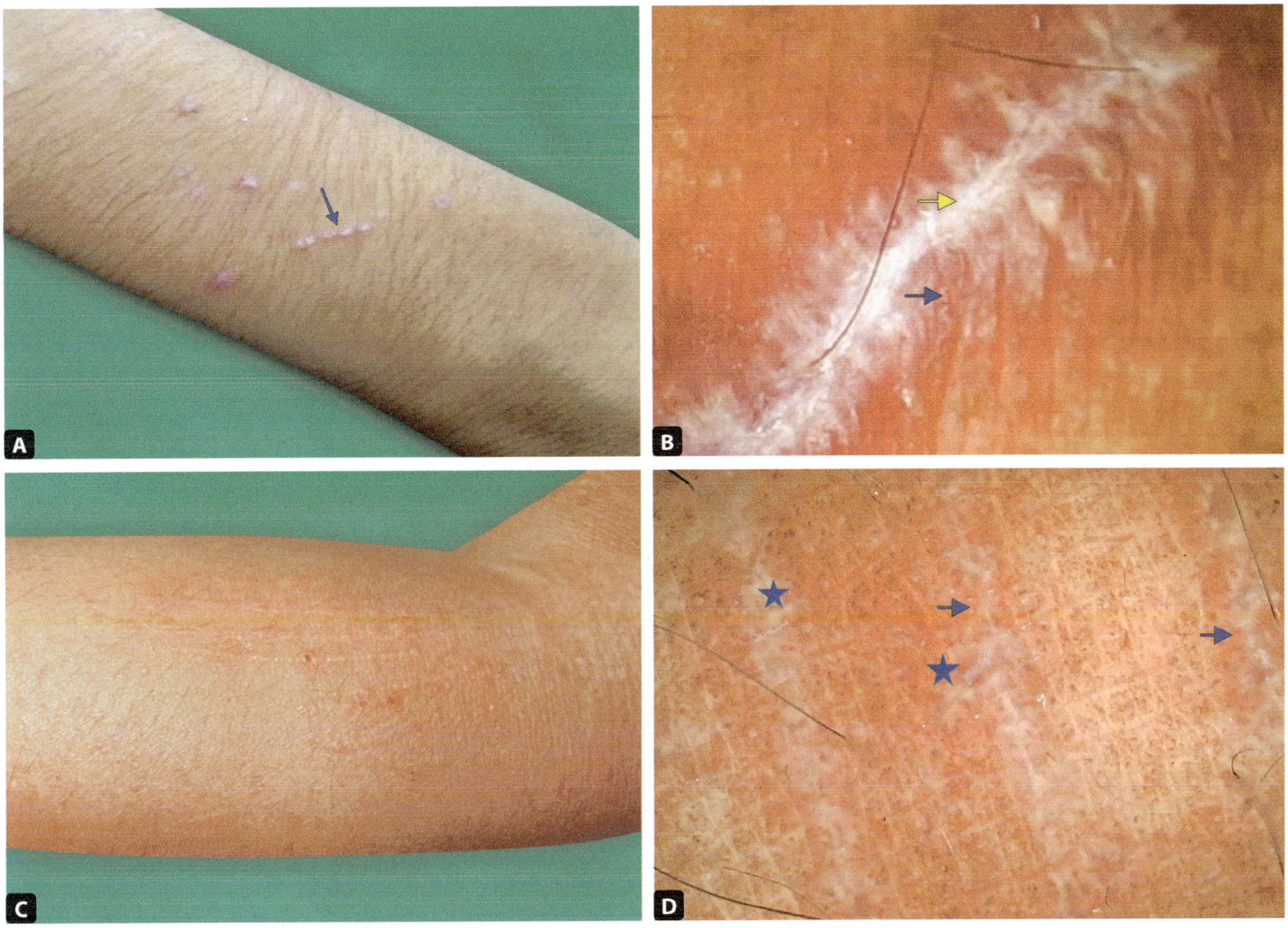

FIGS. 42A TO D: (A) Clinical image of lichen planus showing papules in Koebner's phenomenon (blue arrow); (B) Dermoscopy of lichen planus showing central prominent Wickham's striae (yellow arrow) with perpendicular comb-like secondary projections (blue arrow) from center giving the leaf venation pattern (polarized, Oitez dermoscope, 20×); (C) Clinical image of lichen planus in Koebner's phenomenon showing coalescing violaceous papules in linear fashion along the scratch marks; (D) Dermoscopy of lichen planus showing whitish linear Wickham's striae with lateral projections, few red globules (arrows) and areas of blotchy violaceous pigmentation (stars) (polarized, Oitez dermoscope, 20×).

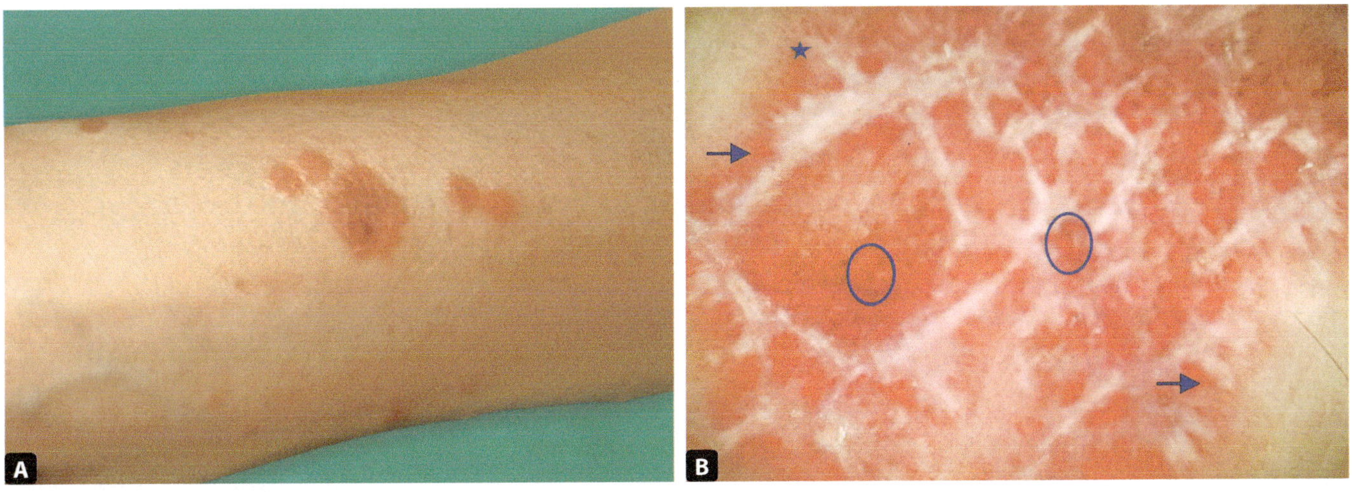

FIGS. 43A TO E: *(Continued)*

(Continued)

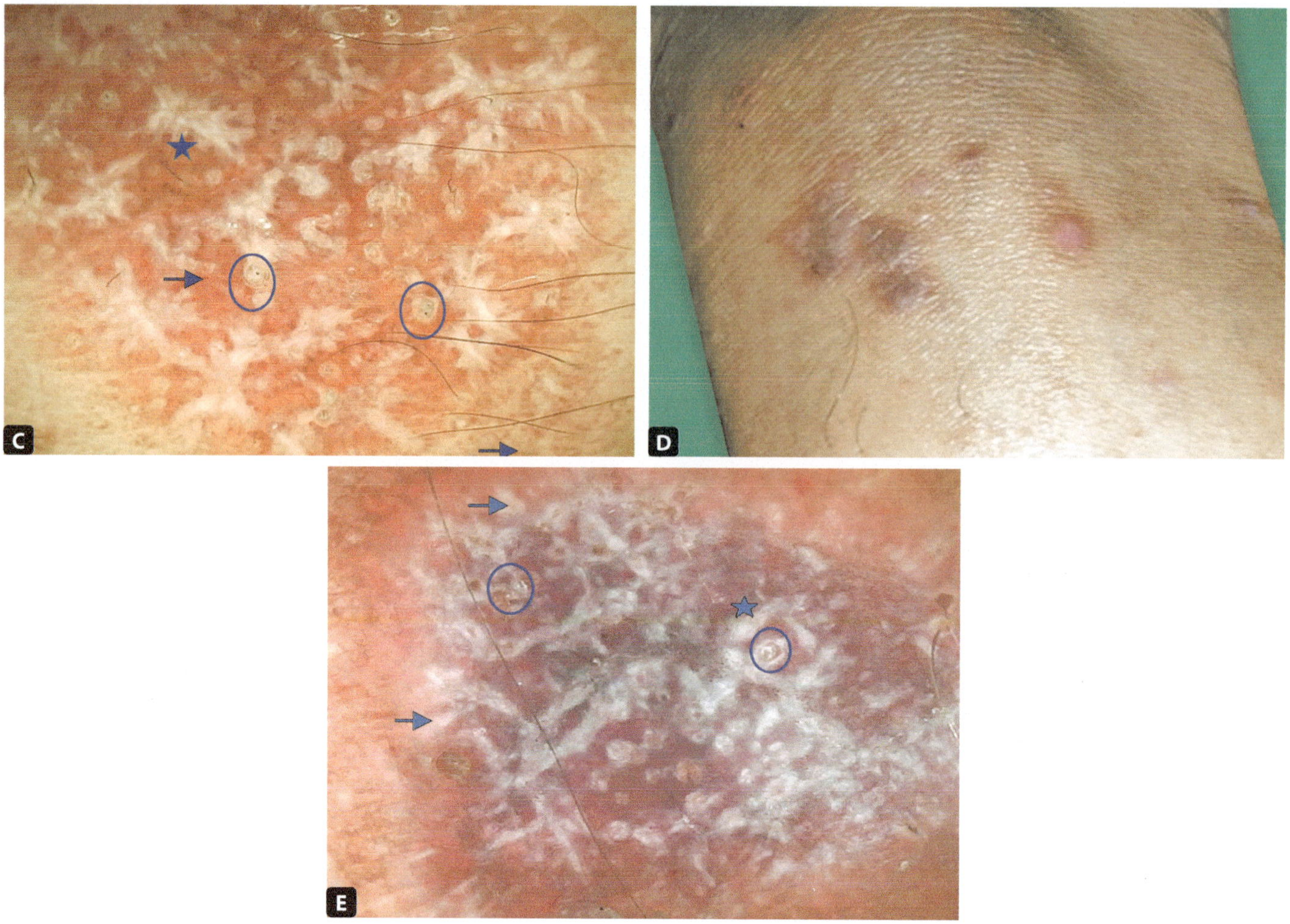

FIGS. 43A TO E: (A) Clinical image of long-standing lesion of lichen planus showing hyperpigmented plaque; (B) Dermoscopy of lichen planus showing arboriform or reticular pattern Wickham's striae with comb-like projections at periphery (star) with linear vessels (arrows) in between the projections, diffuse brown pigmentation in background with grayish dots and globules (circles) (polarized, Oitez dermoscope, 20×); (C) Dermoscopy of lichen planus shows dense reticulate Wickham's striae (star) with grayish dots and globules on a diffuse pale pink background. Few comedo-like openings (circles) and red globules (arrows) are noted (polarized, Oitez dermoscope, 20×); (D) Clinical image of long-standing lesion of lichen planus showing hyperpigmented plaque; (E) Dermoscopy of lichen planus shows dense reticulate Wickham's striae (arrows) and comedo-like openings (circles) on bluish black background (star). Few gray dots are also noted in the center (polarized, Oitez dermoscope, 20×).

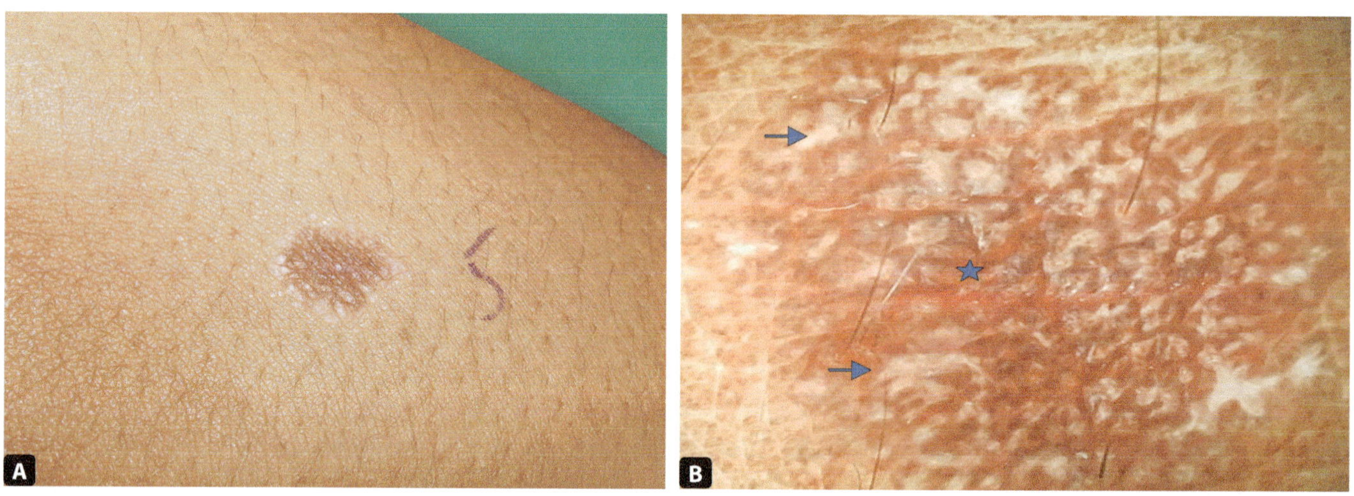

FIGS. 44A AND B: (A) Clinical image of resolving lesion of lichen planus showing hyperpigmented plaque with areas of clearance; (B) Dermoscopy of resolving lesion of lichen planus showing diffuse brownish pigmentation with gray blue globules (star) in the center and few thin reticular and globular Wickham's striae (arrows) mainly at periphery (polarized, Oitez dermoscope, 20×).

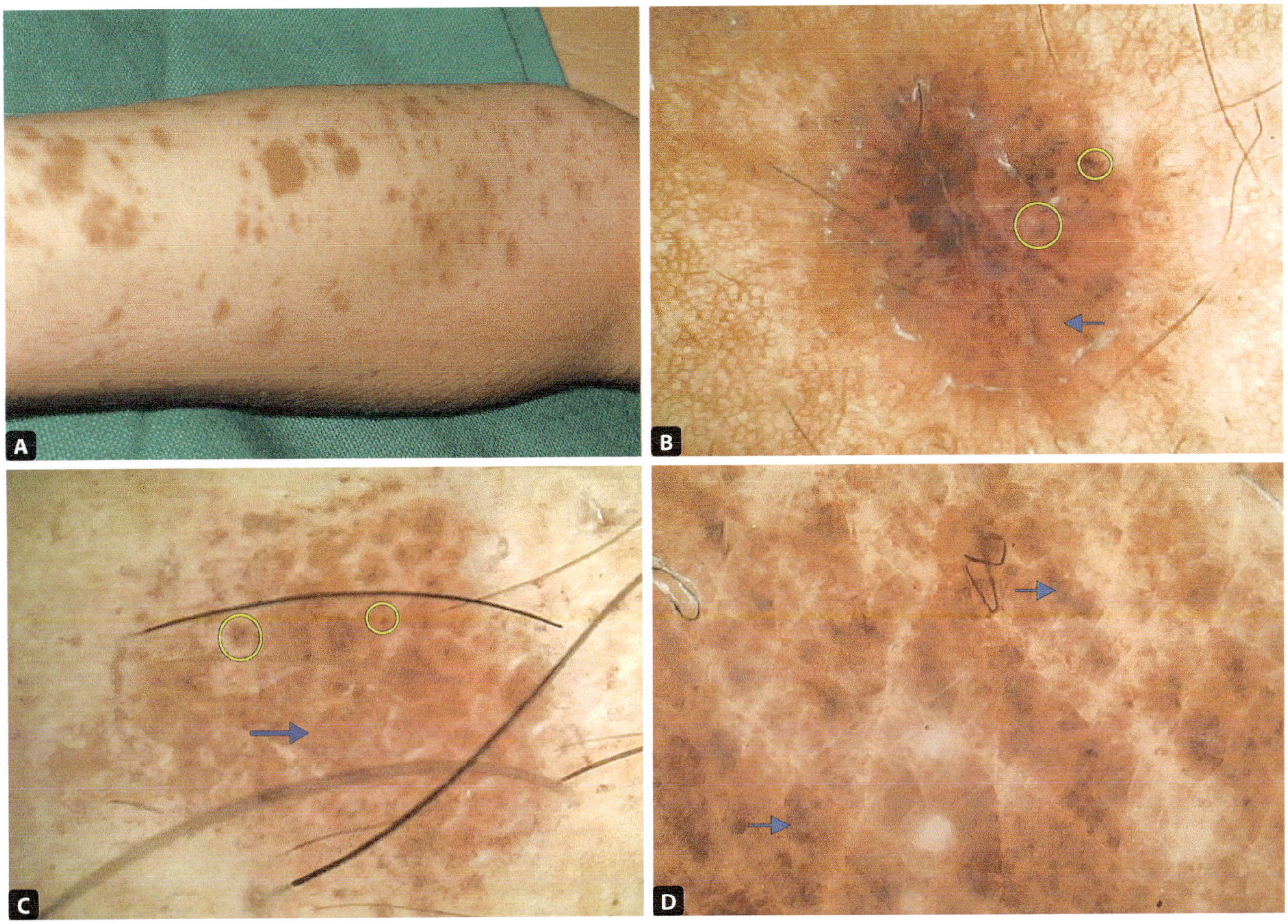

FIGS. 45A TO D: (A) Clinical image of resolved lesion of lichen planus showing hyperpigmented macules and patches; (B) Dermoscopy of resolved lesion of lichen planus showing coarse gray-blue and brown globules (yellow circles) with brownish background (blue arrow) (polarized, Oitez dermoscope, 20×); (C) Dermoscopy of resolved lesion of lichen planus showing diffuse pigmentation (blue arrow) with coarse gray-blue and brown globules (yellow circles) (polarized, Oitez dermoscope, 20×); (D) Dermoscopy of resolved lesion of lichen planus showing gray-blue dots and globules (arrows) of **Figure 45C** in higher magnification with better visualization (polarized, Oitez dermoscope, 200×).

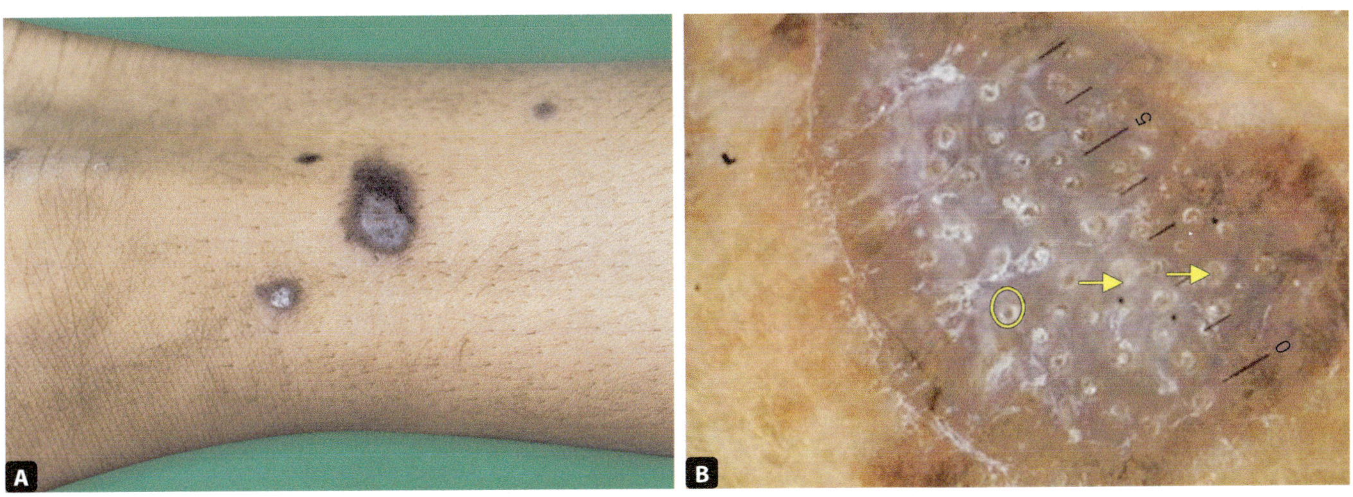

FIGS. 46A TO F: *(Continued)*

(*Continued*)

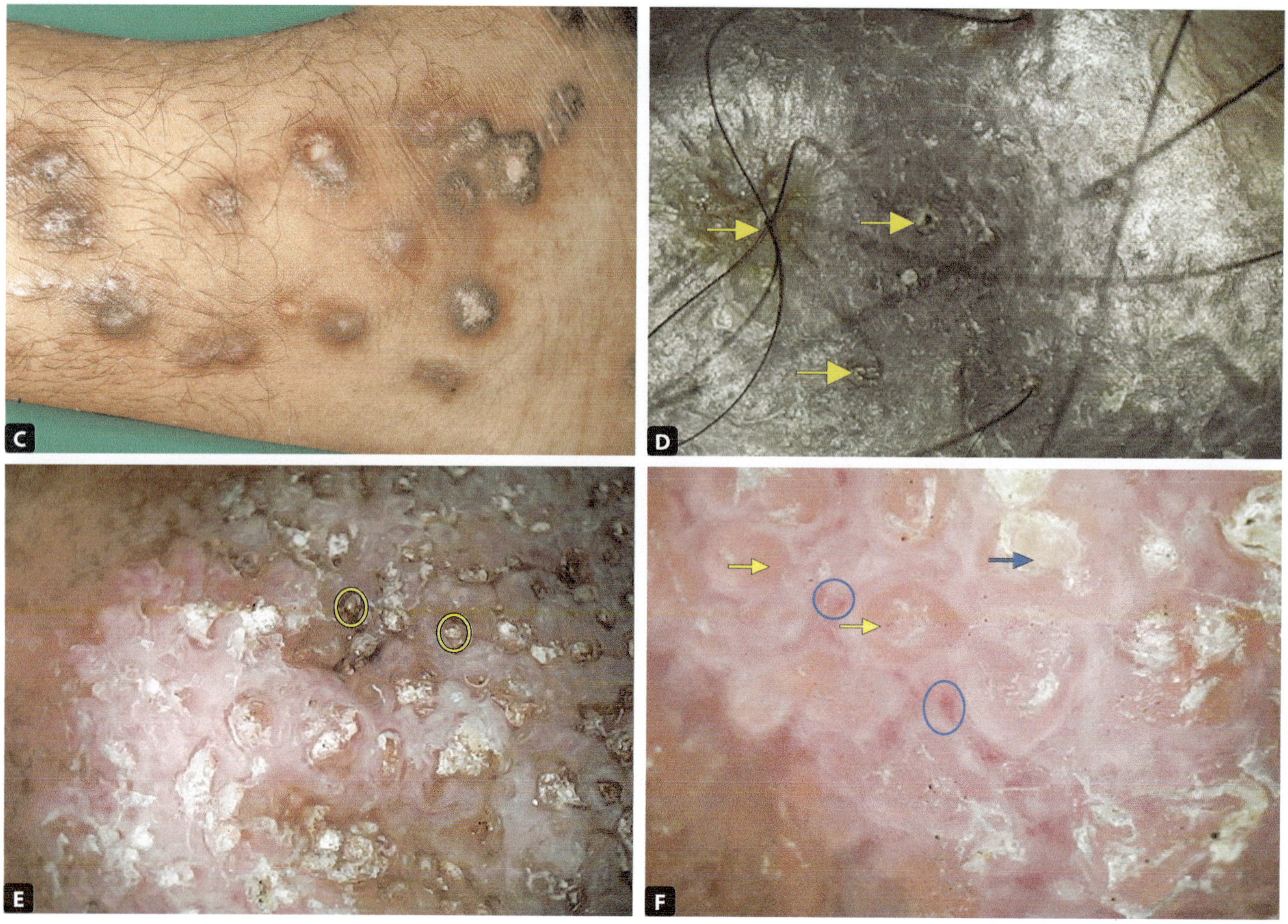

FIGS. 46A TO F: (A) Clinical image of hypertrophic lichen planus showing verrucous hyperpigmented plaques; (B) Dermoscopy of hypertrophic lichen planus showing multiple comedo-like openings (yellow circle) with few keratotic plugs (yellow arrows) with a bluish black background (polarized, Heine Delta 20, 10×); (C) Clinical image of hypertrophic lichen planus showing lichenified plaques on the ankle; (D) Dermoscopy of hypertrophic lichen planus showing keratin-filled crateriform areas or comedo-like structures (arrows) (nonpolarized, Oitez dermoscope, 20×); (E) Dermoscopy of hypertrophic lichen planus showing keratin-filled craters or comedo-like structures (circles) with sparse Wickham's striae (polarized, Oitez dermoscope, 20×); (F) Dermoscopy of hypertrophic lichen planus showing corn pearls (yellow arrows) with comedo-like structures (blue arrow) and few red globules (blue circles) with better visualization (polarized, Oitez dermoscope, 200×).

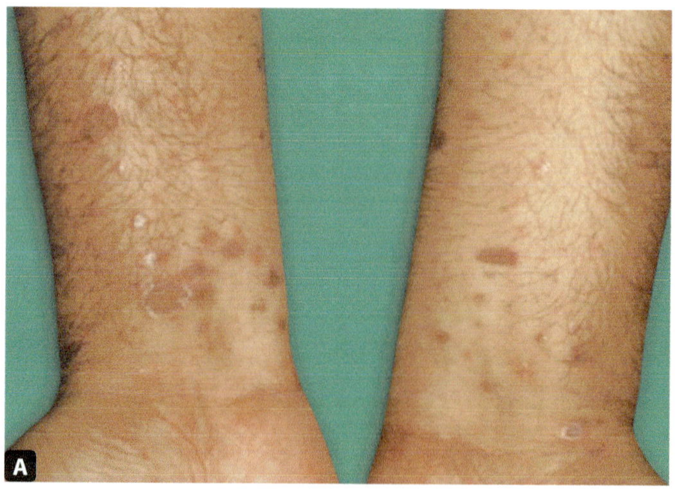

FIGS. 47A TO C: (*Continued*)

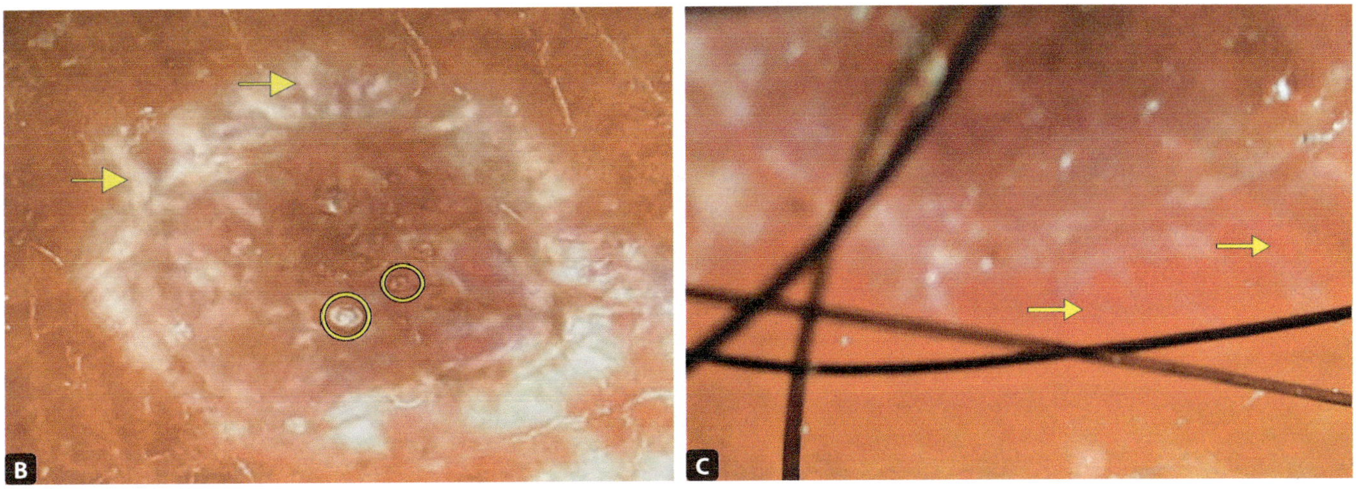

FIGS. 47A TO C: (A) Clinical image of annular lesion of lichen planus showing violaceous ring-shaped lesions with central flattening and raised borders; (B) Dermoscopy of annular lesion of lichen planus showing pigmentation in the center with peripheral ring-shaped Wickham's striae with projections from the ring (arrows) and comedo-like openings (circles) (polarized, Oitez dermoscope, 20×); (C) Radially arranged vessels (arrows) are better visualized in higher magnification (polarized, Oitez dermoscope, 200×).

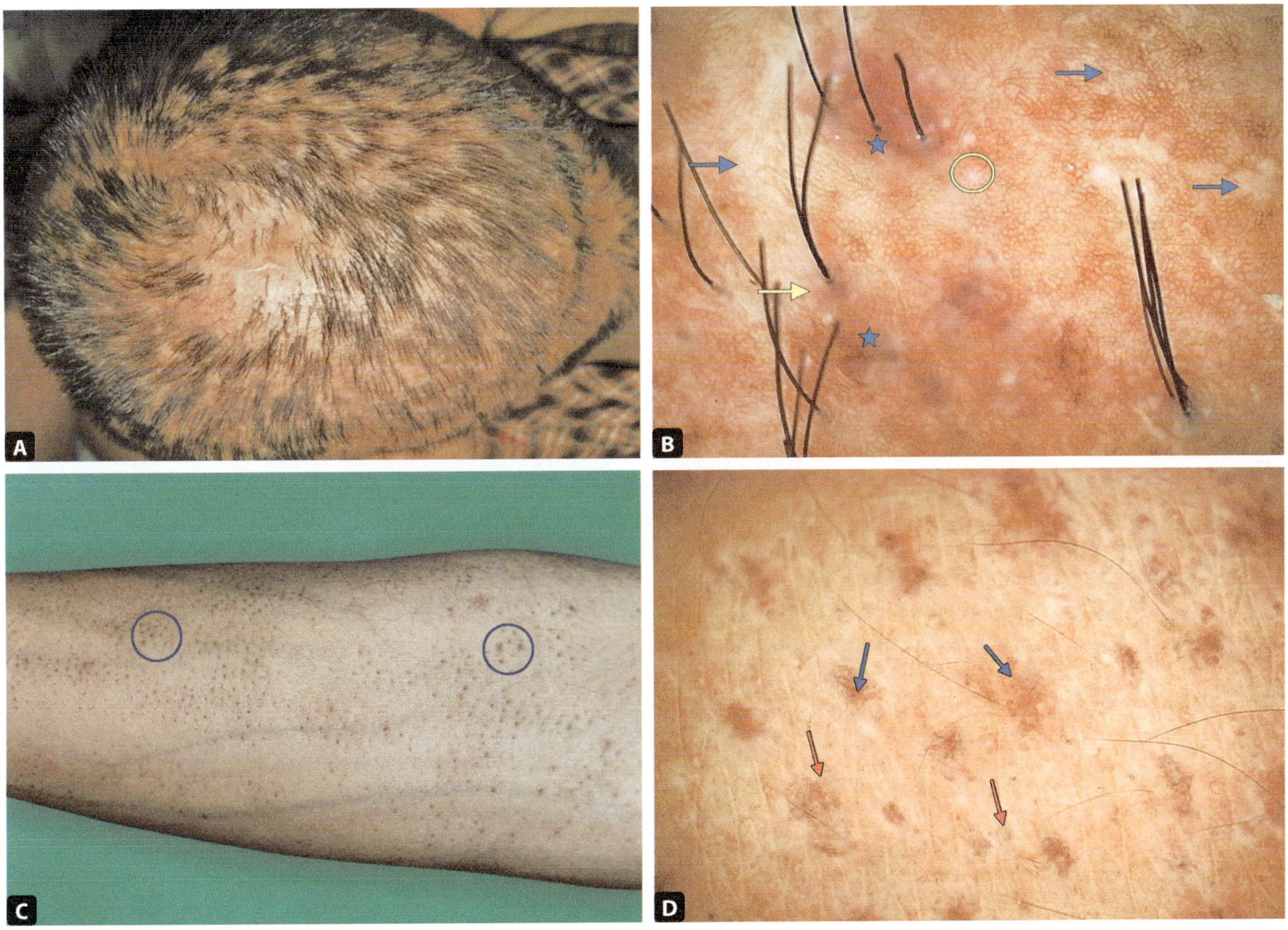

FIGS. 48A TO E: (Continued)

(Continued)

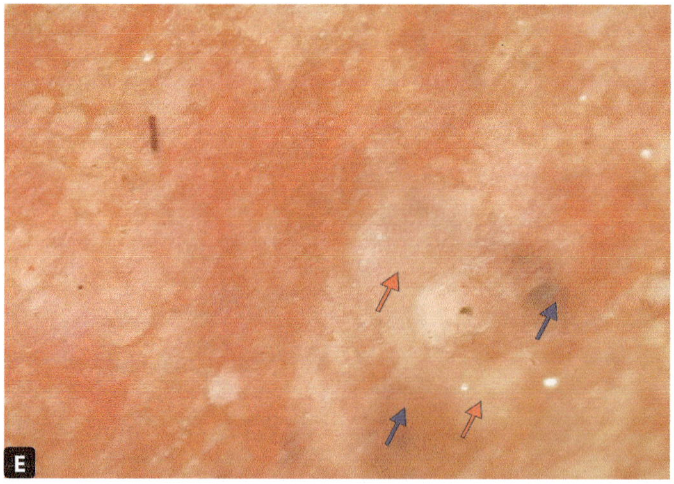

FIGS. 48A TO E: (A) Clinical image of lichen planopilaris showing areas of multiple patches of scarring alopecia on the scalp; (B) Dermoscopy of lichen planopilaris showing absence of follicular openings, white areas (blue arrows), gray-brown dots in targetoid pattern around follicular ostia (blue stars), perifollicular white areas (yellow arrow), and follicular white dots (yellow circle). Note the honeycomb pigmentation (polarized, Oitez dermoscope, 20×); (C) Clinical image of follicular lichen planus showing violaceous follicular papules with keratotic plugs (blue circles) over forearm; (D) Dermoscopy of follicular lichen planus showing white areas (red arrows), perifollicular scale, perifollicular gray-brown dots in targetoid pattern (blue arrows) (polarized, Oitez dermoscope, 20×); (E) Dermoscopy of follicular lichen planus showing perifollicular structureless Wickham's striae (red arrows) and gray-brown pigment dots (blue arrows) (polarized, Oitez dermoscope, 200×).

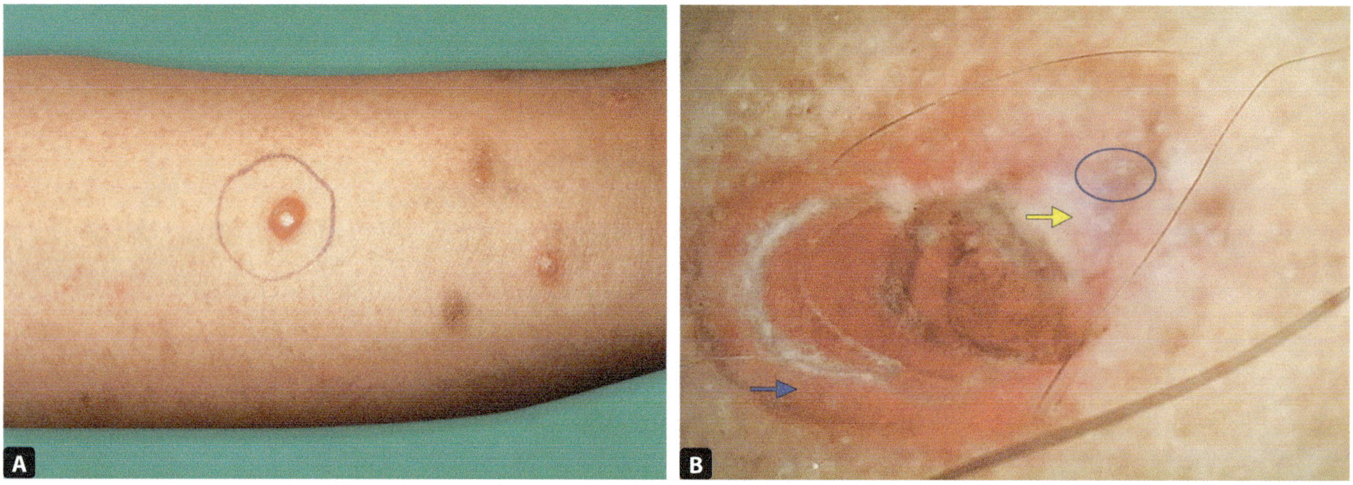

FIGS. 49A AND B: (A) Clinical image of bullous lichen planus showing fluid-filled lesions with purplish hue; (B) Dermoscopy of bullous lichen planus showing reddish structureless area (blue arrow), bluish-white area (blue circle), and whitish structureless Wickham's striae (yellow arrow) on a red background (polarized, Oitez dermoscope, 200×).

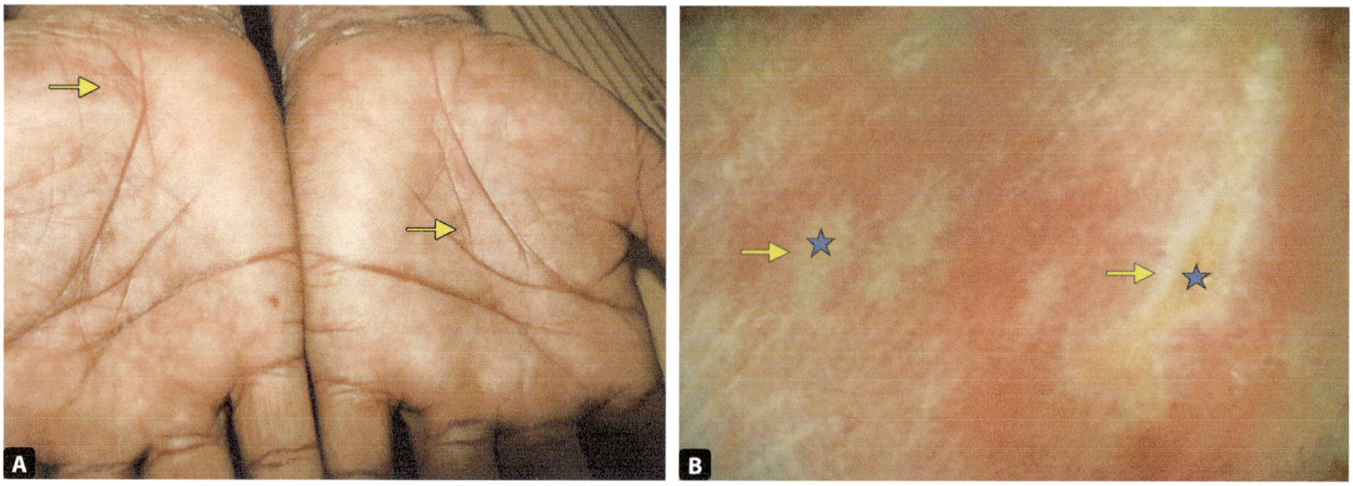

FIGS. 50A TO G: *(Continued)*

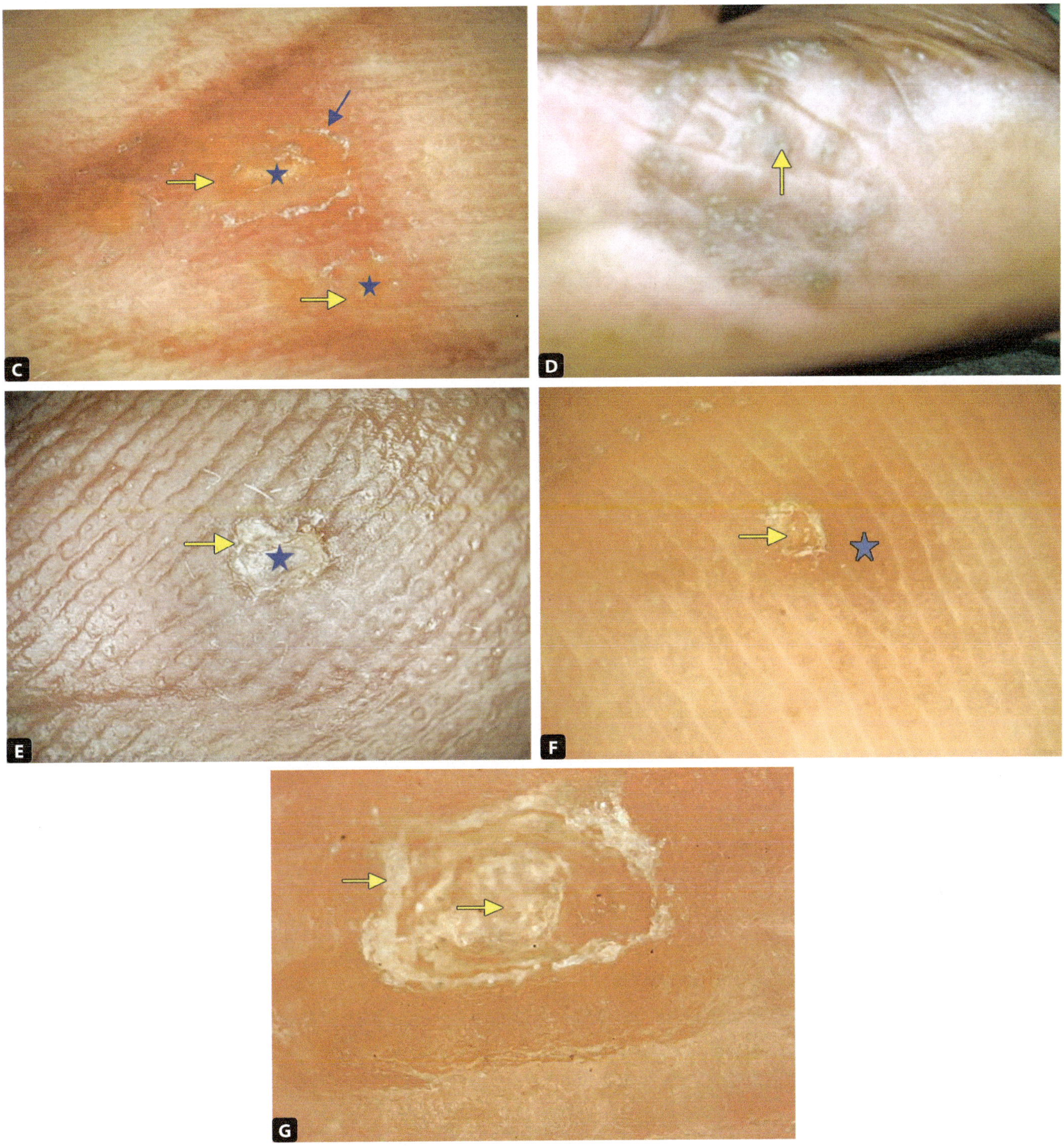

FIGS. 50A TO G: (A) Clinical image of palmoplantar lichen planus with keratotic papules and plaques (arrows) over palms; (B) Dermoscopy of palmar lichen planus shows linear yellowish areas (blue stars) having peripheral whitish halo (yellow arrows) against an erythematous background (polarized, Oitez dermoscope, 20×); (C) Dermoscopy of palmar lichen planus showing round yellowish-brown areas (blue stars) with peripheral whitish halo (yellow arrows) and a collarette of scale (blue arrow) (polarized, Oitez dermoscope, 20×); (D) Clinical image of plantar lichen planus showing yellowish hyperkeratotic papules and plaques; (E) Dermoscopy of plantar lichen planus showing keratin filled with crater (blue star) with scaly border (yellow arrow) (nonpolarized, Oitez dermoscope, 20×); (F) Dermoscopy of plantar lichen planus showing keratin-filled crater (yellow arrow) with a scaly border and perilesional hyperpigmentation (blue star) (polarized, Oitez dermoscope, 20×); (G) Dermoscopy of plantar lichen planus showing concentric layers of white structures and scales (arrows) (polarized, Oitez dermoscope, 200×).

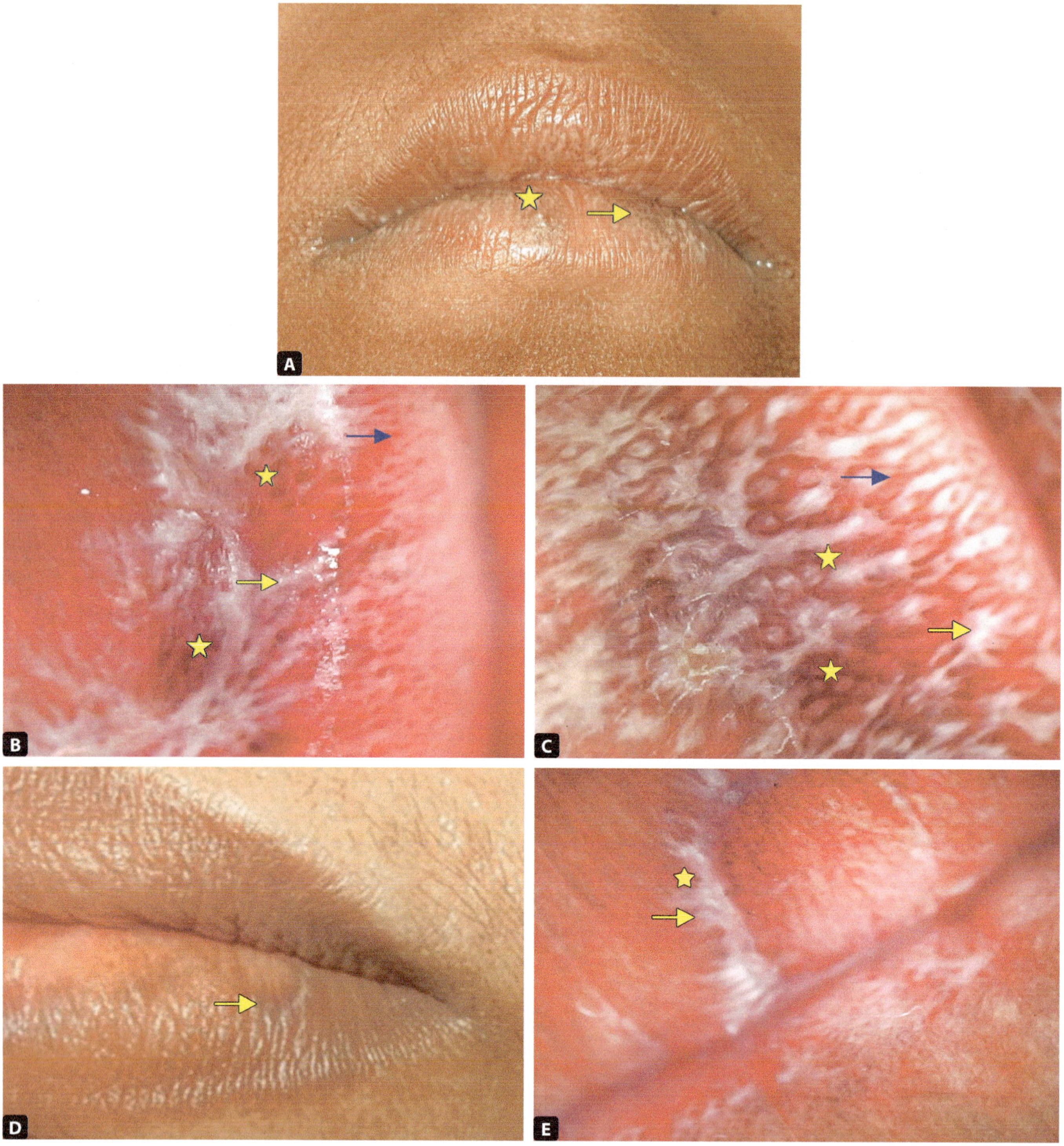

FIGS. 51A TO E: (A) Clinical image of mucosal lichen planus showing violaceous plaque (star) with lacy pattern (arrow) over the lip; (B) Dermoscopy of mucosal lichen planus of lip (from star in **Fig. 51A**) showing linear and reticulate Wickham's striae (yellow arrow) with linear vessels (blue arrow) and bluish-gray pigmentation (yellow stars) in the background (polarized, Oitez dermoscope, 20×); (C) Dermoscopy of mucosal lichen planus of lip showing linear and reticulate Wickham's striae (yellow arrow) with bluish gray pigmentation (yellow stars) and few linear vessels (blue arrow) in between the Wickham's striae (polarized, Oitez dermoscope, 200×); (D) Clinical image of mucosal lichen planus showing annular plaque on lip (arrow); (E) Dermoscopy of mucosal lichen planus of lip showing annular Wickham's striae with peripheral projections (arrow) and bluish-gray pigmentation (star) (polarized, Oitez dermoscope, 20×).

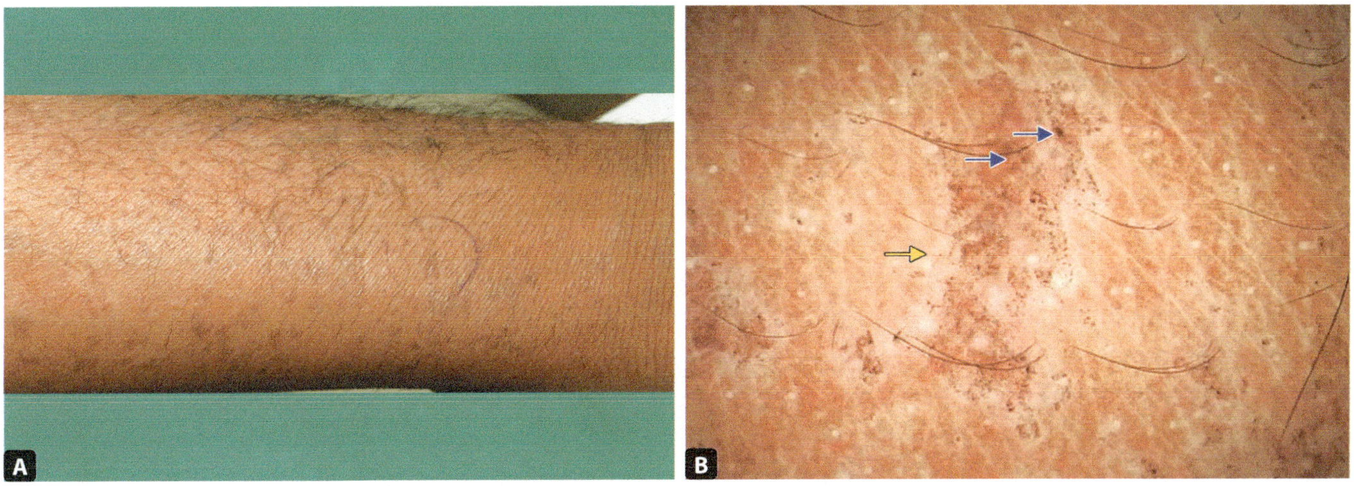

FIGS. 52A AND B: (A) Clinical image of atrophic lichen planus showing multiple violaceous lesions with slight depression in the center and perilesional hypopigmentation; (B) Dermoscopy of atrophic lichen planus showing multiple blue-gray dots and globules (blue arrows) and perilesional white halo (yellow arrow) with diffuse brownish area (polarized, Oitez dermoscope, 20×).

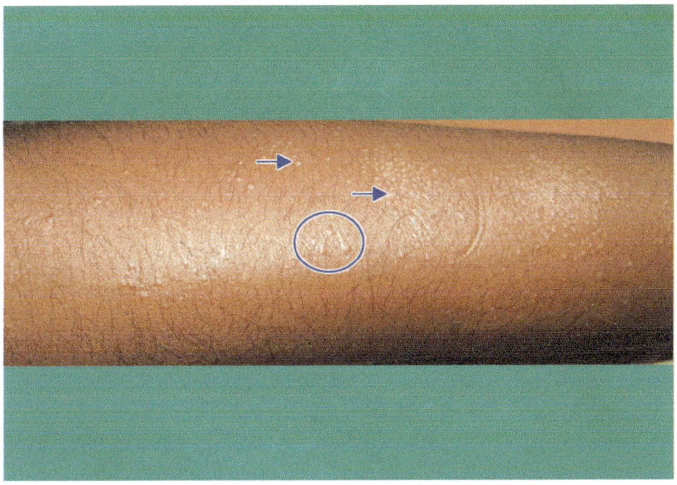

FIG. 53: Clinical image of lichen nitidus showing pinhead-sized skin-colored papules (arrows) and Koebner's phenomenon (circle).

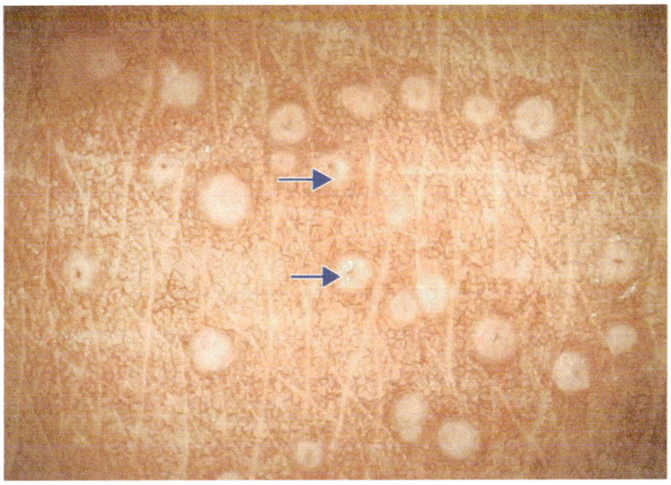

FIG. 54: Dermoscopy of lichen nitidus showing well-circumscribed whitish circular areas with a brown shadow (blue arrows) in the center of few areas (polarized, Oitez dermoscope, 20×).

LICHEN NITIDUS

Clinical Features

Lichen nitidus (LN) is idiopathic inflammatory skin disease clinically characterized by tiny pinpoint to pinhead sized skin colored or hypopigmented papules commonly involving forearms, hands, penis, abdomen, chest, and buttocks but can involve any part of the body (**Fig. 53**).[43]

Dermoscopic Features

Polarized dermoscopy shows well-circumscribed, circular white areas with or without an indistinct brown shadow in the center and linear vessels within the lesion (**Figs. 54** to **57**). Diffuse erythema and peripheral scaling may be seen.[37,44,45]

Nonpolarized dermoscopy reveals a shiny elevated surface with absence of dermatoglyphics over the lesions. Other findings seen in addition are central circular depression and radial ridges radiating from the edges of central depression giving a "sunburst appearance" (**Fig. 58**).[44] Palmoplantar type which clinically presents as hyperkeratotic pits, reveals linear scales in parallel discontinued by oval or elongated well-defined depressions surrounded by ring-shaped, silvery white scales (**Figs. 59** and **60**).[46]

Dermoscopic and histopathologic correlation is described in **Table 5**.

Key Points

- Polarized dermoscopy—white circular areas with or without an indistinct brown shadow in the center and linear vessels within the lesion
- Nonpolarized dermoscopy—ill-defined hypopigmented areas with absence of dermatoglyphics

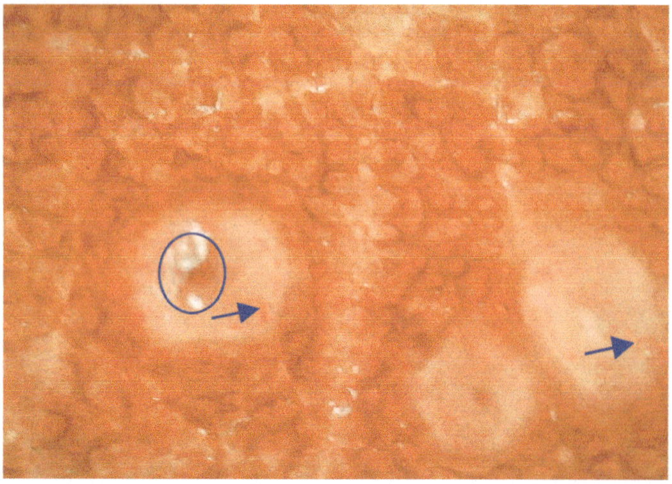

FIG. 55: Dermoscopy of lichen nitidus showing white circular areas with brown shadow (blue circle) in the center and linear vessels (blue arrows) within the lesion (polarized, Oitez dermoscope, 200×).

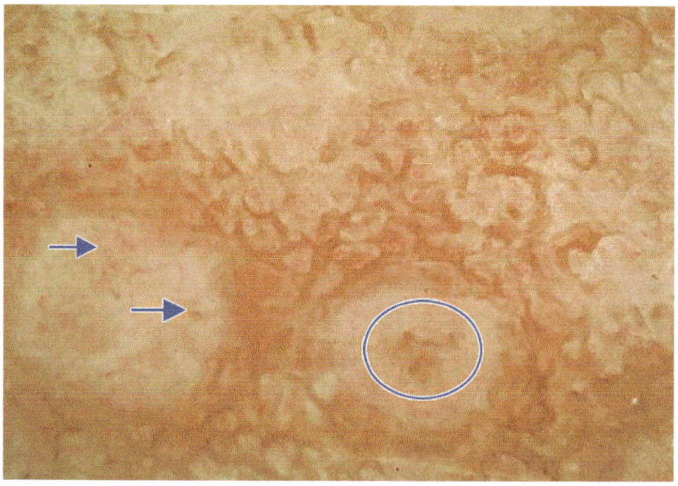

FIG. 56: Dermoscopy of lichen nitidus showing an indistinct brown shadow (blue circle) in the center and red areas (blue arrows) within the lesion (polarized, Oitez dermoscope, 200×).

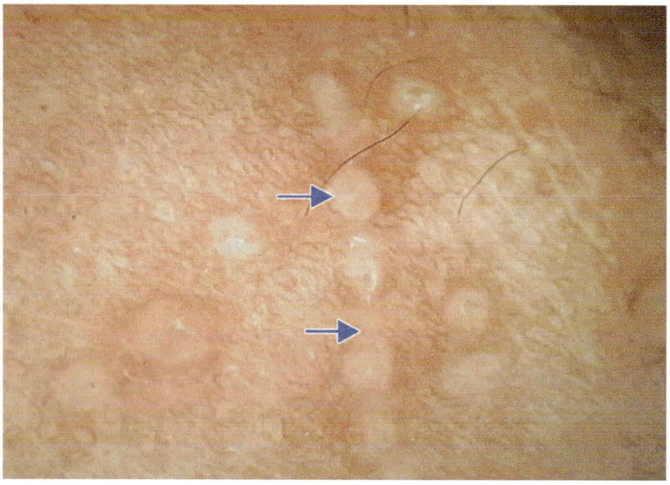

FIG. 57: Dermoscopy of lichen nitidus in Koebner's phenomenon showing white circular areas (arrows) arranged in linear fashion and brown shadow in the center of few lesions. White scale is noted at few places (polarized, Oitez dermoscope, 20×).

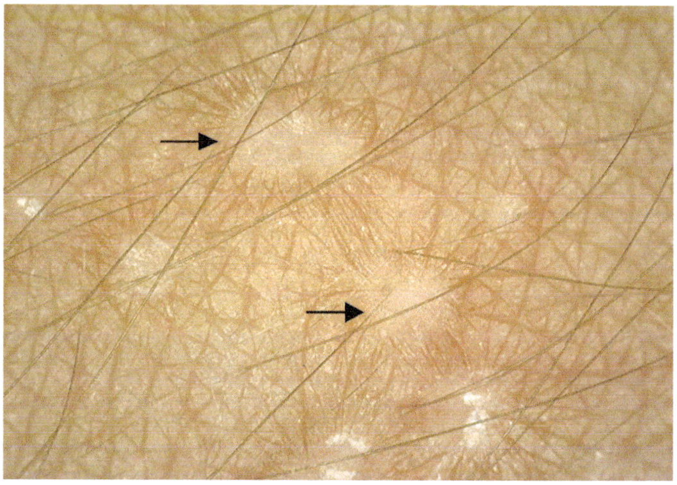

FIG. 58: Dermoscopy of lichen nitidus showing central circular depression with absence of dermatoglyphics and radial ridges giving a sunburst appearance (arrows) (nonpolarized, Oitez dermoscope, 20×).

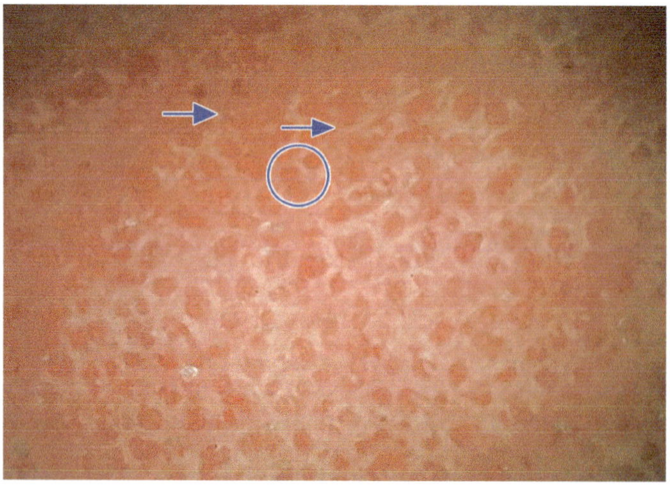

FIG. 59: Dermoscopy of lichen nitidus in palm showing circular red areas (circle) surrounded by thick white lines (arrows) (polarized, Oitez dermoscope, 20×).

TABLE 5: Dermoscopic findings with their histopathological correlation.[37,44]

Dermoscopy finding	Histopathological correlation
White circles	Epidermal acanthosis
Central brownish shadow	Inflammatory infiltrate in the dermal papillae[45]
Central depression	Dense, ball-like inflammatory infiltrate
Radial ridges	Elongated rete ridges at the edge of the lesion
Absence of dermatoglyphics	Flattening of the epidermis overlying the inflammatory infiltrate
Peripheral scaling	Parakeratosis

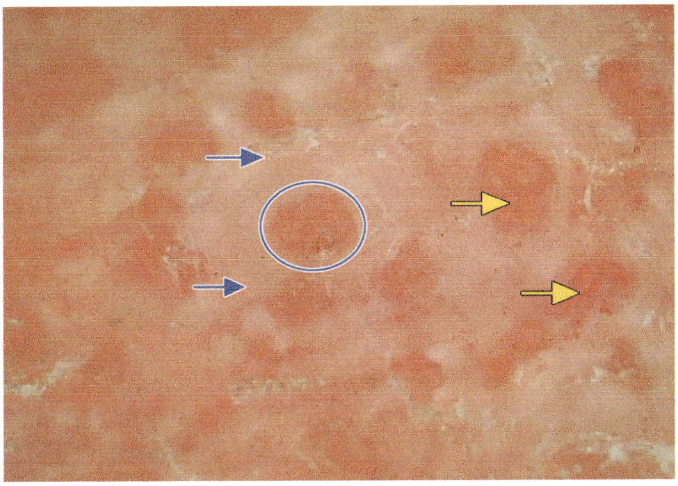

FIG. 60: Dermoscopy of lichen nitidus in palm showing circular red areas (blue circle) surrounded by thick white lines (blue arrows) which are surmounted by scales. Note the short linear vessels (yellow arrows) (polarized, Oitez dermoscope, 200×).

PERFORATING LICHEN NITIDUS

Clinical Features

Perforating lichen nitidus is a rare clinical entity affecting extremities of young individuals characterized by umbilicated grouped papules (**Fig. 61A**).

Dermoscopic Features

Light brown keratin plugs surrounded by whitish annular cloud-like areas (corresponding to acanthotic rete ridges) characterize the dermoscopy of perforating lichen nitidus (**Fig. 61B**).[47] A recent report demonstrated a further peripheral ring of brownish pigmentation.[48]

Key Points

- Concentric rings with central brown keratin plug
- Peripheral whitish annular cloud-like areas
- Central brown keratin plug (corresponding to perforating keratinous material) in perforating lichen nitidus is different from central brown shadows (corresponding to the inflammatory infiltrate) seen in LN among skin of color.

LICHEN STRIATUS

Clinical Features

Lichen striatus appears as an abrupt onset of pink to skin colored asymptomatic papules that soon heal with postinflammatory hypopigmentation, rarely hyperpigmentation. It usually affects children, restricted to one limb as a continuous or interrupted linear band (**Fig. 62A**).

Dermoscopic Features

Characteristic dermoscopy features of lichen striatus include gray granular pigmentation (corresponding to pigment laden macrophages) and white scar-like lines or areas (corresponding to postinflammatory hypopigmentation) (**Fig. 62B**).[49] Onychoscopy of affected nails in lichen striatus[50] shows linear longitudinal fissuring, ridging, and distal splitting involving only one part of the nail corresponding to the periungual lesion of lichen striatus, if present. Background nail bed erythema can also be seen (**Fig. 62C**).

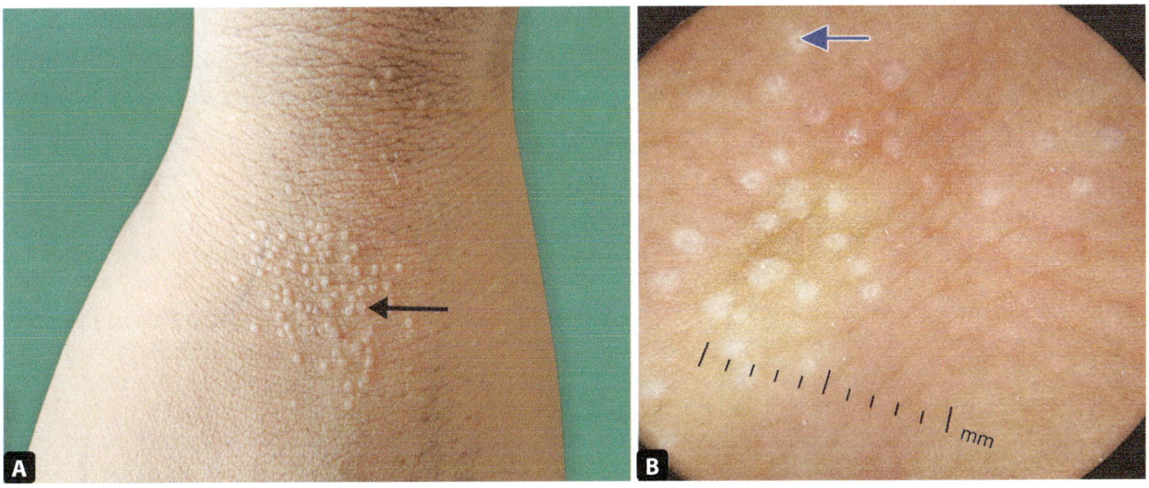

FIGS. 61A AND B: (A) Clinical image of perforating lichen nitidus shows umbilicated papules with occasional central keratotic plugs on the dorsal hand; (B) Dermoscopy revealing concentric rings of central brownish keratin plugs (blue arrow) and peripheral whitish annular cloud-like areas (polarized, DermLite DL4, 3Gen, 10×).

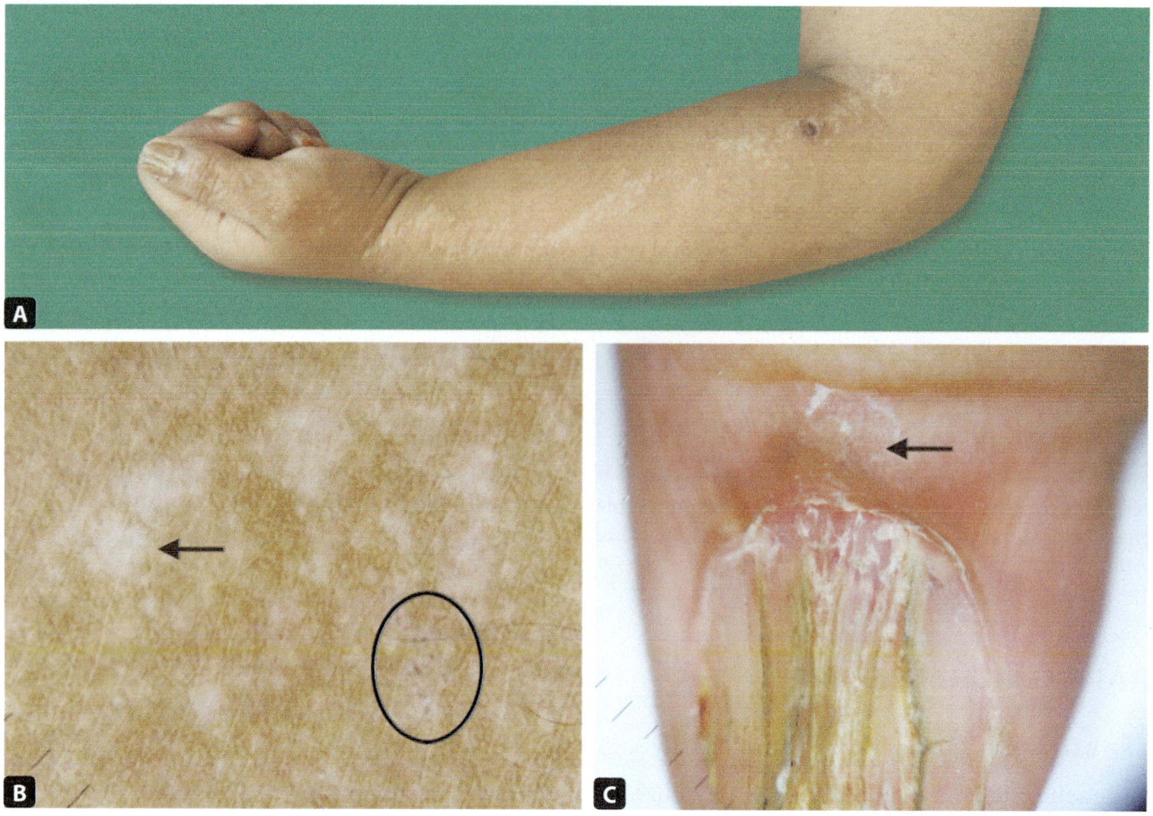

FIGS. 62A TO C: (A) Clinical image of lichen striatus showing linear hypopigmented grouped macules on the forearm extending to the thumb nail in a kid; (B) Dermoscopy of lichen striatus revealing gray granular pigmentation (circle) and white scar-like areas (arrow); (C) Onychoscopy of the involved thumb nail showing linear longitudinal fissuring, ridging, and distal splitting corresponding to the lichen striatus lesion affecting the proximal nail fold (arrow) (polarized, DermLite DL4, 3Gen, 10x).

Key Points

- Cutaneous lesion—gray granular pigmentation and white scar-like areas
- Nail lesion—isolated linear longitudinal fissuring, ridging, and distal splitting

LICHENOID DRUG RASH

Clinical Features

Lichenoid drug rash is characterized by the acute onset of symmetrical scaly plaques on extremities and sun-exposed areas, after intake of certain drugs. They often leave marked postinflammatory pigmentation (**Fig. 63A**). Usually, oral cavity and nails are not affected.

Dermoscopic Features

There is a scarcity in the literature on the dermoscopy of lichenoid drug rash. A report on lichenoid drug rash[51] has mentioned pigment dots on a erythematous background. Presence of scaling and absence of Wickham's striae help to distinguish it from LP (**Fig. 63B**). Subacute eczema can probably be differentiated by the absence of yellow serocrusts and patchy dotted vessels/hemorrhagic spots.

Key Points

- Pigment dots on an erythematous background with scaling
- Absence of Wickham's striae and absence of yellow serocrusts, patchy dotted vessels probably increase the specificity.

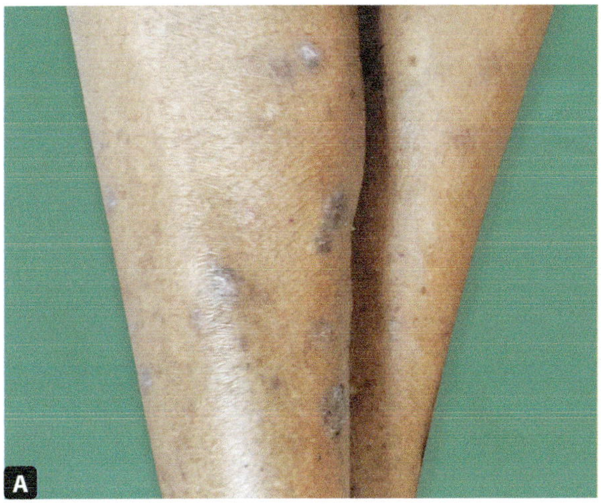

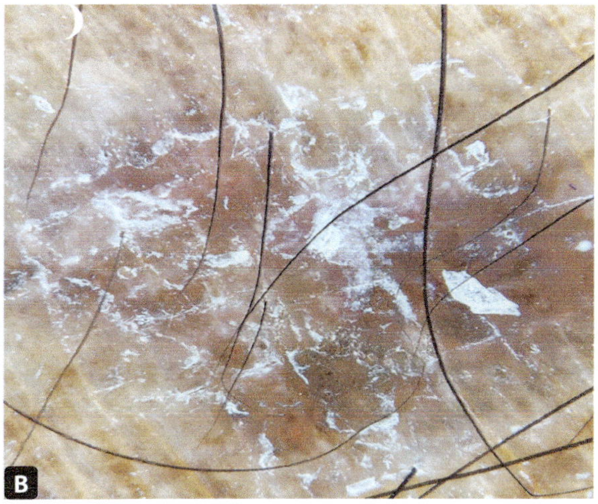

FIGS. 63A AND B: (A) Clinical image of lichenoid drug rash showing well-defined pigmented plaques on both legs after the intake of beta-blockers; (B) Dermoscopy of lichenoid drug rash revealing pigment dots on an erythematous background with white scales. Erythema component was not marked since the dermoscopy was done during the resolving stage of the rash (polarized, DermLite DL4, 3Gen, 10x).

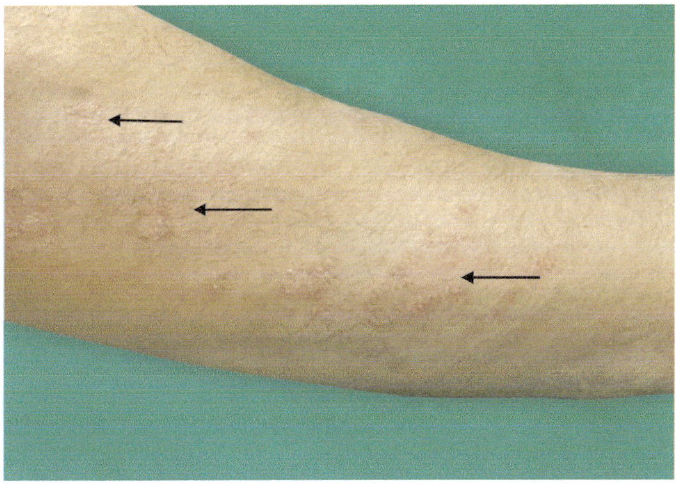

FIG. 64: Clinical image of chronic superficial scaly dermatitis showing multiple erythematous papules and plaques with fine scaling on the forearm (black arrows).

Courtesy: Dr BS Ankad, Bagalkot, Karnataka, India.

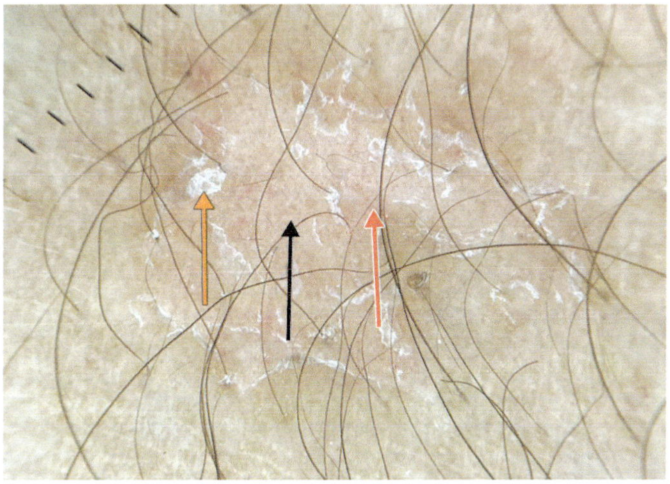

FIG. 65: Dermoscopic image of chronic superficial scaly dermatitis showing red background color (black arrow), nonuniform distribution of dotted blood vessels (red arrow), and fine white scaling (orange arrow) (polarized, Illuco IDS, 10×).

Courtesy: Dr BS Ankad, Bagalkot, Karnataka, India.

CHRONIC SUPERFICIAL SCALY DERMATITIS (SMALL PLAQUE PARAPSORIASIS)

Clinical Features

It is a chronic benign inflammatory condition of unknown etiology, seen more commonly in men. It manifests as round or oval, well-circumscribed erythematous papules or plaques featuring fine scaling scattered over the trunk and extremities, usually < 5 cm in diameter. Symptoms are generally minimal; few patients can have mild itching (**Fig. 64**).[43]

Dermoscopic Features

It includes mainly fine white scaling localized to the skin creases. The background color may range from red to yellow/brown. Dotted blood vessels in a nonuniform pattern may be seen (**Fig. 65**). Scales seen are due to patchy parakeratosis. The red and yellow/brown background color correspond to mild dermal inflammation/vasodilatation and hemosiderin deposits in the dermis.[52]

Key Points

- Fine white scaling localized to the skin creases with a nonuniform pattern of dotted blood vessels is diagnostic of chronic superficial scaly dermatitis.

CONCLUSION

Dermoscopy in papulosquamous diseases is well established in few conditions where it demonstrates specific patterns and in some of the diseases it gives definitive features and in others it is still evolving. One should note that background color, vascular structures, scales, pigmentation, and follicular changes are considered as the parameters in analysis of dermoscopic patterns in papulosquamous lesion.

ACKNOWLEDGMENT

Dr Harshada Mithari, Ex Assistant Professor, Department of Dermatology, Seth GS Medical College and KEM Hospital, Mumbai, Maharashtra, India.

REFERENCES

1. Lallas A, Kyrgidis A, Tzellos TG, Apalla Z, Karakyriou E, Karatolias A, et al. Accuracy of dermoscopic criteria for the diagnosis of psoriasis, dermatitis, lichen planus and pityriasis rosea. Br J Dermatol. 2012;166(6):1198-205.
2. Lallas A, Apalla Z, Argenziano G, Sotiriou E, Di Lernia V, Moscarella E, et al. Dermoscopic pattern of psoriatic lesions on specific body sites. Dermatology. 2014;228(3):250-4.
3. Ankad BS, Beergouder SL. Dermoscopy of inflammatory conditions: the journey so far. EMJ Dermatol. 2017;5:98-105.
4. Vázquez-López F, Manjón-Haces JA, Maldonado-Seral C, Raya-Aguado C, Pérez-Oliva N, Marghoob AA. Dermoscopic features of plaque psoriasis and lichen planus: new observations. Dermatology. 2003;207(2):151-6.
5. Penmetcha Lakshmi C, Praneet A, Madhavi K. A cross-sectional analysis of dermoscopic patterns distinguishing between psoriasis and lichen planus: a study of 80 patients. J Evol Med Dent Sci. 2015;4(105):17017-22.
6. Errichetti E, Stinco G. Dermoscopy in differential diagnosis of palmar psoriasis and chronic hand eczema. J Dermatol. 2016;43(4):423-5.
7. Errichetti E, Lacarrubba F, Micali G, Piccirillo A, Stinco G. Differentiation of pityriasis lichenoides chronica from guttate psoriasis by dermoscopy. Clin Exp Dermatol. 2015;40(7):804-6.
8. Golińska J, Sar-Pomian M, Rudnicka L. Dermoscopic features of psoriasis of the skin, scalp and nails—a systematic review. J Eur Acad Dermatol Venereol. 2019;33(4):648-60.
9. Vázquez-López F, Marghoob AA. Dermoscopic assessment of long-term topical therapies with potent steroids in chronic psoriasis. J Am Acad Dermatol. 2004;51(5):811-3.
10. Lacarrubba F, Pellacani G, Gurgone S, Verzì AE, Micali G. Advances in non-invasive techniques as aids to the diagnosis and monitoring of therapeutic response in plaque psoriasis: a review. Int J Dermatol. 2015;54(6):626-34.
11. Kim GW, Jung HJ, Ko HC, Kim MB, Lee WJ, Lee SJ, et al. Dermoscopy can be useful in differentiating scalp psoriasis from seborrhoeic dermatitis. Br J Dermatol. 2011;164(3):652-6.
12. Khopkar U, Yadav T. Dermoscopy to detect signs of subclinical nail involvement in chronic plaque psoriasis: a study of 68 patients. Indian J Dermatol. 2015;60(3):272.
13. Polat A, Kapıcıoğlu Y. Dermoscopic findings of psoriatic nail and their relationship with disease severity. Turkderm. 2017;51(4):119-23.
14. Errichetti E. Dermoscopy of inflammatory dermatoses (inflammoscopy): an up-to-date overview. Dermatol Pract Concept. 2019;9(3):169-80.
15. Elmas ÖF, Kilitçi A, Acar EM. Dermoscopic profile of pityriasis rosea. Dermatol Sin. 2019;37(4):199-204.
16. Nwako-Mohamadi M, Masenga J, Mavura D, Jahanpour O, Mbwilo E, Blum A. Dermoscopic features of psoriasis, lichen planus, and pityriasis rosea in patients with skin type IV and darker attending the Regional Dermatology Training Centre in Northern Tanzania. Dermatol Pract Concept. 2019;9(1):44-51.
17. Bowers S, Warshaw EM. Pityriasis lichenoides and its subtypes. J Am Acad Dermatol. 2006;55(4):557-72.
18. Ankad BS, Beergouder SL. Pityriasis lichenoides et varioliformis acuta in skin of color: new observations by dermoscopy. Dermatol Pract Concept. 2017;7(1):27-34.
19. Lacarrubba F, Micali G. Dermoscopy of pityriasis lichenoides et varioliformis acuta. Arch Dermatol. 2010;146(11):1322.
20. Clarey DD, Lauer SR, Trowbridge RM. Clinical, dermatoscopic, and histological findings in a diagnosis of pityriasis lichenoides. Cureus. 2020;12(6):e8725.
21. Sonthalia S, Varma S, Khopkar U. Dermoscopy of pityriasis lichenoides chronica in an Indian girl. Indian Dermatol Online J. 2020;11:477-8.
22. Valia R. Etiopathogenesis of seborrheic dermatitis. Indian J Dermatol Venereol Leprol. 2006;72(4):253-5.
23. Errichetti E, Stinco G. Dermoscopy in general dermatology: a practical overview. Dermatol Ther (Heidelb). 2016;6(4):471-507.
24. Lallas A, Argenziano G, Apalla Z, Gourhant JY, Zaballos P, Di Lernia V, et al. Dermoscopic patterns of common facial inflammatory skin diseases. J Eur Acad Dermatol Venereol. 2014;28(5):609-4.
25. Friedman P, Cohen Sabban E, Cabo H. Usefulness of dermoscopy in the diagnosis and monitoring treatment of demodicidosis. Dermatol Pract Concept. 2017;7:35-8.
26. Save S, Malakar S, Mehta P. Recognition of patterns. In: Malakar S (Ed). Dermoscopy: Text and Atlas. New Delhi: Jaypee Brothers Medical Publishers (P) Ltd; 2019. pp. 11-36.
27. Abdel-Azim NE, Ismail SA, Fathy E. Differentiation of pityriasis rubra pilaris from plaque psoriasis by dermoscopy. Arch Dermatol Res. 2017;309(4):311-4.
28. Jha AK, Lallas A, Sonthalia S, Jhakar D, Udayan UK, Chaudhary RK. Differentiation of pityriasis rubra pilaris from plaque psoriasis by dermoscopy. Dermatol Pract Concept. 2018;8(4):299-302.
29. Lewkowicz D, Gottlieb AB. Pediatric psoriasis and psoriatic arthritis. Dermatol Ther. 2004;17(5):364-75.
30. Navarini AA, Feldmeyer L, Töndury B, Fritsche P, Kamarashev J, French LE, et al. The yellow clod sign. Arch Dermatol. 2011;147(11):1350.
31. Güngör Ş, Topal IO, Göncü EK. Dermoscopic patterns in active and regressive lichen planus and lichen planus variants: a morphological study. Dermatol Pract Concept. 2015;5(2):45-53.
32. Tan C, Min ZS, Xue Y, Zhu WY. Spectrum of dermoscopic patterns in lichen planus: a case series from China. J Cutan Med Surg. 2014;18(1):28-32.
33. Friedman P, Cohen Sabban E, Marcucci C, Peralta R, Cabo H. Dermoscopic findings in different clinical variants of lichen planus. Is dermoscopy useful? Dermatol Pract Concept. 2015;5(4):51-5.
34. Vázquez-López F, Alvarez-Cuesta C, Hidalgo-García Y, Pérez-Oliva N. The handheld dermatoscope improves the recognition of Wickham striae and capillaries in lichen planus lesions. Arch Dermatol. 2001;137(10):1376.
35. Vázquez-López F, Maldonado-Seral C, López-Escobar M, Pérez-Oliva N. Dermoscopy of pigmented lichen planus lesions. Clin Exp Dermatol. 2003;28(5):554-5.
36. Vázquez-López F, Pineda FV. Lichen planus. In: Micali G, Lacarrubba F (Eds). Dermatoscopy in Clinical Practice, 2nd edition. Boca Raton: CRC Press; 2016; pp. 79-85.
37. Reddy PS, Sumathy T, Shyamprasad A, Shivaswamy K, Suparna M. Clinical, dermoscopic, and histopathological correlation of lichenoid dermatoses. Indian J Dermatopathol Diagn Dermatol. 2019;6(2):75-82.
38. Arshdeep, Batrani M, Kubba A, Kubba R. Lichen planopilaris beyond scalp: a case series with dermoscopy-histopathology correlation. Int J Dermatol. 2018;57(11):e127-31.
39. Mahajan S. Dermoscopy of lichen planus and differential diagnosis. In: Khopkar US (Ed). Dermoscopy, Trichoscopy and Onychoscopy in Diseases of the Pigmented Skin: An Atlas and Short Text, 2nd edition. New Delhi: Jaypee Brothers Medical Publishers (P) Ltd; 2020. pp. 204-45.
40. Madke B, Gutte R, Doshi B, Khopkar U. Hyperkeratotic palmoplantar lichen planus in a child. Indian J Dermatol. 2013;58(5):405.

41. Mathur M, Acharya P, Karki A, Nisha KC, Shah J, Jha A. Isolated lichen planus of lip: diagnosis and treatment monitoring using dermoscopy. Clin Case Rep. 2019;7(1):146-8.
42. Sonthalia S, Varma S, Jha AK, Jakhar D, Kaliyadan F. Case report: dermoscopic features of oral lichen planus—the evolution of mucoscopy. F1000Res. 2018;7:284.
43. Ingram JR. Eczematous disorders. In: Griffiths C, Barker J, Bleiker T, Chalmers R, Creamer D (Eds). Rook's Textbook of Dermatology, 9th edition. Oxford: Wiley-Blackwell; 2016. pp. 41.21.
44. Jakhar D, Grover C, Kaur I, Sharma S. Dermatoscopic features of lichen nitidus. Pediatr Dermatol. 2018;35(6):866-7.
45. Malakar S, Save S, Mehta P. Brown shadow in lichen nitidus: a dermoscopic marker! Indian Dermatol Online J. 2018;9:479-80.
46. Qian G, Wang H, Wu J, Meng Z, Xiao C. Different dermoscopic patterns of palmoplantar and nonpalmoplantar lichen nitidus. J Am Acad Dermatol. 2015;73(3):e101-3.
47. Martinez-Mera C, Herrero-Moyano M, Capusan TM, Urquía Renke A, Sánchez-Pérez J. Dermoscopy of a perforating lichen nitidus. Australas J Dermatol. 2018;59(1):61-2.
48. LeWitt T, Quan VL, Yazdan P, Zhou XA. Perforating lichen nitidus. JAAD Case Rep. 2020;8:4-8.
49. Kim DW, Kwak HB, Yun SK, Kim HU, Park J. Dermoscopy of linear dermatosis along Blaschko's line in childhood: lichen striatus versus inflammatory linear verrucous epidermal nevus. J Dermatol. 2017;44(12):e355-6.
50. Iorizzo M, Rubin AI, Starace M. Nail lichen striatus: is dermoscopy useful for the diagnosis? Pediatr Dermatol. 2019;36(6):859-63.
51. Rajashekar TS, Shruthi MG, Kuppuswamy SK. Imatinib mesylate induced lichenoid drug eruption masquerading as small plaque parapsoriasis. Int J Res Dermatol. 2018;4(2):262-4.
52. Lallas A, Errichetti E. Papulosquamous disorders. In: Lallas A, Errichetti E, Ioannides D (Eds). Dermoscopy in General Dermatology. London: CRC Press; 2019. pp. 1-48.

6 CHAPTER

Granulomatous Disorders

Vinay Keshavamurthy, Balachandra S Ankad, Soumil Khare

INTRODUCTION

Dermoscopy is increasingly being used to diagnose granulomatous diseases. The dermoscopic features overlap in various granulomatous diseases; the salient features include a yellowish-orange structureless area representing dermal granulomas and vascular response in the form of focused or unfocused vessels. This chapter discusses the dermoscopic features of various granulomatous diseases, highlighting the subtle differences between various dermatoses.

NONINFECTIVE GRANULOMATOUS DISEASES

Sarcoidosis

Clinical Features

Sarcoidosis is a multisystem disease with skin involvement. Clinically, plaque, psoriasiform, hypopigmented, scar sarcoid, ulcerative, subcutaneous, and annular lesions are noted (**Figs. 1A** and **2A**).[1]

Dermoscopic Features

It demonstrates the typical yellowish-orange structureless areas (**Fig. 1B**).[2] In skin of color, brownish-yellow structureless areas are noted (**Fig. 2B**). Well-focused linear and branching telangiectasias, follicular plugs, and scaling are also observed.[3]

Key Points

- Brownish-yellow structureless areas with well-focused linear and branching telangiectasias are characteristically seen in sarcoidosis.

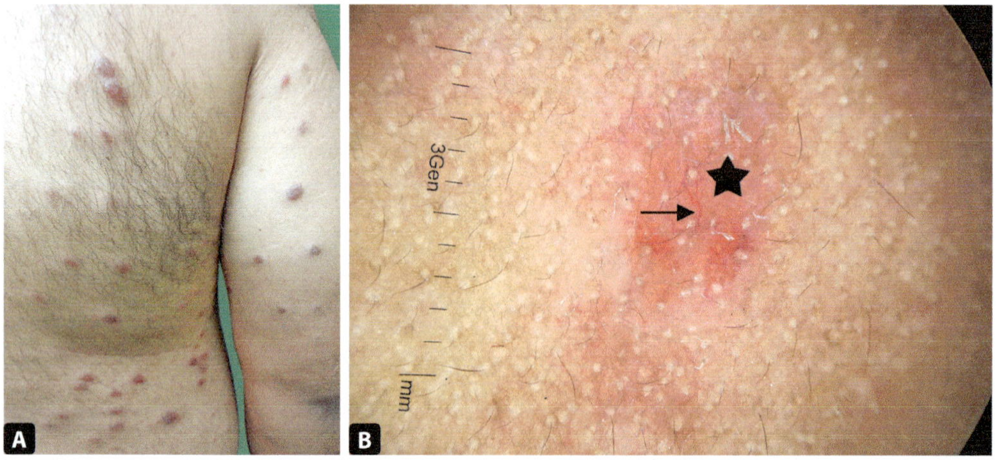

FIGS. 1A AND B: (A) Clinical image of nodular sarcoidosis showing multiple nodules over back; (B) Dermoscopy showing yellowish orange areas (star) and well-focused linear vessels (arrow) (polarized, DermLite DL4, 10×).

Granuloma Annulare

Clinical Features

Granuloma annulare is a common granulomatous dermatitis and manifests as erythematous, annular plaque. Disseminated, actinic, papular, perforating, and subcutaneous are the different variants of granuloma annulare (**Fig. 3A**).[4]

Dermoscopic Features

Dermoscopy reveals yellowish-orange areas with dotted, short linear or branching vessels on a pinkish background (**Fig. 3B**). Vessels are characteristically unfocused. In skin of color, pigmentary changes such as brown dots and globules are prominent instead of yellowish-orange structures (**Fig. 3C**). These pigment structures may be

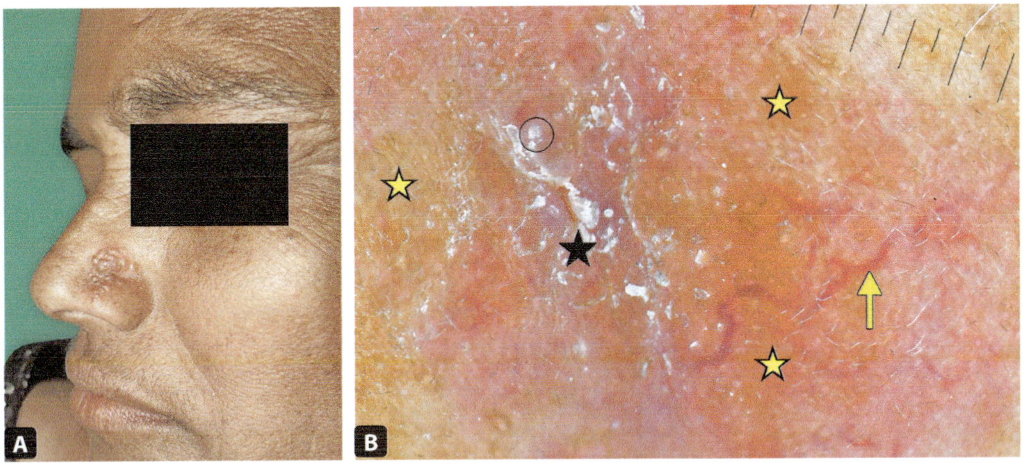

FIGS. 2A AND B: (A) Clinical image of papular sarcoidosis showing coalesced erythematous papules on the side of the nose; (B) Dermoscopy shows well-defined brownish-yellow areas (yellow stars) with well-focused telangiectasia (yellow arrow). Follicular plugging (black circle) and white scales (black star) are well appreciated (polarized, DermLite DL4, 10×).

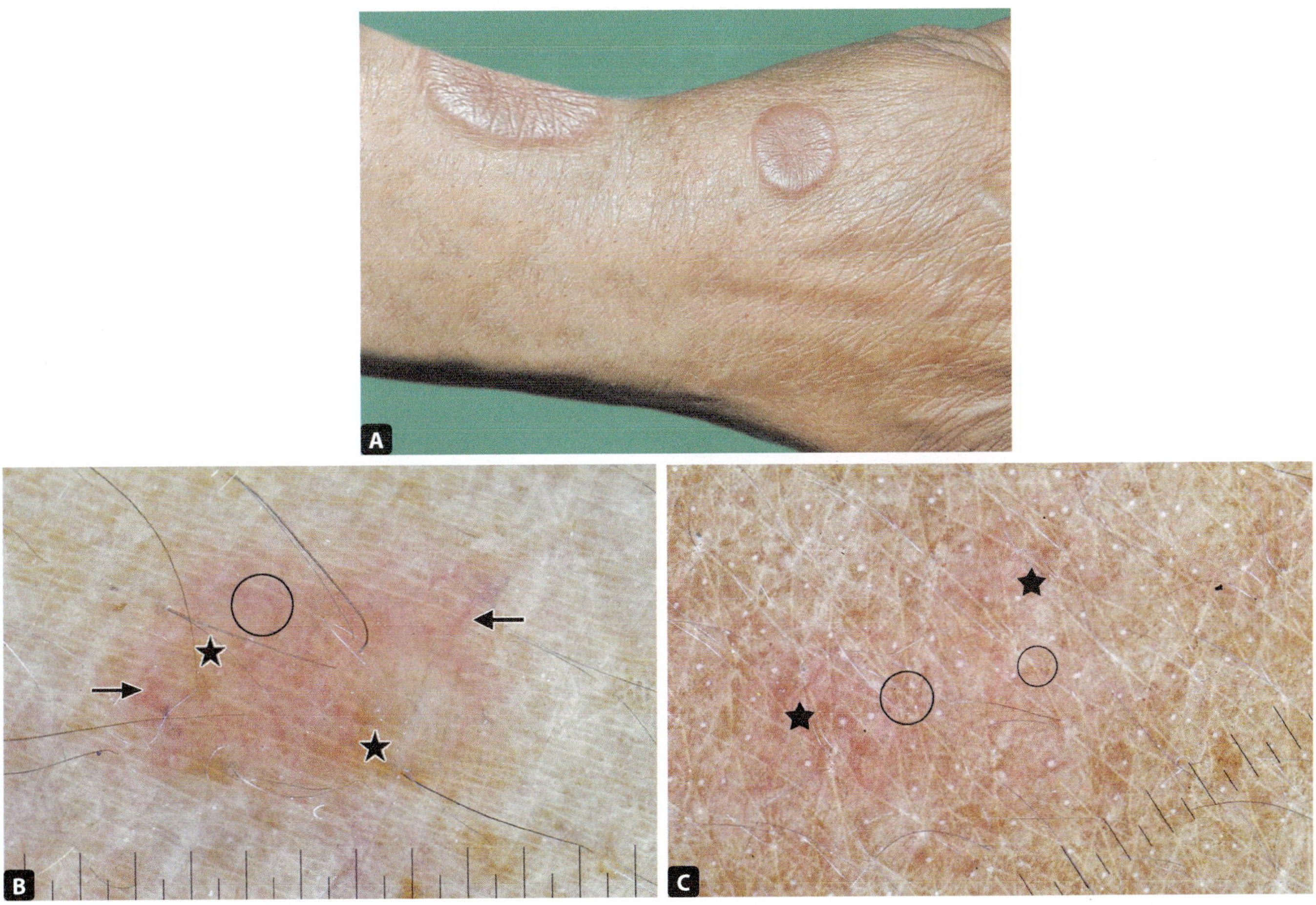

FIGS. 3A TO C: (A) Clinical image of classical granuloma annulare showing erythematous annular plaque on the dorsum of the hand; (B) Dermoscopy image shows brown areas (black stars) with short linear (black arrows) and dotted (black circle) vessels. Note that vessels are unfocused and pinkish background (polarized, DermLite DL4, 10×); (C) In skin of color, dermoscopy image shows brown dots (black circles) on a pinkish background (black stars) (polarized, DermLite DL4, 10×).

physiological rather than being a part of the disease process. In subcutaneous and perforating variants, white crystalline structures, pink and brown areas with scales are noted (**Fig. 4**).[2]

Key Points

- Yellowish orange areas on a pinkish background with dotted and short linear vessels in an unfocused pattern are distinctly seen in granuloma annulare.

Annular Elastolytic Giant Cell Granuloma

Clinical Features

Annular elastolytic giant cell granuloma (AEGCG) is a rare granulomatous condition affecting sun-exposed areas.[5] Skin colored to erythematous, annular, arciform, and polycyclic plaques of varying sizes and central atrophy are found on exposed areas (**Fig. 5A**).

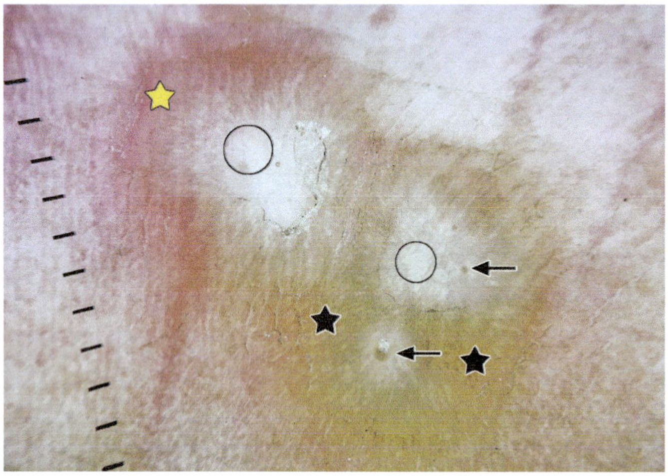

FIG. 4: Dermoscopy of granuloma annulare on the palm shows white crystalline structures (black circles) with brown areas (black stars). Note the pink areas in the periphery of the lesion (yellow star) and few brown globules with scale (black arrows) (polarized, DermLite DL4, 10×).

Dermoscopic Features

Dermoscopy in a reported case showed regular yellowish-orange structureless areas in the peripheral zone associated with whitish-gray scaling and homogeneous, reticular, well-focused vessels over a pale pinkish background were noted in the center.[6] Brownish-yellow or pale yellow structureless areas with branching telangiectasia and erythematous rim are noted in skin of color (**Fig. 5B**).

Key Points

- Yellowish-orange (brownish-yellow) structureless areas with whitish-gray scales and homogeneous, reticular, and well-focused vessels are the characteristics of AEGCG.

Necrobiosis Lipoidica Diabeticorum

Clinical Features

Necrobiosis lipoidica diabeticorum (NLD) is a necrobiotic granulomatous disorder associated with diabetes mellitus which presents as yellowish, atrophic plaques with prominent telangiectasias (**Fig. 6A**).[7] Ulceration can occur in up to one-third of cases.[7]

Dermoscopic Features

Necrobiosis lipoidica diabeticorum shows a diffuse yellowish structureless area representing areas of necrobiosis.[2,8] The vessel are characteristically well focused (**Fig. 6B**). Early and evolving lesions show dotted, comma-shaped and globular vessels, whereas well-established lesions show hairpin-like, branching, and arborizing vessels.[2,8]

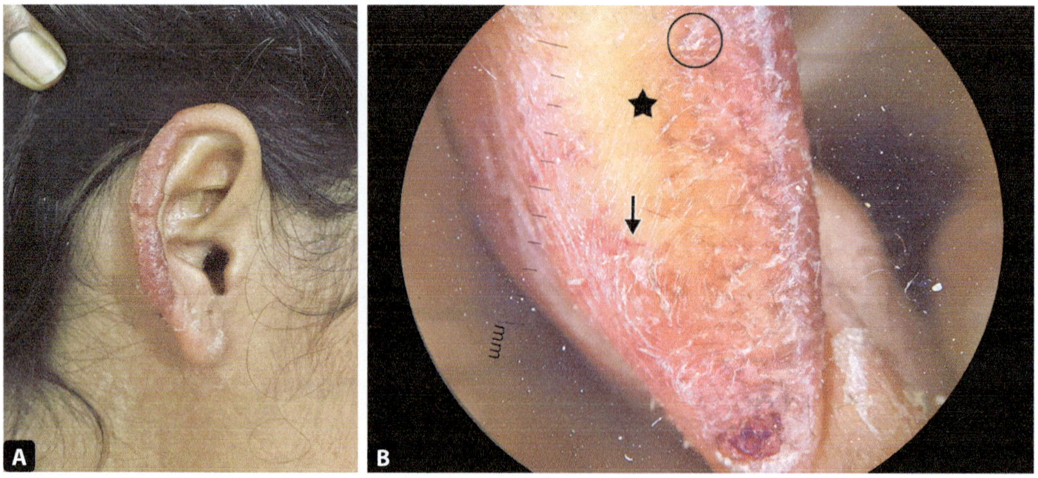

FIGS. 5A AND B: (A) Clinical image of annular elastolytic giant cell granuloma showing erythematous infiltrated nodular plaque on the ear lobule; (B) Dermoscopy image shows brownish-yellow areas (star), short linear vessels (black arrow), and white scales (black circle) (polarized, DermLite DL4, 10×).

Courtesy: Dr Abhijeet Kumar Jha, PMCH, Patna, Bihar, India.

Key Points

- Diffuse yellowish background and well-focused network-like arborizing and hairpin vessels are characteristic of NLD.

Granulomatous Rosacea

Clinical Features

It is an uncommon variant of rosacea and may lack the typical complaints of erythema and flushing.[9,10] Multiple yellowish-brown papules distributed periorally and over the malar area is the most common finding (**Fig. 7A**).

Dermoscopic Features

The dermoscopic features include yellowish-brown structureless areas on a background of erythema and polygonal vessels (vascular polygons) (**Fig. 7B**).[2]

Key Points

- Yellowish orange areas and vascular polygons are typical of granulomatous rosacea.

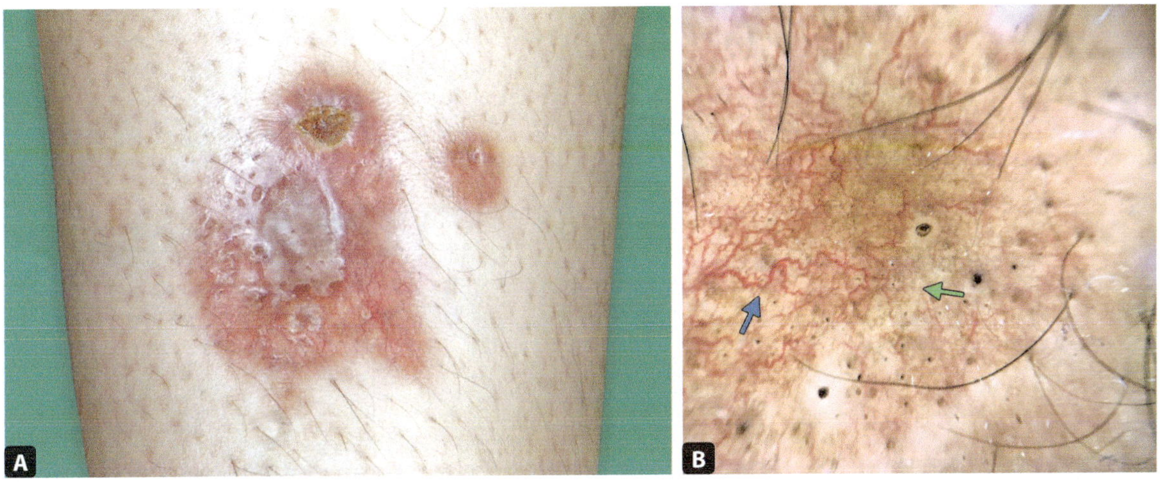

FIGS. 6A AND B: (A) Necrobiosis lipoidica diabeticorum in a patient of type 1 diabetes mellitus showing yellowish atrophic plaques with central ulceration and prominent peripheral telangiectasia over shins; (B) Dermoscopy image shows central yellowish plaque (green arrow) surrounded by well-defined serpentine telangiectatic vessels (blue arrow) (polarized, DermLite DL4, 10×).

Courtesy (Fig. B): Dr Abhijeet Kumar Jha, PMCH, Patna, Bihar, India.

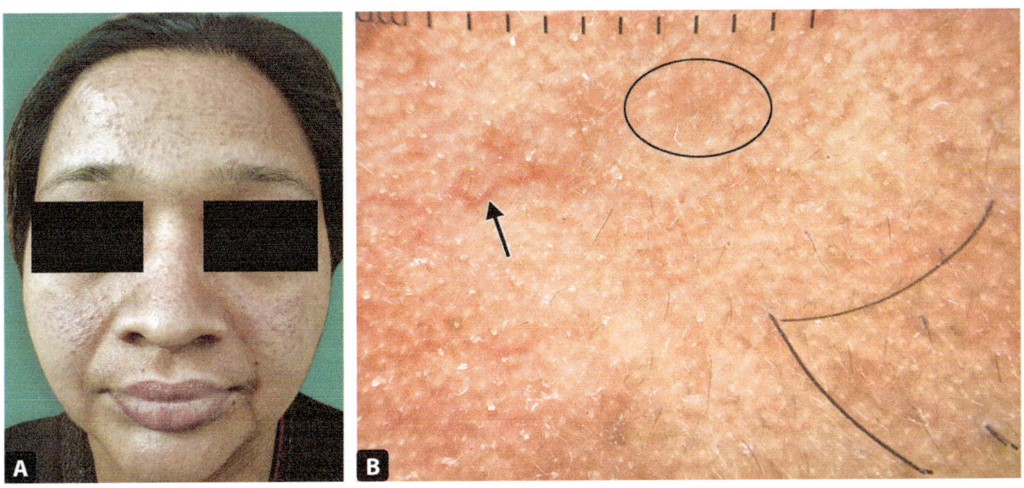

FIGS. 7A AND B: (A) Clinical image of granulomatous rosacea showing erythematous papules over forehead and malar area of the face; (B) Dermoscopic image showing brownish structureless areas (black circle) on a background of erythema and telangiectasia (black arrow) (polarized, DermLite DL4, 10×).

Xanthogranulomatous Diseases

Clinical Features

Xanthogranulomatous diseases may present as juvenile xanthogranuloma (**Fig. 8A**) or xanthoma disseminatum (**Fig. 9A**).

Dermoscopic Features

They exhibit a central orange-yellow structureless area surrounded by an erythematous rim exhibiting linear and branching vessels (setting sun appearance) (**Fig. 9B**).[11,12] Other nonspecific features include discrete pigment network (**Figs. 8B** and **C**), and fine, branched vessels (**Fig. 8D**). Whitish streaks indicating areas of fibrosis can be seen in long-standing lesions (**Fig. 9C**).[13]

Key Points

- "Setting sun" sign is the typical dermatoscopic feature of xanthogranulomatous disorders.
- Discreet pigment network can be appreciated in ethnic skin.

Lupus Miliaris Disseminatus Faciei

Clinical Features

Lupus miliaris disseminatus faciei (LMDF) presents as yellow-red to brown papules on the upper face, ears, and around the eyelids which heals with pock-like scars (**Fig. 10A**).

Dermoscopic Features

Typical dermoscopic findings are ill-defined, discrete, structureless, perifollicular yellow-orange areas (**Fig. 10B**) with keratotic follicular plugs. Other less common findings are central ulceration, linear and hairpin-like vessels, and pink background (**Fig. 10B**).[2,14,15]

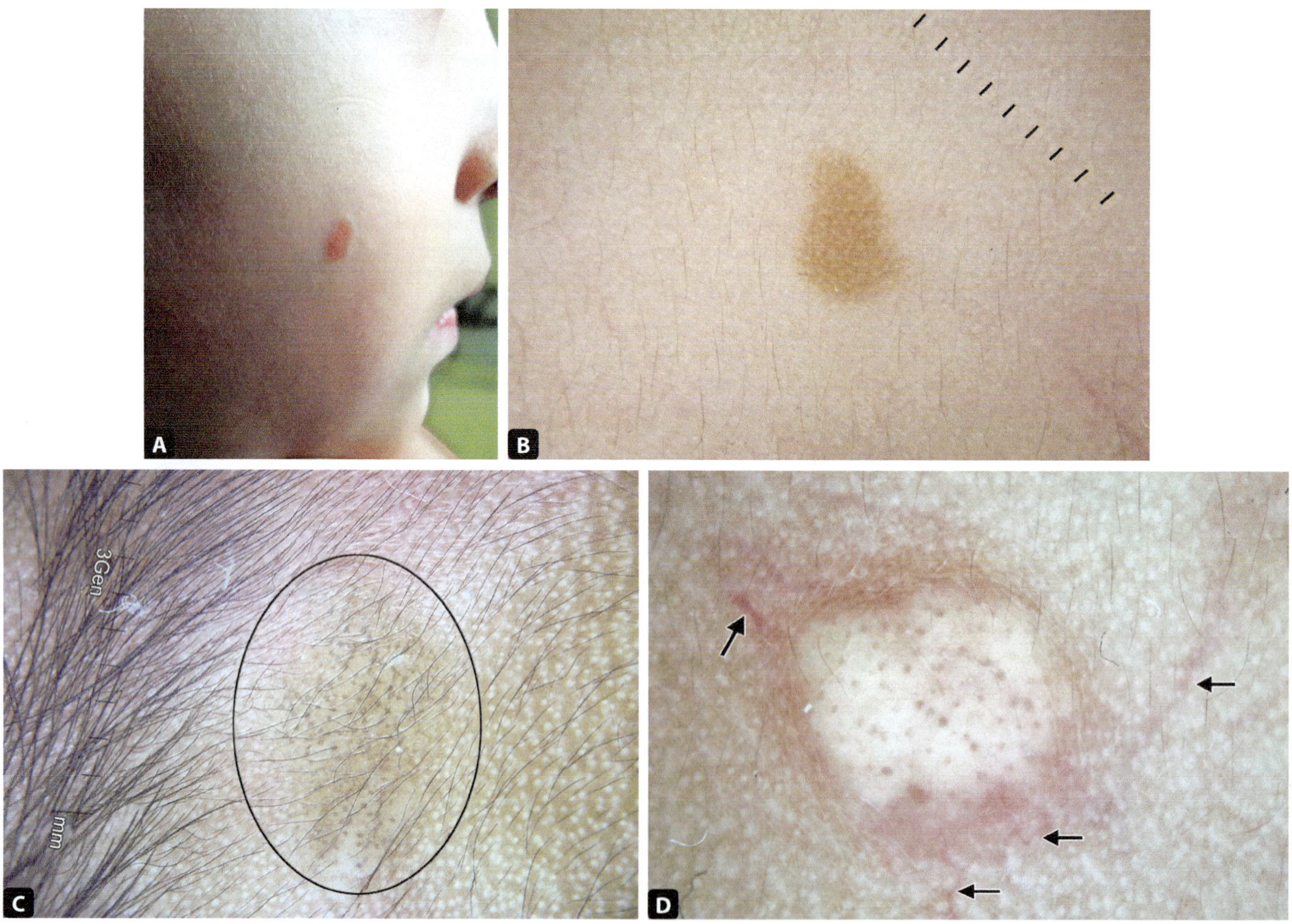

FIGS. 8A TO D: (A) Clinical image of juvenile xanthogranuloma over cheek showing a solitary yellow papule; (B) Dermoscopy image showing yellow globules and accentuated pseudonetwork (polarized, DermLite DL4, 10×); (C) Dermoscopy of juvenile xanthogranuloma in darker skin phototype showing yellowish globules and accentuated pigmentation of appendageal openings (black circle) (polarized, DermLite DL4, 10×); (D) Dermoscopy of another case of juvenile xanthogranuloma showing yellowish globules, prominent appendageal openings and fine branched vessels in the periphery (black arrows) (polarized, DermLite DL4, 10×).

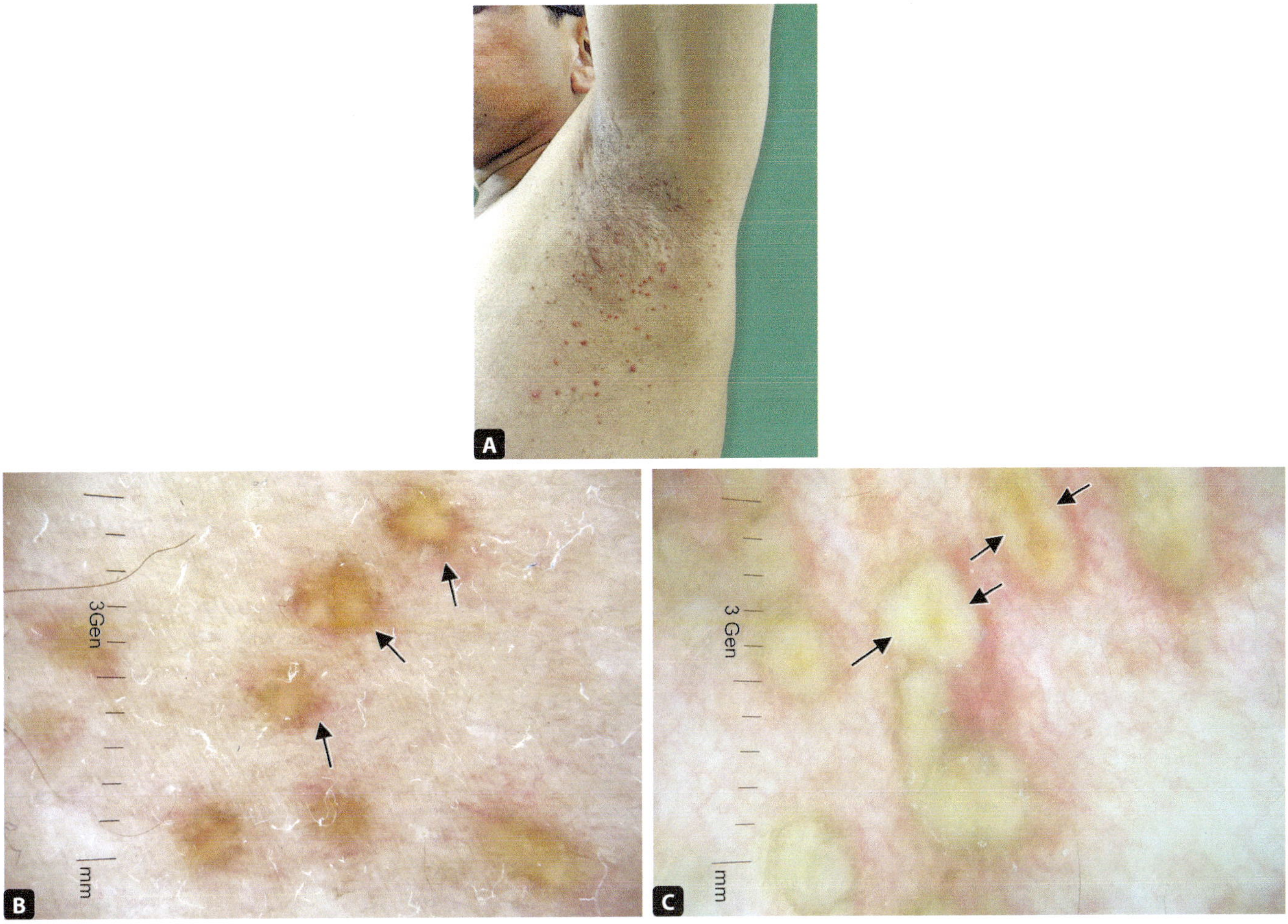

FIGS. 9A TO C: (A) Clinical image of xanthoma disseminatum showing discreet to coalescing yellow papules with flexural predominance; (B) Setting sun sign in a case of xanthoma disseminatum showing central yellowish globules surrounded by a rim of erythema and short fine vessels (black arrows) (polarized, DermLite DL4, 10×); (C) Dermoscopy of late stage of xanthoma disseminatum showing white fibrotic areas (black arrows) surrounded by linear telangiectatic vessels (polarized, DermLite DL4, 10×).

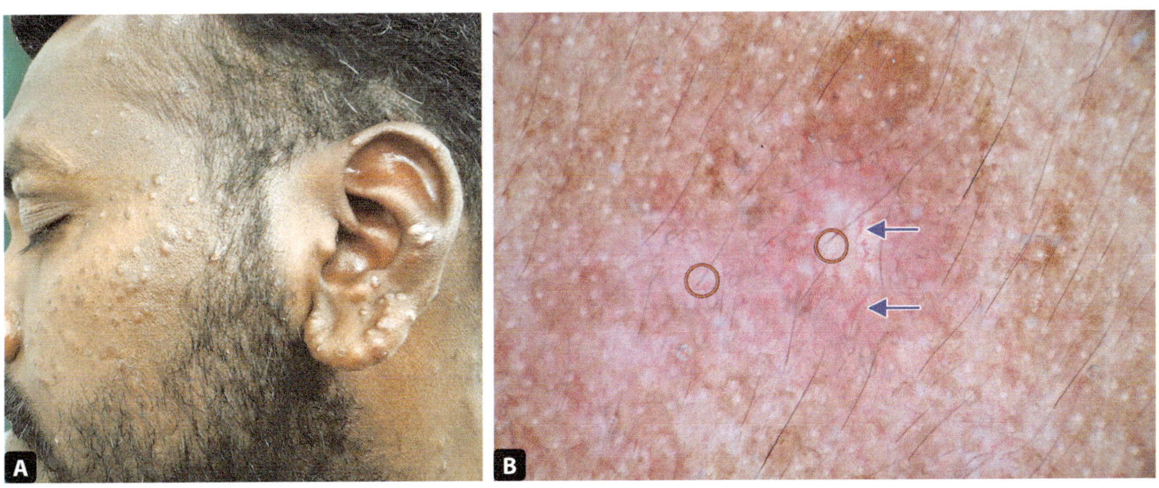

FIGS. 10A AND B: (A) Clinical image of lupus miliaris disseminatus faciei showing brown papules over cheek, periorbital area, and external helix; (B) Dermoscopic image showing perifollicular yellow-orange areas (red circle) with liner vessels (blue arrows) over pink background (polarized, DermLite DL4, 10×).

Litaiem et al. described dermoscopy in various stages of LMDF.[16]

Key Points

- Ill-defined perifollicular yellow-orange areas with keratotic follicular plugs.
- Early lesions show sparse keratotic plugs.
- Fully developed lesions show numerous keratotic plugs, and late lesions show white fibrotic areas.

Tattoo Granuloma

Clinical Features

Tattoos have numerous potential complications, including granulomatous tissue reaction. It may present clinically as pruritus, focal edema, papules, nodules, and plaques (**Fig. 11A**).

Dermoscopic Features

Focal orange structureless areas with crystalline structures, yellow scales, and greenish areas, which are accentuation of the tattoo ink (**Fig. 11B**).[17]

Key Points

- Yellow-orange areas with crystalline structures
- Accentuation of the color of tattoo ink

INFECTIVE GRANULOMATOUS DISEASES

Leprosy

Clinical Features

The disease occurs in a spectrum from tuberculoid leprosy to lepromatous leprosy (**Figs. 12A, 13A,** and **14A**), with some special forms like histoid leprosy. Lepra reactions occur during, before, or after multidrug therapy (**Figs. 13A** and **14A**).[18]

Dermoscopic Features

As other granulomatous dermatoses, leprosy also shows yellowish-orange areas and linear vessels (**Fig. 12B**).[19] Brownish-yellow areas are noted in skin of color. Distinctively, there is paucity of appendages in the lesional skin in the form of reduced number of white dots of eccrine and follicular openings as compared to

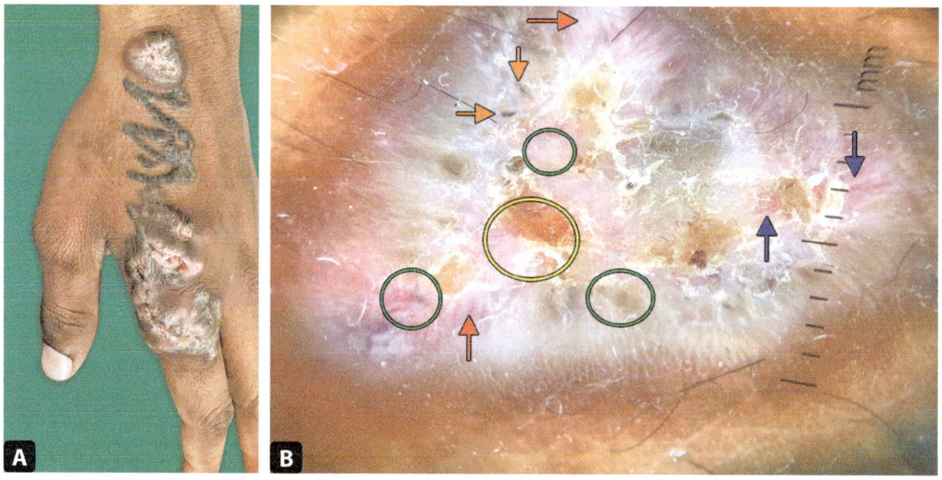

FIGS. 11A AND B: (A) Clinical image of granulomatous tattoo reaction showing infiltrated ulcerative plaques overlaying the tattoo site; (B) Dermoscopic image showing multiple yellow-orange structureless areas (green circles), whitish streaks (red arrows), yellow scales (yellow circle), out of focus vessels (blue arrows) and greenish blue dots and clods (orange arrow) present in and at the margin of the lesion (polarized, DermLite DL4, 10×).

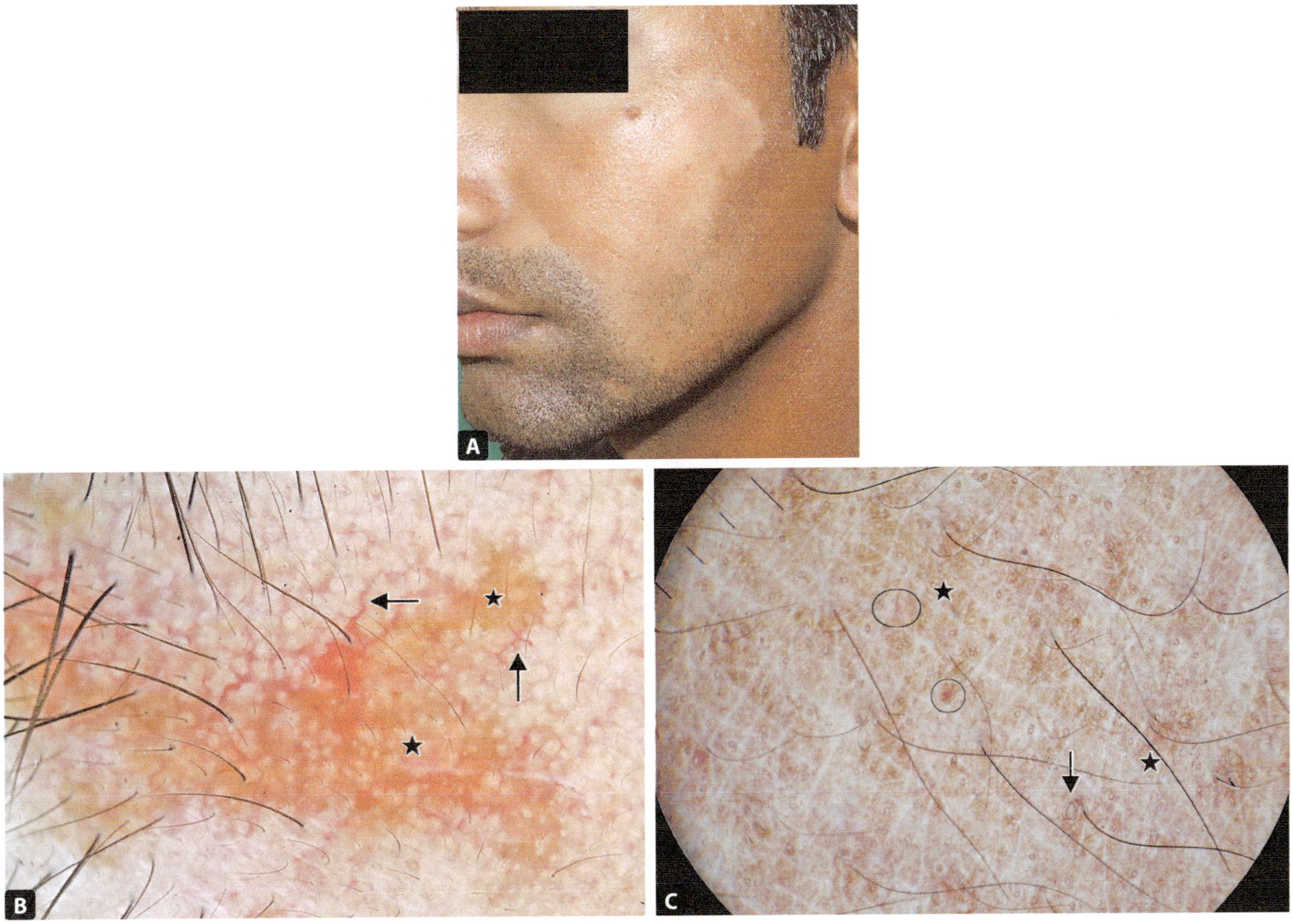

FIGS. 12A TO C: (A) Clinical image of tuberculoid leprosy shows well-defined hypopigmented plaque on the face; (B) Dermoscopy of tuberculoid leprosy shows brownish-yellow areas (black stars) and arborizing vessels (black arrows) (polarized, DermLite DL4, 10×); (C) Dermoscopy of tuberculoid leprosy shows distorted pigment network (black stars) with dotted and short linear vessels (black circles). Note the pigtail hairs (black arrow). Decreased follicular and eccrine openings are well appreciated (polarized, DermLite DL4, 10×).

uninvolved skin (**Figs. 12C** and **13B**).[19-21] Other features include broken pigment network and hair changes such as pigtail hairs (**Fig. 12C**). Hypopigmented lesions of lepromatous spectrum show white chrysalis-like structures and white shiny lines (**Fig. 14B**).[19] Type 1 reactions are characterized by lesional erythema, arborizing vessels, occurrence of scaling, and follicular plugs (**Fig. 13C**).[19,22] In type 2 reactions, milky-red areas and dotted vessels are seen (**Fig. 14C**). Lepromatous nodules reveal yellow globular structures and arborizing crown vessels on a pinkish background. Brown pigment is conspicuously present at the periphery of the nodule (**Fig. 15A**), whereas histoid leprosy shows yellowish globular areas and crown vessels (**Fig. 15B**).[19,23]

Key Points

- Yellowish-orange (brownish-yellow) areas, linear and branching telangiectatic vessels, and appendageal loss are characteristic of tuberculoid lesions.
- White shiny structures are typically observed in borderline lepromatous, histoid, and lepromatous lesions.
- Crown vessels are classically seen in nodular lesions of lepromatous leprosy and histoid leprosy.
- Reactional lesions demonstrate milky-red areas, pronounced follicular changes, scales, and predominant vascular elements.

Lupus Vulgaris

Clinical Features

Lupus vulgaris (LV) is the most common form of cutaneous tuberculosis, manifesting at unusual sites with atypical features. Clinically, an infiltrated plaque, which tends to progress from one end and heals from the other, is seen (**Figs. 16A, 17A,** and **18A**).

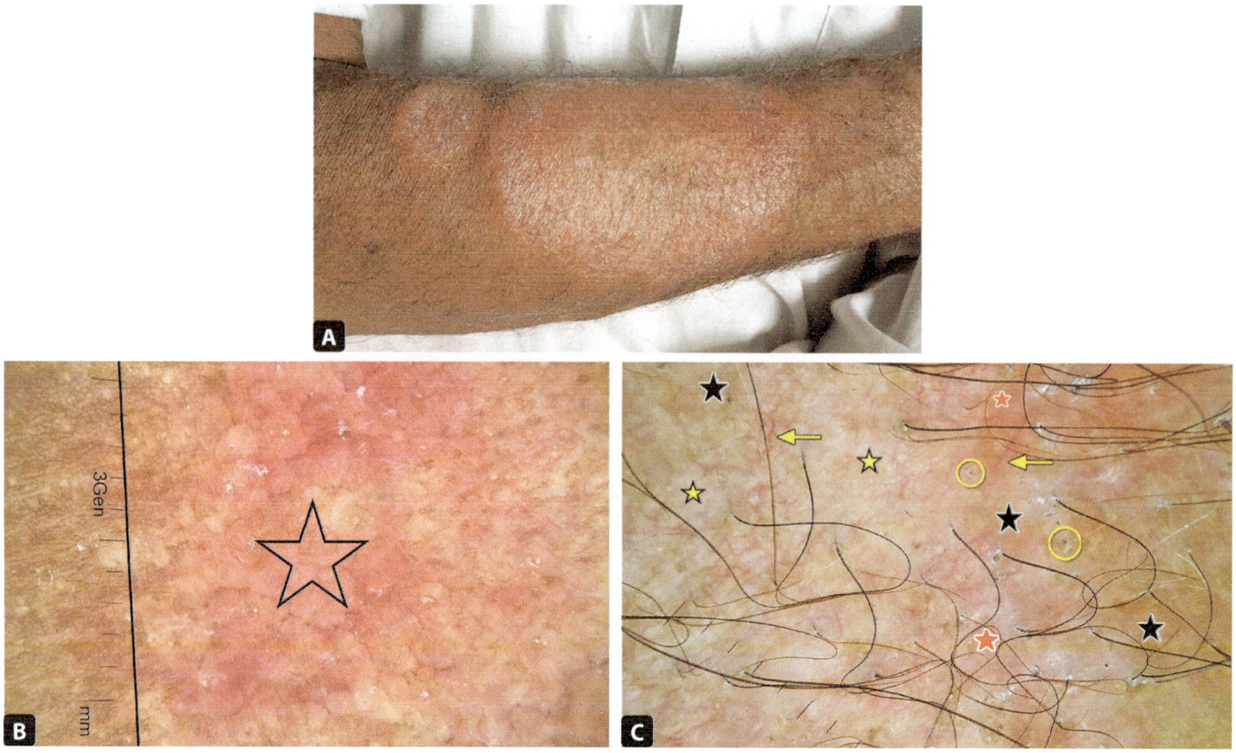

FIGS. 13A TO C: (A) Clinical image of borderline tuberculoid leprosy with type 1 reaction showing erythematous plaque and satellite lesion with desquamation; (B) Dermoscopy of borderline tuberculoid leprosy showing distorted pigment network and paucity of appendageal structures compared to normal skin on the left. Yellowish-orange areas representing dermal granulomas are well appreciated (star) (polarized, DermLite DL4, 10×); (C) Dermoscopy of borderline tuberculoid leprosy with type 1 reaction shows arborizing vessels (yellow arrows), brownish-yellow globules (black stars) with milky-red (red stars) and white (yellow stars) areas. Note the broken hairs (yellow circles) and white scales on a pinkish-white background (polarized, DermLite DL4, 10×).

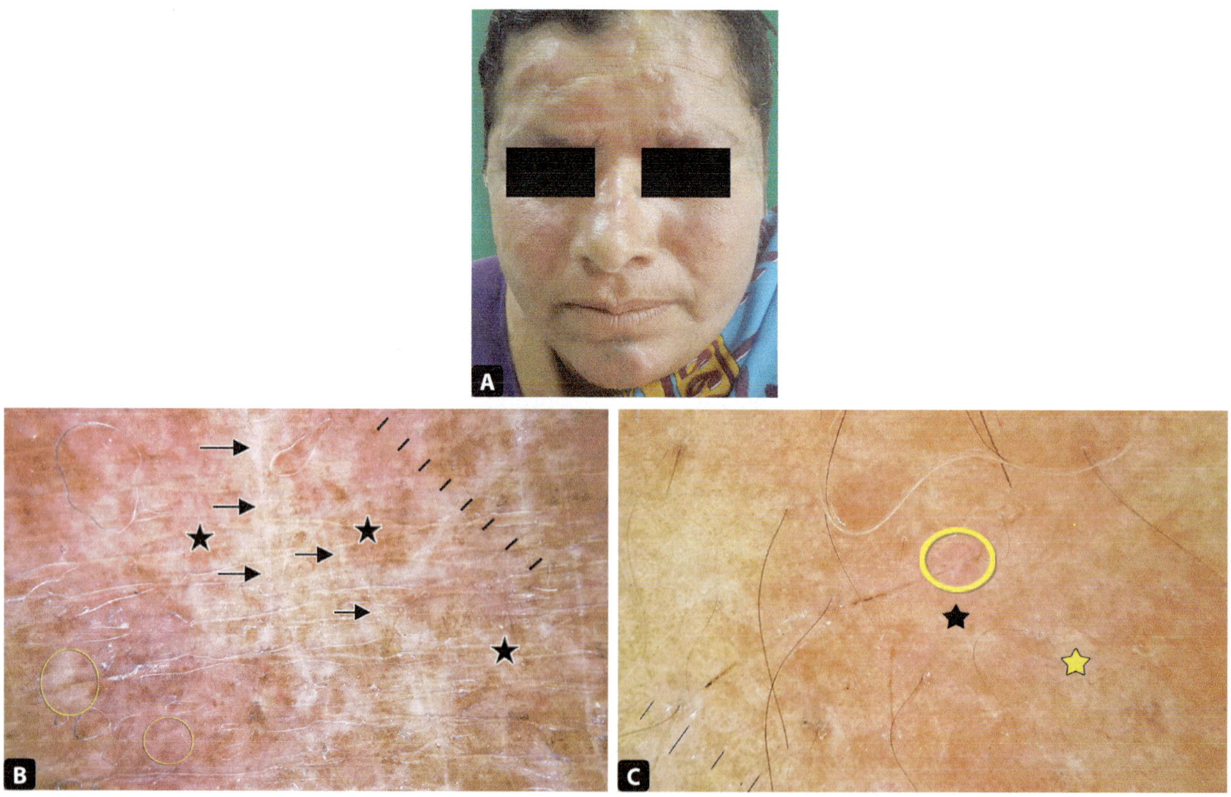

FIGS. 14A TO C: (A) Clinical image of lepromatous leprosy with type 2 reaction showing erythematous and indurated plaques on the face; (B) Dermoscopy of borderline lepromatous leprosy shows distorted pigment network (black stars) with decreased follicular and eccrine openings and white shiny lines (black arrows). Note the pinkish background and chrysalis-like structures (white shiny streaks) (yellow circles) (polarized, DermLite DL4, 10×); (C) Dermoscopic image showing milky-red structures (black star) and white areas (yellow star). Note the dotted vessels (yellow circle) on a pinkish background (polarized, DermLite DL4, 10×).

Dermoscopic Features

Dermoscopic features of LV include yellow-orange areas and well-focused vessels, including linear branching, linear and arborizing vessels (**Figs. 16B, 17B,** and **18B**). Other findings include whitish reticular streaks (**Figs. 16B** and **17B**), milia-like cyst, erosions, white scales, pigment structures, and follicular plugs (**Fig. 18B**).[1,24] Yellow-orange areas, which become more prominent on contact polarized dermoscopy, are similar to "apple-jelly" sign in diascopy (**Fig. 17B**).[2] Erosions and ulceration can occur with LV but are uncommon in sarcoidosis.[25]

Key Points

- The yellow-orange area with well-focused vessels is the most consistent feature and yellowish hue is more prominent on contact polarized dermoscopy.
- Whitish reticular streaks with scales and pigment dots are a frequent finding in the Indian population.

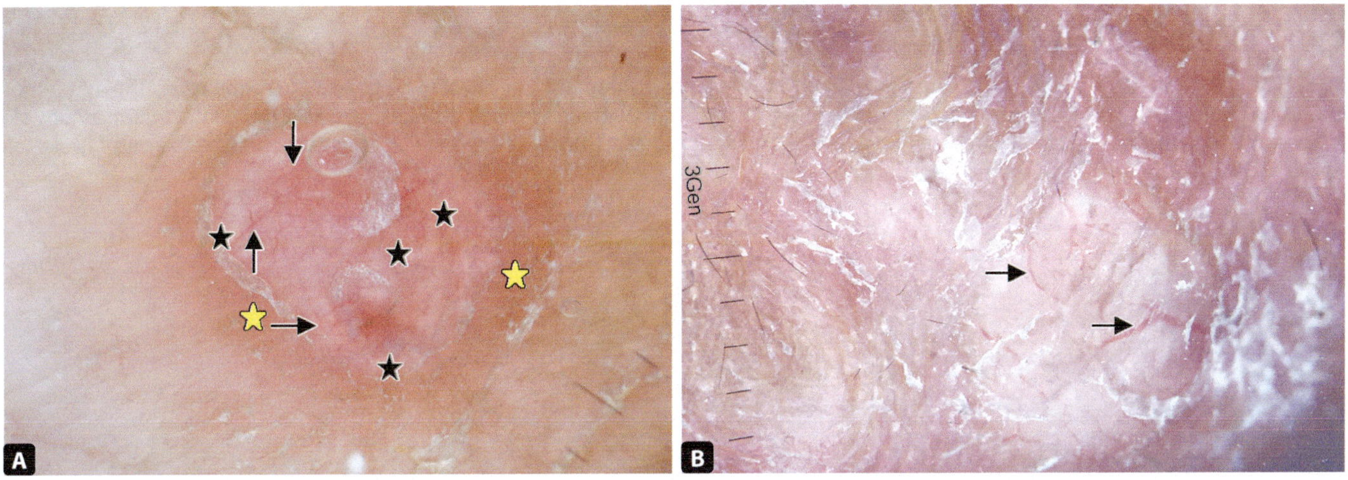

FIGS. 15A AND B: (A) Dermoscopy of lepromatous leprosy shows yellow globular structures (black stars) and arborizing crown vessels (black arrows). Note the brown pigmentation in the periphery (yellow stars) (polarized, DermLite DL4, 10×); (B) Dermoscopy of histoid nodule showing yellowish globular areas and crown vessels (black arrows) (polarized, DermLite DL4, 10×).

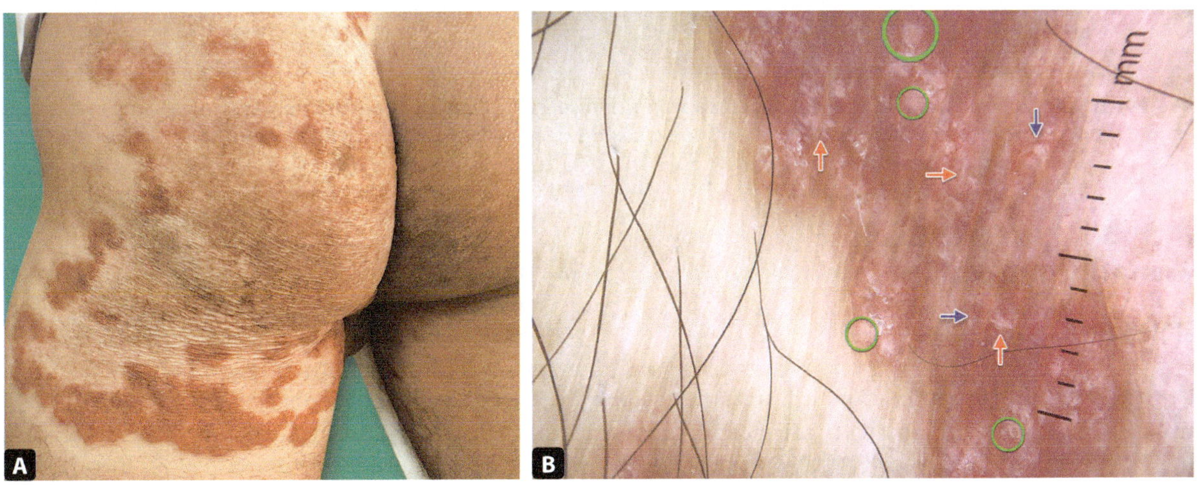

FIGS. 16A AND B: (A) Clinical image of lupus vulgaris over left buttock showing erythematous infiltrated papules to plaques over the margins and central scarring; (B) Dermoscopic image showing yellow-orange areas (green circles), whitish reticular streaks (red arrows), and fine-focused linear and dotted vessels (blue arrows) over pink background (polarized, DermLite DL4, 10×).

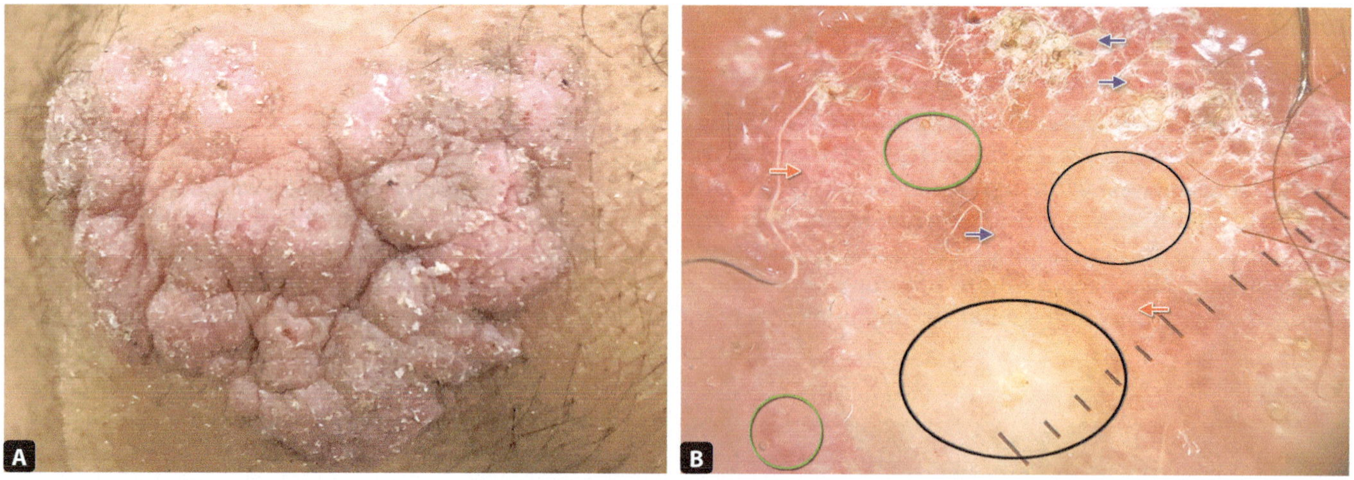

FIGS. 17A AND B: (A) Clinical image of lupus vulgaris showing erythematous infiltrated verrucous plaque over the left elbow; (B) Dermoscopic image showing yellow-orange areas (green circles), prominent yellow hue (black circles) at site of contact dermoscopy akin to diascopy, whitish reticular streaks (red arrows), focused linear and dotted vessel (blue arrows), scales and pink background (polarized, DermLite DL4, 10×).

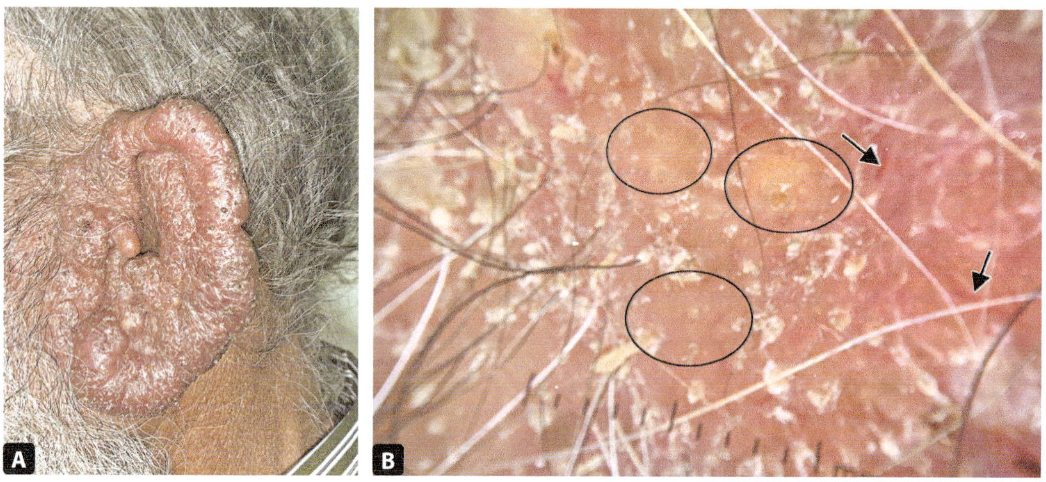

FIGS. 18A AND B: (A) Clinical image of lupus vulgaris showing diffuse infiltration with destruction of the ear architecture resulting in Turkey ear; (B) Dermoscopic image showing yellowish orange globules (black circles), linear unfocused vessels (black arrows), and scaling and follicular plugging (polarized, DermLite DL4, 10×).

Cutaneous Leishmaniasis

Clinical Features

Clinically, it starts as an erythematous infiltrated papule or nodule, which later develops into ulcer and crusts (**Fig. 19A**). The mucosal surface can rarely be involved in old-world leishmaniasis (**Fig. 20A**). Post-kala-azar dermal leishmaniasis (PKDL) commonly affects adolescents and young adults (**Fig. 21A**).

Dermoscopic Features

Although cutaneous leishmaniasis (CL) is a granuloma, the "orange areas" are observed only in 15% of cases.[26,27] The most consistent features described with CL are diffuse erythema and vascular structures, followed by white/yellow follicular keratotic plugs and white peripheral projections in a white starburst pattern (**Figs. 19B** and **C**).

Vascular elements observed are hairpin-like, comma, linear, dotted, glomerular, and corkscrew vessels.[26-28] Yellow hue, ulceration/erosion, scales, thrombotic vessels, white scar-like areas, milia-like cysts, pustules, and a perilesional hypopigmented halo are the other observed findings.[29,30]

Yellow tears are ellipsoid, oval, targetoid (rarely round) follicular plugs filled with keratin surrounding a crust or ulcer in the middle with asymmetrical, radially arranged polymorphic vessels.[30] Yellow tears are more commonly seen in early lesions distributed over the face and neck.

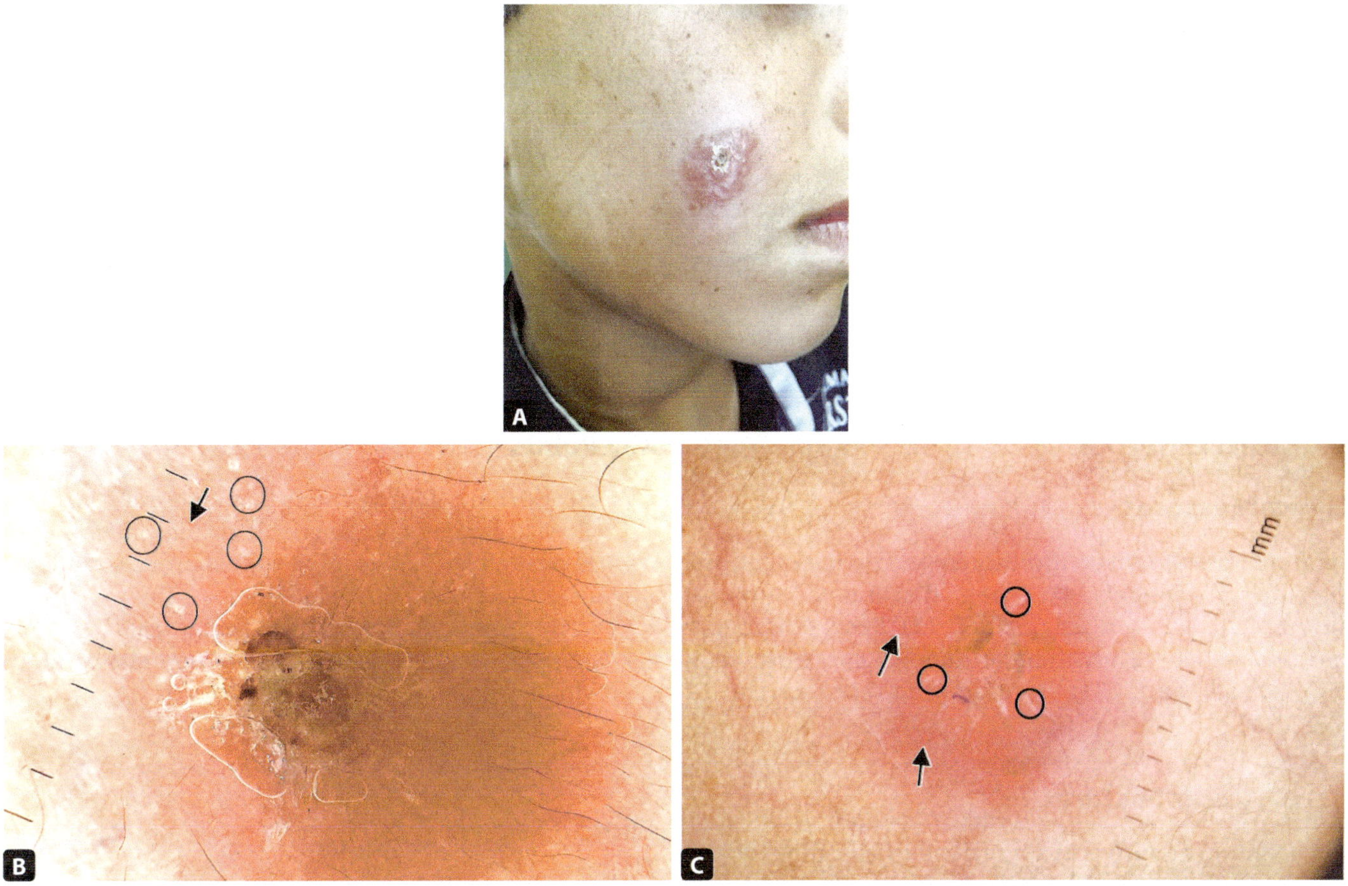

FIGS. 19A TO C: (A) Clinical image of cutaneous leishmaniasis showing erythematous succulent plaque with central ulceration and crusting over right cheek; (B) Dermoscopic image showing diffuse erythema, comma vessels (black arrow), yellow tears (black circles), and central erosion and crusting (polarized, DermLite DL3N, 10×); (C) Another case of cutaneous leishmaniasis showing central crusting, diffuse erythema, peripheral linear unfocused vessels (black arrows), and white chrysalis-like structures in a starburst pattern (black circles) (polarized, DermLite DL3N, 10×).

Courtesy (Fig. C): Dr Yasmeen J Bhat, Government Medical College, Srinagar, Jammu and Kashmir, India.

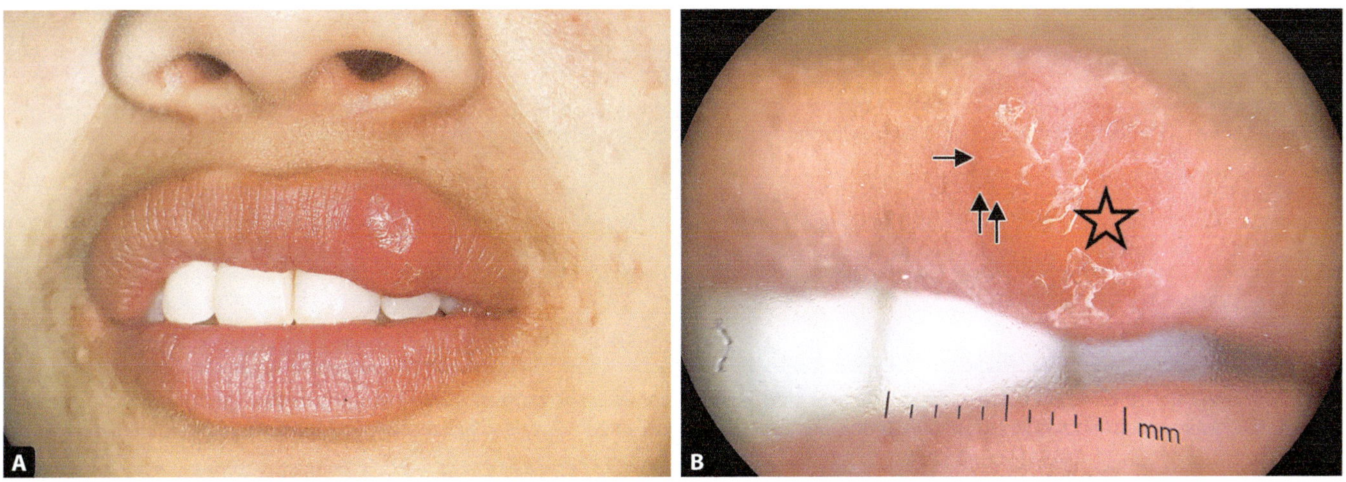

FIGS. 20A AND B: (A) Clinical image of cutaneous leishmaniasis involving the lips shows a crateriform papulonodular lesion with surface scaling; (B) Dermoscopic image showing yellowish-orange areas (black star), linear vessels (black arrows), and superficial scaling (polarized, DermLite DL4, 10×).

Yellow tears correspond histopathologically to follicular plugs, and a "white starburst-like pattern" may be attributed to the parakeratotic hyperkeratosis located around the erosion.[27]

Llambrich et al. described four dermoscopic patterns in Cutaneous leishmaniasis.[27] Initial lesions show pattern 1, consisting of with yellow-orange areas, irregular linear and comma vessels (**Fig. 20B**). Advanced lesions reveal pattern

2 with hairpin, irregular linear vessels (**Fig. 19B**).[31] PKDL shows a broken pigment network, yellowish-orange areas, and arborizing vessels (**Fig. 21B**).

Key Points

- Site and duration of the lesion are essential factors in determining the dermoscopic features of CL.
- Polymorphic vascular patterns and pink background are universally seen.
- Yellow tears and white starburst pattern, when present, are more characteristic of CL.

Sporotrichosis

Clinical Features

Sporotrichosis is a deep mycosis caused by the organism *Sporothrix schenckii.*[32] Three distinct cutaneous morphologies described include (1) fixed cutaneous sporotrichosis, (2) lymphocutaneous sporotrichosis (**Fig. 22A**), and (3) disseminated sporotrichosis (**Fig. 23A**).[32]

Dermoscopic Features

The common feature is scattered yellowish-orange areas corresponding to the dermal granulomas.[33] Early and evolving lesions show diffuse background erythema (representing ongoing inflammation), yellowish-orange areas, and variable telangiectatic vessels (**Fig. 22B**). Healing lesions show white fibrotic strands and linear telangiectatic vessels (**Fig. 22C**). Facial lesions, in addition, show "yellow tears" akin to those seen in CL (**Fig. 24**).[33]

Disseminated sporotrichosis shows generalized erythema, yellowish structureless areas surrounded by arborizing telangiectasias (representing inflammation and neovascularization), white scar-like areas (representing fibrosis), and white roundish structures (correspond to epidermal micropustules (microabscesses) (**Fig. 23B**).[34]

Key Points

- Early lesions show diffuse background erythema, yellowish-orange areas, variable telangiectatic vessels, and healing lesions showing white fibrotic strands and linear telangiectatic vessels.
- Facial lesions in addition show "yellow tears".
- Disseminated sporotrichosis, in addition, shows intense erythema and roundish white structures.

Chromoblastomycosis

Clinical Features

Lesions present with erythematous papule/nodule with overlying scales and crusts (**Fig. 25A**).[35]

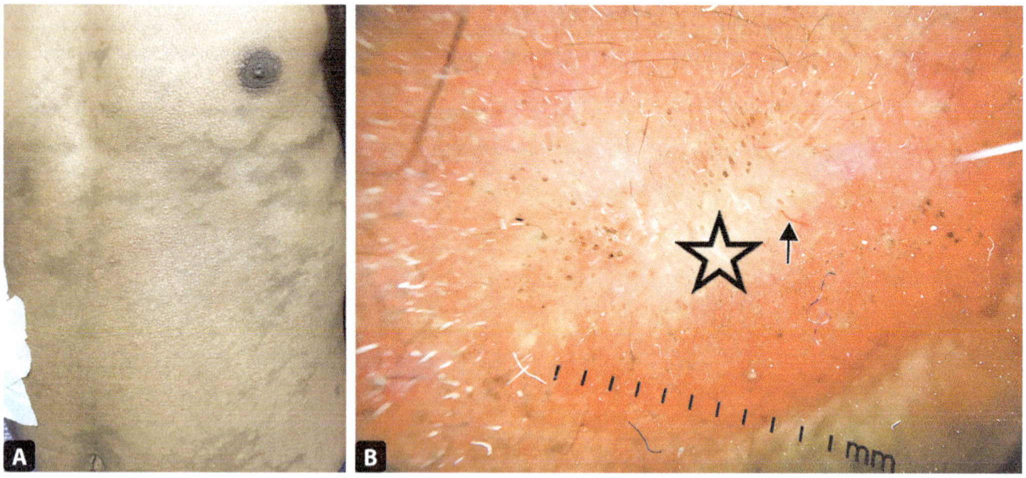

FIGS. 21A AND B: (A) Clinical image of post-kala-azar dermal leishmaniasis showing multiple hypopigmented geographic plaques over trunk; (B) Dermoscopic image showing yellowish-orange areas (black star), linear vessels (black arrow), and follicular plugs (polarized, Dermlite DL200, 10×).

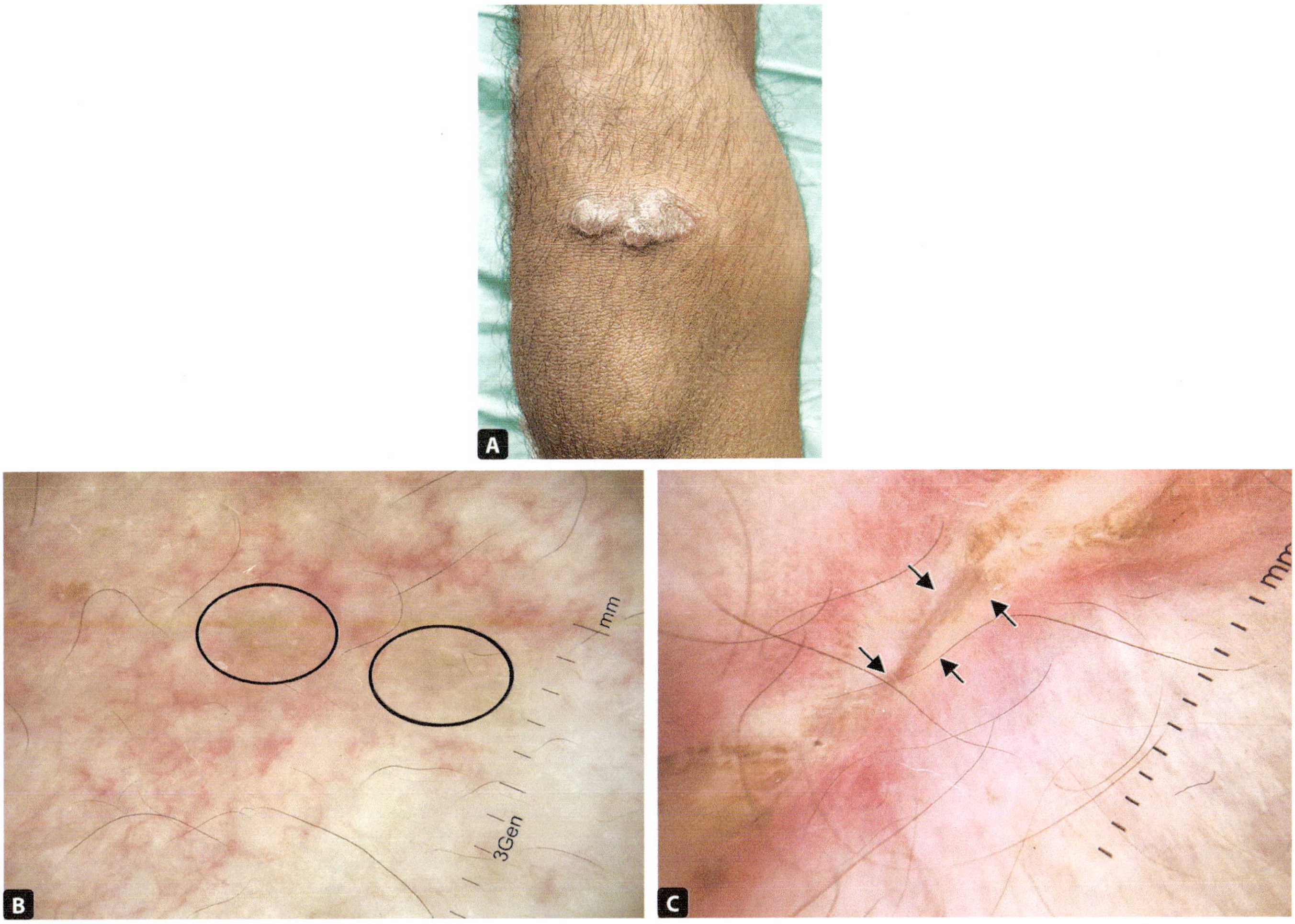

FIGS. 22A TO C: (A) Clinical image of lymphocutaneous sporotrichosis showing vegetative plaque over left knee; (B) Dermoscopy image of early lesion of sporotrichosis reveals yellowish-brown areas (black circles) surrounded by arborizing vessels. Yellowish-brown areas represent dermal granuloma (polarized, DermLite DL4, 10×); (C) Dermoscopy of healed lesions of sporotrichosis showing fibrotic streams (black arrows) surrounded by dotted and comma-shaped vessels (polarized, DermLite DL4, 10×).

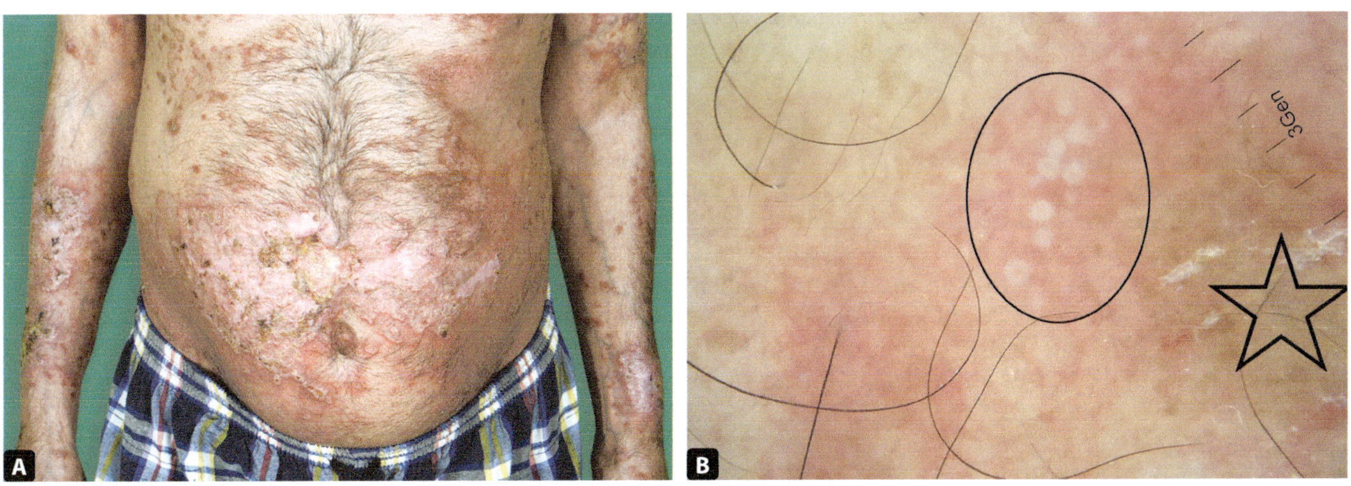

FIGS. 23A AND B: (A) Clinical image of disseminated cutaneous sporotrichosis showing erythematous and ulcerative plaque with satellite lesions involving the abdomen and limbs; (B) Dermoscopy of disseminated sporotrichosis showing multiple white roundish structures (black circle) on a background of erythema and arborizing vessels. Yellowish-brown areas representing dermal granulomas are seen (black star) (polarized, DermLite DL4, 10×).

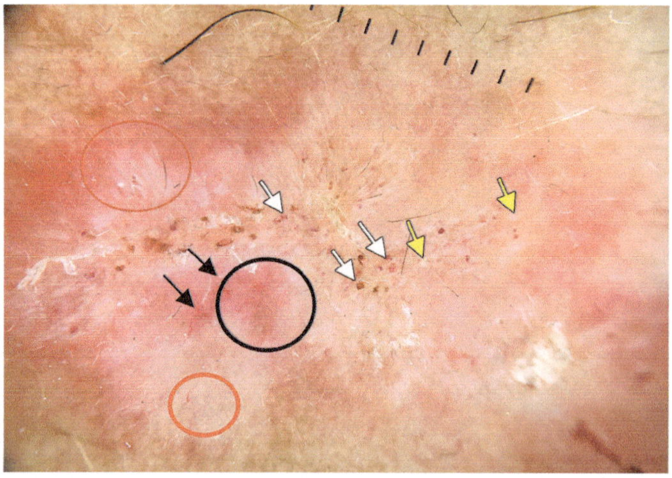

FIG. 24: Fixed cutaneous sporotrichosis over face showing yellow tears (yellow arrows), whitish crystalline structures (red circles), and superficial hemorrhagic spots (white arrows). Yellowish-orange areas (black circle) and ill-focused vessels (black arrows) can also be appreciated (polarized, DermLite DL4, 10×).

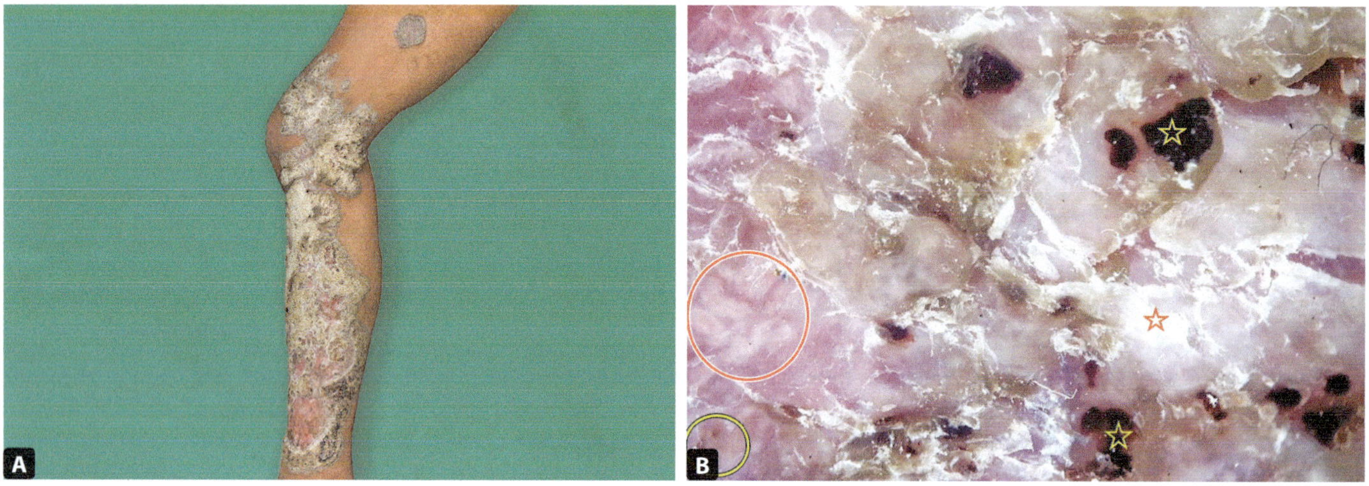

FIGS. 25A AND B: (A) Clinical image of chromoblastomycosis showing erythematous crusted plaque with slight atrophy and scaling; (B) Dermoscopy of chromoblastomycosis shows brownish-yellow areas (red circle), dotted vessels (yellow circle), and white scales (red star). Characteristic black dots and globules are well appreciated (yellow stars) (polarized, DermLite DL4, 10×).

Courtesy (Fig. B): Dr Keshavmurthy A Adya, SBMP MCHRC, Vijayapur, Karnataka, India.

Dermoscopic Features

Multiple yellow-orange ovoid structures with interspersed brown dots, crusts, and scales on reddish or white-pink background are observed.[35] In skin of color, brownish globular structures are seen.[36] Multiple blackish-red dots are most characteristic (**Fig. 25B**). Resolution of blackish-red dots corresponds to the clinical clearance of the lesion.[37]

Key Points

- Multiple yellow-orange (brownish-yellow) ovoid structures on the reddish or white-pink background and interspersed brown dots, crusts, and scales.

Mycetoma

Clinical Features

It is a neglected tropical disease characterized by painless, woody hard swelling and multiple discharging sinuses (**Fig. 26A**).[38]

Dermoscopic Features

Black granules are highly suggestive of eumycotic mycetoma (**Fig. 26B**).[39] Deep-seated fungal colonies appear as bluish-white structureless areas surrounded by a white halo.[39] Yellow globules, white superficial scales, telangiectasia, and dotted vessels are also noted.[40]

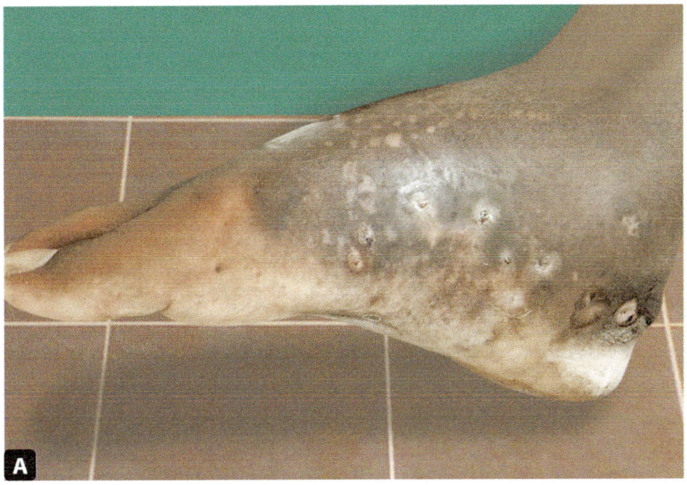

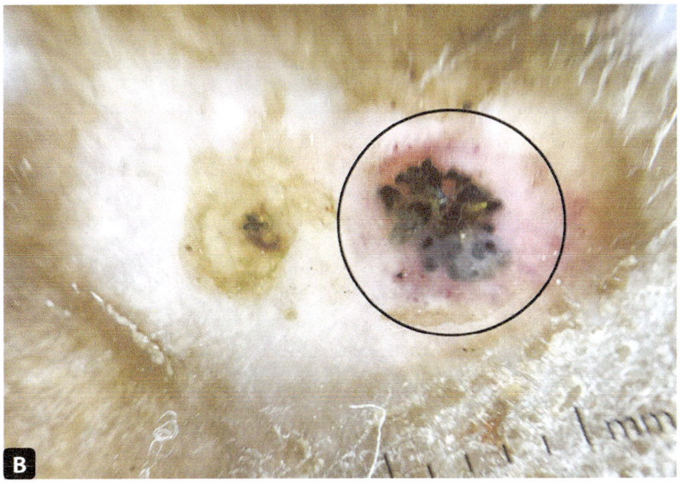

FIGS. 26A AND B: (A) Clinical image of mycetoma of the right foot showing diffuse swelling and multiple discharging sinuses; (B) Dermoscopy of one of the sinus showing multiple black dots representing fungal grains (black circle). Bluish white veil can be appreciated from 5 o'clock to 8 o'clock position, representing deep-seated grains covered by thin layer of epidermis. A rim of erythema with dotted vessels surrounds these sinuses (polarized, DermLite DL4, 10×).

Courtesy: Dr Gitesh Sawatkar, AIIMS, Nagpur, Maharashtra, India.

Key Points

- Black-colored granules over sinus opening are diagnostic of eumycotic mycetoma.
- Yellow globules representing dermal granulomas and dotted vessels are other features.

KEY POINTS

- Brownish yellow areas are characteristic feature of granuloma in skin of color.
- Different arrangement and morphology of vessels can point towards the diagnosis.
- Additional features like follicular changes, scales and pigmentation can vary according to the duration and site of the lesion.

CONCLUSION

Dermoscopy can aid in the early diagnosis, staging, prognosis as well as improve the yield of histopathology for the diagnosis of granulomatous disorders.

REFERENCES

1. Lallas A, Argenziano G, Apalla Z, Gourhant J, Zaballos P, Di Lernia V, et al. Dermoscopic patterns of common facial inflammatory skin diseases. J Eur Acad Dermatol Venereol. 2014;28:609-14.
2. Errichetti E, Stinco G. Dermatoscopy of granulomatous disorders. Dermatol Clin. 2018;36:369-75.
3. Chauhan P, Meena D, Hazarika N. Dermoscopy of sarcoidosis: a useful clue to diagnosis. Indian Dermatol Online J. 2018;9:80-1.
4. Errichetti E, Lallas A, Apalla Z, Di Stefani A. Stinco G. Dermoscopy of granuloma annulare: a clinical and histological correlation study. Dermatology. 2017;233:74-9.
5. Gutiérrez-González E, Pereiro M Jr, Toribio J. Elastolytic actinic giant cell granuloma. Dermatol Clin. 2015;33:331-41.
6. Errichetti E, Cataldi P, Stinco G. Dermoscopy in annular elastolytic giant cell granuloma. J Dermatol. 2019;46:e66-7.
7. Sibbald C, Reid S, Alavi A. Necrobiosis lipoidica. Dermatol Clin. 2015;33: 343-60.
8. Lallas A, Zaballos P, Zalaudek I, Apalla Z, Gourhant JY, Longo C, et al. Dermoscopic patterns of granuloma annulare and necrobiosis lipoidica. Clin Exp Dermatol. 2013;38:425-7.
9. Alexis AF, Callender VD, Baldwin HE, Desai SR, Rendon MI, Taylor SC. Global epidemiology and clinical spectrum of rosacea, highlighting skin of color: review and clinical practice experience. J Am Acad Dermatol. 2019;80:1722-9.e7.
10. Lee GL, Zirwas MJ. Granulomatous rosacea and periorificial dermatitis: controversies and review of management and treatment. Dermatol Clin. 2015;33:447-55.
11. Vinay K, Sawatkar GU, Saikia UN, Dogra S. Dermatoscopic features of xanthoma disseminatum. Int J Dermatol. 2017;56:1175-6.
12. Litaiem N, Zeglaoui F. Is the setting sun dermoscopic pattern specific to juvenile xanthogranuloma? J Am Acad Dermatol. 2018;78:e49.
13. Oliveira TE, Tarlé RG, Mesquita LA. Dermoscopy in the diagnosis of juvenile xanthogranuloma. An Bras Dermatol. 2018;93:138-40.
14. Chauhan P, Jindal R, Shirazi N. Dermoscopy of lupus miliaris disseminatus faciei: a step closer to diagnosis. Dermatol Pract Concept. 2020;10:e2020055.
15. Ayhan E, Alabalik U, Avci Y. Dermoscopic evaluation of two patients with lupus miliaris disseminatus faciei. Clin Exp Dermatol. 2014;39:500-2.
16. Litaiem N, Chamli A, Bacha T, Jones M, Goucha S, Rammeh S, et al. Dermoscopic features of lupus miliaris disseminatus faciei: distinct aspects depending on disease stage. Clin Case Rep. 2020;8:1793-6.
17. Bombonato C, Argenziano G, Lallas A, Moscarella E, Ragazzi M, Longo C. Orange color: a dermoscopic clue for the diagnosis of granulomatous skin diseases. J Am Acad Dermatol. 2015;72:S60-3.
18. Kumar B, Naafs B, Dogra S. Leprosy. Lepr Rev. 2007;78:5-6.
19. Vinay K, Kamat D, Chatterjee D, Narang T, Dogra S. Dermatoscopy in leprosy and its correlation with clinical spectrum and histopathology: a prospective observational study. J Eur Acad Dermatol Venereol. 2019;33:1947-51.
20. Ankad BS, Sakhare PS. Dermoscopy of borderline tuberculoid leprosy. Int J Dermatol. 2018;57:74-6.
21. Chopra A, Mitra D, Agarwal R, Saraswat N, Talukdar K, Solanki A. Correlation of dermoscopic and histopathologic patterns in leprosy—a pilot study. Indian Dermatol Online J. 2019;10:663-8.

22. Jha AK, Zeeshan MD, Tiwary P, Singh A, Roy PK, Chaudhary RK. Dermoscopy of type 1 lepra reaction in skin of color. Dermatol Pract Concept. 2020;10:e2020083.
23. Acharya P, Mathur MC. Clinicodermoscopic study of histoid leprosy: a case series. Int J Dermatol. 2020;59:365-8.
24. Errichetti E, Stinco G. Dermoscopy in general dermatology: a practical overview. Dermatol Ther (Heidelb). 2016;6:471-507.
25. Pellicano R, Tiodorovic-Zivkovic D, Gourhant JY, Catricalà C, Ferrara G, Caldarola G, et al. Dermoscopy of cutaneous sarcoidosis. Dermatology. 2010;221:51-4.
26. Yücel A, Günaşti S, Denli Y, Uzun S. Cutaneous leishmaniasis: new dermoscopic findings. Int J Dermatol. 2013;52:831-7.
27. Llambrich A, Zaballos P, Terrasa F, Torne I, Puig S, Malvehy J. Dermoscopy of cutaneous leishmaniasis. Br J Dermatol. 2009;160:756-61.
28. Bhat YJ, Yaseen A, Sheikh S, Hassan I. Dermoscopy of two cases of cutaneous leishmaniasis. Indian J Dermatol. 2020;65:232-4.
29. Taheri AR, Pishgooei N, Maleki M, Goyonlo VM, Kiafar B, Banihashemi M, et al. Dermoscopic features of cutaneous leishmaniasis. Int J Dermatol. 2013;52: 1361-6.
30. Ayhan E, Ucmak D, Baykara SN, Akkurt ZM, Arica M. Clinical and dermoscopic evaluation of cutaneous leishmaniasis. Int J Dermatol. 2015;54:193-201.
31. Caltagirone F, Pistone G, Arico M, Vitale F, Sorbello D, Rizzo D, et al. Vascular patterns in cutaneous leishmaniasis: a videodermatoscopic study. Indian J Dermatol Venereol Leprol. 2015;81:394-8.
32. Mahajan VK. Sporotrichosis: an overview and therapeutic options. Dermatol Res Pract. 2014;2014:272376.
33. Vinay K, Bhattacharjee R, Bishnoi A, Chatterjee D, Rudramurthy S, Dogra S. Dermatoscopic features of cutaneous sporotrichosis. J Eur Acad Dermatol Venereol. 2020;34:e718-20.
34. Dabas G, Kaur H, Vinay K, Kumaran MS, Shivaprakash MR, Saikia UN, et al. Dermoscopy in disseminated sporotrichosis. J Eur Acad Dermatol Venereol. 2019;33:e33-5.
35. Chauhan P, Jindal R, Shirazi N. Dermoscopy of chromoblastomycosis. Indian Dermatol Online J. 2019;10:759-60.
36. Jayasree P, Malakar S, Raja H, Gopinathan N. Dermoscopic features in nodular chromoblastomycosis. Int J Dermatol. 2018;58:e107-9.
37. Subhadarshani S, Yadav D. Dermoscopy of chromoblastomycosis. Dermatol Pract Concept. 2017;7:23-4.
38. Verma P, Jha A. Mycetoma: reviewing a neglected disease. Clin Exp Dermatol. 2019;44:123-9.
39. Litaiem N, Midassi O, Zeglaoui F. Detecting subclinical mycetoma's black grains using dermoscopy. Int J Dermatol. 2019;58:231-2.
40. Ankad BS, Manjula R, Tejasvi T, Nikam BP. Dermoscopy of eumycotic mycetoma: a case report. Dermatol Pract Concept. 2019;9:297-9.

7 CHAPTER

Infectious Diseases

Manas Chatterjee, Kinjal D Rambhia, Debjit Kar

INTRODUCTION

Dermoscopy is a noninvasive, efficient, and quick tool for diagnosis of dermatological conditions. Dermoscopy of infections always carries a risk of transmission which can be reduced by using noncontact dermoscopes or appropriate barriers such as ice caps or other methods such as cling films/wraps.

BACTERIAL INFECTIONS

Impetigo

Clinical Features

Impetigo is a contagious, superficial pyogenic infection of the skin caused by *Staphylococcus* and less frequently, *Streptococcus*. It can occur in two main clinical forms, i.e., nonbullous and bullous impetigo (**Fig. 1A**).

Dermoscopic Features

Peripheral scaling, yellow crusts, and dotted vessels in cases with crusted lesions (**Figs. 1B** and **C**).[1]

Key Points

- Peripheral scaling, yellow crusts, and dotted vessels

Folliculitis

Clinical Features

Infective folliculitis can be bacterial, viral, parasitic, and fungal in origin (**Fig. 2A**). Dermoscopy provides important findings for the diagnosis of folliculitis such as Demodex folliculitis (demodex tail), dotted vessels in Malassezia folliculitis, corkscrew-like hair, zigzag hair and black dot in

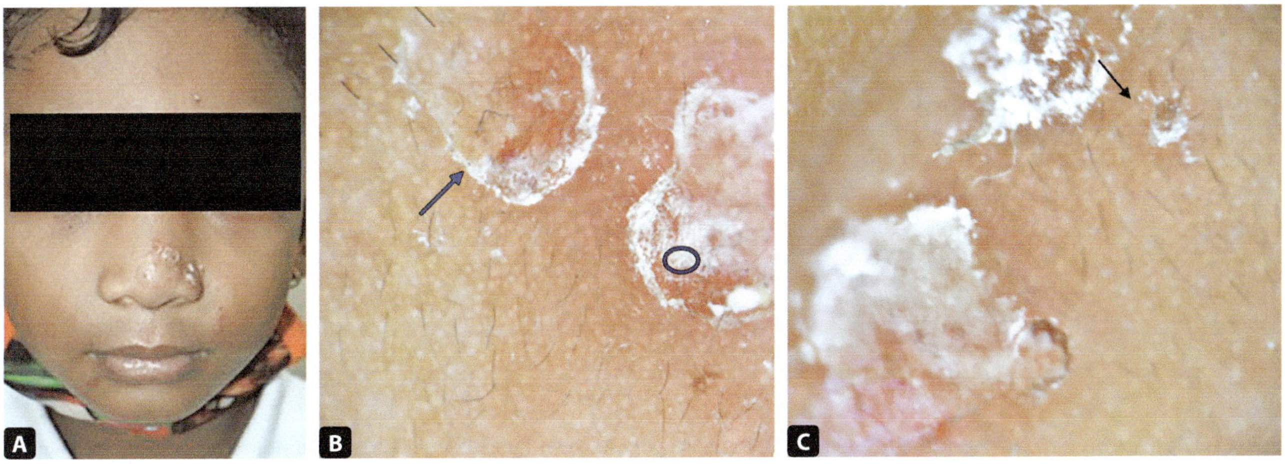

FIGS. 1A TO C: (A) Multiple, erythematous crusted papules and ruptured vesicles in a young child with impetigo; (B) Peripheral scaling (blue arrow), yellowish scale-crust (blue circle) seen on dermoscopy (polarized, DermLite DL3, 10×); (C) Whitish-yellow scale-crust (black arrow) seen on dermoscopy (polarized, DermLite DL3, 10×).

dermatophytic folliculitis, hair tuft in folliculitis decalvans, and ingrown hair in pseudofolliculitis.

Dermoscopic Features

Folliculocentric lesion with pustule around hair follicle (**Fig. 2B**). Peripheral sparse dotted vessels and clods (**Fig. 2B**). Folliculocentric white lines with white and gray dots and globules on gray background indicating chronic inflammatory process leading to perifollicular fibrosis in chronic lesions (**Figs. 2C** and **2D**).[2]

Key Points

- Micropustule
- Dotted or globular vessels
- White lines

Furuncle

Clinical Features

It is defined as the infection of a hair follicle with *Staphylococcus aureus.*

Dermoscopic Features

Erythema and white structureless area can be seen in all cases (**Fig. 3**). Hazy yellow structures can be seen in few cases.[3,4]

Key Points

- Erythema and white structureless area
- Hazy yellow structures

Pseudofolliculitis Barbae

Clinical Features

It is a subacute or chronic pyogenic infection involving the whole depth of the follicle and usually refers to the disease in the beard area. It is also referred to as sycosis barbae (**Fig. 4A**). Stretching the skin while using razors and infrequent shaving might be important risk factors along with racial predisposition in races with curly hairs (**Fig. 4D**).

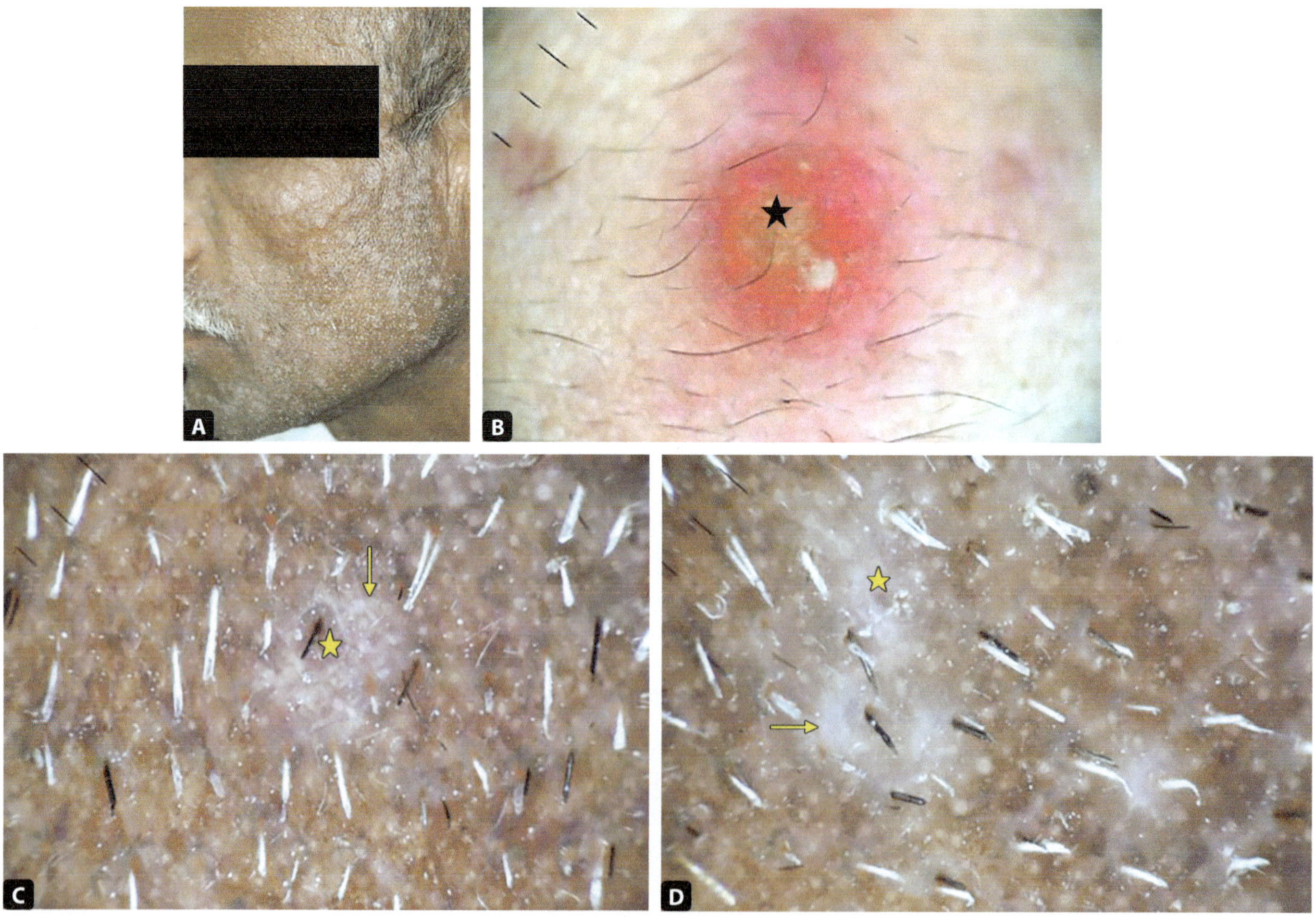

FIGS. 2A TO D: (A) Chronic pityrosporum folliculitis with multiple papules over face; (B) Folliculocentric yellowish homogenous area (star) with few linear and dotted vessels (polarized, DermLite DL3, 10×); (C) Folliculocentric white lines (arrow), gray-white dots and globules on gray background (star) indicating perifollicular fibrosis (polarized, DermLite DL3, 10×); (D) Folliculocentric white lines (yellow arrow) on gray background (yellow star) indicating perifollicular fibrosis (polarized, DermLite DL3, 10×).

Dermoscopic Features

"Handle bar" sign showing curved hair attached to the skin on both ends. White areas (possibly indicating fibrosis) and scaling, underlying linear bluish pigmentation (indicating the buried hair shaft), are characteristic. Linear vessels with occasional areas of hemorrhage may be seen (**Figs. 4B, 4C**, and **4E**).[5,6]

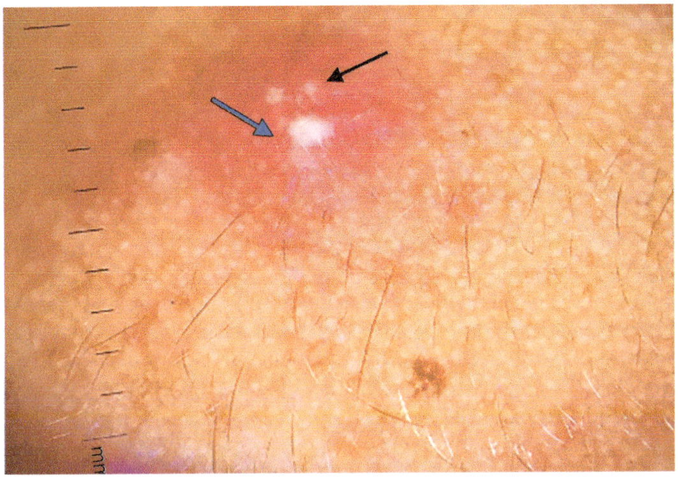

FIG. 3: Erythema and white globule (blue arrow) along with hazy yellow globule (black arrow) seen in furuncle (polarized, DermLite DL3, 10×).

Key Points

- "Handle bar" sign showing curved hair attached to the skin on both ends.

Trichomycosis Axillaris

Clinical Features

Trichomycosis axillaris is a superficial bacterial infection that is typically caused by *Corynebacterium tenuis*. Patient presents with discoloration of the axillary or beard/ moustache hair associated with bad odor. On examination, the adherent concretions on the hair shaft may be yellow, black, or red and there is typically an associated rancid or acidic odor (**Fig. 5A**).

Dermoscopic Features

On dermoscopy, yellowish hair casts around hairs are found (**Fig. 5B**).[7]

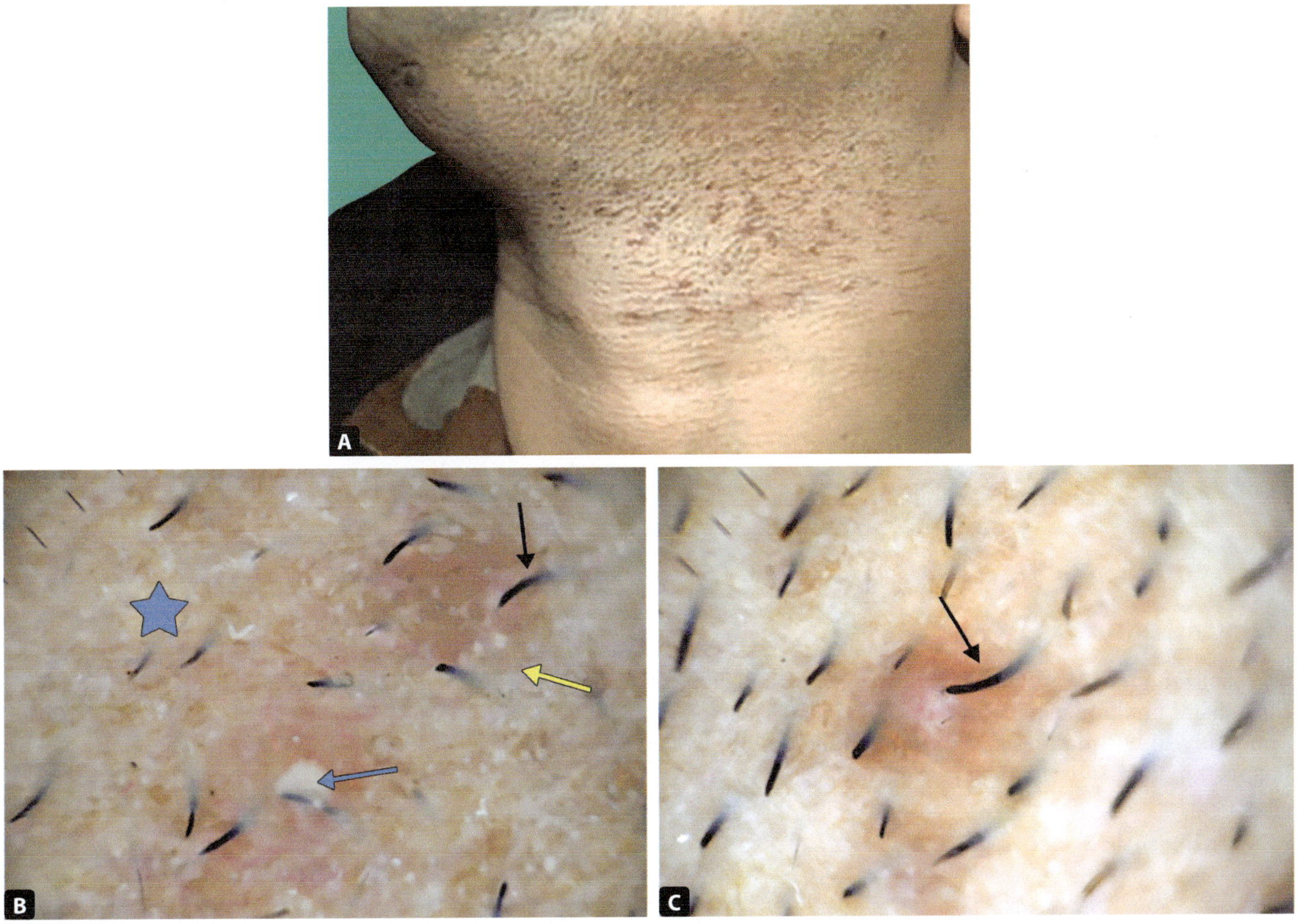

FIGS. 4A TO E: *(Continued)*

(Continued)

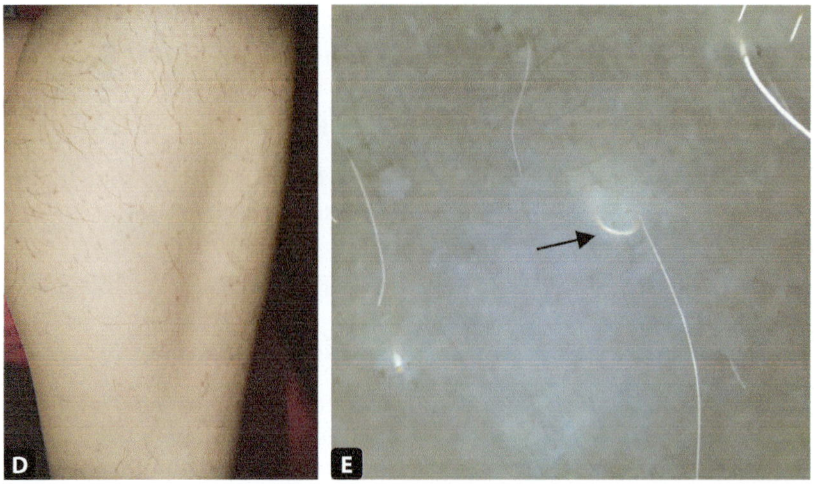

FIGS. 4A TO E: (A) Multiple erythematous papules in the beard region in sycoses barbae; (B) Dermoscopy of the papules reveal "handle bar" sign showing curved hair attached to the skin on both ends (black arrow), yellowish globule around the hair (blue arrow), white areas (yellow arrow), and underlying linear bluish pigmentation (blue star) (polarized, DermLite DL3, 10×); (C) "Handle bar" sign showing curved hair attached to the skin on both ends (black arrow) (polarized, DermLite DL3, 10×); (D) Pseudofolliculitis of the leg; (E) "Handle bar" sign showing curved hair attached to the skin on both ends (black arrow) (polarized, DermLite DL3, 10×).

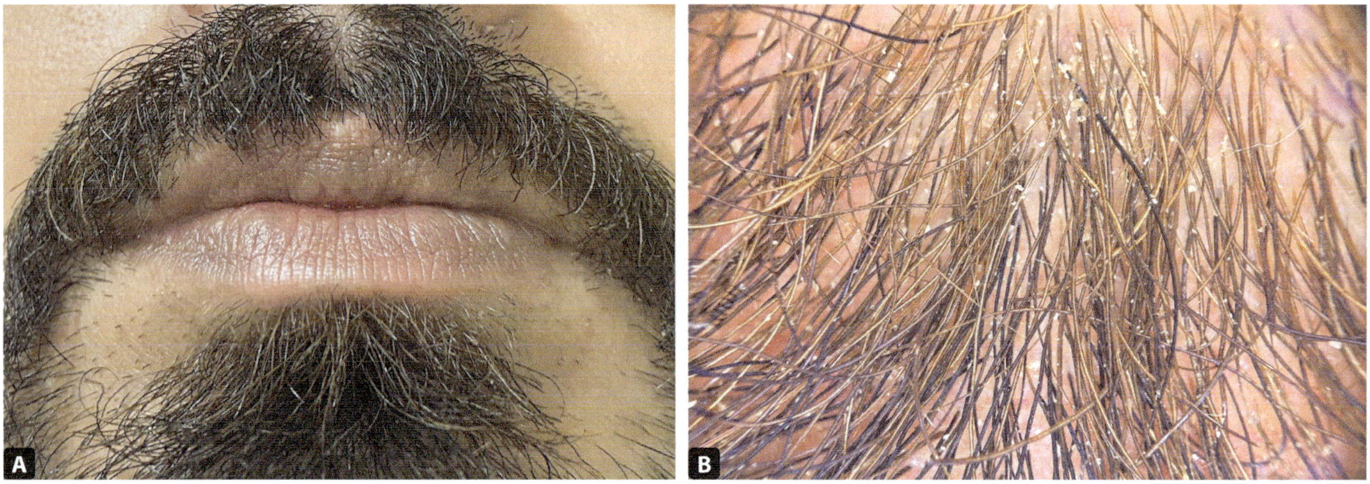

FIGS. 5A AND B: (A) Beard hair demonstrating yellowish discoloration in trichomycosis; (B) Dermoscopy shows yellowish hair casts around the hair shaft (polarized, DermLite DL3, 10×).

Key Points

- Yellowish hair casts around hairs

Blistering Distal Dactylitis

Clinical Features

A localized group A β-hemolytic *Streptococcus* infection of the distal phalanx usually in a child, typically between 2 and 16 years. It manifests as multiple bullae on the volar aspects of the hands and fingers (**Fig. 6A**).

Dermoscopic Features

Dermoscopic features reveal yellow homogeneous areas which are lakes of pus under the epidermis. Prominent dermatoglyphic pattern of the fingers is seen. Prominent desquamation showing yellowish scales may be seen in the regression phase (**Fig. 6B**).

Key Points

- Yellow homogeneous areas
- Prominent desquamation showing yellowish scales may be seen in the regression phase.

Pitted Keratolysis

Clinical Features

Pitted keratolysis is a superficial bacterial infection by coryneforms that commonly affect the weight-bearing areas of soles in hot and humid climates. Conspicuous, discrete, hollow, circular lesions with a punched-out appearance coalesce in places to produce irregular erosions (**Fig. 7A**).

Dermoscopic Features

Dermoscopy of the pits reveals better visualization of shallow crater-like irregular pits (**Fig. 7B**). Heterogeneous architecture of the pit wall according to random dissolution of stratum corneum by bacterial colonies can be seen at higher magnification.[1,8,]

Key Points

- Shallow crater-like irregular pits

Hansen's Disease

Clinical Features

Leprosy is a chronic granulomatous condition caused by *Mycobacterium leprae* presenting as hypopigmented patches, plaques, or nodules (**Fig. 8A**).

Dermoscopic Features

Yellowish-orange structureless areas, vascular structures, broken/reduced pigment network, and paucity of appendageal structures are findings common to all subtypes. However, two most common dermoscopic findings are white areas (corresponding to a decreased number of melanocytes) and decreased density of hair (**Fig. 8B**).[9,10]

Key Points

- Yellowish-orange structureless areas, vascular structures, broken/reduced pigment network, and paucity of appendageal structures

Lupus Vulgaris

Clinical Features

It is a chronic, progressive, paucibacillary form of cutaneous tuberculosis, occurring in a previously sensitized individual with a high degree of immunity to tuberculin.

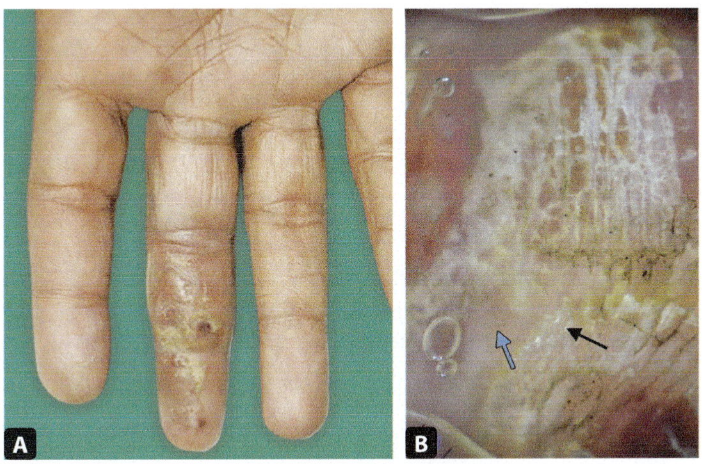

FIGS. 6A AND B: (A) Blistering distal dactylitis in an adult (healing) with multiple pustules on middle and distal phalanx; (B) Dermoscopy showing yellow homogenous areas (blue arrow) with yellowish scales (black arrow) (areas of desquamation) (polarized, DermLite DL3, 10×).

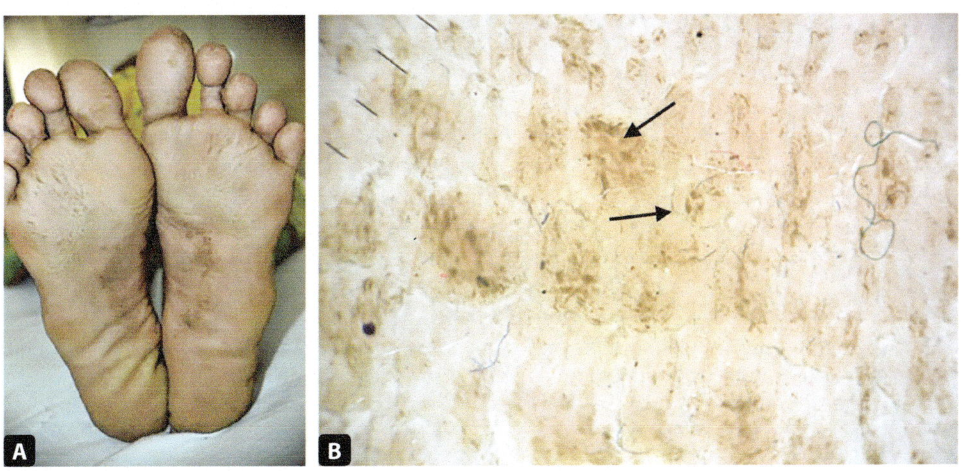

FIGS. 7A AND B: (A) Multiple, well-defined, shallow circular pits over the weight-bearing areas of the sole in pitted keratolysis; (B) Dermoscopy shows shallow crater-like irregular pits (black arrow) (polarized, DermLite DL3, 10×).

The characteristic lesion is a plaque, composed of soft, reddish brown papules, which resemble apple jelly on diascopy (**Fig. 9A**).

Dermoscopic Features

Yellowish-orange structureless areas which correspond to the granulomas are found (**Fig. 9B**). The appearance is similar to as seen in sarcoidosis, although the yellowish hue is deeper in lupus vulgaris lesions. Linear branching vessels can also be seen.[11, 12]

Key Points

- Yellowish-orange structureless areas
- Linear branching vessels

FUNGAL INFECTION

Superficial Fungal Infections

Pityriasis Versicolor

Clinical Features

Hypopigmented or hyperpigmented perifollicular macules with fine branny scales, which gradually coalesce.

Dermoscopic Features

Alteration in background pigmentation in both the hyperpigmented and hypopigmented variant, with folliculocentric lesion. Fine branny scales mostly localized to the skin cleavage lines, in achromic or hyperchromic well-defined lesion. Additionally, perifollicular scaling may also be

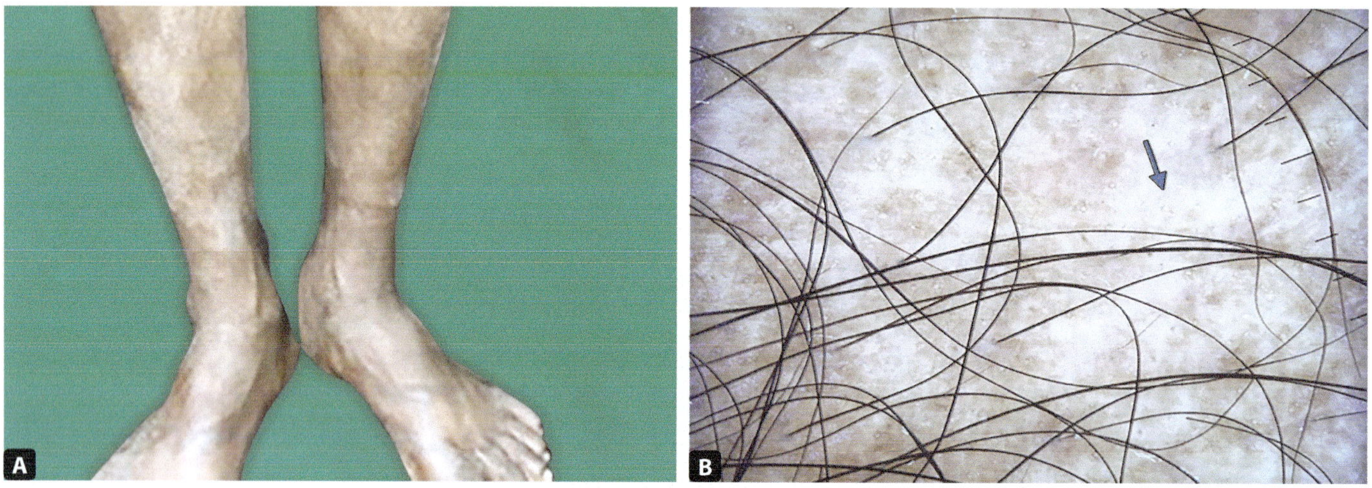

FIGS. 8A AND B: (A) Multiple, hypopigmented, hypoesthetic patches with decreased hairs over lower limbs in leprosy; (B) Focal white areas and decreased density of hair on dermoscopy (arrow) (polarized, DermLite DL3, 10×).

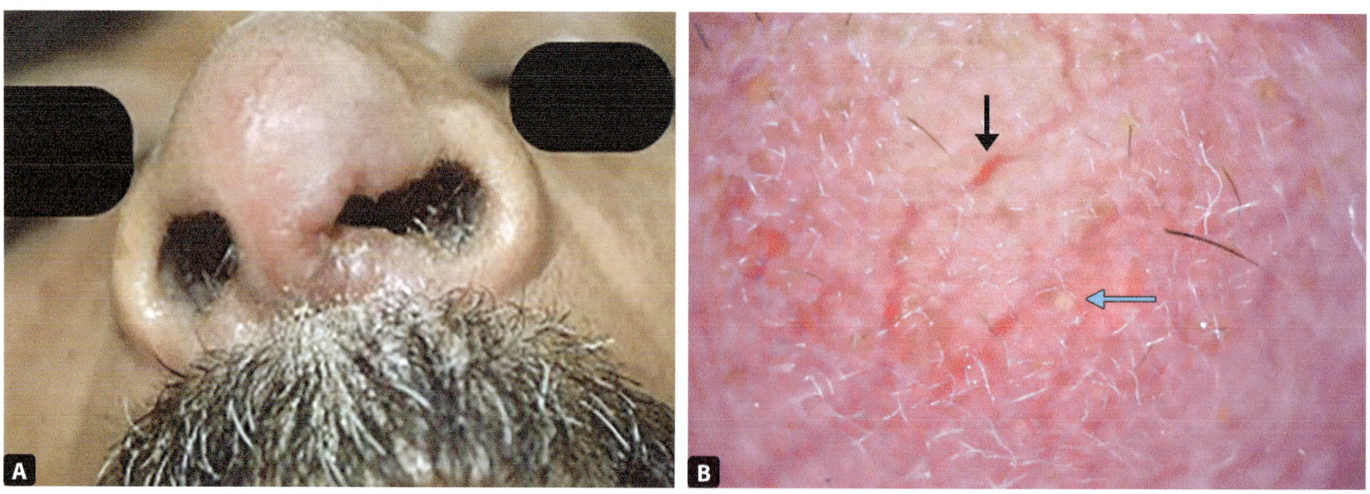

FIGS. 9A AND B: (A) Firm, erythematous irregular nodules present over the nose (apple jelly nodules) in a histopathologically confirmed case of lupus vulgaris; (B) Yellowish-orange structureless areas (blue arrow) seen along with linear branching vessels (black arrow) on dermoscopy (polarized, DermLite DL3, 10×).

present. Contrast pigmentary ring around the primary hypopigmented lesion surrounded by a ring of increased pigmentation and vice versa is metaphorically described as contrast halo sign (**Fig. 10**).[13]

Key Points

- Fine/Branny white scales on an altered pigmentary network
- Prominent scales in skin cleavage lines
- Contrast pigmentary ring around the lesion

Tinea Capitis

Clinical Features

Discoid patch of partial hair loss, with varying degree of inflammation and easily pluckable hairs.

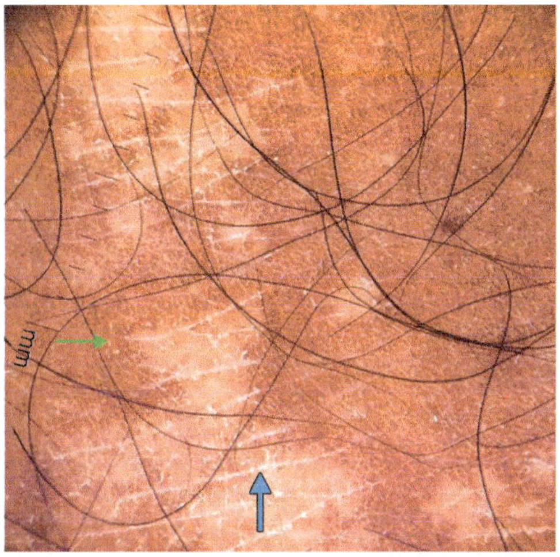

FIG. 10: Fine branny scales (blue arrow) and "contrast halo" sign with rim of contrast pigmentation around the hypochromic lesion (green arrow) in pityriasis versicolor (polarized, DermLite DL3, 10×).

Dermoscopic Features[14-20]

- *Comma hairs*: Bending of short or broken hairs due to partial damage to hair shafts by ectothrix parasitization. These hairs retain their normal thickness and color.
- *Corkscrew hairs*: Present as short hairs with multiple twists, indicate endothrix infection. First described by Hughes et al. in black patients affected by *Trichophyton schoenleinii.*

Other Features

- Interfollicular scales
- Broken or dystrophic hairs
- Black dot
- *Hair casts*: Whitish scale around proximal hair shaft
- *Morse code hairs*: Transverse horizontal white bands present in regular distribution along hair shaft (horizontal bands correspond to localized areas of fungal infection, which result in hair perforation).
- *Cigarette ash hair*: Irregularly disrupted and incompact appearance of hair end, giving the appearance of cigarette ash. It indicates response to treatment after starting antifungals, as the endothrix spores are eliminated causing breakage of hair shaft. These represent the broken corkscrew hairs (**Figs. 11A** and **B**).
- *"i" hair*: Short broken hairs look like the letter "i." Represents localized area of fungal infection, resulting in hair perforation
- *Block hair*: Very short hairs with a transverse horizontal distal end
- *Zig zag hair*: Hair with numerous bends at sharp angles

Key Points

- Bending or twisting of terminal hairs, i.e., comma and corkscrew hairs are the characteristic dermoscopic feature.

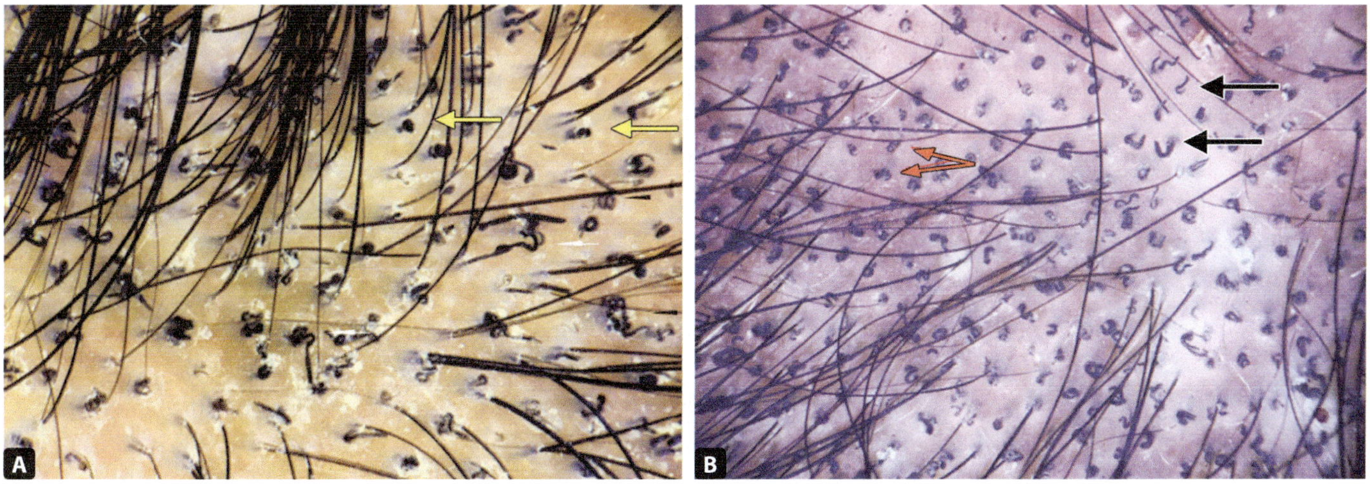

FIGS. 11A AND B: (A) Comma hair, short bent hairs, hairs with multiple twists, cork screw hair (white arrow), and "i" hairs (yellow arrows) in tinea capitis (polarized, DermLite DL3, 10×); (B) Comma hairs (black arrows) and cork screw hairs (red arrows) in tinea capitis (polarized, DermLite DL3, 10×).

- Constellation of other features (as described above) in various combination

Tinea Corporis/Cruris

Clinical Features

Annular plaques with relative central clearing and a slightly raised advancing edge.

Dermoscopic Features

Thin rim of superficial scale at the periphery of annular plaque, not normally visible to naked eye (**Fig. 12**). Scaling is a sign of active disease, which may represent inadequate clearance or recurrence (usually absent in steroid modified tinea). A rim of erythema may extend beyond the scales. Older lesions may show intermittent black dots in between the scales (scale crusts/crusts). Crusting may be there because of repeated scratching or as an early sign of secondary eczematization.[21]

Follicular micropustules and brown spots surrounded by a white-yellowish halo around a hair follicle suggest invasion of hair follicle. The follicular micropustules are mostly seen in vellus hairs and the inflammation can lead to loss of the vellus hair. The postinflammatory pigmentation in the form of brown hypopigmentation or even mild scarring results into white halo formation.

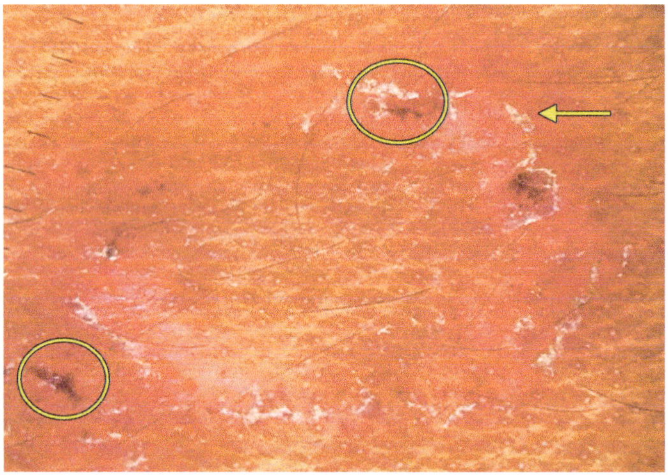

FIG. 12: White scales (arrow) and brown globules (circles) at periphery in tinea corporis (polarized, DermLite DL3, 10×).

Key Points

- Well-defined lesion, with rim of fine scales and mild erythema
- Chronic lesions with crust, intense erythema and hair follicle involvement evident on dermoscopy

Tinea Manuum/Pedis

Clinical Features

Unilateral plaques with well-defined thicker scale at periphery. Erythema is relatively rare (**Fig. 13A**).

Dermoscopic Features

White scales are present in early stages; more prominent in palmar and plantar creases. In steroid modified versions, erythema would be present at the borders unrelated to psoriasis and eczema. It is a diagnosis of exclusion on dermoscopy (**Fig. 13B**).

Key Points

- White scales more prominent in skin creases

Tinea Incognito

Clinical Features

Atypical lesions with varied morphology. They are poorly defined lesions with more erythema and papulovesicles.[22]

Dermoscopic Features

Vellus hair involvement and follicular pustules may be present. Concentric areas of erythema separated by scales are present (**Fig. 14**). Translucent easily deformable hairs that look weakened and transparent, and show bends, are likely due to massive fungal invasion involving the whole hair shaft. Dotted vessels and telangiectasia are also seen on prolonged use of topical steroid.[22]

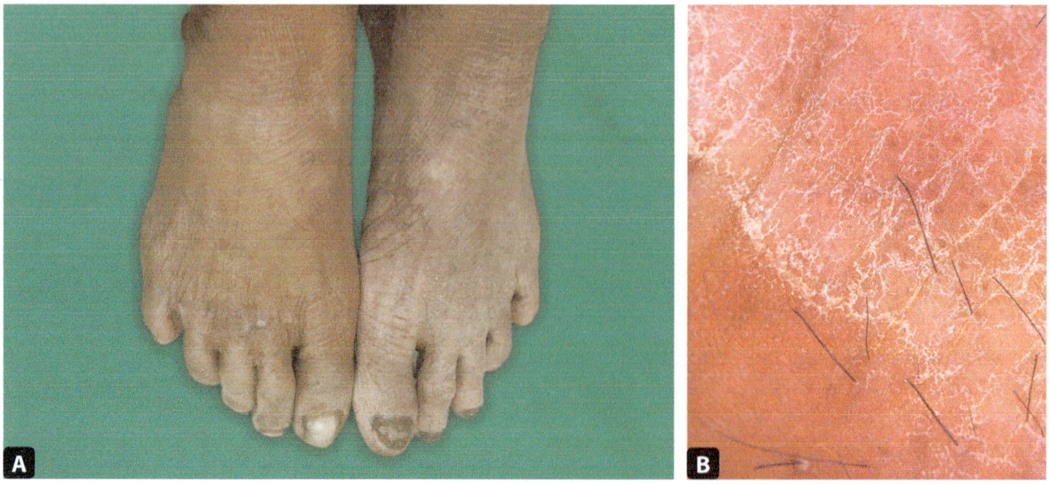

FIGS. 13A AND B: (A) Scaly plaques over the left foot in a case of tinea pedis; (B) Accentuation of scales in the creases in case of tinea.

Key Points

- Vellus hair involvement and follicular pustules
- Concentric areas of erythema, separated by scales

Tinea Unguium

Clinical Features

It may be unilateral or affects few nails. Yellow brown discoloration of nail plate with tunneling may be seen (**Fig. 15A**). Friable debris under nail plate with separation of nail plate from nail bed may be present.[23]

Dermoscopic Features

Spikes and longitudinal striations of different colors (the Aurora Borealis pattern). Proximal jagged edge or frayed distal border of onycholysis is seen versus linear proximal edge in traumatic onycholysis.[23] Ruin-like appearance of subungual hyperkeratosis and debris may be seen (**Fig. 15B**). Pseudoleukonychia with melanonychia and black dots may also be seen.

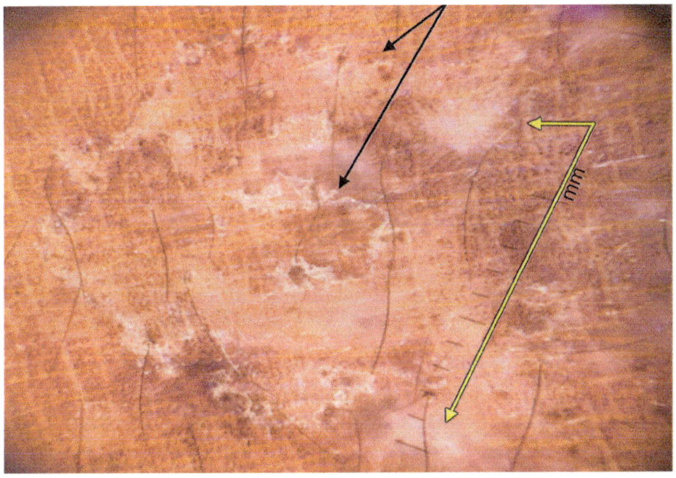

FIG. 14: Chronic steroid modified tinea corporis shows loss of annular definition, concentric areas of erythema and scaling (black arrows), black dots in between and white halo (yellow arrows) (polarized, DermLite DL3, 10×).

Key Points

- Longitudinal striations of different colors
- Jagged distal border

Subcutaneous Fungal Infection

Mycetoma

Clinical Features

It is a chronic infection of subcutaneous tissue caused by fungi (eumycetoma) or filamentous bacteria (actinomycetoma) in which patient presents with minimally painful, gradually progressive swelling involving feet with presence of discharging sinus and grains (**Fig. 16A**).

Dermoscopic Features

Dermoscopy of actinomycetoma shows yellow globules, white scales, red globules, and white structureless areas. Dermoscopy of eumycotic mycetoma shows yellow globules, red structureless areas, white superficial scales, and dotted vessels (**Figs. 16B** and **C**). It is usually difficult to differentiate the two on dermoscopy.[24,25]

Key Points

- Yellow globules, white scales, red globules, and white structureless areas

Sporotrichosis

Clinical Features

Sporotrichosis is a subcutaneous mycosis caused by dimorphic fungus Sporothrix schenckii. It presents with erythematous papules and plaques with or without central ulceration in a sporotrichoid distribution (**Fig. 17A**).

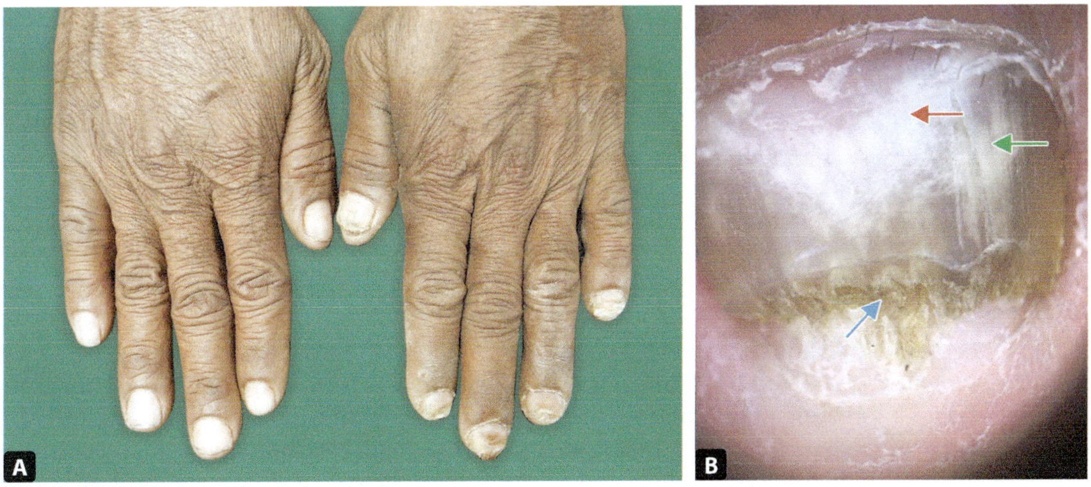

FIGS. 15A AND B: (A) Clinical image of tinea unguium; (B) Dermoscopy of tinea unguium shows jagged edge of proximal margin of onycholytic area (red arrow), white fluffy or cloudy shadow, longitudinal lamellar splitting and micro splitting (green arrow), and subungual hyperkeratosis (blue arrow) (polarized, DermLite DL3, 10×).

Courtesy (Fig. A): Dr Balachandra Ankad, SN Medical College, Bagalkot, Karnataka, India.

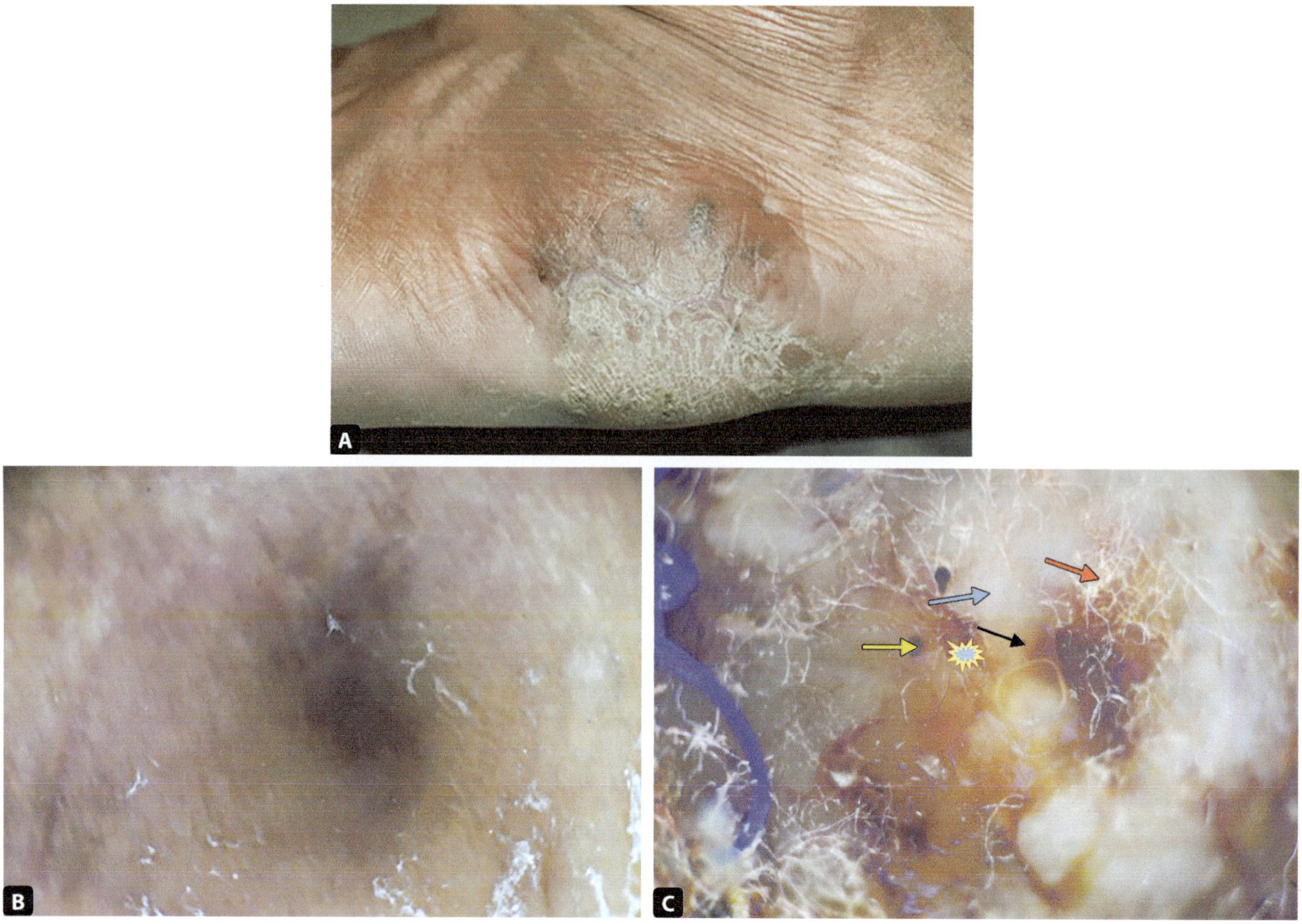

FIGS. 16A TO C: (A) A case of early eumycotic mycetoma on lateral aspect of left foot with superadded hyperkeratosis; (B) Small black grains are clearly visible as structureless blue-gray area related to subcutaneous compact masses of pigmented fungi (polarized, DermLite DL3, 10×); (C) Yellow globules (black arrow), whitish structureless areas (blue arrow), black grains (yellow arrows), white superficial scales (red arrows), and blood spots (yellow and blue star) are seen (polarized, DermLite DL3, 10×).

Dermoscopic Features

Dermoscopy shows yellowish structureless areas, arborizing telangiectasia, and white scar-like areas. Peripheral rim of erythema and red dots (orange arrow) and central ulceration can be seen (**Fig. 17B**).[26]

Key Points

- Yellowish structureless areas, arborizing telangiectasia, and white scar-like areas

Chromoblastomycosis

Clinical Features

It is a chronic cutaneous fungal infection commonly caused by *Fonsecaea* and *Cladophialophora species.* Clinically, it presents as an erythematous papule and nodule progressing to form a verrucous plaque with central clearing usually at the site of inoculation by foreign material (**Fig. 18A**).

Dermoscopic Features

Irregular blackish red dots which correspond to the black dots observed clinically. These represent transepithelial elimination of the inflammatory cells and fungal elements along with hemorrhage. White and pink areas, and scale and crust with white background with yellowish-orange ovoid structures representing the granulomas are found (**Fig. 18B**).[27,28]

Key Points

- White background with yellowish-orange ovoid structures, and scale and crust

Protozoal Infections

Cutaneous Leishmaniasis

Clinical Features

Leishmaniasis is a protozoal disease caused by Leishmania sp. and transmitted by sand fly vectors. The typical evolution of cutaneous leishmaniasis (CL) begins with reddish infiltrated papules that can evolve to form tender nodules (**Fig. 19A**). Nodules can progress to form ulcerative lesions with a central depression and raised indurated border which can finally heal with an atrophic scar.

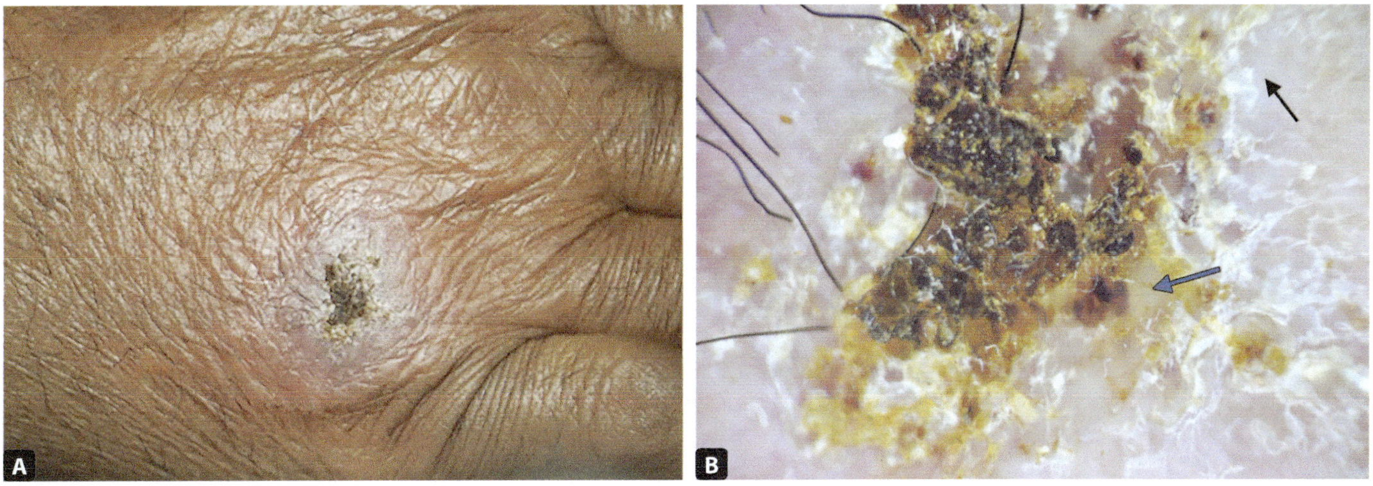

FIGS. 17A AND B: (A) Fixed cutaneous sporotrichosis showing hyperkeratotic crusted erythematous plaque on dorsum of hand; (B) Yellowish structureless areas (blue arrow), crusting, and white scar-like areas (black arrow) (polarized, DermLite DL3, 10×).

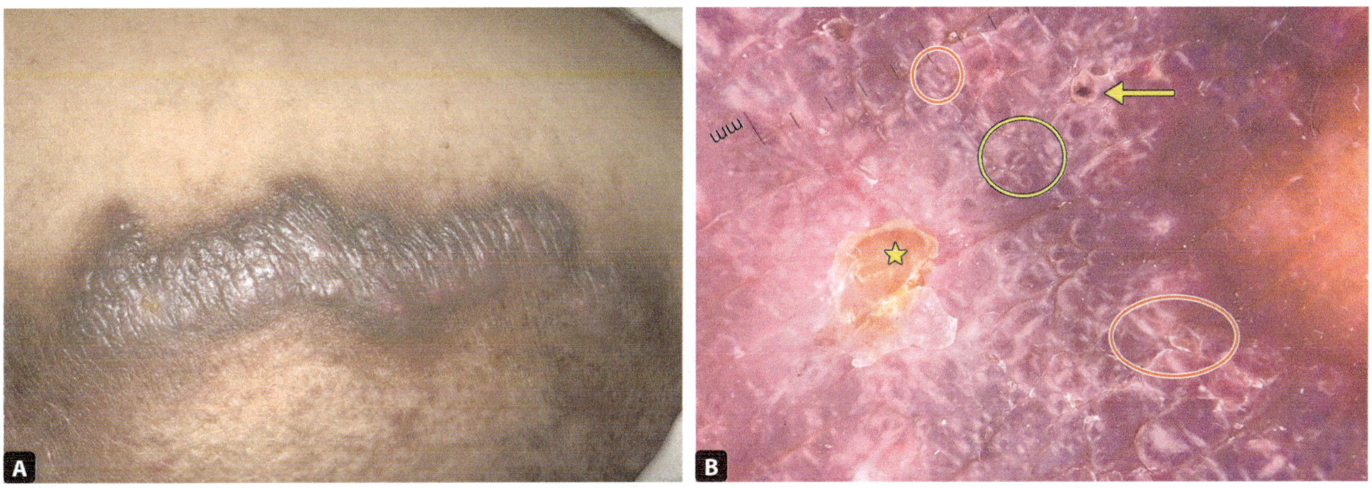

FIGS. 18A AND B: (A) Clinical image of chromoblastomycosis showing infiltrated and verrucous plaque; (B) Dermoscopy shows white chrysalis-like structures (red circles), black dots (yellow arrow), and crusting (yellow star) and dotted vessels (yellow circle) (polarized, DermLite DL4, 10×).

Courtesy: Dr Sneha Gandhi, Consultant Dermatologist, Karnal, Haryana, India.

Dermoscopic Features

Most common dermoscopic feature seen in almost 100% cases is generalized erythema. Vascular structures comprising of linear irregular, hairpin, and comma-shaped patterns can be seen. "Yellow tears" which are yellow structures with an oval and/or tear-drop form correspond histopathologically to follicular plugs due to the lateral compression of follicular openings from the tumoral lesion growth (**Fig. 19B**). White starburst-like pattern due to the parakeratotic hyperkeratosis surrounding the erosion can be seen in lesions with central ulceration.[29,30]

Parasitic Infections

Scabies

Clinical Features

It is a condition caused by mite, *Sarcoptes scabiei*, and is characterized by excoriations and papules over the axilla, groins, wrists, nipples, periumbilical areas, and web spaces of the fingers and toes (**Figs. 20A** and **C**).

Dermoscopic Features

The characteristic dermoscopic signs of classical scabies are as follows:[31-33]

- Delta wing jet with contrail sign (triangle sign, delta glider, delta wing jet, jet plane, jet liner with trail)[1,2]

  Dermoscopic examination at higher magnification of 40X shows small black triangular structures with a linear segment below the base of the triangular structure resembling a jet with contrail. Microscopically, the jet-shaped triangular structure corresponds to the anterior part of the mite (mouth and anterior pair of legs). The contrail represents the burrow containing eggs and feces of the mite (**Figs. 20B** and **D**).
- *Classic S-shaped burrow*: A curvilinear trail of whitish-yellow scale with multiple brown dots which represent mites' fecal pellets[2]

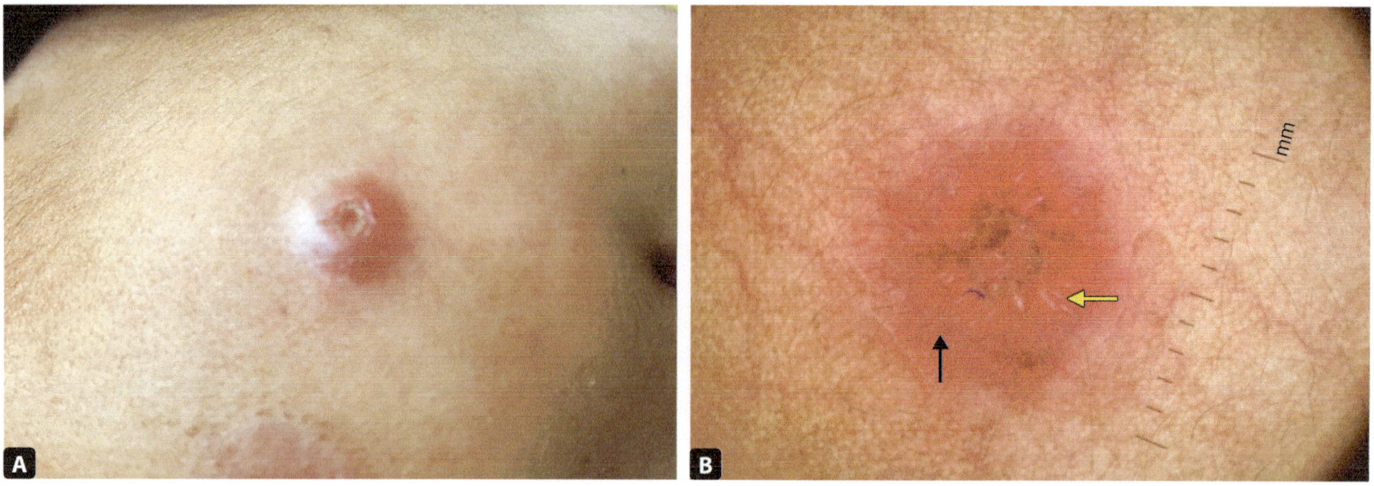

FIGS. 19A AND B: (A) Infiltrated nodule on face in a case of cutaneous leishmaniasis; (B) Dermoscopy shows linear vessels (black arrow), white starburst like pattern (yellow arrow) in a background of erythema (polarized, DermLite DL3, 10×).
Courtesy: Dr Yasmeen J Bhat, Associate Professor, Department of Dermatology, GMC, Srinagar, Jammu and Kashmir, India.

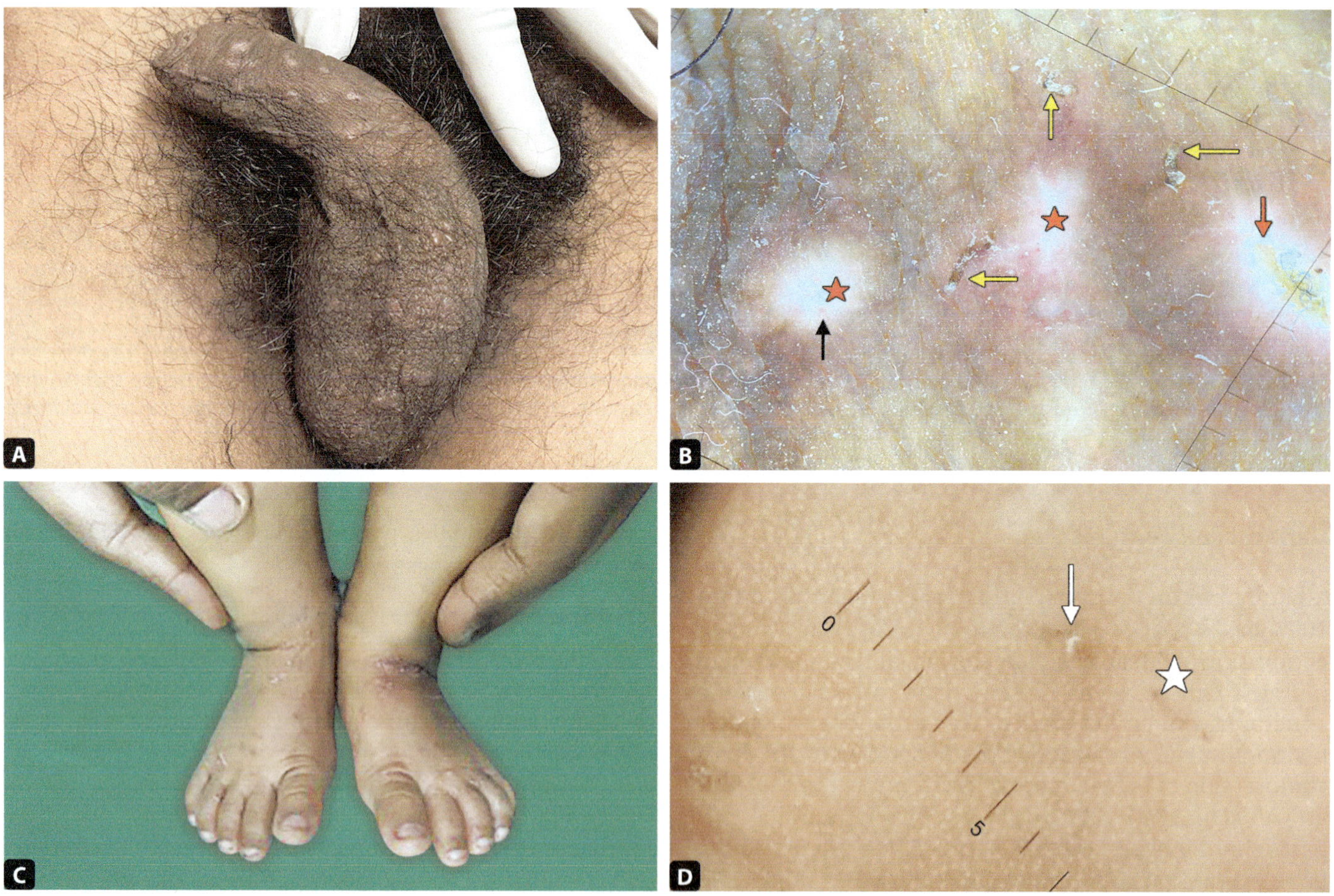

FIGS. 20A TO D: (A) Excoriated papules and nodules on the genital area in scabies; (B) Dermoscopic image of scabies showing burrow as curvilinear structures (yellow arrows), white areas (red stars), mild scaling (red arrow), and red dots (black arrow) (polarized, FotoFinder Handyscope, 10×); (C) Multiple excoriated and scaly papules, few pustules over the foot in a case of scabies; (D) Dermoscopic image showing delta wing jet with contrail appearance (arrow) and the classic S-shaped burrow (star) (polarized, Heine Delta 20T, 10×).
Courtesy (Figs. A and B): Dr Balachandra Ankad, SN Medical College, Bagalkot, Karnataka, India.

- *Mini triangle sign*: Mature scabetic eggs showing minute heads of maturing mite within the eggs
- *Noodle sign*: Characterized by presence of several (hundreds) of burrows seen in the same dermoscopic field in a noodle-like pattern[3] in crusted scabies

Limitations of Dermoscopy in the Diagnosis of Scabies

- Differentiation of jetliner sign from excoriations and artefacts caused as a result of scratching is difficult especially while using lower magnification.
- It is not possible to visualize eggs and feces of the mite in low magnification
- Typical jetliner sign is usually not visible in heavily pigmented skin or in hairy body areas

Key Points

- Delta wing jet with contrail sign (the jet-shaped triangular structure corresponds to the anterior part of the mite and the contrail represents the burrow filled with eggs and feces of the mite)
- Classic S-shaped burrow is represented by a curvilinear trail of scale.

Pediculosis

Clinical Features

Pediculosis capitis caused by pediculus humanus var capitis is characterized by focal erythema, excoriations, and erosions and crusting over the scalp. Pthirus pubis (crab louse) infestation presents with slate gray to bluish irregularly shaped macules known as maculae ceruleae.

Dermoscopic Features

Identification of nits attached to the hair shafts. The different stages of identification of nits are as follows:[34]

- Active viable nits appear as ovoid whitish brown structures with tense convex wall and intact closed operculum containing viable eggs. They are found close to the scalp surface (**Fig. 21A**).
- Abortive nits appear as ovoid, relatively translucent structure which is nonviable.
- Empty nits are seen as whitish crystalline translucent structure without an operculum and are located furthest from the scalp.[1]

Nits must be differentiated from pseudonits (dandruff, hair casts, and hair spray or gel residues) which appear as bizarre whitish structures not attached to the hair shafts. Identification of adult lice is easy with dermoscopy (**Fig. 21B**).

Key Points

- Dermoscopy helps in the diagnosis of pediculosis by identification of nits and lice.
- Aids in the assessment of treatment efficacy, treatment compliance, and for screening household contacts

Demodicidosis or Demodicosis

Clinical Features

Demodicidosis is caused by an obligate human ectoparasite demodex mite. The different clinical manifestations of demodicidosis include diffuse erythema, nut-meg grater-like appearance (**Fig. 22A**), follicular scales, rosacea-like lesions, perioral dermatitis, pustular eruptions, and blepharitis.

Dermoscopic Features

"Demodex tails" are creamy whitish gelatinous thread-like structures which occur due to the presence of mites and keratotic material in the follicle (**Fig. 22B**). "Demodex follicular openings" are characterized by dilated follicular openings with grayish brown plugs surrounded by erythematous halo. Other nonspecific findings include reticular dilated blood vessels, diffuse erythema, scaling, and pustules depending on the clinical subtype of demodicidosis.[35,36]

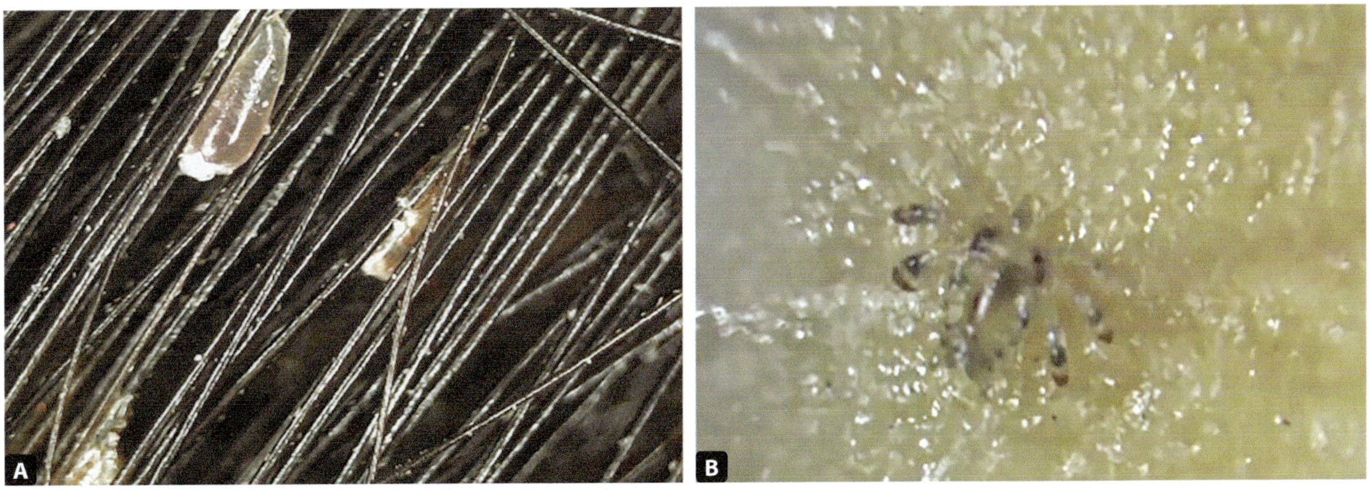

FIGS. 21A AND B: (A) Dermoscopic image showing brownish nits attached to the hair shaft (polarized, Escope Oitez, 10×); (B) Dermoscopic image of adult louse (polarized, Escope Oitez, 10×).

Courtesy (Fig. B): Dr Sweta Rambhia, Consultant Dermatologist, Just Care Skin Clinic, Malad, Mumbai, Maharashtra, India.

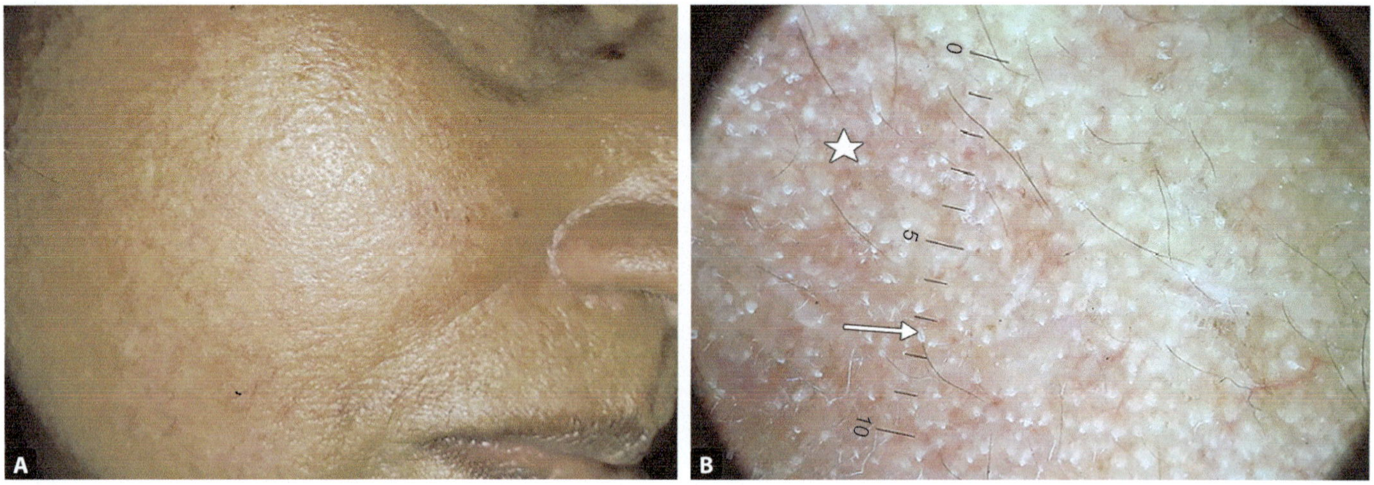

FIGS. 22A AND B: (A) Clinical picture showing nutmeg grater appearance of the face in demodicidosis; (B) Dermoscopic picture showing creamy white gelatinous thread-like structures emanating from the follicle (arrow). Note the diffuse erythema and dilated vessels (star) (polarized, Heine Delta 20T, 10×).

Key Points

- Demodex tails are visualized as creamy white thread-like structures emanating from the follicle.
- Dilated follicular openings with plugging, diffuse erythema, scaling, and pustules may be seen in demodicidosis.

VIRAL INFECTIONS

Viral Warts

Common Warts (or Verruca Vulgaris)

Clinical Features

Circumscribed firm papules with verrucous surface[15,37-39]

Dermoscopic Features

Well-defined group of whitish or off-white or skin-colored densely packed papilla, with central black or red dots (normal or thrombosed vessels). These dots and haloes are surrounded by an off-white or light brown band or rim. This rim represents the keratotic halo we see on naked eye examination (**Fig. 23**). This rim represents papillomatosis on histopathology.[15,37-39]

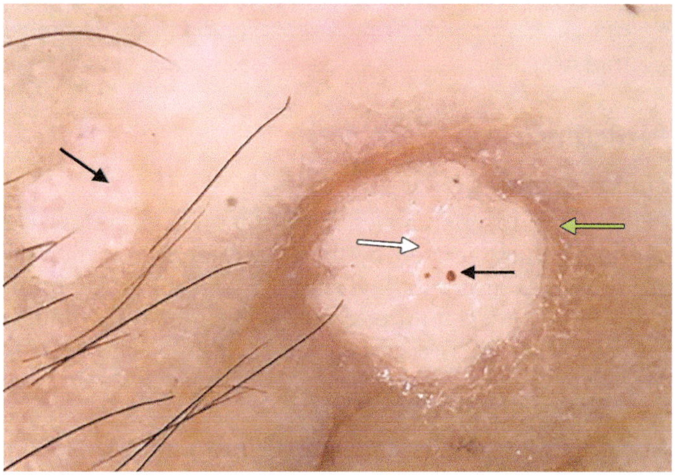

FIG. 23: Common wart shows group of densely packed papilla (white arrow), containing thrombosed vessels (black arrows) surrounded by keratotic halo (green arrow) (polarized, DermLite DL3, 10×).

Filiform Warts

Clinical Features

Thin elongated firm projections arising from a horny base (**Fig. 24A**).[15,37-39]

Dermoscopic Features

Fingerlike or knoblike projections. Each projection with a whitish or off-white top represents hyperkeratosis on histopathology, and a flesh-colored or translucent base or stalk-containing hairpin vessels (**Fig. 24B**). It presents as one of the most beautiful pictures on dermoscopy tempting us to name it as the "*Viral cauliflower.*"[15,37-39]

Verruca Plana

Clinical Features

Skin-colored to hyperpigmented flat smooth papules with a velvety surface.[15,37-39]

Dermoscopic Features

Reddish brown dots over a well-defined light brown or flesh-colored background and irregular pseudo-sieve appearance, typically sparing hair follicles. Red dots represent apices of capillaries in the papillary dermis (**Fig. 25**).[15,37-39]

Genital Warts

Clinical Features

Varied clinical presentation varying from sessile flat papules resembling verruca plana to grouped soft to firm finger-like projections.[15,37-39]

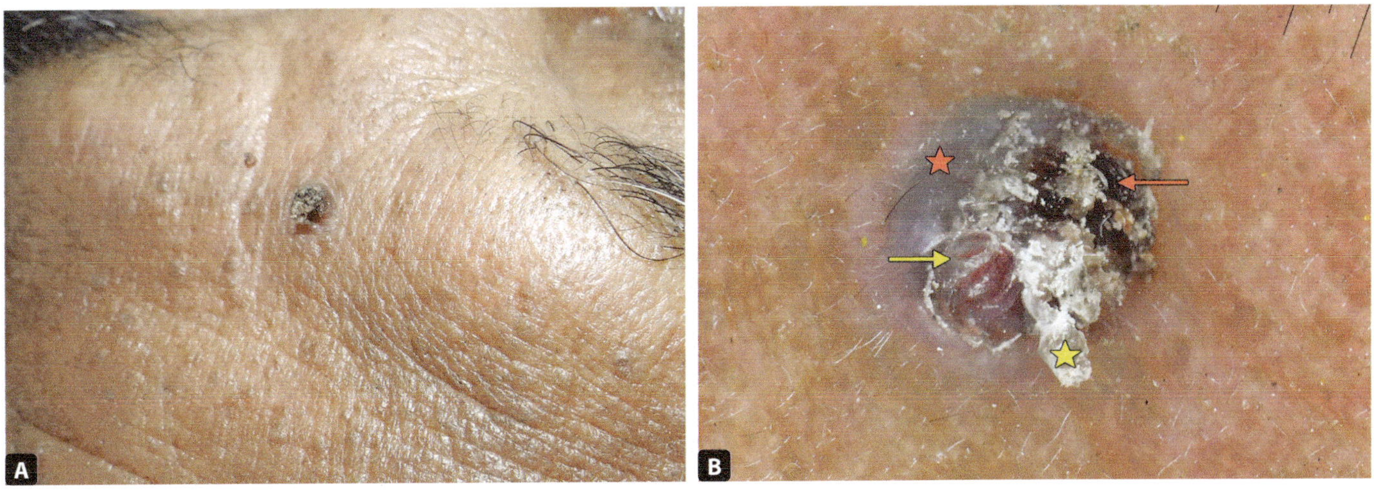

FIGS. 24A AND B: (A) Clinical image of filiform wart shows finger-like projections from a single base; (B) Dermoscopy of filiform wart shows linear vessels with halo (yellow arrow), grayish base (red star), white scale (yellow star), and dried hemorrhage (red arrow) (polarized, DermLite Foto II Pro, 10×).

Courtesy: Dr Balachandra Ankad, SN Medical College, Bagalkot, Karnataka, India.

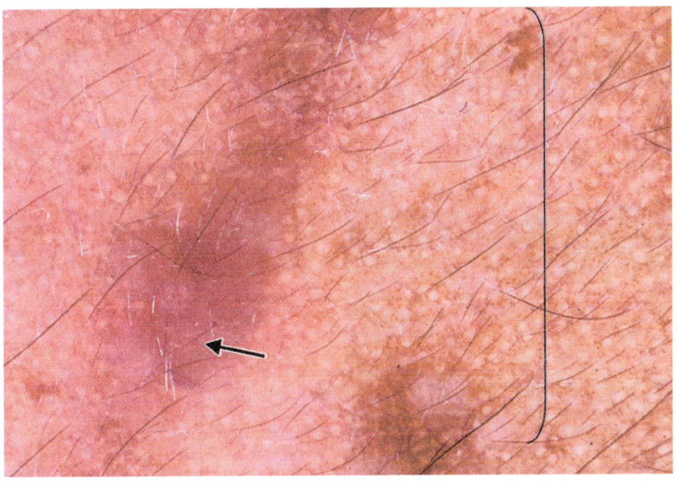

FIG. 25: Verruca plana shows regularly placed red/black dots (black arrow), on a flesh-colored background. Note the linearly placed homogenous structures, interrupted in between by normal skin (bracket: depicting the pseudo Koebner phenomenon) (polarized, DermLite DL3, 10×).

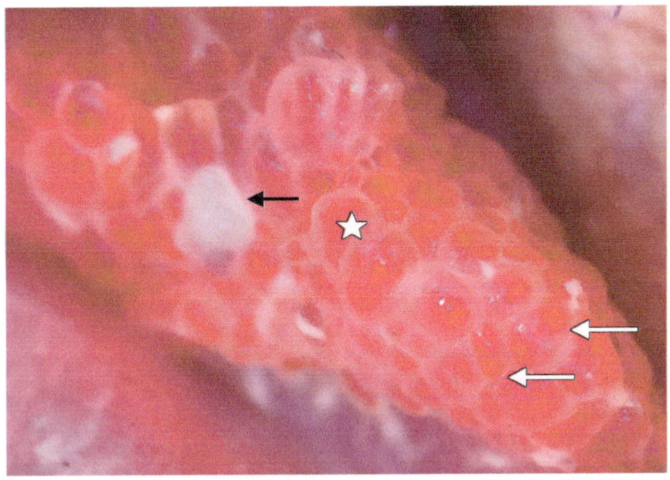

FIG. 26: Knob-like projections (white star) containing glomerular (white arrows) and hair pin vessels with keratotic top "Stalactites" (black arrow) (polarized, DermLite DL3, 10×).

Dermoscopic Features

Mosaic knoblike or fingerlike projections with combination of glomerular and hairpin vessels inside these projections (vs. dotted or pin point vessels in other types of viral warts). The keratotic top can be described as showing a "stalactite appearance" (author's own metaphor to describe the lesions) (**Fig. 26**).[15,37-39]

Plantar Warts

Clinical Features

Well-defined hyperkeratotic papules and plaques with multiple small tightly packed warts, surrounded by a horny collar and interspersed by reddish-black dots in between.[15,37-39]

Dermoscopy

Irregularly distributed and grooved reddish-black dots (due to high pressure on plantar vasculature) with yellow halo (**Fig. 27**).

Dermoscopic Differential

Corn: Translucent central core surrounded by white rim without any hemorrhagic dots without any breakage of dermatoglyphics. Callosity: Yellow homogeneous opacity.[15,37-39]

Key Points

- Finger-like or papillomatous structures
- Reddish-black dots
- Glomerular or hair pin-like vessels in genital warts

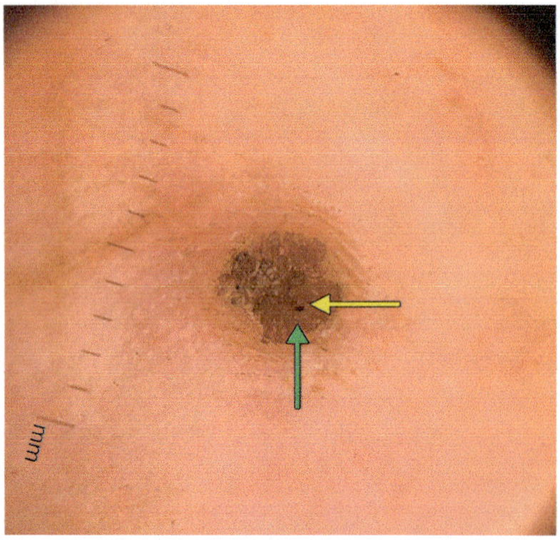

FIG. 27: Plantar wart shows irregularly distributed reddish-black dots (yellow arrow) surrounded by keratotic halo (green arrow) with distinct disruption of dermatoglyphics (polarized, DermLite DL3, 10×).

Molluscum Contagiosum

Clinical Features

Smooth dome-shaped pearly white papule mostly with a central umbilication (**Fig. 28A**).

Dermoscopic Features

Central pore on a whitish to yellowish amorphous area often surrounded by thin crown vessels (represents inverted lobules of hyperplastic squamous epithelium occupied by molluscum bodies). Crown vessels are blood vessels arranged radially or peripherally which do not cross the midline (**Figs. 28B** and **C**) (represents dermal vessels which do not cross the midline).[40]

Always examine a few lesions as they are in different stages of development and a single lesion may not have all the features. Three types of central white structures in relation to size, duration and histopathology; (1) Classic central roundish white area, (2) small and young lesions:

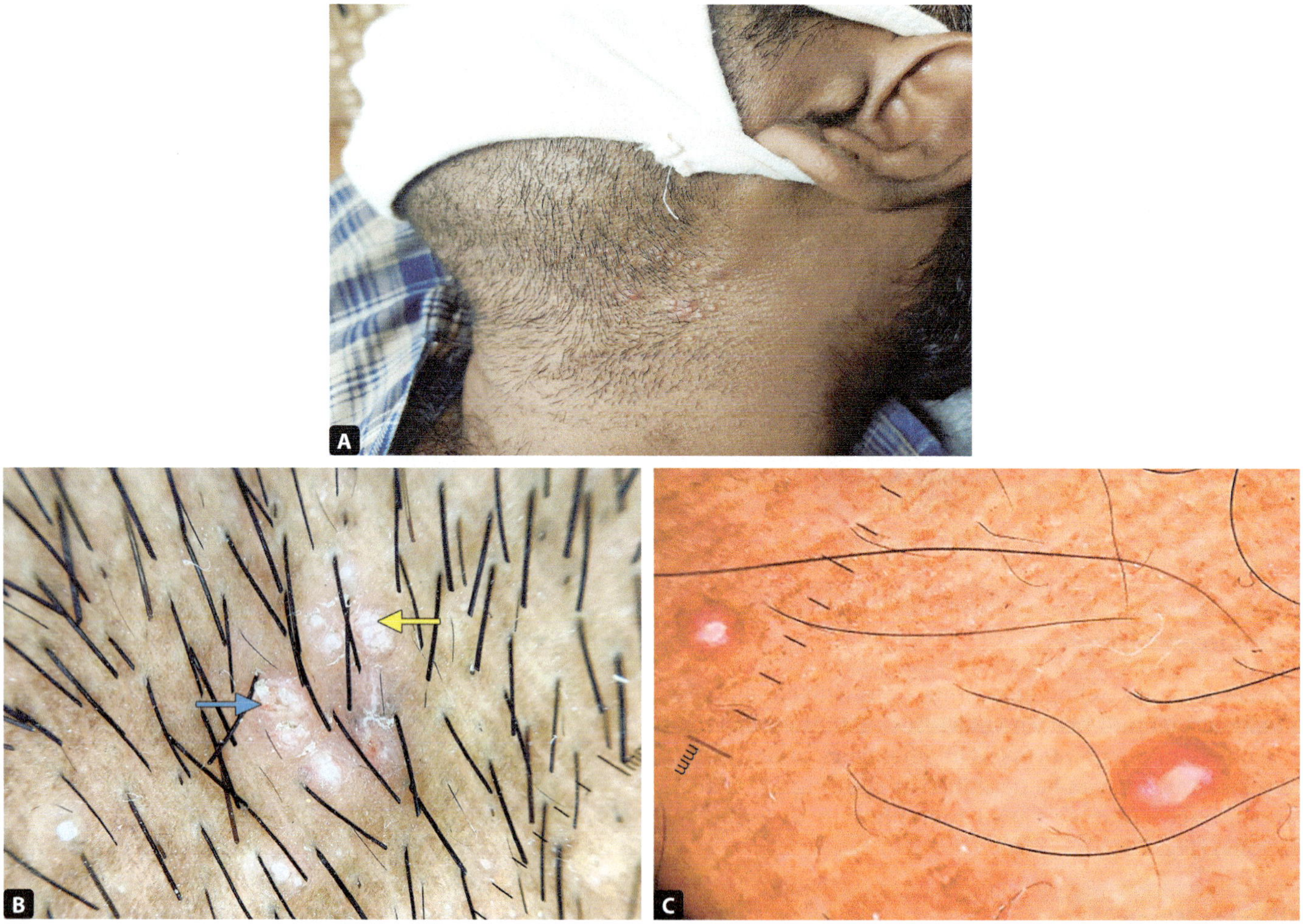

FIGS. 28A TO C: (A) Multiple skin-colored and whitish papules over the mandibular area in a case of molluscum contagiosum; (B) Dermoscopy of molluscum contagiosum shows white globular structures (yellow arrow) and peripheral linear vessels (blue arrow) (polarized, Illuco, ×10); (C) Central pore on a whitish amorphous area. Crown vessels arranged peripherally which do not cross the midline (polarized, DermLite DL3, 10×).

Courtesy (Figs. A and B) : Dr Balachandra Ankad, SN Medical College, Bagalkot, Karnataka, India.

4 clover leaf-like structural appearance (rosettes), and (3) large and old lesions: Polylobular.

Key Points

- Central white amorphous area
- Surrounded by crown vessels which do not cross the midline

KEY POINTS

- Dermoscopy is a noninvasive, quick tool for the diagnosis of dermatological infections.
- It is a reliable method to monitor response to treatment especially in conditions like scabies and pediculosis.

CONCLUSION

Dermoscopy is a useful tool for the diagnosis of infections and infestations, especially scabies and pediculosis. Routine dermoscopic examination at every visit may also be used for monitoring response to treatment.

ACKNOWLEDGEMENT

Dr Major Richa Kumar, Graded Specialist (Dermatology), Command Hospital (Eastern Command), Kolkata, West Bengal, India.

REFERENCES

1. Chatterjee M, Neema S. Dermatoscopy of infections and infestations. Indian Dermatol Online J. 2021;12(1):14-23.
2. Durdu M, Errichetti E, Eskiocak AH, Ilkit M. High accuracy of recognition of common forms of folliculitis by dermoscopy: An observational study. J Am Acad Dermatol. 2019;81(2):463-71.
3. Nayak SS, Mehta HH, Gajjar PC, Nimbark VN. Dermoscopy of general dermatological conditions in Indian population: A descriptive study. Clin Dermatol Rev. 2017;1:41-51.
4. Sharma S, Verma KK. Skin and soft tissue infection. Indian J Pediatr. 2001;68 Suppl 3:S46-50.
5. Kaliyadan F, Kuruvilla J, Al Ojail HY, Quadri SA. Clinical and dermoscopic study of pseudofolliculitis of the beard area. Int J Trichology. 2016;8(1):40-2.
6. Chuh A, Zawar V. Epiluminescence dermatoscopy enhanced patient compliance and achieved treatment success in pseudofolliculitis barbae. Australas J Dermatol. 2006;47(1):60-2.
7. Rojas Mora E, Freites Martínez A, Hernández-Núñez A, Actas BMJ. Trichomycosis axillaris: Clinical, Wood lamp, and dermoscopic diagnostic images. Dermosifiliogr 2017;108(3):264-66.
8. Lockwood LL, Gehrke S, Navarini AA. Dermoscopy of pitted keratolysis. Case Rep Dermatol. 2010;2(2):146-8.
9. Ankad BS, Sakhare PS. Dermoscopy of borderline tuberculoid leprosy. Int J Dermatol. 2018;57(1):74-6.
10. Errichetti E, Stinco G. Dermatoscopy of granulomatous disorders. Dermatol Clin. 2018;36(4):369-75.
11. Brasiello M, Zalaudek I, Ferrara G, Gourhant JY, Capoluongo P, Roma P, et al. Lupus vulgaris: a new look at an old symptom--the lupoma observed with dermoscopy. Dermatology. 2009;218(2):172-4.
12. Lallas A, Argenziano G, Apalla Z, Gourhant JY, Zaballos P, Di Lernia V, et al. Dermoscopic patterns of common facial inflammatory skin diseases. J Eur Acad Dermatol Venereol. 2014;28(5):609-14.
13. Kaur I, Jakhar D, Singal A. Dermoscopy in the evaluation of pityriasis versicolor: A cross sectional study. Indian Dermatol Online J. 2019;10(6):682-5.
14. Malakar S, Pal A. Infectious dermatoses. In: Dermoscopy Text and Atlas, 1st edition. New Delhi: Jaypee Brothers Medical Publishers; 2019. pp. 148-81.
15. Mapelli ET, Gualandri L, Cerri A, Menni S. Comma hairs in tinea capitis: a useful dermatoscopic sign for diagnosis of tinea capitis. Pediatr Dermatol. 2012;29(2):223-4.
16. Hughes R, Chiaverini C, Bahadoran P, Lacour JP. Corkscrew hair: a new dermoscopic sign for diagnosis of tinea capitis in black children. Arch Dermatol. 2011;147(3):355-6.
17. Lin YT, Li YC. The dermoscopic comma, zigzag and barcode like hairs markers of fungal infection of the hair follicles. Dermatologica Sinica. 2014;32:160-3.
18. Wang HH, Lin YT. Barcode-like hair: Dermoscopic marker of taenia capitis and taenia of the of the eyebrow. J Am Acad Dermatol. 2015;72(1 Suppl):S41-2.
19. Lu M, Ran Y, Dai Y, Lei S, Zhang C, Zhuang K, et al. An ultrastructural study on corkscrew hairs and cigarette-ash-shaped hairs observed by dermoscopy of tinea capitis. Scanning. 2016;38(2):128-32.
20. Rudnicka L, Szepietowski JC, Slowinska M, Lukomska M, Maj M, Pinheiro AMC. Tinea capitis. In: Rudnicka L, Olszewka M, Ralowska A, (eds). Atlas of Trichoscopy. London: Springer; 2012. p. 367.
21. Bhat Y, Keen A, Hassan I, Latif I, Bashir S. Can dermoscopy serve as a diagnostic tool in dermatophytosis? A pilot study. Indian Dermatol Online J. 2019;10(5):530-5.
22. Ankad BS, Reshme AS, Nikam BP, Drago ND. Dermoscopic differentiation of pustular psoriasis and tinea incognito. Clin Dermatol Rev. 2020;4(2):136-40.
23. Piraccini BM, Balestri R, Starace M, Rech G. Nail digital dermoscopy (onychoscopy) in the diagnosis of onychomycosis. J Eur Acad Dermatol Venerol. 2013;27(4):509-13.
24. Ankad BS, Manjula R, Tejasvi T, Nikam BP. Dermoscopy of eumycotic mycetoma: A case report. Dermatol Pract Concept. 2019;9(4):297-9.
25. Ankad BS, Beergoudar SL, Nikam BP. Dermatoscopy in actinomycetoma: An observation. Indian Dermatol Online J. 2019;10(3):330-31.
26. Dabas G, Kaur H, Vinay K, Kumaran MS, Shivaprakash MR, Saikia UN, et al. Dermoscopy in disseminated sporotrichosis. J Eur Acad Dermatol Venereol. 2019;33(1):e33-5.
27. Subhadarshani S, Yadav D. Dermoscopy of chromoblastomycosis. Dermatol Pract Concept. 2017;7(4):23-24.
28. Chauhan P, Jindal R, Shirazi N. Dermoscopy of chromoblastomycosis. Indian Dermatol Online J. 2019;10(6):759-60.
29. Llambrich A, Zaballos P, Terrasa F, Torne I, Puig S, Malvehy J. Dermoscopy of cutaneous leishmaniasis. Br J Dermatol. 2009;160(4):756-61.
30. Serarslan G, Ekiz Ö, Özer C, Sarıkaya G. Dermoscopy in the diagnosis of cutaneous leishmaniasis. Dermatol Pract Concept. 2019;9(2):111-18.
31. Grover C, Jakhar D. Dermoscopy in the diagnosis of scabies. Int J Dermoscope. 2017;1(2):67-8.
32. Park JH, Kim CW, Kim SS. The diagnostic accuracy of dermoscopy for scabies. Ann Dermatol. 2012;24(2):194-9.
33. Chavez-Alvarez S, Villarreal-Martinez A, Argenziano G, Ancer-Arellano J, Ocampo-Candiani J. Noodle pattern: a new dermoscopic pattern for crusted scabies (Norwegian scabies). J Eur Acad Dermatol Venereol. 2018;32(2): e46-7.
34. Gupta V, Sonthalia S, Bhat YJ, Langar S, Bossiela M. Inflammatory and infectious conditions. In: Lallas A, Errichetti E, Ionnides D, (eds). Dermoscopy in general Dermatology, 1st edition. London: CRC Press; 2018. pp. 295-309.
35. Sonthalia S, Agrawal M, Bhatia J, Zeeshan M, Elsamanoudy S, Tiwary P et al. Entomodermoscopy update: A contemporary review on dermoscopy of cutaneous infections and infestations. Indian Dermatol Online J. 2021;12(2):220-36.
36. Segal R, Mimouni D, Feuerman H, Pagovitz O, David M. Dermoscopy as a diagnostic tool in demodicidosis. Int J Dermatol. 2010;49(9):101-23.
37. Dong H, Shu D, Campbell TM, Frühauf J, Soyer HP, Hofmann-Wellenhof R. Dermatoscopy of genital warts. J Am Acad Dermatol. 2011;64(5):859-64.
38. Marcucci C, Sabban EC, Friedman P, Peralta R, Calb I, Cabo H. Dermoscopic findings in Bowenoid papulosis: report of two cases. Dermatol Pract Concept. 2014;4(4):61-3.
39. Bañuls J, Arribas P, Berbegal L, DeLeón FJ, Francés L, Zaballos P. Yellow and orange in cutaneous lesions: clinical and dermoscopic data. J Eur Acad Dermatol Venereol. 2015;29(12):2317-25.
40. Piccolo V. Update on dermoscopy and infectious skin diseases. Dermatol Pract Concept. 2019;10(1):e2020003.

8 CHAPTER

Hyperpigmented Dermatoses

Niti Khunger, Anuradha Bishnoi, Anuradha Jindal, Aswath Rajan

INTRODUCTION

Basics of Dermoscopy of Pigmentary Lesions

The two most important features in dermoscopy are color and structures.[1] Color indicates the depth of the lesion and structure indicates the development of the lesion. Structures can be arranged in various patterns.[2]

Color

Melanin is the most important chromophore in depicting the color of pigmented skin lesions. Depending on the concentration of melanin and its anatomic location, the colors range from black, dark brown, light brown, gray and blue secondary to Tyndall effect (**Fig. 1**).

Structural Elements

The basic structural elements are lines, dots, globules, blotches, clods, streaks that include pseudopod and radial streaming, circle and structureless areas.[3] Pattern is defined as the multiple repetition of single basic structure/element in a particular fashion. Pattern of lines can be reticular, branched, parallel, radial, and curved to name a few (**Fig. 2**).[4]

Patterns

Structural elements arranged in various patterns can be a clue to diagnosis. The pigment network consists of intersecting pigmented lines forming a honeycomb-like appearance (**Fig. 3A**).[3] It may be interrupted by skin markings as seen on the dorsa of the hands. Pseudonetwork

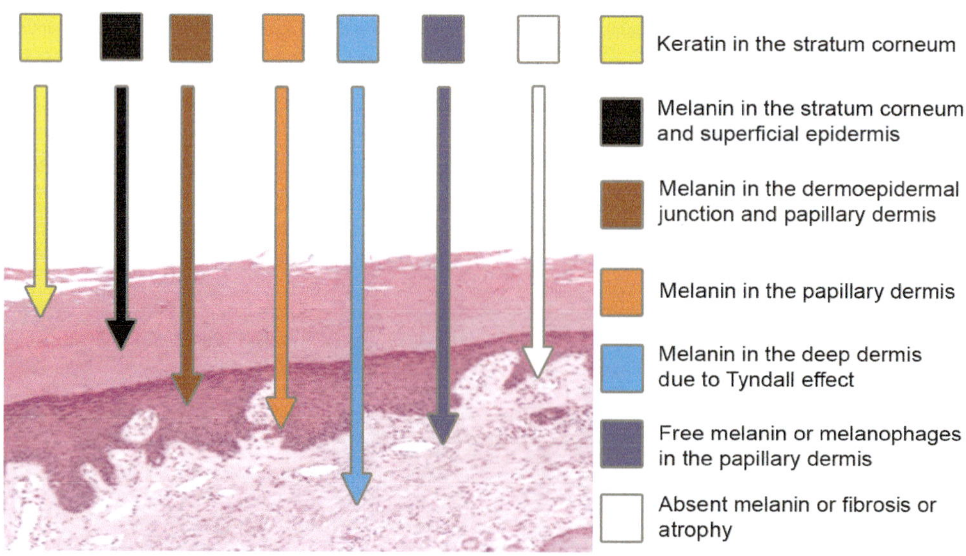

FIG. 1: Color of pigmented lesions depends on the location of melanin in the skin. Black (stratum corneum), dark brown (superficial epidermis), light brown (dermoepidermal junction), gray (papillary dermis), and blue (reticular dermis).

is the normal pattern observed on the face. As the rete ridges are absent or blunted on the face, the true network pattern is not seen but a reticular-like pattern is observed secondary to the adnexal opening of hair follicles and sweat glands appearing as holes (hypomelanotic areas) on the background of diffuse pigmentation forming pseudonetwork (**Fig. 3B**).[4] In the reverse network, relatively lighter areas comprise the grid, filled with relatively darker areas. Parallel pattern is seen in acral lesions and can be of various types such as parallel furrow, fibrillar, lattice-like and parallel ridge pattern (**Fig. 4**).[4]

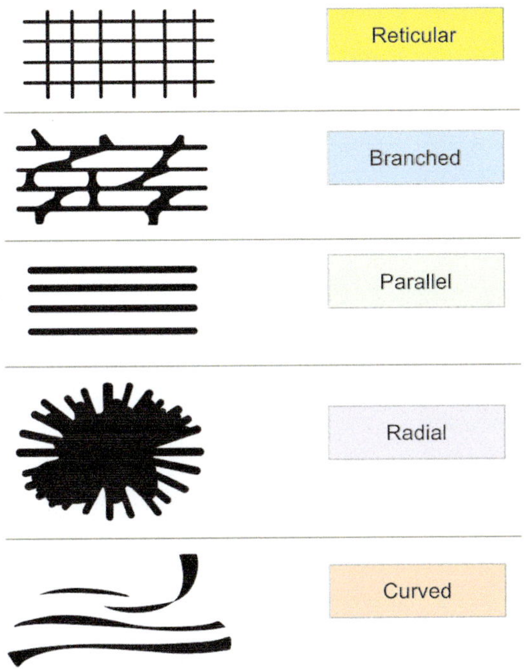

FIG. 2: Schematic diagram of various patterns of lines.

DERMOSCOPIC FEATURES OF HYPERPIGMENTED DERMATOSES

Hyperpigmented dermatoses are common in darker skin types and dermoscopy plays a valuable role not only in diagnosis, but also in selection of therapy, follow-up, and prognosis. This chapter deals with common hyperpigmented disorders.[5]

Pigmented lesions can be clinically divided into focal, patterned, and diffuse pigmented dermatoses for a systematic approach.

FOCAL PIGMENTATION

Freckles

Clinical Features

The term ephelides is derived from Greek word "epi" (upon) and "helios" (sun), depicting inevitable role of sunlight as causative factor. They are most commonly seen as circumscribed, small macules, usually around 5 mm in diameter, pale brown in color solely on the sun-exposed skin, with a clear demarcation line between the freckle and the normal skin (**Fig. 5**).

Dermoscopic Features

Dermoscopy of freckles shows brown uniform pigmented network and pseudonetwork with moth-eaten edges at the border (**Fig. 6**). The color and pattern are more subtle as compared to lentigines.[6] In histopathology, mild hyperpigmentation of basal keratinocytes is seen with normal architecture, without increase in number of melanocytes.

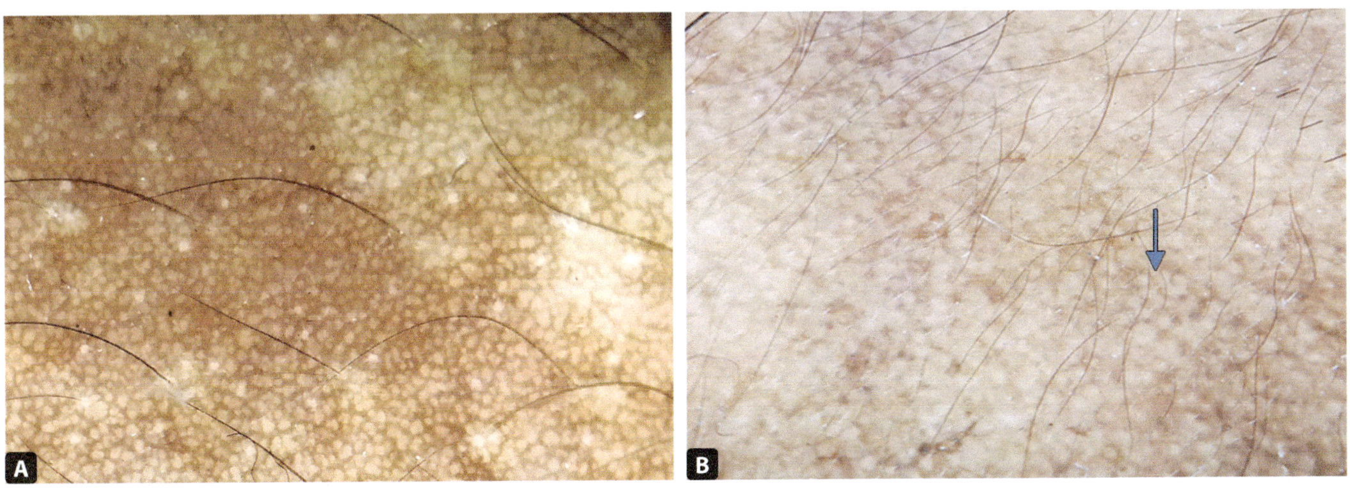

FIGS. 3A AND B: (A) Dermoscopic image of normal skin over dorsum of hand showing the interrupted reticular pattern by skin markings (polarized, Heine Delta T20, 10×); (B) Pseudonetwork on the face with a pseudo reticular pattern, secondary to the adnexal opening of follicles and eccrine glands appearing as holes (polarized, Heine Delta T20, 10×).

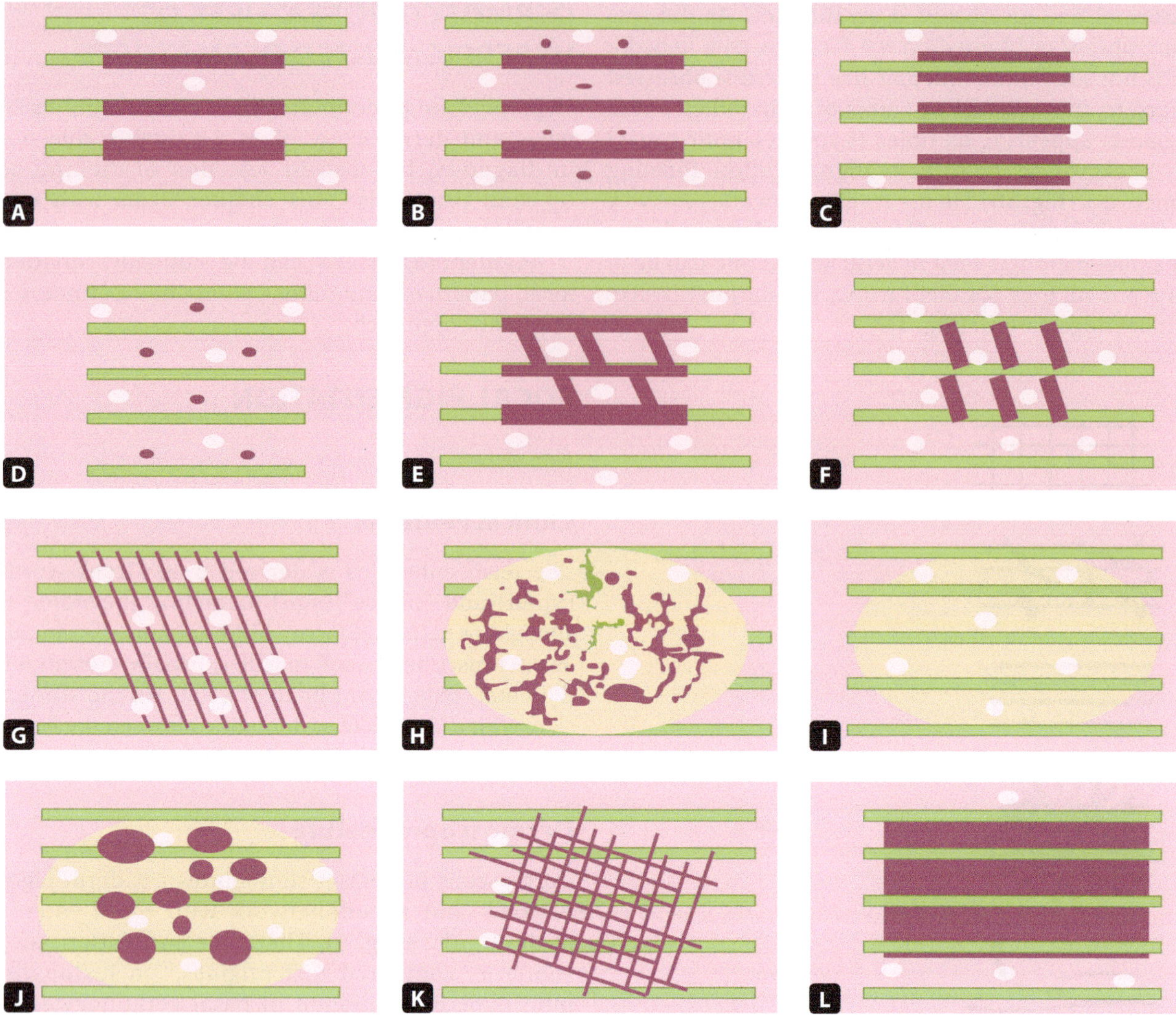

FIGS. 4A TO L: Pigment patterns in acral lesions: (A) Parallel furrow; (B) Fibrillar; (C) Lattice-like; (D) Parallel ridge; (E) Lattice like; (F) Fibrillar; (G) Filamentous; (H) Non typical; (I) Homogenous; (J) Globular; (K) Acral reticular; and (L) Parallel ridge pattern.

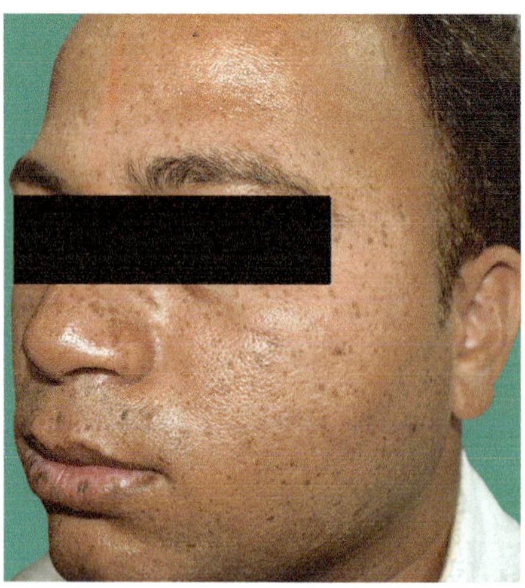

FIG. 5: Clinical image of freckles seen as circumscribed, small brown macules.

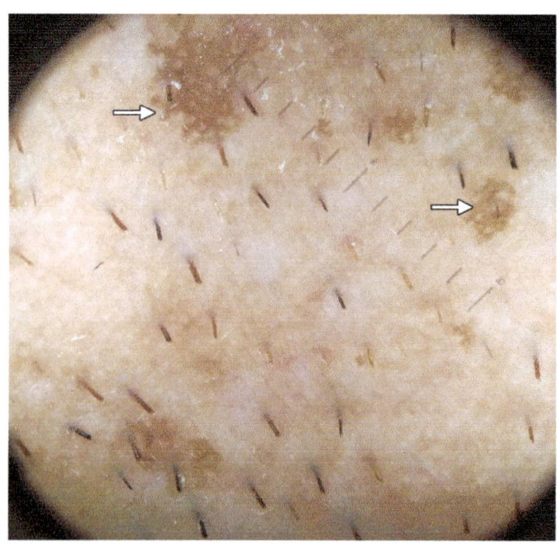

FIG. 6: Dermoscopic image of freckles showing well-defined localized exaggerated pseudonetwork with moth-eaten edges at the border (white arrows) with a clear demarcation line between the freckle and the normal skin (polarized, Heine Delta T20, 10×).

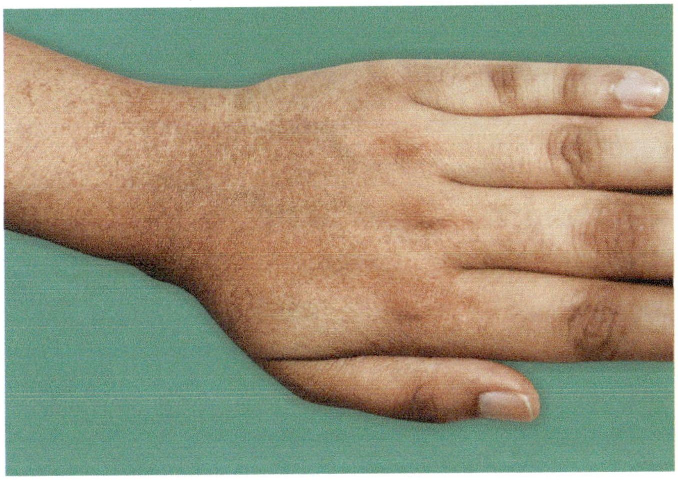

FIG. 7: Clinical image of lentigines over hand.

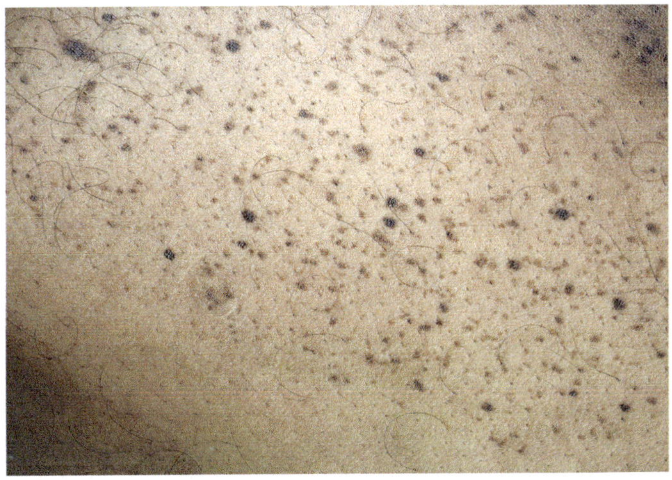

FIG. 8: Clinical image of lentigines over upper trunk showing brown-black well-defined macules.

Key Points

- Exaggerated pseudonetwork with moth-eaten border.

Lentigines

Clinical Features

Lentigo is a well-circumscribed small brown to black-pigmented macule secondary to increase in the number of melanocytes at dermoepidermal junction without any focal nest of proliferation. Lentigo simplex is the most prevalent form of lentigo, both on sun-exposed and nonexposed areas (**Figs. 7** and **8**). When they occur on the exposed areas, they are called as solar lentigines. An ink spot lentigo is jet black in color.

Dermoscopic Features

In lighter skin tones, regularly arranged fine delicate pigmented network (fingerprint-like areas) corresponding to pigmented rete ridges are observed (**Fig. 9**).

In darker skins, a regularly arranged reticular network with sharply demarcated irregular curved borders giving a moth-eaten border are seen or homogeneous brown pigmentation (**Fig. 10**).[7] The lesions on the face depict the pseudoreticular pattern with "moth-eaten border" at the periphery seen as concave areas at the periphery of the lesion (**Figs. 11** and **12**). In contrast to acquired melanocytic nevus, the pigmentation does not tend to fade away at the periphery (**Fig. 13**).[8]

Key Points

- Moth-eaten borders
- Fingerprint-like areas
- Pseudonetwork on face

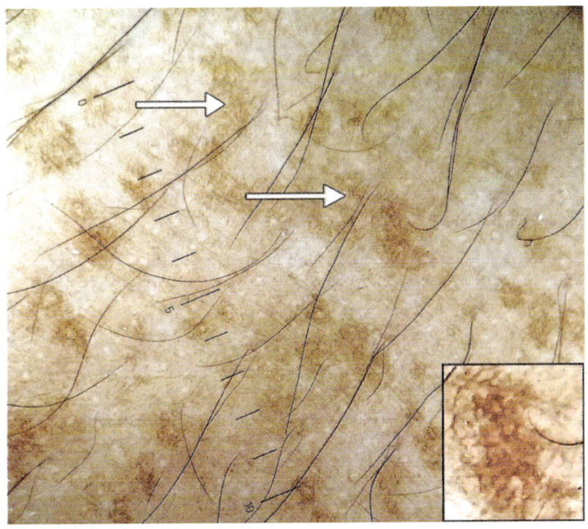

FIG. 9: Dermoscopic image of solar lentigines characterized by irregular but sharply demarcated brown, delicate pigment network with fingerprint-like areas (white arrows) (inset) (polarized, Heine Delta T20, 10×).

Flat Seborrheic Keratosis

Flat seborrheic keratoses are common, benign, pigmented epidermal tumors, occurring commonly after 50 years of age.[9] They can evolve from a lentigo.

Clinical Features

Seborrheic keratosis can occur at any location, but the common areas of involvement are face and trunk. The lesions are usually well-circumscribed, dull, flat, tan, or brown patches that later become raised with a waxy verrucous or "stuck-on" appearance (**Fig. 14**).[10]

Dermoscopic Features

Typical dermoscopic features of seborrheic keratosis include comedo-like openings and milia-like cysts (**Fig. 15**) which can be tiny white starry dots or large yellow clods with

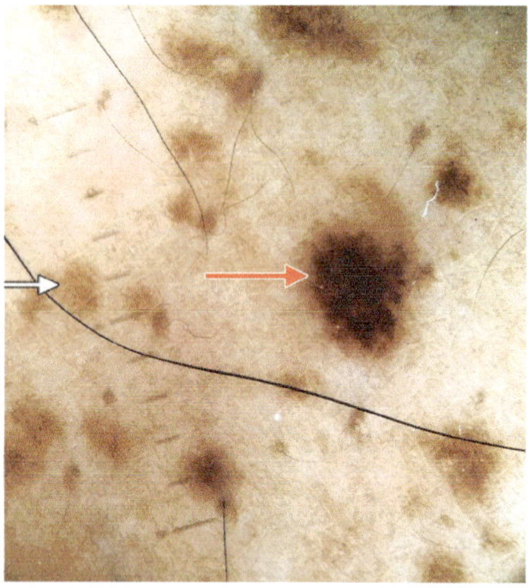

FIG. 10: Dermoscopic image of lentigines showing light brown delicate pigmented network with fingerprint-like areas (white arrow) and dark brown pigmentary network with moth-eaten border (red arrow) (polarized, Heine Delta T20, 10×).

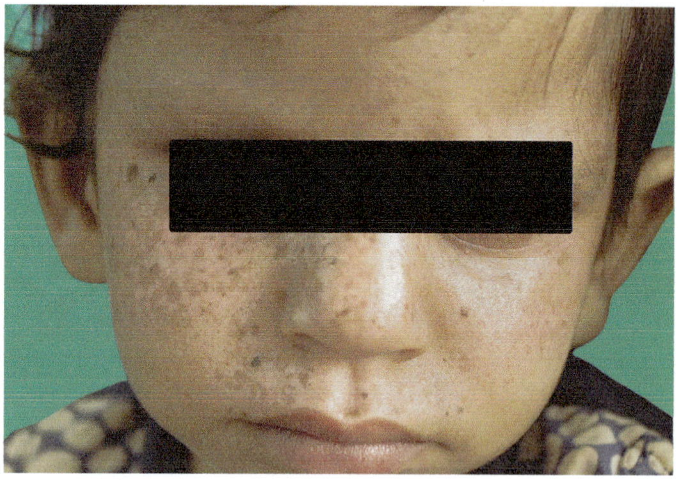

FIG. 11: Clinical image of lentigines over face.

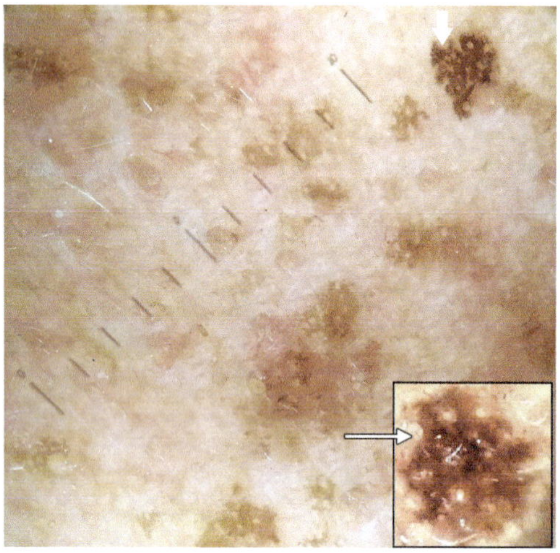

FIG. 12: Dermoscopic image of lentigines showing brownish accentuation of pigmentary pseudonetwork with moth-eaten border (white arrow, inset), with uniform center and margin (polarized, Heine Delta T20, 10×).

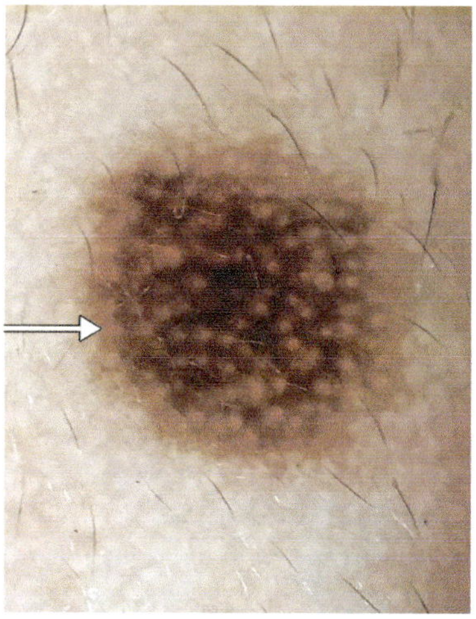

FIG. 13: Dermoscopic image of acquired melanocytic nevus showing the fading of pigmentation at the periphery (white arrow) (polarized, Heine Delta T20, 10×).

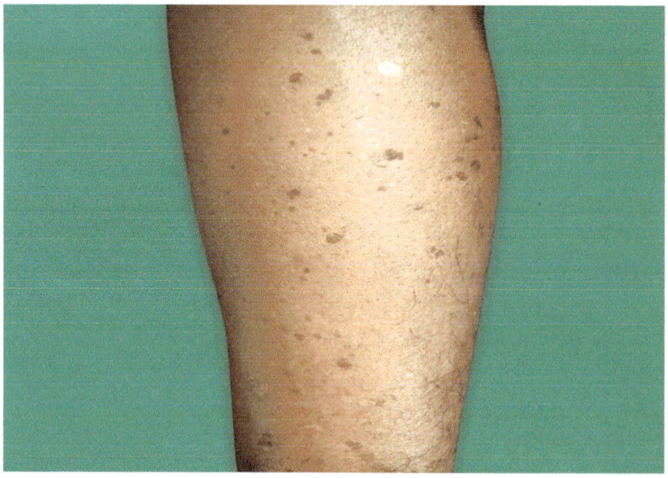

FIG. 14: Clinical photograph of early seborrheic keratosis shows sharply defined and slightly raised brown oval papules or polypoidal lesions with velvety stuck on appearance.

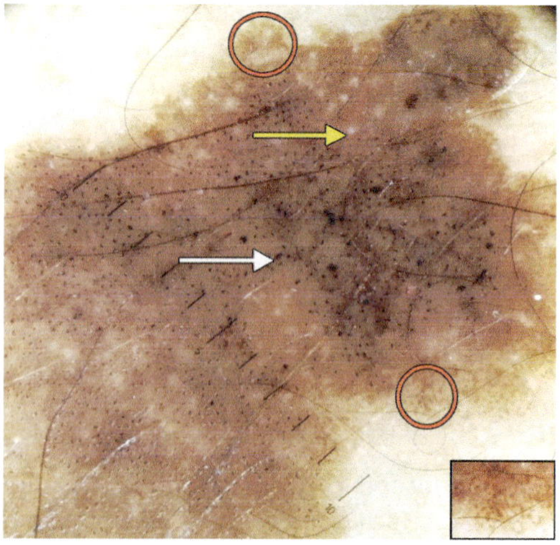

FIG. 15: Dermoscopy of seborrheic keratosis shows comedo-like openings with keratinous plugging (white arrow), milia-like cyst (yellow arrow), and marginal fat fingers (red circles) (inset) (polarized, Heine Delta T20, 10×).

irregular crypts and fissures on the surface. Border shows a sharp demarcation with moth-eaten appearance. Light brown fingerprint-like structures are seen (**Fig. 16**). Rarely, capillaries might be seen as hairpin loops surrounded by a white halo.[11]

On histopathology, acanthosis with proliferation of small cuboidal keratinocytes is seen with multiple "horn pseudocysts" with "string sign".

Key Points

- Sharply demarcated border with or without moth-eaten appearance
- Comedo-like opening, milia-like cysts
- Irregular crypts and fissures

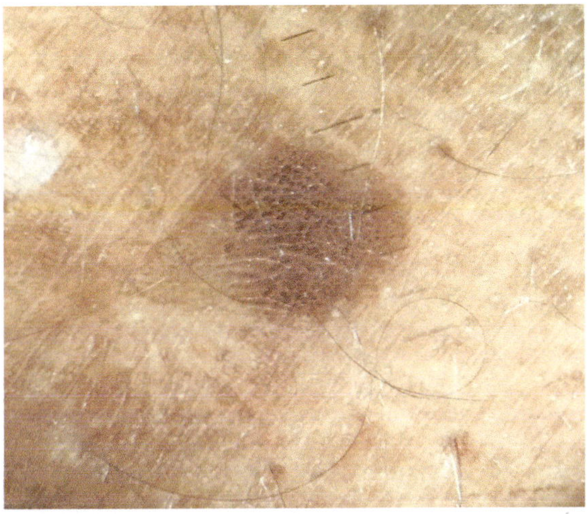

FIG. 16: Dermoscopic image showing brownish clods finger-like pattern at the margin (polarized, Heine Delta T20, 10×).

Dowling–Degos Disease (Reticulate Pigmented Anomaly of the Flexures)

It is an autosomal dominant hereditary disorder due to mutations in keratin 5 gene, manifesting in early adult life, mostly seen in females.[12]

Clinical Features

It is characterized by multiple spotted and reticulate pigmentation more over the flexures of neck, submammary folds, axilla, elbows, knees, and groin. The other salient features classically seen in this condition are pitted perioral scars and comedo-like follicular hyperkeratotic papules on the upper back and neck (**Fig. 17**).[13]

Dermoscopic Features

Dermoscopy of the macules shows irregular brownish projections known as brown star appearance (**Fig. 18**). Histopathologically, it corresponds to the elongated antler-like branching of rete ridges with pigmentation at the tip. The center of lesion is paler or hypopigmented representing the epidermal atrophy with lack of pigment or the follicular infundibulum (**Fig. 19**).[14] Dermoscopy also helps to highlight the follicular pits on the skin surface, the comedo-like openings, keratinous plugging and breaks in the dermatoglyphic pattern (**Figs. 20** and **21**).[15]

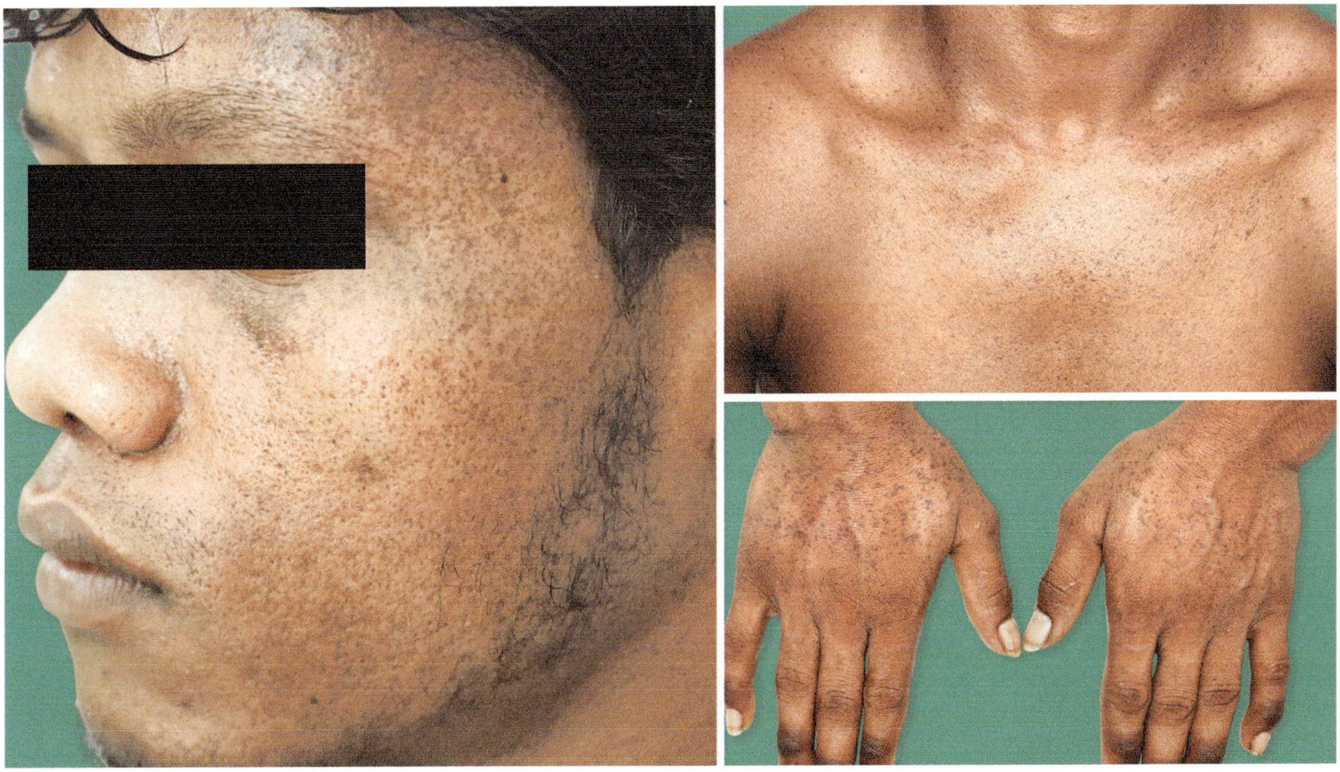

FIG. 17: Clinical image of Dowling–Degos disease showing multiple spotted and reticulate pigmentation more over the face, body, and dorsum of hands with perioral pitted scars.

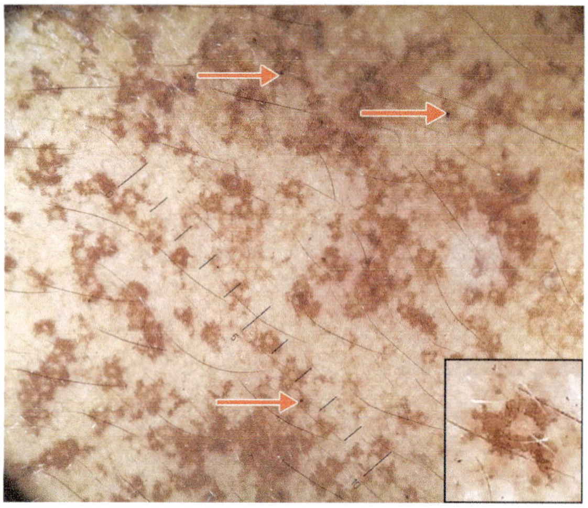

FIG. 18: Dermoscopic image of Dowling–Degos disease on the face showing irregular brownish projections—star appearance of brown globules pale or hypopigmented center (inset) and multiple black globules indicating keratinous plugging (red arrows) (polarized, Heine Delta T20, 10×).

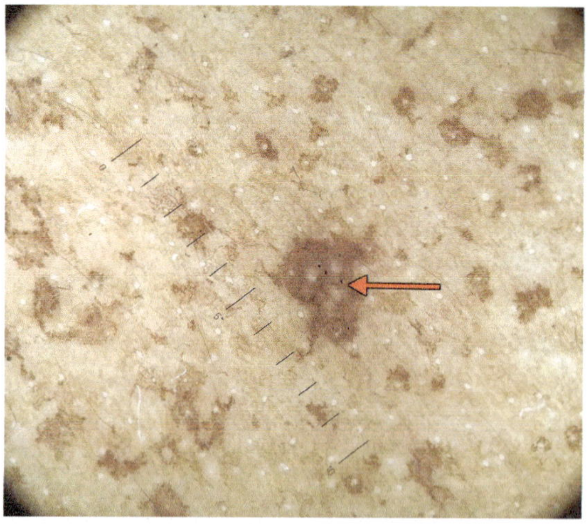

FIG. 19: Dermoscopic image of Dowling–Degos disease showing star appearance of brown globules with keratinous plugging (red arrow) (polarized, Heine Delta T20, 10×).

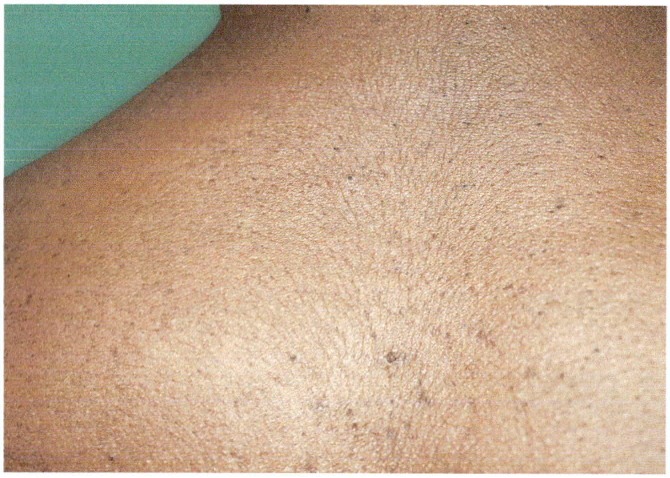

FIG. 20: Clinical image of Dowling–Degos disease showing multiple pigmented macules and papules with comedo-like lesions on the back.

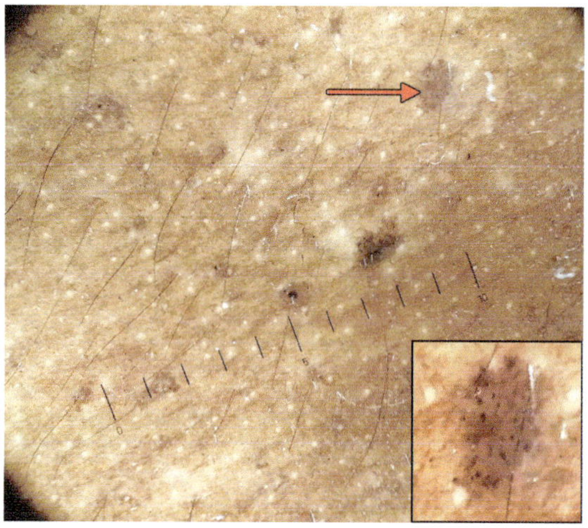

FIG. 21: Dermoscopic image of Dowling–Degos disease on the back showing numerous comedones with plugging over the lesion (red arrow) (close-up view) (polarized, Heine Delta T20, 10×).

Key Points

- Irregular brownish projections (brown star appearance) surrounding the pale and hypopigmented center
- Follicular pits and keratinous plugging

Café-au-Lait Macules

Clinical Features

Café-au-lait macules (CALMs) appear as well-defined circumscribed light brown oval to round macules with irregular or serrated margins. Isolated CALMs are commonly < 3 in number, ranging from 0.5 to 1.5 cm and can be seen in 10–20% of normal individuals. Six or more café-au-lait spots > 5 mm in greatest diameter in prepubertal individuals and > 15 mm in greatest diameter in postpubertal individuals are included in the diagnostic criteria for neurofibromatosis (**Figs. 22** to **24**).[16]

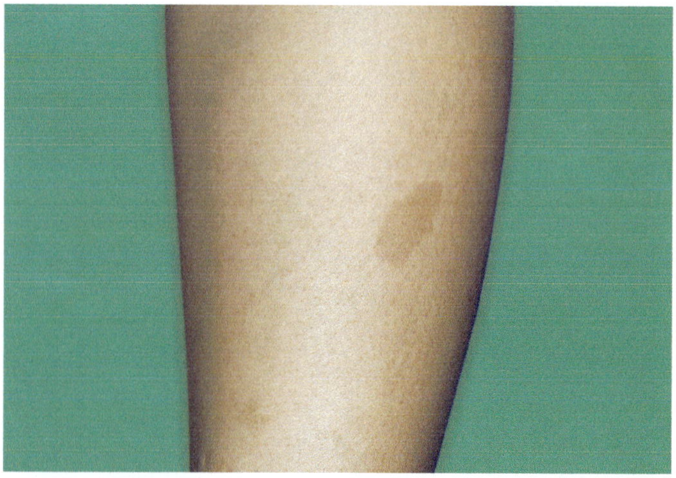

FIG. 22: Clinical image of café-au-lait macule over the forearm in a normal individual.

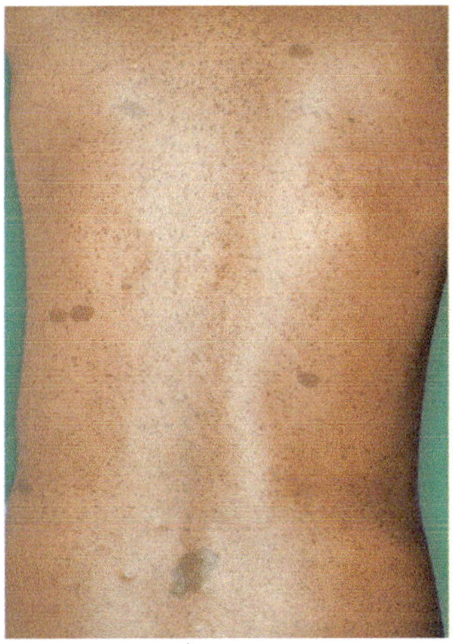

FIG. 23: Multiple café-au-lait macules in patient with neurofibromatosis.

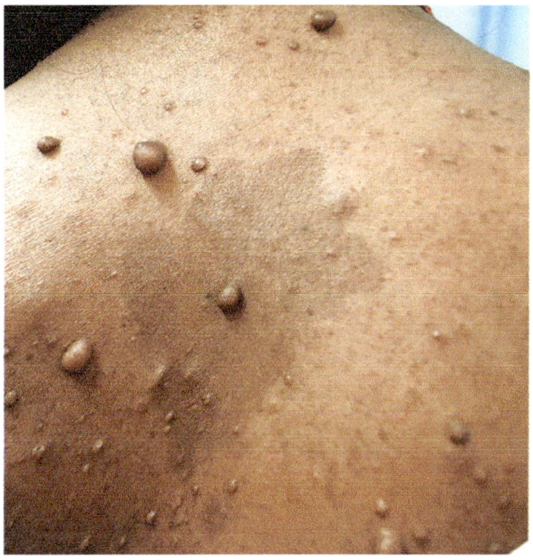

FIG. 24: Giant café-au-lait macule in patient with neurofibromatosis.

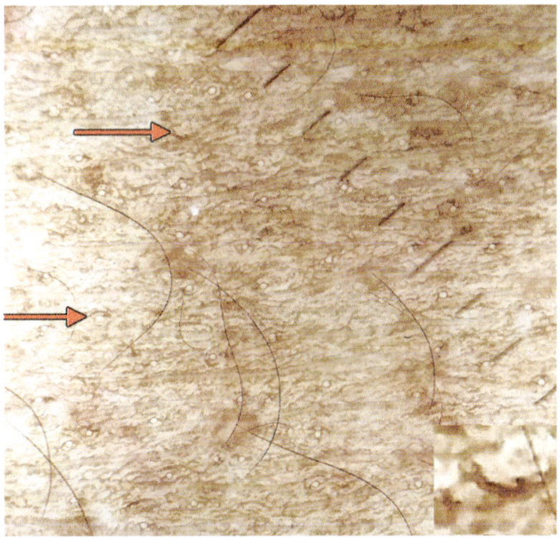

FIG. 25: Dermoscopic image of café-au-lait macule with accentuation of reticular pattern with focal thickening of pigmented lines in arcuate pattern (red arrows) (close-up view) (polarized, Heine Delta T20, 10×).

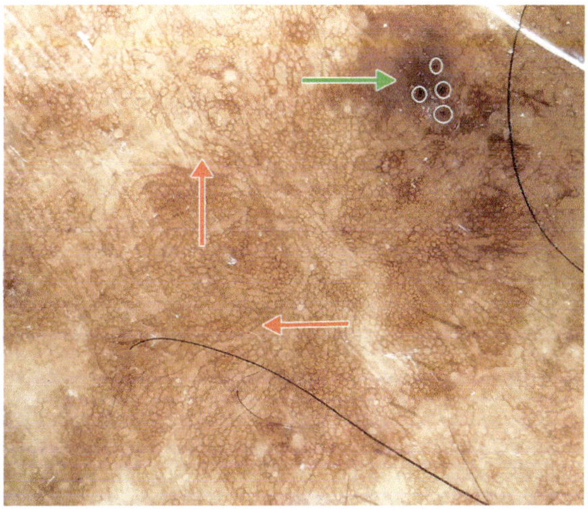

FIG. 26: Dermoscopic image of café-au-lait macule with thickened parallel lines (red arrows) forming a snail track appearance with coexisting seborrheic keratosis (green arrow) with multiple comedo-like openings with follicular plugging (white circles) (polarized, Heine Delta T20, 10×).

Dermoscopic Features

Café-au-lait macules present as darker pigment network with irregular focal thickening of reticular lines (**Fig. 25**).[17] The appearance varies with skin color. In lighter tones, the focal thickening appears as multiple arcuate and parallel lines. In darker pattern, the focal thickened lines join to form a snail track-like pattern (**Figs. 26** and **27**). In darkest tones, there is uniform dark brown accentuation of reticular pattern with few light brown areas in the center of the lesion (**Figs. 28** and **29**).[18]

On histopathology, an increased amount of melanin in the basal layer along with giant melanosomes can be seen.

Key Points

- Normal reticular pattern with irregular focal thickening of reticular lines
- Snail track-like pattern

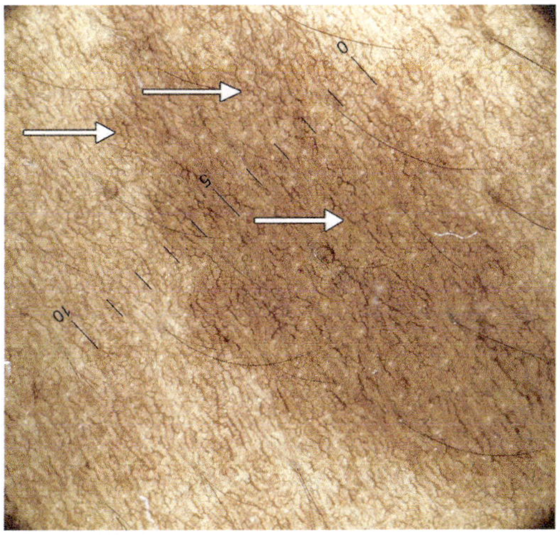

FIG. 27: Dermoscopic image of café-au-lait macule in skin of color showing the thickened lines join to form a snail track-like pattern (white arrows) (polarized, Heine Delta T20, 10×).

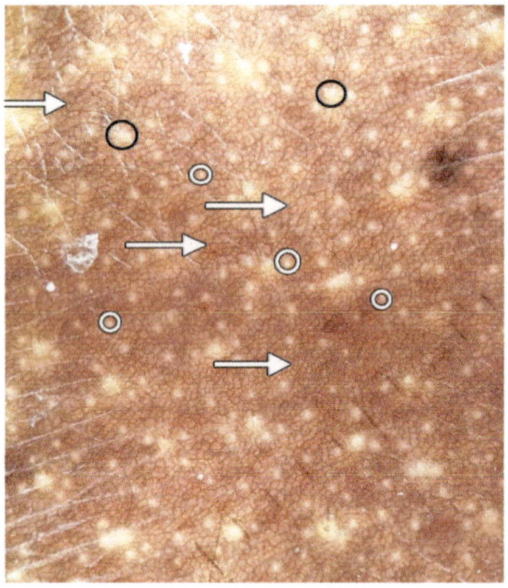

FIG. 28: Dermoscopic image of café-au-lait macule with uniform accentuation of reticular pattern (white arrows) sparing the follicular opening (black circles) and ductal openings (white circles) (polarized, Heine Delta T20, 10×).

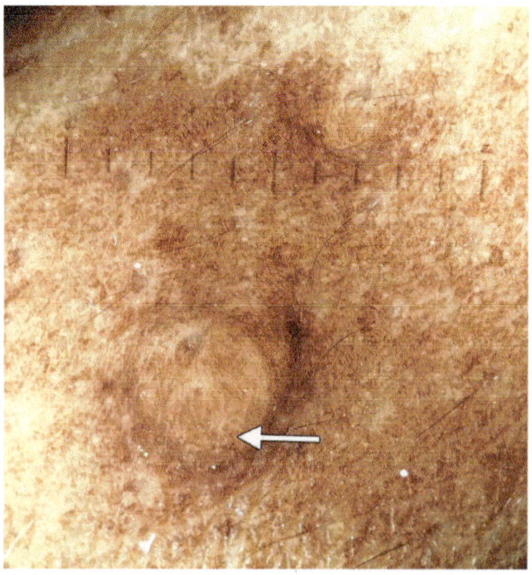

FIG. 29: Dermoscopic image of café-au-lait macule with multiple arcuate lines (white arrow) and reticular pattern over the neurofibroma (polarized, Heine Delta T20, 10×).

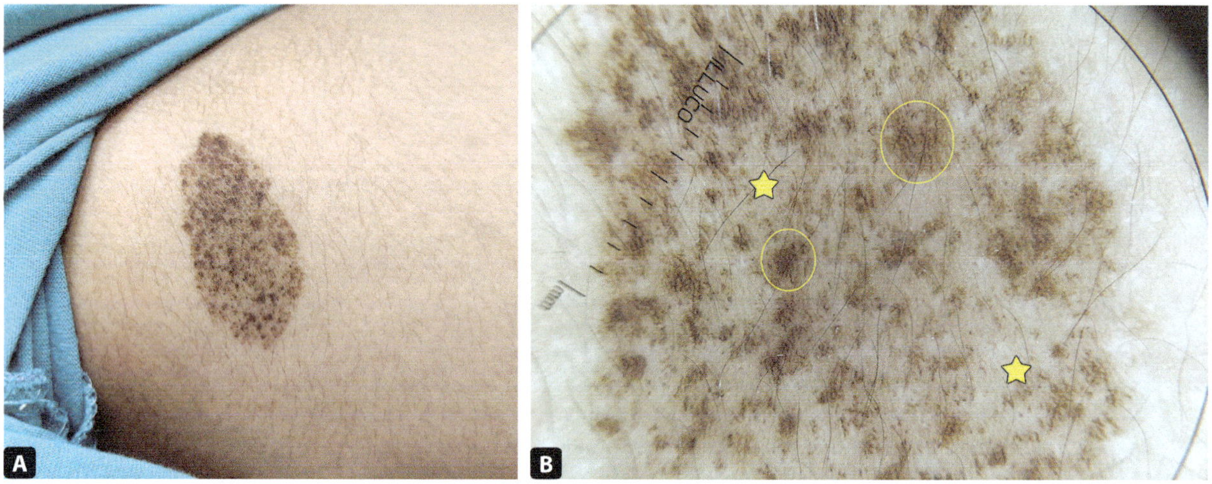

FIGS. 30A AND B (A) Clinical image of nevus spilus; (B) Dermoscopy of nevus spilus shows darker reticular pattern (circles) in the pigmented spots on a faint brownish background (stars) (polarized, Illuco IDS 1100, 10×).

Courtesy (Fig. B): Dr Balachandra Ankad, SN Medical College, Bagalkot, Karnataka, India.

Nevus Spilus

Clinical Features

Nevus spilus is characterized by a tan-colored patch covered with multiple small speckled pigmented macules or papules measuring 1–3 mm in size. Most common location is upper limb and trunk but it can occur anywhere on the body (**Fig. 30A**).[19]

Dermoscopic Features

Dermoscopy of nevus spilus reveals number of focal, homogeneous, brownish, hyperpigmented reticuloglobular structures over a light brown color background with reticular pattern (**Fig. 30B**).[20]

On histopathology, hyperpigmented base shows histological features of CALM or lentigo simplex while the speckled lesions on the top show histopathological features of nevi—junctional, compound, intradermal dysplastic, Spitz or blue nevi.

Key Points

- Background—light brown color with reticular pattern (lattice-like)
- Speckled lesions—reticuloglobular brownish structures

Fixed Drug Eruption

Clinical Features

Fixed drug eruption (FDE) is an adverse drug reaction manifesting as well-defined round-oval, dusky red-violaceous hyperpigmented patch that characteristically

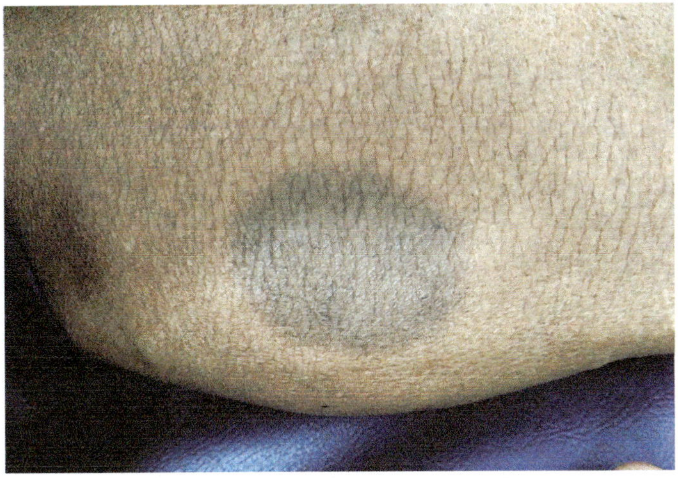

FIG. 31: Clinical image of fixed drug eruption showing oval, well-defined hyperpigmented patch.

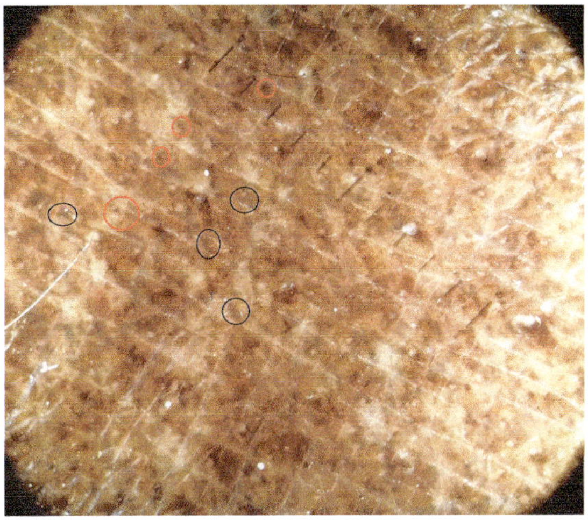

FIG. 32: Dermoscopic image of fixed drug eruption showing coarse ill-defined brown (red circles) and gray (black circles) dots, and globules in mixed shades of gray-brown or gray-blue (polarized, Heine Delta T20, 10×).

recurs or darkens at the same site following repeated drug exposure (**Fig. 31**).

Dermoscopic Features

The dermoscopy of FDE shows coarse ill-defined dots and globules with mixed shades of color, i.e., gray-brown or gray-blue (**Fig. 32**). The variability in color is due to pigment incontinence at various levels in the dermis.[21]

Histopathology shows interface dermatitis in an early lesion with scattered apoptotic keratinocytes and superficial perivascular infiltrate, while a late lesion shows dermal melanophages.

Key Points

- Ill-defined dots and globules with mixed shades of color.

PATTERNED PIGMENTATION

Melasma

Clinical Features

Melasma is a chronic, acquired, localized, bilateral, symmetrical, macular hypermelanosis of skin, clinically characterized by blotchy hyperpigmentation of the face particularly on the forehead and malar eminences and to a lesser degree involving the lower portion of the cheeks, chin, the upper lip and the sides of the neck and rarely the neck and forearm (**Fig. 33**).[22]

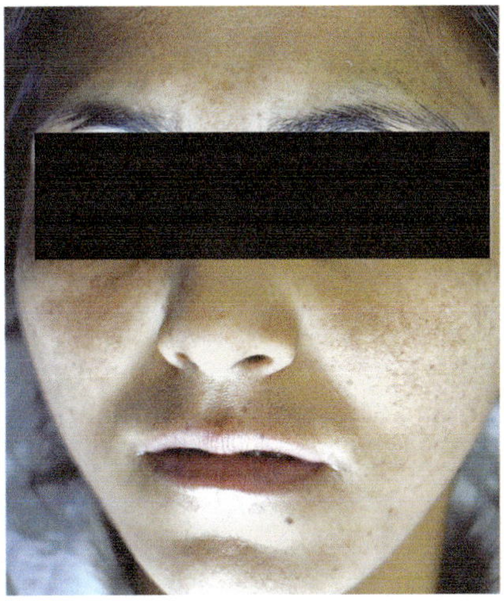

FIG. 33: Clinical photograph of epidermal melasma shows the scattered brown pigmented macules.

Role of dermoscopy in melasma:

- In determining the depth of melasma, whether epidermal or mixed, epidermal and dermal
- Early identification of complications of treatment such as exogenous ochronosis, depigmentation, and atrophy
- To visualize telangiectasia or increased vascularity due to steroid abuse
- Therapeutic and prognostic significance

Dermoscopic Features

The characteristic feature of melasma is exaggeration of pseudonetwork pattern with sparing of the sweat duct and follicular opening.[23]

- Early epidermal melasma shows exaggerated pseudonetwork with scattered islands of brown pigmentation predominantly light brown in color with few scattered granules (**Fig. 34**).
- Established epidermal melasma shows diffuse exaggerated pseudonetwork, predominantly brown in color (**Fig. 35**). Fine brown granules can be superimposed on the reticular network sparing the follicular and sweat duct opening and with concave borders—"jelly sign".[24]

- Mixed melasma shows heterogeneous irregular dark brown hyperpigmentation in shades of brown and gray, forming certain patterns (**Figs. 36A** and **B**). Various dermoscopic patterns observed are honeycomb-like reticular pattern, arcuate pigmented lines (**Fig. 36C**), granular pigmented, perifollicular grayish circles and blotches (**Fig. 36D**) and gray-brown concentric circles around the follicular and ductal opening (**Figs. 36E** to **G**).[25] Melasma with prolonged steroid abuse shows extensive telangiectasia comprising bright red superficial vessels, dull red deep vessels, and white atrophic areas (**Figs. 37A** and **B** and **Figs. 38A** and **B**).
- Dermal melasma shows diffuse pseudoreticular pattern with predominant blue-gray pigmented granules and blue-gray perifollicular accentuation (**Figs. 39A** and **B**).[26]

Dermoscopy also helps in monitoring the response to the treatment. Reduction in thickness of the lines, decreased perifollicular pigmented deposition, and changing color pattern form gray-blue to brown indicated response to the treatment in mixed melasma (**Fig. 40**).

Key Points

- Epidermal melasma—exaggerated pseudonetwork, dispersed brown areas
- Mixed melasma—diffuse irregular dark brown-gray hyperpigmentation with honeycomb-like reticular pattern
- Dermal melasma—predominant blue-gray pigmented granules and blue-gray perifollicular accentuation

Exogenous Ochronosis

Clinical Features

Exogenous ochronosis clinically presents as grayish-brown macules with interspersed "confetti-like" hypopigmented

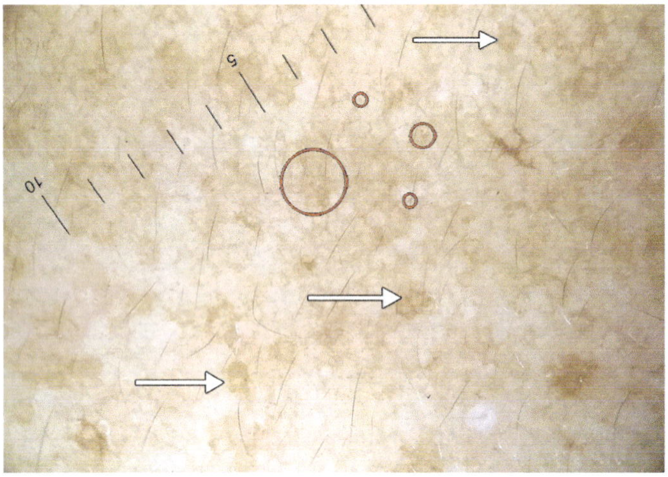

FIG. 34: Dermoscopic image of early epidermal melasma shows exaggerated pseudonetwork with scattered islands of brown pigmentation (white arrow) predominantly light brown in color with few dispersed granules (red circles) (polarized, Heine Delta T20, 10×).

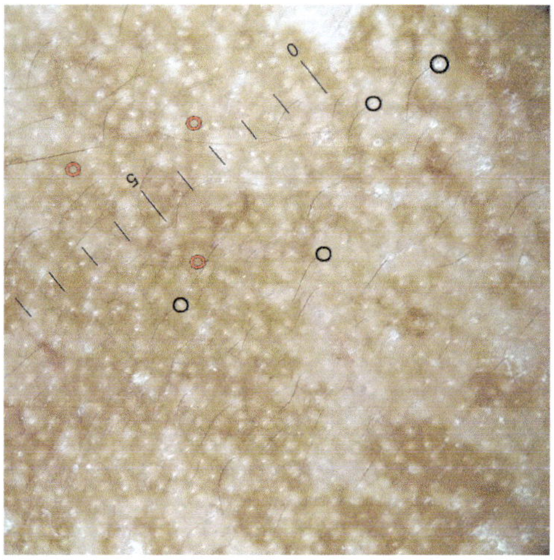

FIG. 35: Dermoscopic image of established epidermal melasma exaggerated pseudonetwork, brown pigmentation sparing the follicular openings (black circles) and sweat duct opening (red circles) (polarized, Heine Delta T20, 10×).

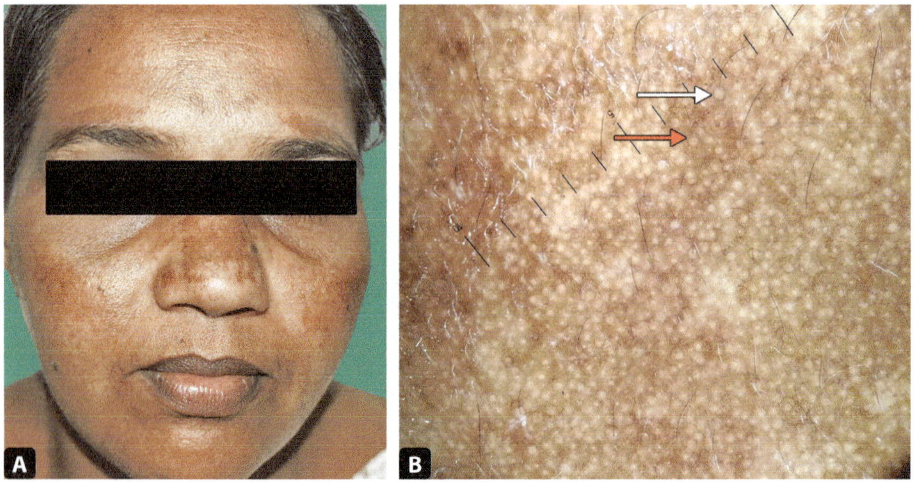

FIGS. 36A TO G: *(Continued)*

(Continued)

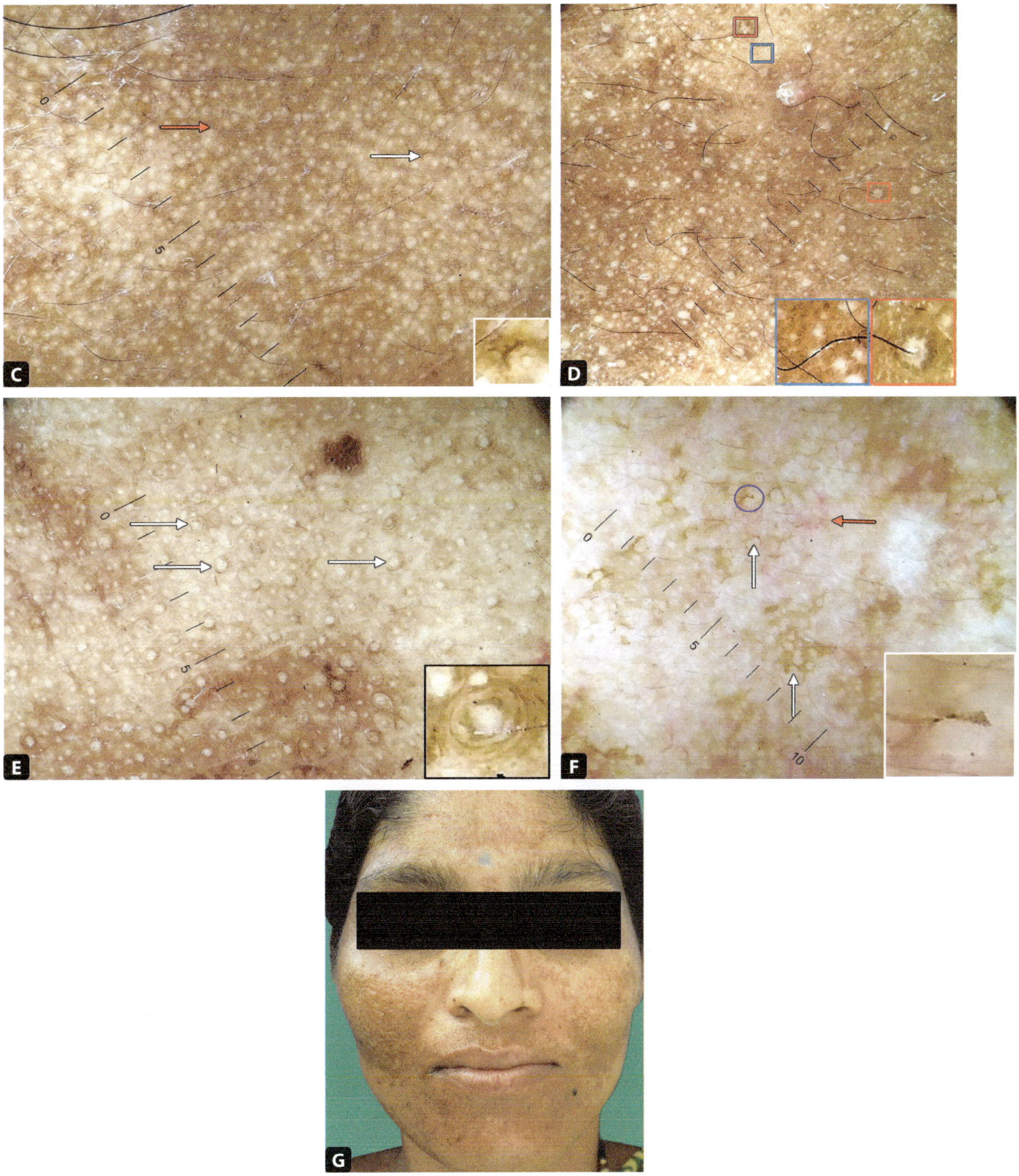

FIGS. 36A TO G: (A) Clinical image of mixed melasma shows dark brown hyperpigmented patches; (B) Dermoscopic image of mixed melasma shows diffuse dark brown honeycomb-like reticular pattern (red arrow) and perifollicular grayish circles (white arrow) (polarized, Heine Delta T20, 10×); (C) Dermoscopic image of mixed melasma shows diffuse dark brown honeycomb-like reticular pattern (red arrow) and arcuate pigmented lines (white arrow and close-up view) (polarized, Heine Delta T20, 10×); (D) Dermoscopic image of mixed melasma with multiple arcuate pigmented lines (blue box), perifollicular grayish blotches (red box). The close-up view helps in better visualization of gray-brown pigmented arcuate lines (blue box) and aggregation of gray-brown pigmented globules around the follicles (red box) (polarized, Heine Delta T20, 10×); (E) Dermoscopic image of mixed melasma showing gray-brown concentric circles around the follicular and ductal opening (white arrows, close-up view) (polarized, Heine Delta T20, 10×); (F) Dermoscopic image of mixed melasma exaggerated pseudonetwork, dispersed brown areas in heterogeneous brown pigmentation sparing the follicular and sweat duct opening. The borders are concave—jelly sign (white arrows) with scattered slate-gray arcuate pigmentation (blue circle) made of fine granules (inset) and telangiectasia (red arrow) (polarized, Heine Delta T20, 10×); (G) Clinical image of mixed melasma with dark brown to grayish patch of hyperpigmentation.

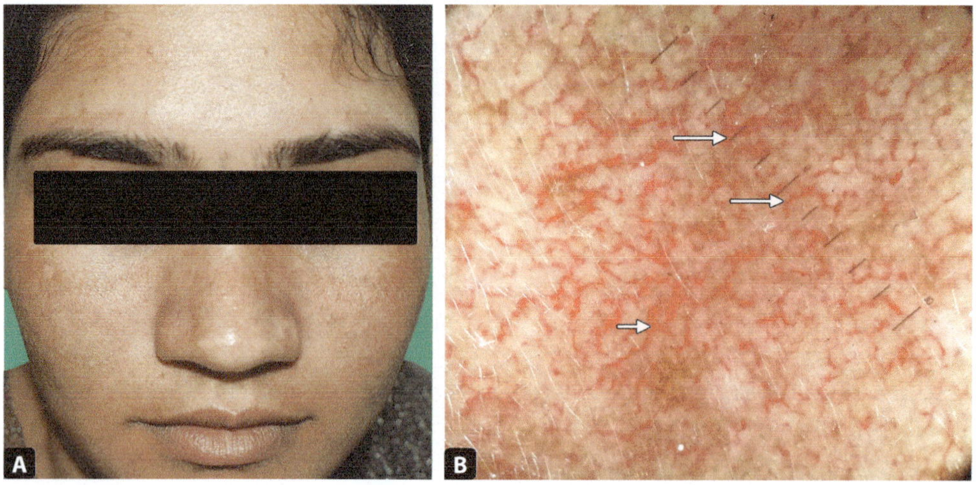

FIGS. 37A AND B: (A) Clinical image of epidermal melasma with scattered islands of light brown pigmentation; (B) Dermoscopic image of epidermal melasma shows exaggerated pseudonetwork with predominant telangiectasia secondary to steroid misuse (white arrows) (polarized, Heine Delta T20, 10×).

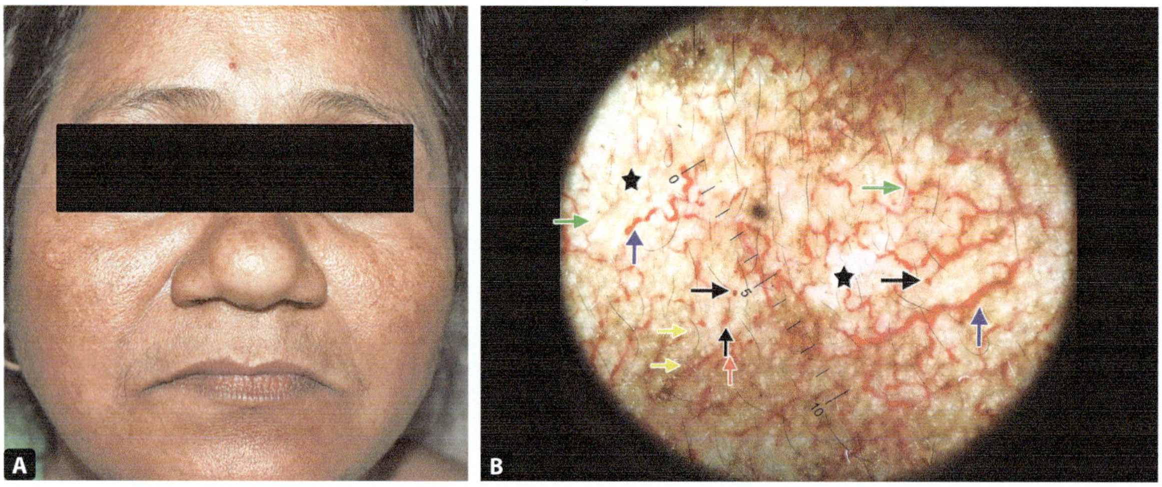

FIGS. 38A AND B: (A) Clinical image of mixed melasma with telangiectasia; (B) Dermoscopic image of mixed melasma with prolonged steroid abuse showing extensive, bright red and sharply focused telangiectasia (blue arrows), and poorly focused, dull or milky red deep vessels (green arrows). Part of short linear vessels (black arrows), white areas suggest fibrosis (black stars) and white dots indicating eccrine openings (yellow arrows) are also found (polarized, Heine Delta T20, 10×).

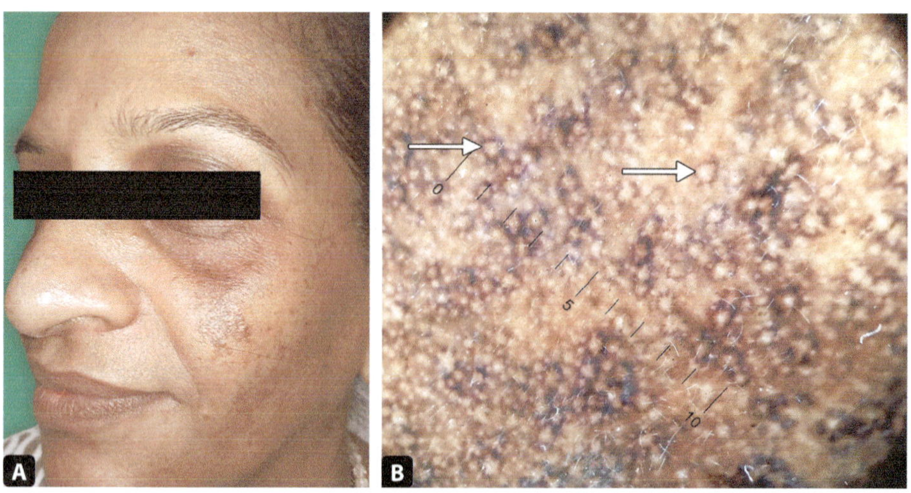

FIGS. 39A AND B: (A) Clinical image of dermal melasma with dark brown to grayish patch of hyperpigmentation with periorbital pigmentation; (B) Dermoscopic image of dermal melasma showing exaggerated pseudoreticular pattern with predominant blue circles (white arrows) around the follicular and ductal opening (polarized, Heine Delta T20, 10×).

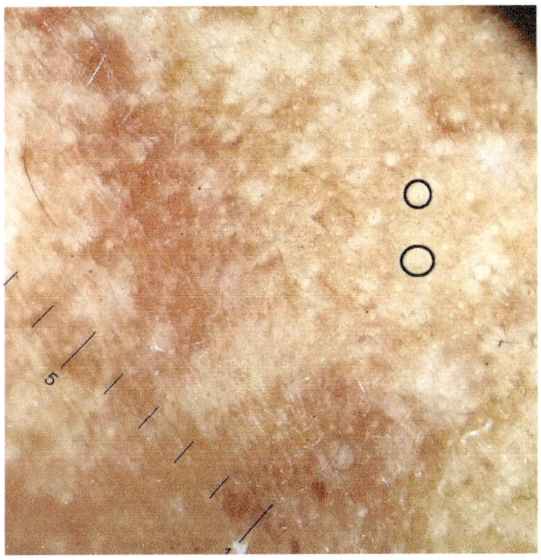

FIG. 40: Dermoscopic image with positive response to the treatment as compared to **Figure 36D** showing changing color from the previous gray-brown pigmentation to light brown pigmentation, with clearance of perifollicular pigment deposition (black circles) (polarized, Heine Delta T20, 10×).

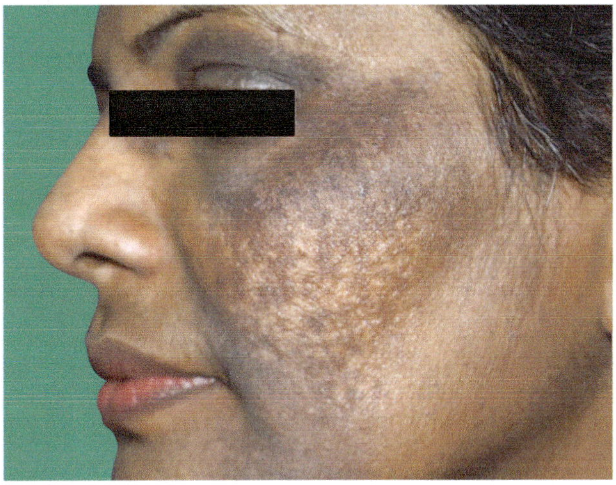

FIG. 41: Clinical image of exogenous ochronosis showing grayish-brown macules with interspersed "confetti-like" depigmented macular areas with tiny brown papules.

macular areas in the early stages, progressing to tiny brown caviar-like papules, erythema, telangiectasia, and specks of pigmentation (**Fig. 41**).[27]

Dermoscopic Findings

The characteristics of exogenous ochronosis are irregular thick brown-gray amorphous areas obliterating the follicular opening, appearing as "worm-like" curvilinear areas.[27] Other features are confetti-like depigmented patches seen as white areas, multiple dark brown-gray globular, annular or arciform structures over the melasma patches (**Fig. 42**).[28]

Key Points

- Irregular thick brown-gray amorphous worm-like areas
- Obliteration of the follicular opening
- Confetti-like depigmented patches

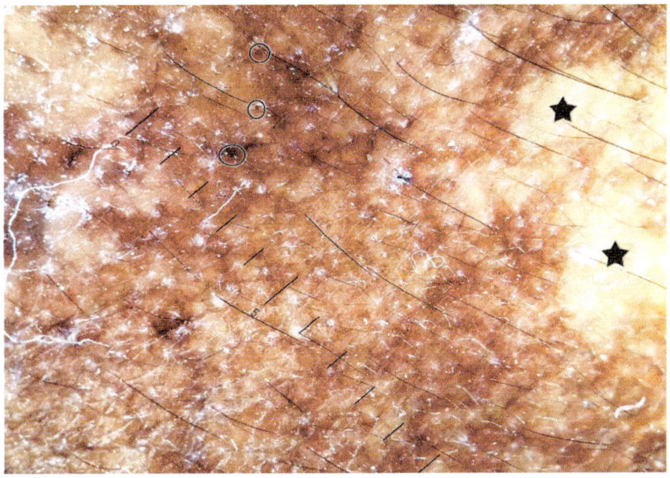

FIG. 42: Dermoscopic image of exogenous ochronosis showing irregular thick brown-gray amorphous areas ("worm-like" curvilinear structures) with obliterating the follicular opening. Other findings are confetti-like depigmented patches seen as white areas (black stars), multiple dark brown-gray globules (black circles) over the melasma patches with fine scales (polarized, Heine Delta T20, 10×).

Pigmentary Demarcation Lines

Pigmentary demarcation lines (PDLs) are also known as Futcher's or Voigt's lines.

Clinical Features

Pigmentary demarcation lines refer to the border of abrupt transition of skin color from hyperpigmented outer surfaces to hypopigmented or normal inner surface. They are most commonly seen in dark individuals over the face, limbs, and trunk.[29] Eight demarcation lines are named according to the alphabets A to H of which F, G and H are seen on the face. PDL-F and G type lines are seen over the outer aspect of the eye presenting as V and W-shaped patches, respectively (**Figs. 43A** and **44A**).[30] PDL-H is a band of hyperpigmentation extending from angle of mouth to outer aspect of chin.[31]

Dermoscopic Features

Dermoscopy of PDL shows an exaggerated pseudoreticular pattern with scattered globules and granules. The features closely resemble melasma, and can be differentiated by predominant brownish patterned pigmentation confined only to the lesional skin in contrast to melasma involving both the lesional and normal looking skin.[32] PDLs show well-defined borders, in contrast to melasma with diffuse involvement extending to the normal skin (**Figs. 43B** and **44B**).[33]

Key Points

- Exaggerated pseudonetwork pattern
- Scattered blotchy globules and granules

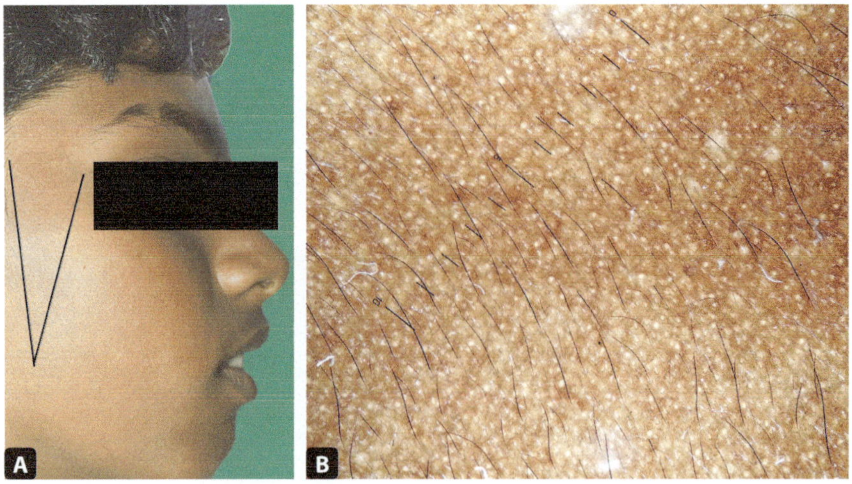

FIGS. 43A AND B: (A) Clinical image of pigmentary demarcation line—F; (B) Dermoscopic image of pigmentary demarcation line—F showing exaggerated pseudoreticular pattern.

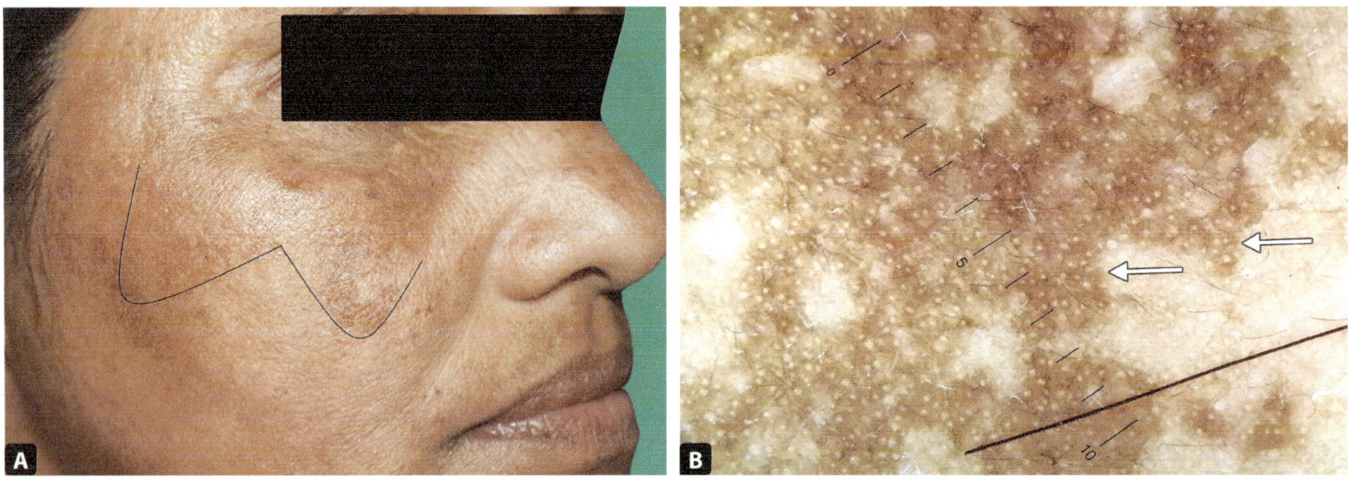

FIGS. 44A AND B: (A) Clinical image of pigmentary demarcation line—G showing W-shaped patch; (B) Dermoscopic image of pigmentary demarcation line—G accentuation of pseudoreticular pattern with well-defined borders (white arrows) (polarized, Heine Delta T20, 10×).

Periorbital Hyperpigmentation

Clinical Features

Periorbital hyperpigmentation (POH), also called "dark circles", is a commonly encountered problem in the outpatient clinic. POH appears as bilateral, round, or semi-circular ill-defined homogeneous pigmented macules and patches primarily involving the infraorbital region. It can also extend to upper eyelid, malar regions, eyebrows, temporal region, and lateral nasal root.[34] Huang et al. classified POH into pigmented, vascular, structural, and mixed types. Pigmented type is seen as an infraorbital brown hue (**Fig. 45A**).[35] Vascular type appears as infraorbital blue, purple or pink hue with or without periorbital puffiness. Structural type appears as structural shadows secondary to loss of fat with bony prominence, infraorbital palpebral bags, and blepharoptosis. The most common is the mixed type that can be further classified into pigmented-vascular, pigmented-structural, and vascular-structural (**Fig. 46A**).

Dermoscopy not only helps in identifying the type of POH but also aids in determining the therapeutic modalities, as the different types of POH require different modalities of approach.

Dermoscopic Features

The dermoscopic patterns of pigmented POH can be either pseudoreticular or reticuloglobular. The epidermal type of pigmentation presents as uniform brownish accentuation of pseudonetwork (**Fig. 45B**)[36] with perifollicular and perieccrine pigmentation (**Fig. 45C**). Mixed pigmentation shows irregular accentuation of pseudonetwork with multiple arcuate lines and perifollicular and perieccrine pigment deposition (**Fig. 46B**).[37]

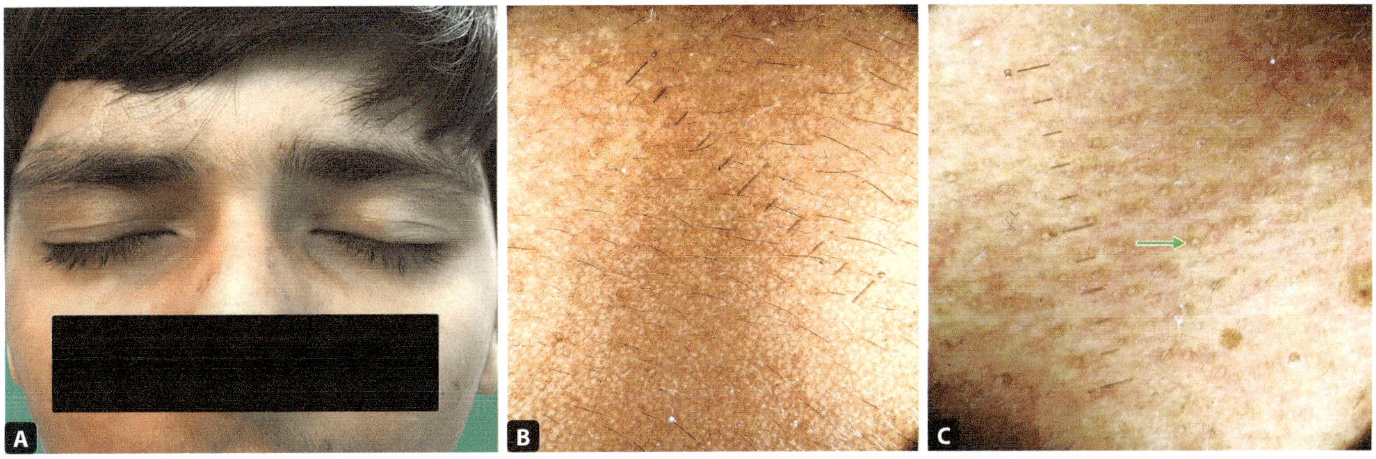

FIGS. 45A TO C: (A) Clinical photograph of pigmented periorbital hyperpigmentation; (B) Dermoscopic image of periorbital hyperpigmentation showing epidermal type with uniform brownish accentuation of pseudonetwork (polarized, Heine Delta T20, 10×); (C) Dermoscopic image of periorbital hyperpigmentation with perifollicular and perieccrine brown epidermal pigmentation (green arrow) with ill-defined pinkish hue indicating deep dermal vessels (polarized, Heine Delta T20, 10×).

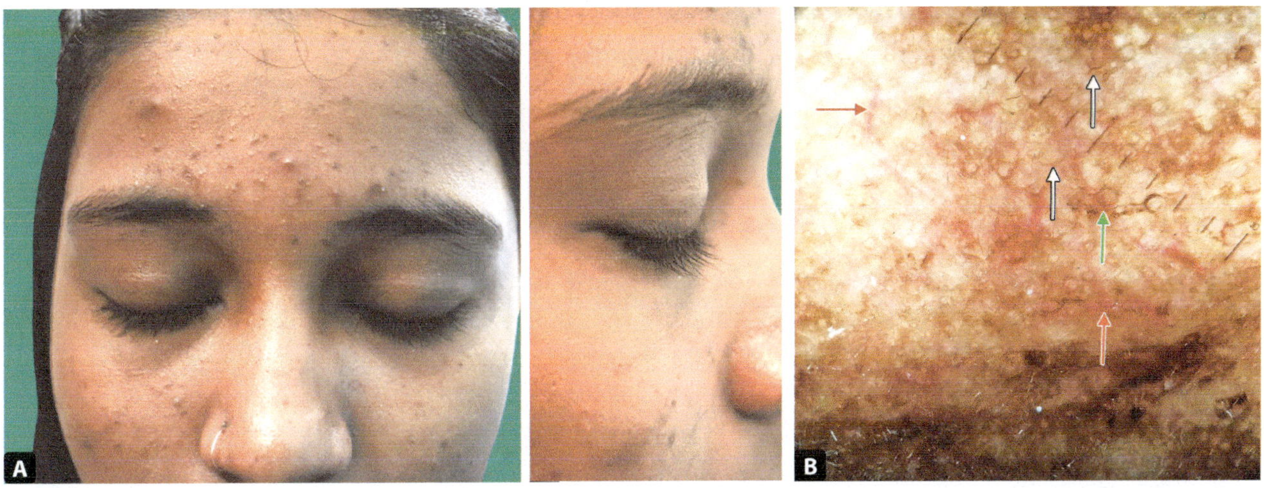

FIGS. 46A AND B: (A) Clinical image of pigmented-vascular periorbital hyperpigmentation; (B) Dermoscopic image of pigmented and vascular periorbital hyperpigmentation showing mixed type of pigmentation—irregular accentuation of pseudonetwork pattern, perifollicular pigmentation (green arrow), arcuate lines (white arrows), out of focus dermal vessels (red arrows) (polarized, Heine Delta T20, 10×).

The vascular type of POH shows either diffuse erythema or multiple thin branched superficial vessels present as bright red well-defined vessels or deep dermal vessels appearing as dull red erythematous lines. The structural component changes include atrophy and exaggerated skin markings (**Figs. 47A** and **B**).

Key Points

- Epidermal pigmented POH shows as uniform brownish accentuation of pseudonetwork.
- Mixed pigmented POH reveals irregular accentuation of pseudonetwork, arcuate lines.
- Vascular type of POH shows diffuse erythema or superficial or dermal vessels.
- Structural type shows atrophy and exaggerated skin markings.

Nevus of Ota

Clinical Features

Nevus of Ota clinically presents as unilateral macules of blue-gray discoloration of the face in the region of maxillary and ophthalmic division of trigeminal nerve, i.e., periocular area, forehead, temple, malar region, and nose. The ipsilateral eye may also show bluish discoloration of sclera and conjunctiva (**Fig. 48A**). Rarely, it may be bilateral.[38]

Dermoscopic Findings

The dermoscopic characteristics are structureless ill-defined bluish to slate-gray homogeneous area in a patchy distribution (**Fig. 48B**).[39] Other findings are scattered brown dots, fine scales, white clods in a "four dots clod"

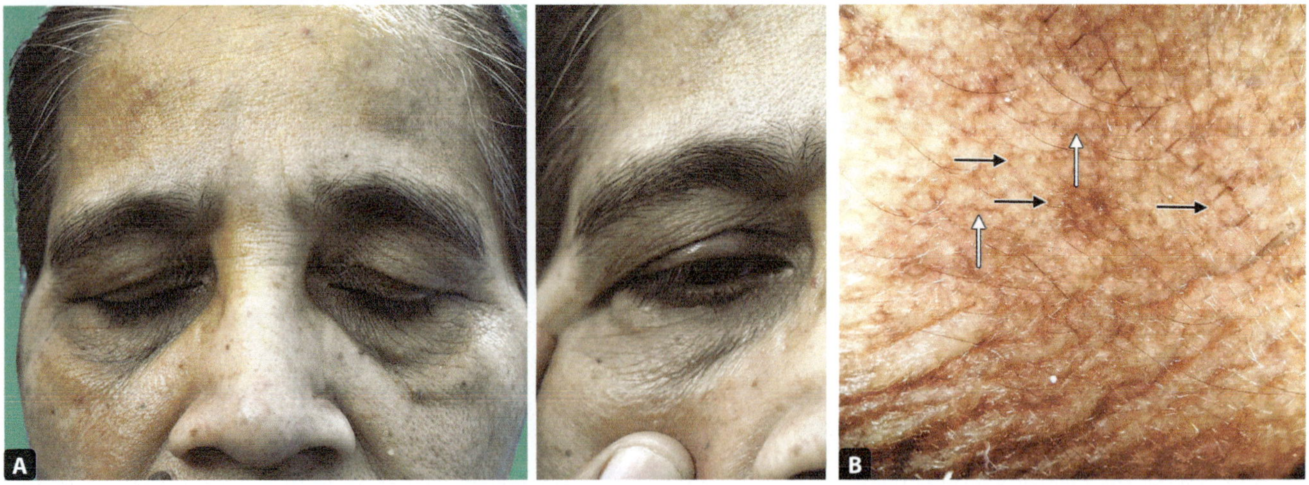

FIGS. 47A AND B: (A) Clinical image of periorbital hyperpigmentation with, infraorbital palpebral bag, retention of pigmentation on stretch test; (B) Dermoscopic image of pigmented and structural periorbital hyperpigmentation showing picture similar to mixed melasma with irregular accentuation of pseudoreticular pattern, arcuate lines (black arrows), irregular thickened lines (white arrows) with underlying laxity of skin (polarized, Heine Delta T20, 10×).

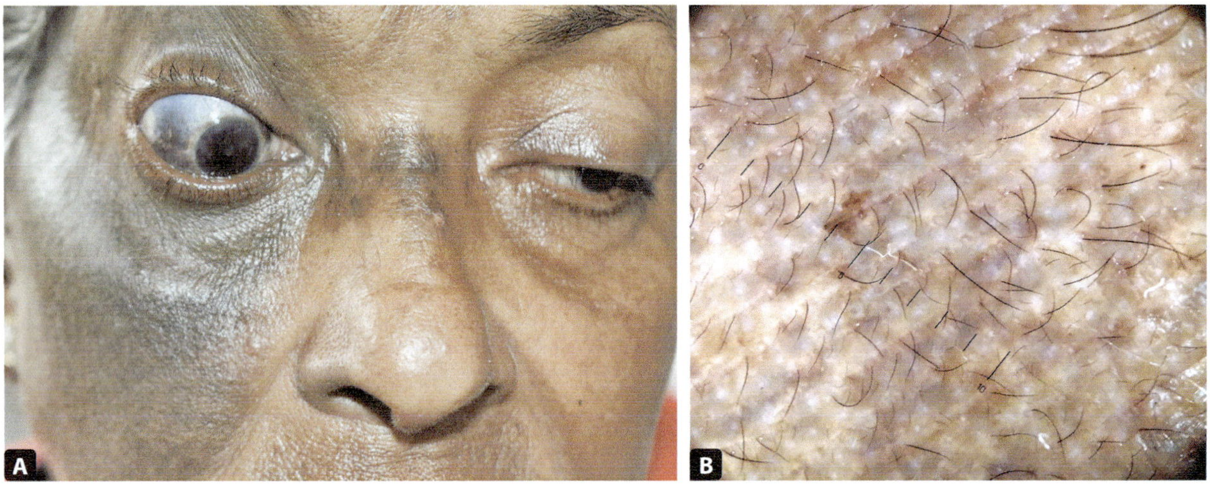

FIGS. 48A AND B: (A) Clinical image of nevus of Ota with unilateral patch of blue-gray discoloration of face with the ipsilateral eye showing bluish discoloration of conjunctiva; (B) Dermoscopic image of nevus of Ota shows ill-defined bluish to slate-gray globules in a patchy distribution (polarized, Heine Delta T20, 10×).

arrangement, perifollicular hypopigmentation, yellowish structureless areas.[39]

Becker's Nevus

Clinical Features

Becker's nevus is a cutaneous hamartoma, an epidermal nevus of organoid type with late onset. It clinically presents as a hyperpigmented macule or patch, most commonly seen on the anterior chest, shoulder or scapular region, that later becomes corrugated and acquires terminal hair (**Fig. 49A**).[40]

Dermoscopic Features

Dermoscopy of Becker's nevus differs from center and periphery. The center of the lesion shows dense pigmentation with uniformly thickened reticular lines (**Fig. 49B**). There may be blotchy hyperpigmented globules with perifollicular hyperpigmentation and multiple terminal hairs.[41]

In the periphery, there is blunted or normal reticular pigmentary network with less terminal hairs and less perifollicular pigmentation. The margin may even show focal or perifollicular hypopigmentation (**Fig. 50**). Advanced lesions may show furrows, hypertrophic hair follicles and rarely few dilated vessels.[42]

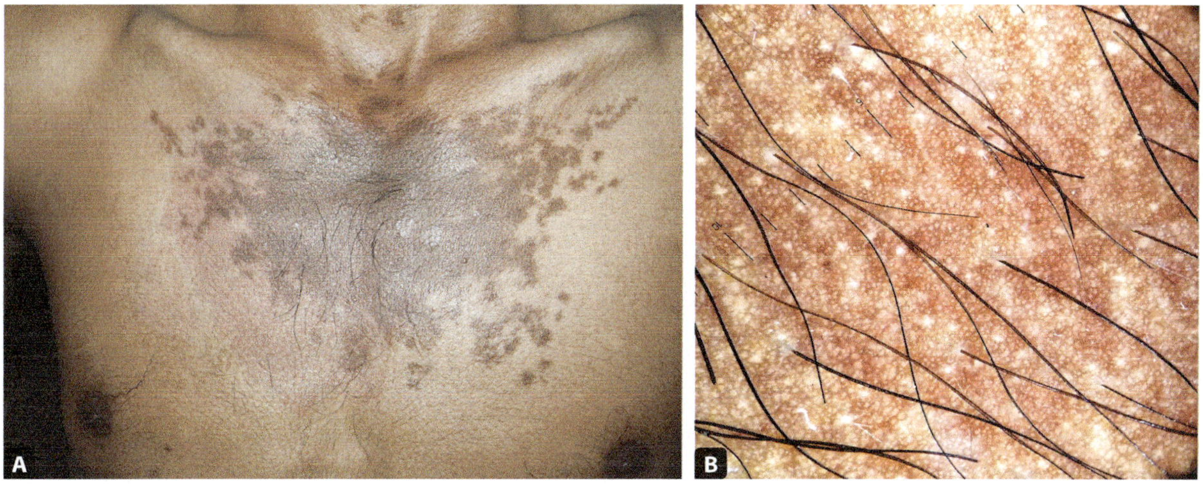

FIGS. 49A AND B: (A) Clinical image of Becker's nevus presenting as hyperpigmented patch on anterior chest with thick and dark hair; (B) Dermoscopic image of Becker's nevus show dense pigmentation with uniformly thickened reticular lines in the center of the lesion (polarized, Heine Delta T20, 10×).

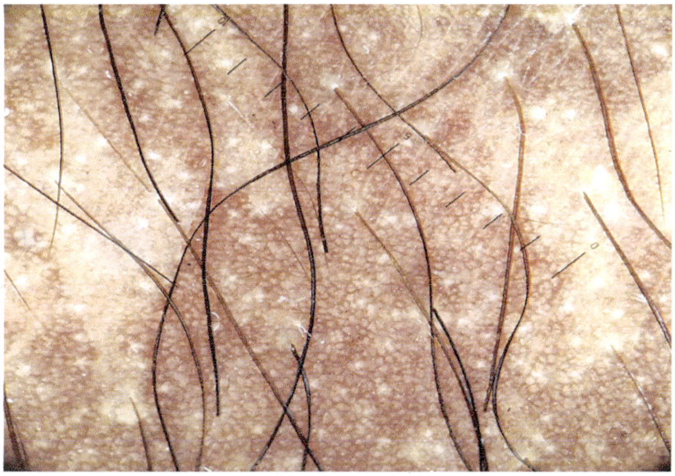

FIG. 50: Dermoscopic image of Becker's nevus at periphery shows hypopigmented areas with blunted reticular pattern, and terminal hairs and few areas of at the periphery of the lesion (polarized, Heine Delta T20, 10×).

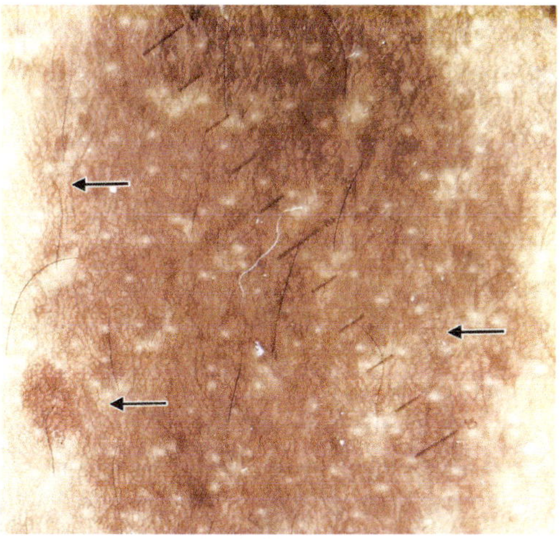

FIG. 51: Dermoscopic image of Becker's nevus showing dense thick pigmented lines in the centre and the periphery showing blunted fine delicate lines (black arrows) with few hypopigmented areas, terminal hairs and few areas of at the periphery of the lesion (polarized, Heine Delta T20, 10×).

Isolated CALM is one of the close differential diagnoses to Becker's nevus. Unlike Becker's nevus, CALM shows multiple focal thickening of reticular lines both at center and periphery forming a snail track-like pattern with multiple arcuate lines (**Fig. 51**). The central blotches, globules, focal hypo- or hyperpigmentation, terminal hairs are not seen in dermoscopy of CALM.[43]

Key Points

- Uniform dense reticular pattern at the center with terminal hair
- Blunted reticular pigmentation at periphery
- Blotchy hyperpigmented globules and perifollicular pigmentation

DIFFUSE PIGMENTATION

Acquired Dermal Macular Hyperpigmentation

Clinical Features

This particular entity encompasses few hyperpigmentary conditions which show dermal melanin in histopathology including lichen planus pigmentosus (LPP), erythema dyschromicum perstans (EDP), and pigmented contact dermatitis (PCD). All of these disorders are characterized by the development of virtually noninflammatory, hyperpigmented macules of varying shades coalescing to form diffuse patches. Histopathology is essentially similar with significant dermal melanin incontinence, usually accompanied by interface dermatitis, which may be minimal to nonexistent in quiescent cases. In view of the clinicopathological similarities, the term "acquired dermal macular hyperpigmentation (ADMH)" is being recently used to describe the dermoscopic features of these entities.[44-46]

Dermoscopic Features

The major dermoscopic finding is gray-blue pigmented dots, globules, and blotches. The size of dots is <0.1 mm by definition, and that of globules is >0.1 mm. Structures that occupy > 10% of the lesional surface area and obscure details underneath are referred to as blotches (**Fig. 52**). The color of these dots and globules depends upon their location, and varies from black, brown, gray, and blue (when present in the superficial epidermis, epidermis, papillary dermis, reticular dermis, respectively). The normal pigment distribution on the face appears to be distributed around the appendageal openings, imparting a pseudoreticular network, which gets accentuated in both melasma and ADMH affecting the face.[43] On the neck and other body areas, the dots and globules are distributed around the creases, sparing the creases themselves. Individual dots and globules can further be arranged into various global patterns and grades correlating with the magnitude of melanin incontinence observed on histopathology. These global patterns were defined for the facial skin, especially the temple and the preauricular area.[47,48]

Grade I ADMH has scattered sparsely distributed blue-gray dots forming no specific pattern, known as peppering (**Figs. 53** and **54**). This is seen in LPP.

Grade II demonstrates blue-gray dots coalescing to form linear/broken-linear and arcuate/semiarcuate structures (Chinese letter pattern or hem-like pattern) (**Figs. 55** and **56**). This pattern is observed in LPP. Hem-like arrangement of pigment globules is definitive of LPP (**Fig. 57**).

Grade III demonstrates blue-gray globules coalescing around numerous pilosebaceous units and sweat glands to form pseudoreticular pattern (**Figs. 58** to **60**). These patterns are predominately seen in PCD, EDP, and LPP.

Grade IV demonstrates massive melanin incontinence characterized by the presence of big globules and blotches, which appear as diffuse deposition of pigment just sparing the appendageal orifices and obliterating the underlying normal pigment network completely (**Figs. 61** and **62**). This particular pattern in found in LPP.

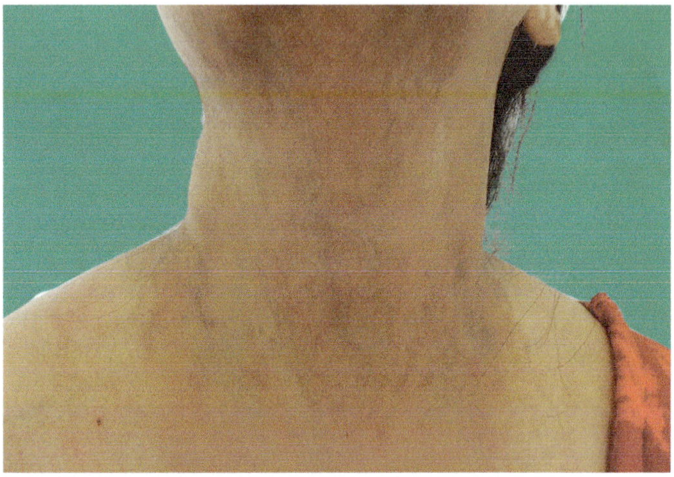

FIG. 53: Ill-defined, blotchy patches on the neck of a patient with acquired dermal macular hyperpigmentation.

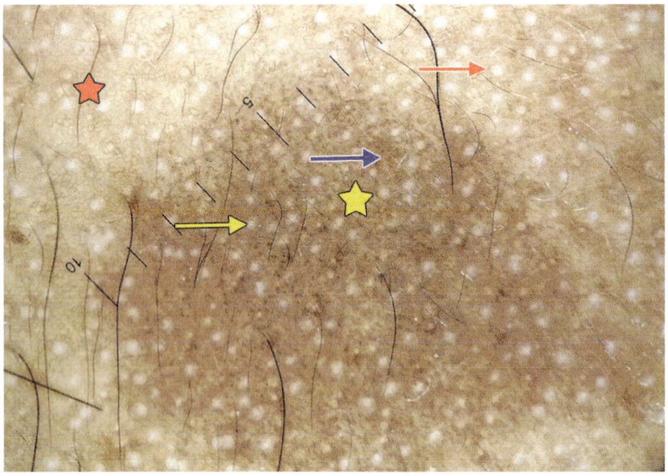

FIG. 52: Normal background pseudoreticular pigmentation of ethnic skin in background (red star) with spared eccrine openings (red arrow). The affected area demonstrates an accentuation of normal pseudoreticular pattern (yellow star) with eccrine openings still spared (yellow arrow). The melanin incontinence characteristic of acquired dermal macular hyperpigmentation is visible in the form of dots (blue arrow) (polarized, DermLite II Hybrid M, 10×).

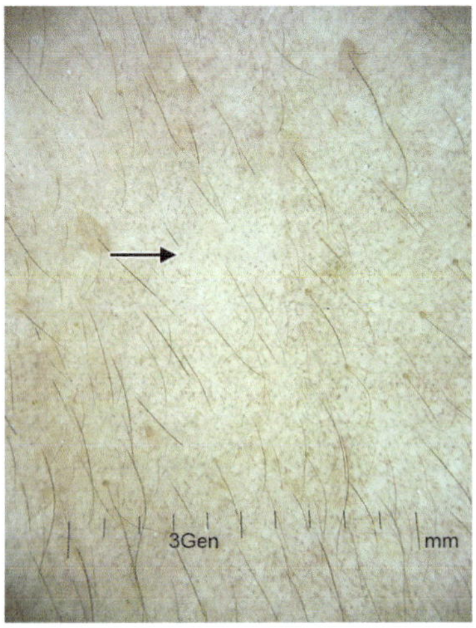

FIG. 54: Grade I acquired dermal macular hyperpigmentation has scattered sparsely distributed blue-gray dots forming no specific pattern, known as peppering (black arrow) (polarized, DermLite II Hybrid M, 10×).

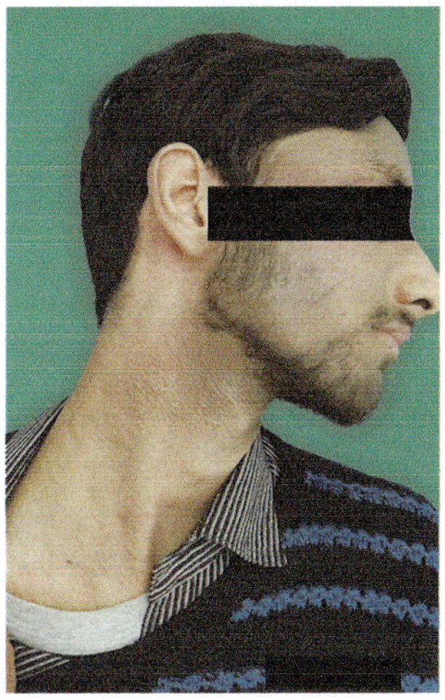

FIG. 55: Diffuse hyperpigmentation on the neck of a patient with acquired dermal macular hyperpigmentation.

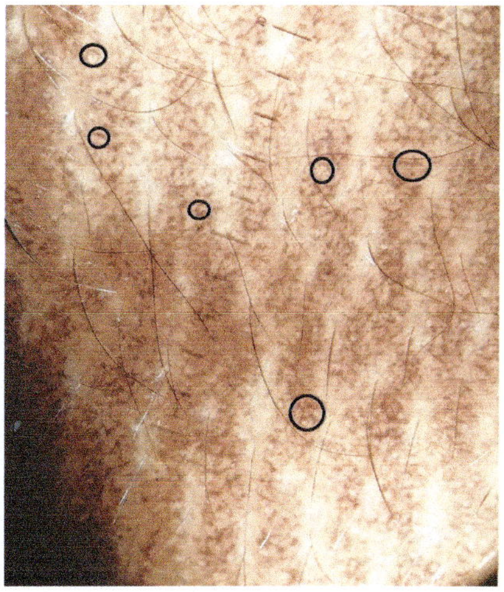

FIG. 56: Grade II acquired dermal macular hyperpigmentation demonstrates prominent Chinese letter pattern or hem-like pattern (black circles) (polarized, DermLite II Hybrid M, 10×).

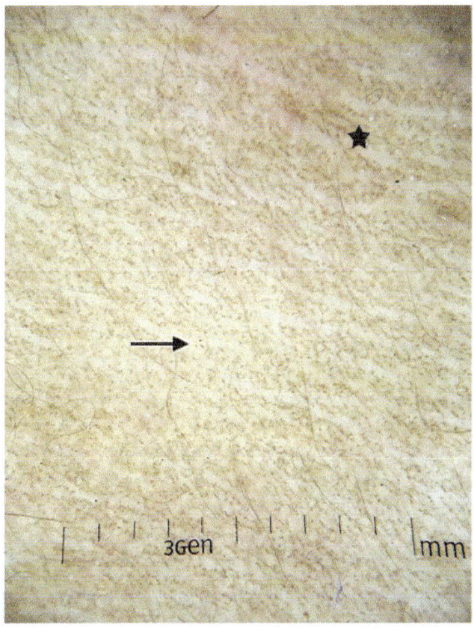

FIG. 57: Another picture showing grade II pigmentation with blue-gray dots (black arrow) coalescing to form linear/broken-linear (black star) and arcuate/semiarcuate structures. Chinese letter pattern or hem-like pattern (polarized, DermLite II Hybrid M, 10×).

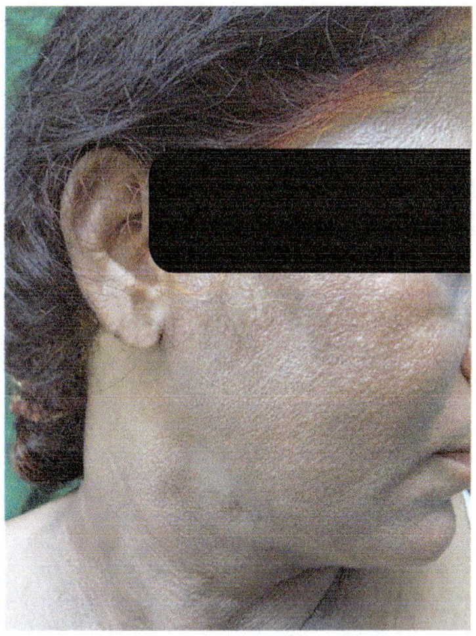

FIG. 58: Diffuse hyperpigmentation on the lateral face and neck of a patient with acquired dermal macular hyperpigmentation.

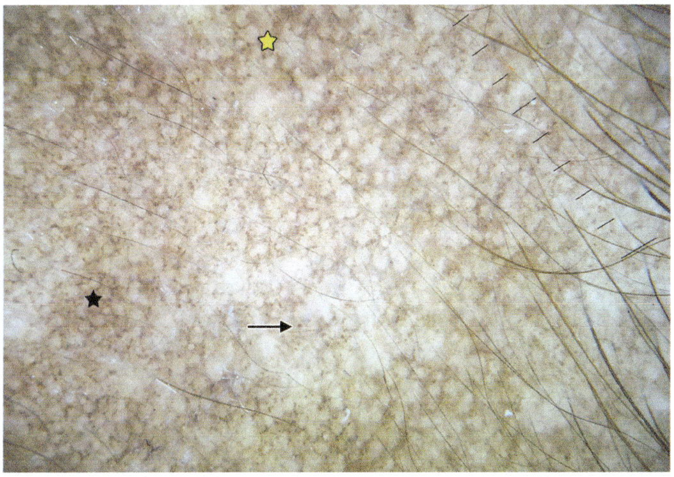

FIG. 59: Grade III demonstrates blue-gray dots (black arrow) and globules (yellow star) coalescing around numerous white dots of follicular and eccrine openings to form pseudoreticular pattern (black arrow) (polarized, DermLite II Hybrid M, 10×).

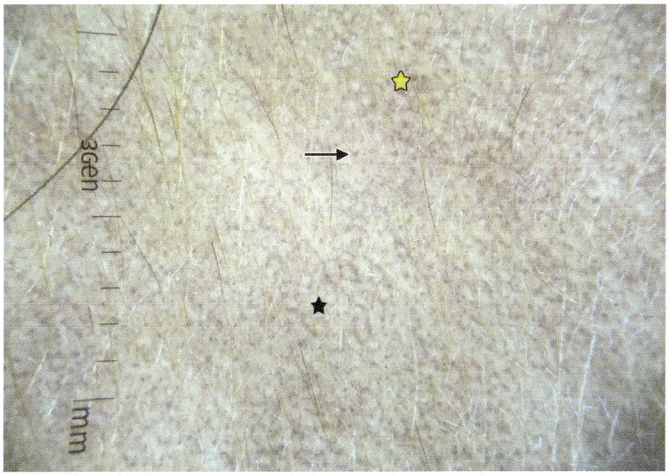

FIG. 60: Another picture showing grade III pigmentation with blue-gray dots (black arrow) and globules (yellow star) coalescing around numerous white dots of follicular and eccrine openings to form pseudoreticular pattern (black arrow) (polarized, DermLite II Hybrid M, 10×).

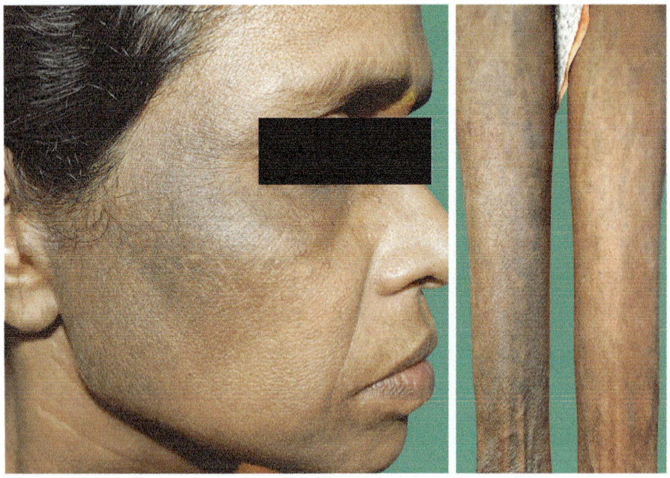

FIG. 61: Dense diffuse hyperpigmentation on the face and upper limbs of a patient with acquired dermal macular hyperpigmentation.

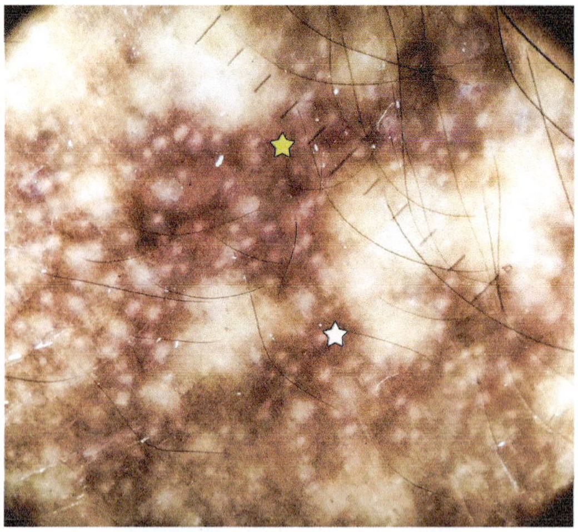

FIG. 62: Grade IV demonstrates massive melanin incontinence characterized by the presence of big globules (white star) and blotches (yellow star) which appear as diffuse deposition of pigment just sparing the appendageal orifices and obliterating the underlying normal pigment network completely (polarized, DermLite II Hybrid M, 10×).

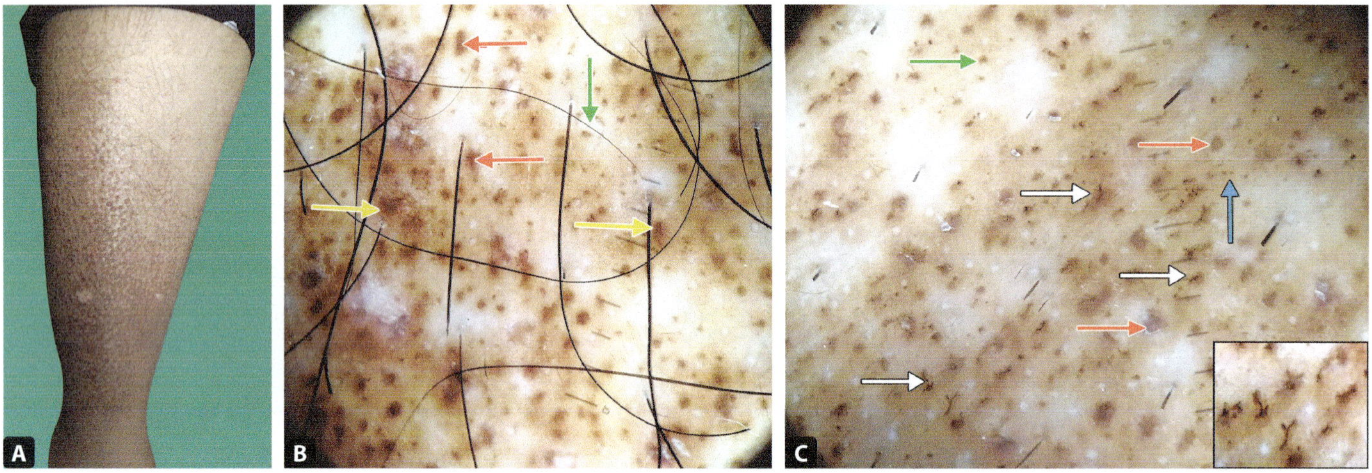

FIGS. 63A TO C: (A) Clinical image of biphasic amyloidosis showing reticulate hyperpigmented papules and macules; (B) Dermoscopic image of amyloid macules showing irregular hyperpigmented blotches (yellow arrows) and central brown clod (red arrows) or white area (green arrow) with surrounding streaks or brown dots in hub and spoke pattern (polarized, DermLite DL4, 10×); (C) Dermoscopic image of amyloid macules showing brown clods and the radiating brown lines described as hub and spoke pattern (white arrows, inset), gray blotches (red arrows), brown blotches (green arrow), scattered brown dots (blue arrow) (polarized, DermLite DL4, 10×).

Key Points

- Acquired diffuse bluish-gray macular disorders such as LPP, ashy dermatosis, Riehl's melanosis can be grouped together as they show similar dermoscopic and histopathological features.
- Dermoscopy of ADMH predominantly features gray-blue dots, globules, and blotches.
- Distributed in various patterns including peppering, hem-like, reticular/pseudoreticular and diffuse.

Primary Localized Cutaneous Amyloidosis

Three clinicopathological types of primary localized cutaneous amyloidosis are (1) macular, (2) lichen, and (3) nodular amyloidosis.[49]

Macular Amyloidosis

Clinical Features

It is clinically characterized by small, brown to gray macules distributed symmetrically over arms and upper back associated with pruritus. The most striking clinical presentation is the reticulated or the rippled pattern (**Fig. 63A**).[49] Histopathology, it is characterized by abnormal extracellular deposition of amyloid proteins in the skin, especially in the superficial papillary dermis.

Dermoscopic Features

Dermoscopy of macular amyloidosis shows the central hub encircled by brown streaks of pigmentation, leaf-like extensions, noncircular thick projections and a smooth border called as "hub and spoke pattern" (**Figs. 63B and C**).[50,51] The central hub can be brown or white or both, and corresponds to basket-weave orthokeratosis. The brown pigment corresponds to histopathologically increased basal cell pigmentation and melanin granules within the amyloid deposits in the papillary dermis.

Lichen Amyloidosis

Clinical Features

It mostly presents as intensely pruritic, lichenoid hyperkeratotic papules with fine scaling and hyperpigmentation.[49] The shins are the most common site of involvement (**Fig. 64A**).

Dermoscopic Features

Dermoscopy of lichen amyloidosis demonstrates that most of the central hub seen in macular amyloidosis is replaced by white scar-like tissue, which is surrounded by a rim of brown dots resembling a volcanic crater.[50] The scar-like area corresponds to pathological change of acanthosis and compact orthokeratosis.[51,52] As the horny layer gets thicker, the structure less areas become predominant. Other features are gray-brown blotches and scattered brown granules (**Fig. 64B**). Additional dermoscopic findings described in the literature are horseshoe pattern, cart-wheel pattern, and amorphous pigmented globular pattern.[52]

Key Points

- Central hub encircled by brown streaks of pigmentation—hub and spoke pattern
- Scar-like pattern

Acanthosis Nigricans

Clinical Features

Acanthosis nigricans clinically presents as hyperpigmentation and thickening with papillomatous elevations distributed symmetrically on the neck and other flexural areas such as axillae, antecubital and popliteal fossa, groins, umbilicus, and perianal areas, usually in the setting of diabetes mellitus, polycystic ovarian disease, malignancy, etc.[53] It may also present as facial and periocular pigmentation, with a velvety texture (**Fig. 65A**). Histopathology, demonstrates prominent papillomatosis instead of acanthosis.

Dermoscopic Features

The most common dermoscopic findings are the presence of linear crista cutis and sulcus cutis that corresponds to the papillomatosis with interspersed rete ridges histopathologically. Multiple focal brown to black hyperpigmented dots can also be routinely seen representing the focal melanin accumulation in epidermis (**Fig. 65B**).[43] Other clues that can be appreciated are exophytic papillary structures (**Fig. 65C**), multiple asymmetric blotches, milia-like cysts, and perieccrine pigment deposition.[43]

Key Points

- Linear crista cutis and sulcus cutis pattern
- Multiple focal hyperpigmented dots

The dermascopic approach to hyperpigmented lesions is presented in **Figure 66**.

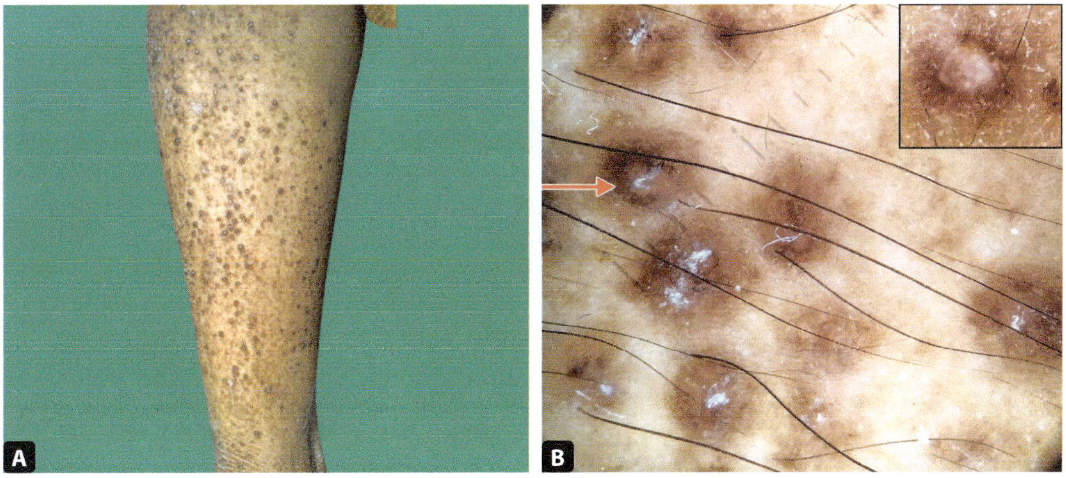

FIGS. 64A AND B: (A) Clinical image of lichen amyloidosis showing multiple hyperpigmented scaly papules; (B) Dermoscopic image of lichen amyloidosis showing central scar-like hub surrounded by brownish rim resembling horseshoe pattern (red arrow) and a volcanic crater (inset) (polarized, DermLite DL4, 10×).

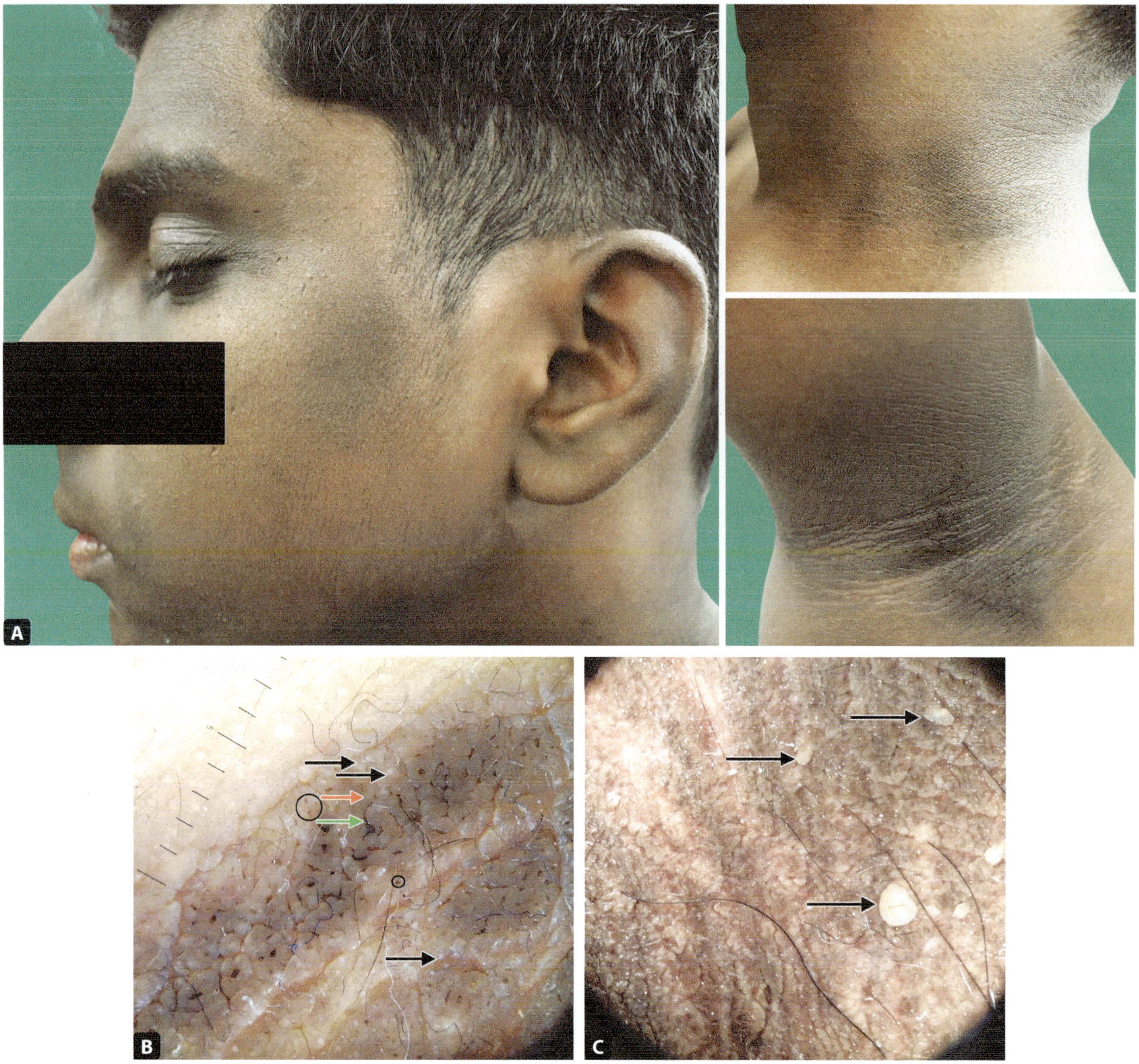

FIGS. 65A TO C: (A) Clinical picture of acanthosis nigricans over the face, neck, and axilla; (B) Dermoscopic image of acanthosis nigricans showing the presence of linear crista cutis (red arrow) and sulcus cutis (green arrow), with focal pigmented dots (black circles), exophytic papillary structures (black arrows) (polarized, DermLite DL4, 10×); (C) Dermoscopic image of acanthosis nigricans showing the presence of linear crista cutis, sulcus cutis with exophytic papillary structures (black arrows) (polarized, DermLite DL4, 10×).

CONCLUSION

Dermoscopy is a valuable addition in the diagnosis and management of hyperpigmented skin lesions. A systematic algorithmic approach is useful in diagnosis. It can assist clinical diagnosis; play a role in selection of treatment as in periocular melanosis and melasma and also help in selecting the site of biopsy as in exogenous ochronosis. In addition, it is a useful modality to detect early complications as in melasma and decide endpoint of treatment as in laser treatment of nevus of Ota. Dermoscopy is no longer an optional skill but an essential tool for the dermatologist.

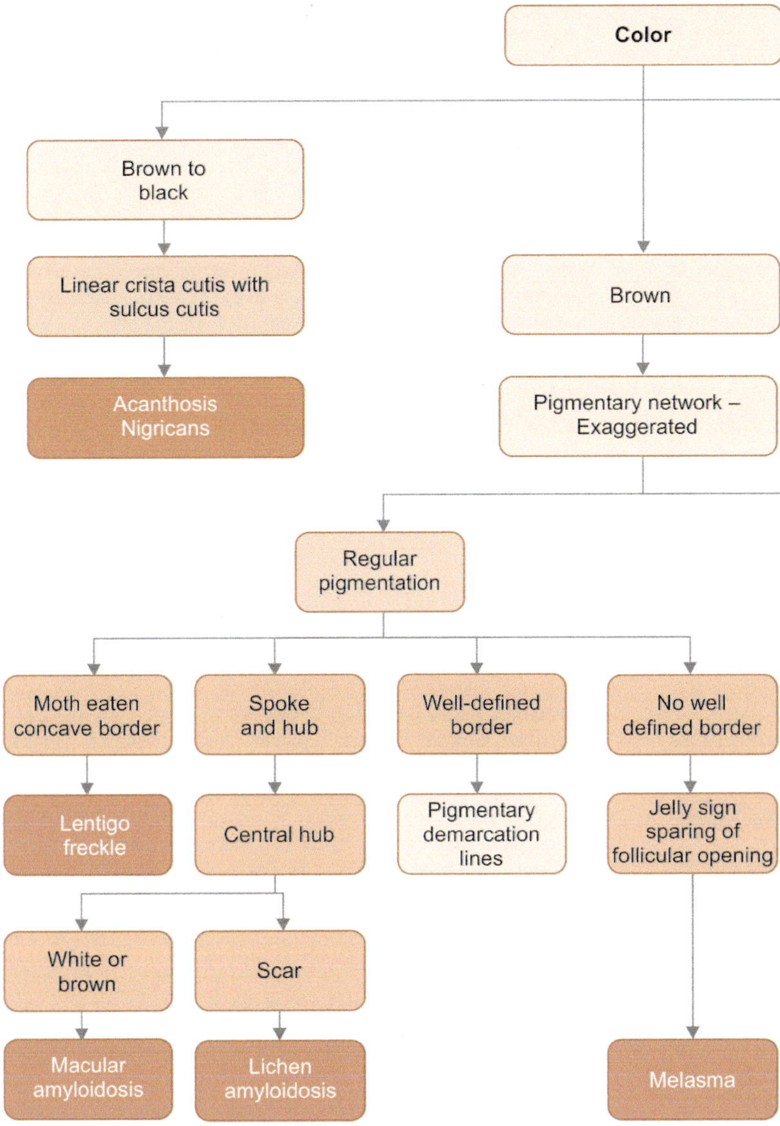

FIG. 66: Algorithmic approach to pigmented lesions.

REFERENCES

1. Kittler H, Pehamberger H, Wolff K, Binder M. Diagnostic accuracy of dermoscopy. Lancet Oncol. 2002;3:159-65.
2. Soyer HP, Argenziano G, Chimenti S, Ruocco V. Dermoscopy of pigmented skin lesions. Eur J Dermatol. 2001;11:270-6.
3. Nischal KC, Khopkar US, Haldar SS. Dermoscopy: applications and patterns in diseases of the brown skin. In: Khopkar US (Ed). Dermoscopy and Trichoscopy in Diseases of the Brown Skin: Atlas and Short Text. New Delhi: Jaypee Brothers Medical Publishers (P) Ltd; 2012. pp. 13-7.
4. Kittler H, Marghoob AA, Argenziano G, Carrera C, Curiel-Lewandrowski C, Hofmann-Wellenhof R, et al. Standardization of terminology in dermoscopy/dermatoscopy: results of the third consensus conference of the International Society of Dermoscopy. J Am Acad Dermatol. 2016;74:1093-106.
5. Argenziano G, Soyer HP, Chimenti S, Talamini R, Corona R, Sera F, et al. Dermoscopy of pigmented skin lesions: results of a consensus meeting via the Internet. J Am Acad Dermatol. 2003;48:679-93.
6. Elgart GW. Seborrheic keratoses, solar lentigines, and lichenoid keratoses. Dermatoscopic features and correlation to histology and clinical signs. Dermatol Clin. 2001;19:347-57.
7. Tanaka M, Sawada M, Kobayashi K. Key points in dermoscopic differentiation between lentigo maligna and solar lentigo. J Dermatol. 2011;38:53-8.
8. Argenziano G. Interactive Atlas of Dermoscopy. Milan: Edra Medical Publishing and New Media; 2000.
9. Jackson JM, Alexis A, Berman B, Berson DS, Taylor S, Weiss JS. Current understanding of seborrheic keratosis: prevalence, etiology, clinical presentation, diagnosis, and management. J Drugs Dermatol. 2015;14:1119-25.
10. Rajesh G, Thappa DM, Jaisankar TJ, Chandrashekar L. Spectrum of seborrheic keratoses in South Indians: a clinical and dermoscopic study. Indian J Dermatol Venereol Leprol. 2011;77:483-8.
11. Alapatt GF, Sukumar D, Bhat MR. A clinicopathological and dermoscopic correlation of seborrheic keratosis. Indian J Dermatol. 2016;61:622-7.
12. Brown WG. Reticulate pigmented anomaly of the flexures. Case reports and genetic investigation. Arch Dermatol. 1982;118:490-3.
13. Schwartz RA, Birnkrant AP, Burgess GH, Stoll HL Jr, Yaqub M, Fox MD. Reticulate pigmented anomaly. Cutis. 1980;26:380-1.
14. Nirmal B, Dongre AM, Khopkar US. Dermatoscopic features of hyper and hypopigmented lesions of Dowling-Degos disease. Indian J Dermatol. 2016;61:125.
15. Geissler S, Dyall-Smith D, Coras B, Guther S, Peters B, Stolz W. Unique brown star shape on dermatoscopy of generalized Dowling-Degos disease. Australas J Dermatol. 2011;52:151-3.
16. Thappa DM, Jeevankumar B, Karthikeyan K. Giant café-au-lait macule in neurofibromatosis type 1. J Dermatol. 2001;28:60-1.
17. Luk DC, Lam SY, Cheung PC, Chan BH. Dermoscopy for common skin problems in Chinese children using a novel Hong Kong-made dermoscope. Hong Kong Med J. 2014;20:495-503.

18. Nischal KC, Khopkar US. Principles and technique of dermoscopy and videodermoscopy. In: Khopkar US. Dermoscopy and Trichoscopy in Diseases of the Brown Skin: Atlas and Short Text. New Delhi: Jaypee Brothers Medical Publishers (P) Ltd; 2012. pp. 1-9.
19. Corradin MT, Cacitti V, Giulioni E, Patriarca MM, Vettorello A. Nevus spilus: a review of the literature. SM Dermatolog J. 2015;1:1003.
20. Kami⊠ska-Winciorek G. Dermoscopy of nevus spilus. Dermatol Surg. 2013;39:1550-4.
21. Errichetti E, Ankad BS, Sonthalia S, Jha AK, Keshavmurthy V, Kyrgidis A, et al. Dermoscopy in general dermatology (non-neoplastic dermatoses) of skin of colour: a comparative retrospective study by the International Dermoscopy Society. Eur J Dermatol. 2020;30:688-98.
22. Manjunath KG, Kiran C, Sonakshi S, Agrawal R. Melasma: through the eye of a dermoscope. Int J Res Dermatol. 2016;2:113.
23. Nanjundaswamy BL, Joseph JM, Raghavendra KR. A clinico dermoscopic study of melasma in a tertiary care center. Pigment Int. 2017;4:98-103.
24. Chatterjee M, Neema S. Dermoscopic characteristics of melasma in Indians: a cross-sectional study. Int J Dermoscopy. 2017;1:6-10.
25. Sonthalia S, Jha AK, Langar S. Dermoscopy of melasma. Indian Dermatol Online J. 2017;8:525.
26. Manjunath KG, Kiran C, Sonakshi S, Ashwini N, Agrawal R. Comparative study of Wood's lamp and dermoscopic features of melasma. J Evid Based Med Health. 2015;2:9012-5.
27. Khunger N, Kandhari R. Dermoscopic criteria for differentiating exogenous ochronosis from melasma. Indian J Dermatol Venereol Leprol. 2013;79:819.
28. Charlin R, Barcaui CB, Kac BK, Soares DB, Rabello-Fonseca R, Azulay-Abulafi L. Hydroquinone induced exogenous ochronosis: a report of four cases and usefulness of dermatoscopy. Int J Dermatol. 2008;47:19-23.
29. Somani VK, Razvi F, Sita VN. Pigmentary demarcation lines over the face. Indian J Dermatol Venereol Leprol. 2004;70:336-41.
30. Malakar S, Lahiri K, Banerjee U, Mondal S, Sarangi S. Periorbital melanosis is an extension of pigmentary demarcation line-F on face. Indian J Dermatol Venereol Leprol. 2007;73:323-5.
31. Antony A, Kumar P. Pigmentary demarcation lines: a clinical profile of 50 subjects and report of new pattern of pigmentation observed. Int J Res Dermatol. 2018;4:323-7.
32. Khunger N, Kandhari R, Singh A, Ramesh V. A clinical, dermoscopic, histopathological and immunohistochemical study of melasma and facial pigmentary demarcation lines in the skin of color. Dermatol Ther. 2020;33:e14515.
33. Chatterjee M, Neema S. Dermoscopy of pigmentary disorders in brown skin. Dermatol Clin. 2018;36:473-85.
34. Sarkar R, Ranjan R, Garg S, Garg VK, Sonthalia S, Bansal S. Periorbital hyperpigmentation: a comprehensive review. J Clin Aesthet Dermatol. 2016;9:49-55.
35. Huang YL, Chang SL, Ma L, Lee MC, Hu S. Clinical analysis and classification of dark eye circle. Int J Dermatol. 2014;53:164-70.
36. Jage M, Mahajan S. Clinical and dermoscopic evaluation of periorbital hyperpigmentation. Indian J Dermatopathol Diagn Dermatol. 2018;5:42-7.
37. Ahuja SK, Deshmukh AR, Khushalani SR. A study of dermatoscopic pattern of periorbital hypermelanosis. Pigment Int. 2017;4:29-34.
38. Zinoune S, Douhi Z, Baybay H, Elloudi S, Mernissi FZ. Bilateral nevus of Ota: an unusual presentation. Madridge J Case Rep Stud. 2019;3:1000137.
39. Elmas ÖF, Kilitçi A. Dermoscopic findings of nevus of Ota. Balkan Med J. 2020;37:116-8.
40. Nair PA, Modasia K, Bhavsar N, Navadiya R. Dermatoscopy of Becker's nevus. Egypt J Dermatol Venerol. 2019;39:37-9.
41. Ingordo V, Iannazzone SS, Cusano F, Naldi L. Dermoscopic features of congenital melanocytic nevus and Becker nevus in an adult male population: an analysis with a 10-fold magnification. Dermatology. 2006;212:354-60.
42. Thomas M, Khopkar US. Becker's nevus vs café-au-lait macules (CALMS): a dermoscopic analysis. In: Khopkar US (Ed). Dermoscopy and Trichoscopy in Diseases of the Brown Skin: Atlas and Short Text. New Delhi: Jaypee Brothers Medical Publishers (P) Ltd; 2012. pp. 81-90.
43. Ankad BS, Drago N, Koti V, Nikam B. Dermoscopic approach to hyperpigmented lesions in skin of color. Clin Dermatol Rev. 2020;4:84-91.
44. Bishnoi A, Vinay K, Kumaran SM, Parsad D. Everything is in the name: macular hyperpigmentation of uncertain etiology or acquired dermal macular hyperpigmentation of varied etiologies? Indian J Dermatol Venereol Leprol. 2019;85:85-7.
45. Pirmez R, Duque-Estrada B, Donati A, Campos-do-Carmo G, Valente NS, Romiti R, et al. Clinical and dermoscopic features of lichen planus pigmentosus in 37 patients with frontal fibrosing alopecia. Br J Dermatol. 2016;175:1387-90.
46. Errichetti E, Angione V, Stinco G. Dermoscopy in assisting the recognition of ashy dermatosis. JAAD Case Rep. 2017;3:482-4.
47. Sharma VK, Gupta V, Pahadiya P, Vedi KK, Arava S, Ramam M. Dermoscopy and patch testing in patients with lichen planus pigmentosus on face: a cross-sectional observational study in fifty Indian patients. Indian J Dermatol Venereol Leprol. 2017;83:656-62.
48. Vinay K, Bishnoi A, Parsad D, Saikia UN, Sendhil Kumaran M. Dermatoscopic evaluation and histopathological correlation of acquired dermal macular hyperpigmentation. Int J Dermatol. 2017;56:1395-9.
49. Weidner T, Illing T. Primary localized cutaneous amyloidosis: a systematic treatment review. Am J Clin Dermatol. 2017;18:629-42.
50. Chuang YY, Lee DD, Lin CS, Chang YJ, Tanaka M, Chang YT, et al. Characteristic dermoscopic features of primary cutaneous amyloidosis: a study of 35 cases. Br J Dermatol. 2012;167:548-54.
51. Kumar P, Neema S, Pathak N. Macular amyloidosis in a middle-aged woman. Pigment Int. 2018;5:57-8.
52. Sharma RK. Dermoscopic study of primary cutaneous amyloidosis: new cartwheel and horse-shoe pattern revealed. JDA Indian J Clin Dermatol. 2018;1:68-70.
53. Phiske MM. An approach to acanthosis nigricans. Indian Dermatol Online J. 2014;5:239-49.

9 CHAPTER

Hypopigmentary Disorders

Nirmal B, Vishal Gupta, Savitha L Beergouder, Ashwini PK

INTRODUCTION

Hypopigmentary disorders constitute a large and heterogenous group of diseases that are clinically characterized by hypo- or depigmented macules. Dermoscopy is a noninvasive imaging technique that allows for examination of all lesions and appreciation of subtle distinctive features invisible to naked eye to aid in the differential diagnosis of hypopigmentary disorders. In this chapter, we discuss the dermoscopic findings of the common hypopigmentary disorders.

VITILIGO

Clinical Features

Vitiligo is an acquired disorder of depigmentation characterized by white macules and patches (**Fig. 1**) because of loss of melanocytes. Stability in vitiligo is an important concept in guiding patient management and an important prerequisite for surgery. Dermoscope is a useful auxiliary handheld tool to diagnose and evaluate the activity of vitiligo. It is imperative to differentiate stable vitiligo from unstable vitiligo from a therapeutic point of view.

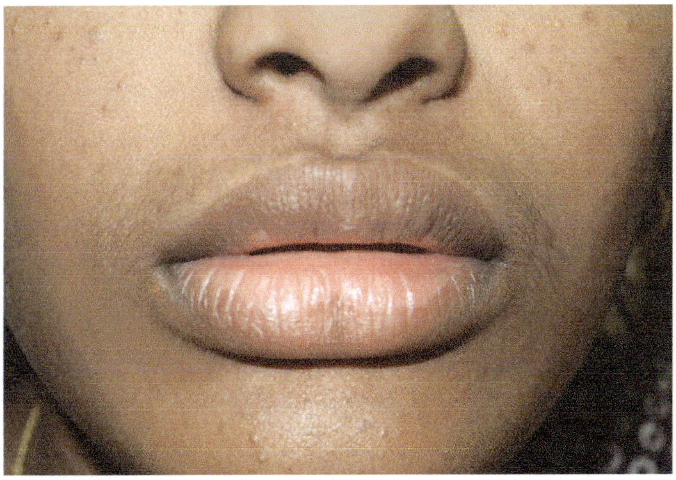

FIG. 1: Clinical photograph of vitiligo shows depigmented macules over lips.

Dermoscopic Features

The role of dermoscopy in vitiligo is:

- Assessment of disease activity
- Pattern of repigmentation (**Fig. 2**)
- Extent of repigmentation[1]
- To differentiate from other disorders with decreased pigmentation.

The major dermoscopic features of vitiligo include diffuse white glow, alteration in the pigment network, perifollicular pigment changes, satellite lesions, micro-Koebnerization, and leukotrichia. White structureless areas or absent pigment network appear to glow due to total loss of melanocytes in the epidermis. Diffuse white glow is due to reflection of incident light completely by collagen in the upper dermis.

Characteristic dermoscopic findings to assess disease activity of vitiligo can be grouped under the following parameters denoted by the acronym *BPLeFoSK* criteria[2] and scored (**Table 1**):

- *B*order: Sharp, ill-defined, trichrome (**Fig. 3**)
- *P*igment network within the patch: Absent, reticular, reduced, reverse[3] (**Fig. 4**). Absent and reticular are stable pigment networks. Reverse pigmentary network is white reticulate pattern with pigmentation in between, indicates evolving vitiligo.
- Peri*le*sional hyperpigmentation (**Fig. 5**)
- Peri*fo*llicular hyperpigmentation (**Fig. 6**)
- *S*atellite lesion (**Fig. 7**)
- Micro-*K*oebner phenomenon (**Fig. 8**)

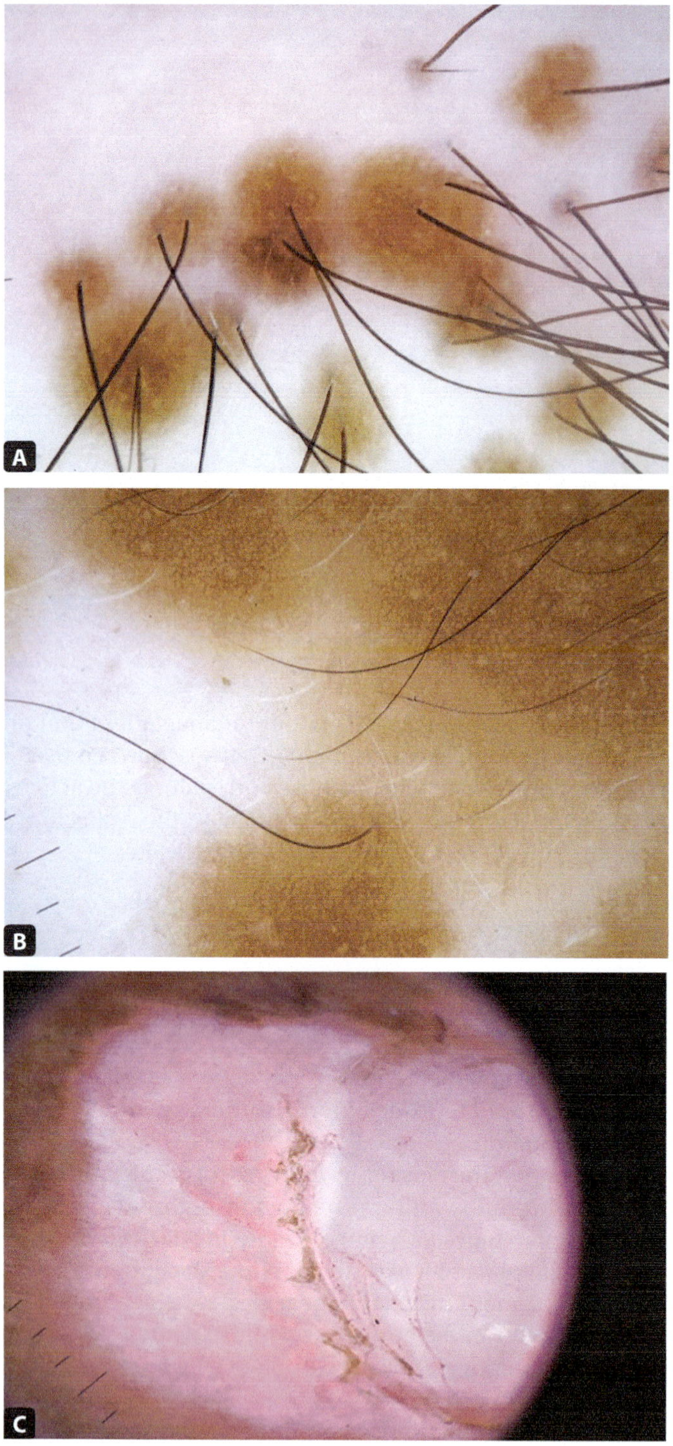

FIGS. 2A TO C: Dermoscopic image of patterns of repigmentation: (A) Perifollicular, (B) marginal, and (C) diffuse (polarized, DermLite DL3, 10×).

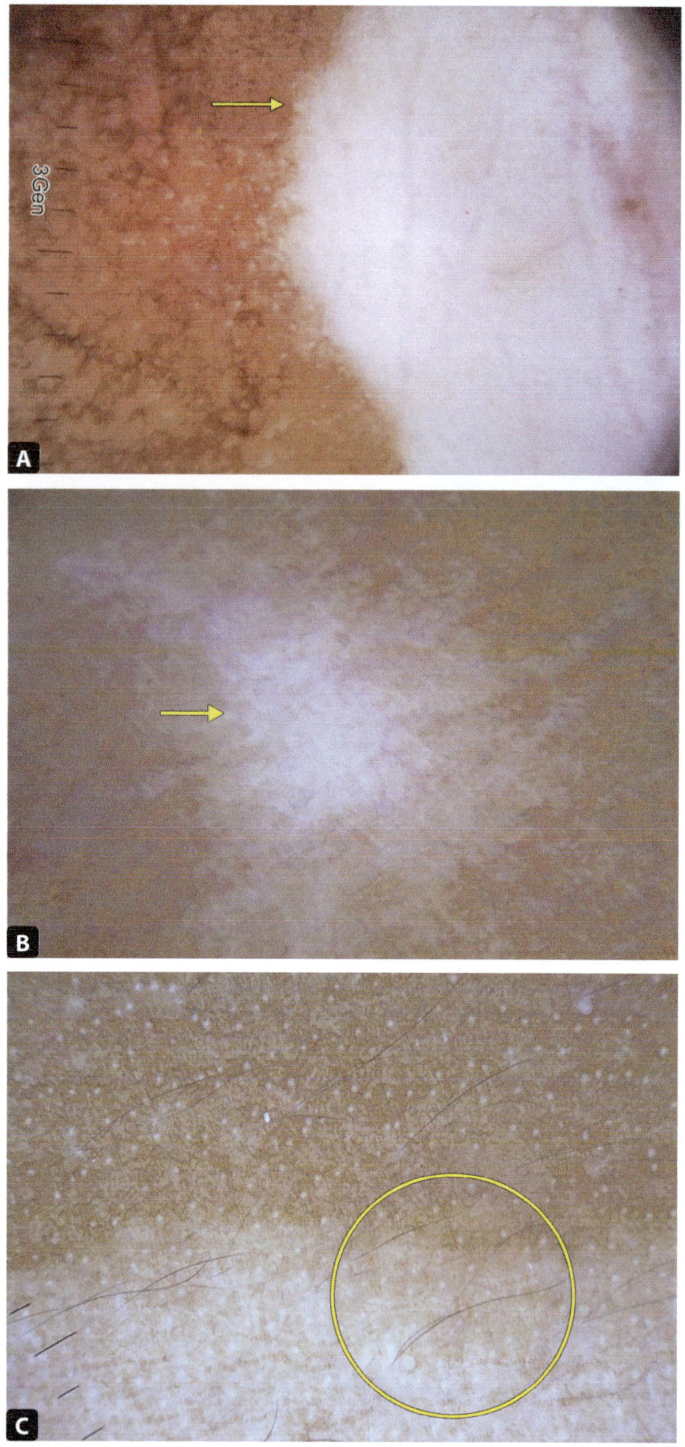

FIGS. 3A TO C: Dermoscopic image of border of vitiligo lesion: (A) Sharp, (B) ill-defined, and (C) trichrome. Sharp border represents stable vitiligo (polarized, DermLite DL3, 10×).

TABLE 1: Scoring for stability in vitiligo: BPLeFoSK criteria.

S. No.	Dermatoscopic parameters	Score
1	*B*order (Sharp)	+1
2	*P*igment network (Absent/Reticulate)	+1
3	Peri*le*sional pigmentation	+1
4	Peri*fo*llicular pigmentation	+1
5	*S*atellite lesion	−1.5
6	Micro-*K*oebner phenomenon	−2

Vitiligo patch is considered stable in the presence of sharp border, absent pigment network, reticulate pigment network, perilesional hyperpigmentation, and perifollicular pigmentation and in the absence of satellite lesions and micro-Koebner phenomenon. A cutoff score of ≥1.5 (sensitivity 90% and specificity 94.37%) using the "BPLeFoSK criteria" indicates stability of a lesion of vitiligo. Progressive vitiligo patterns on dermoscopy include: Trichrome, comet-tail, polka dot, confetti-like, starburst, nebulous, salt and pepper patterns.[4]

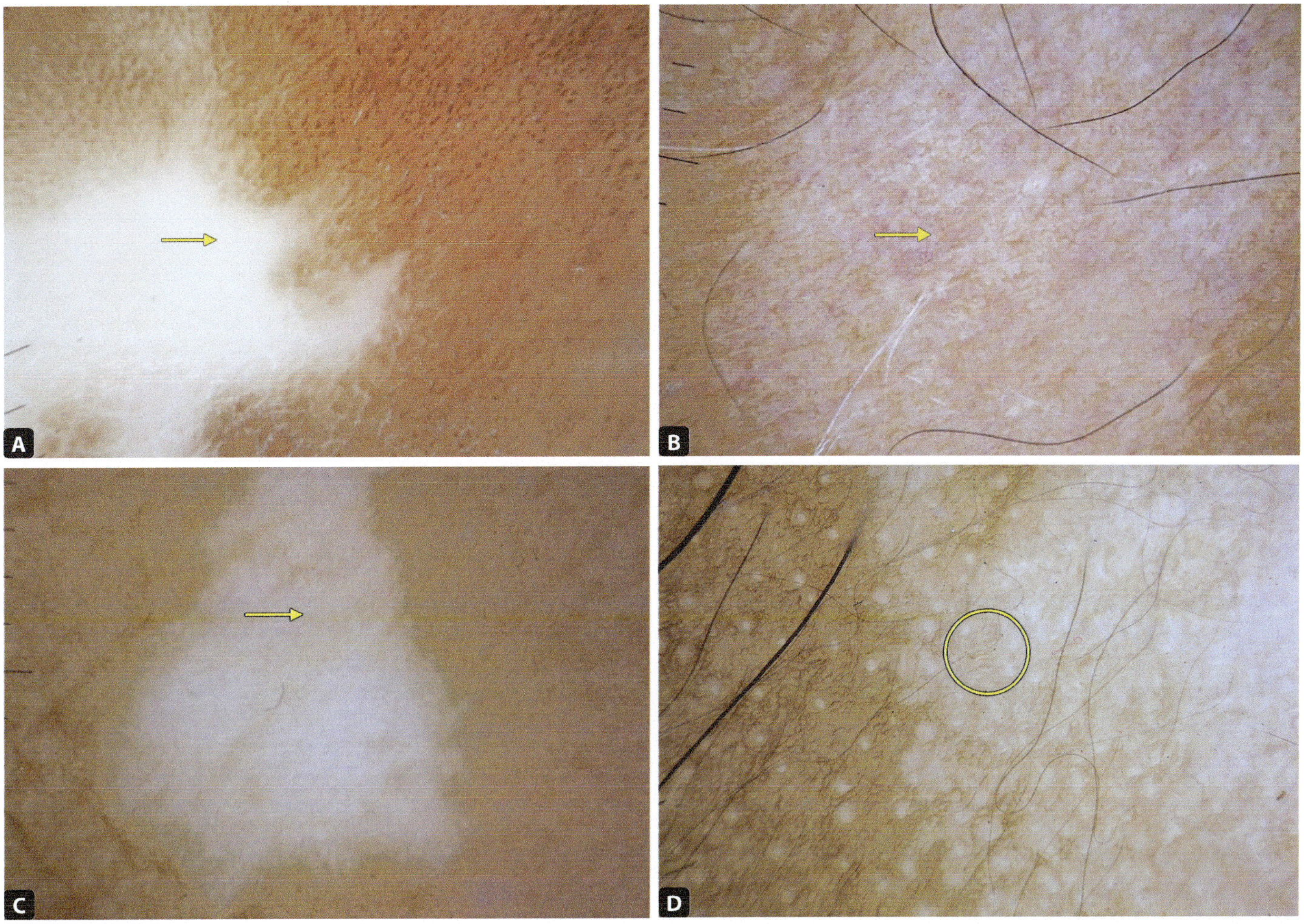

FIGS. 4A TO D: Dermoscopic image of pigment network within the vitiligo lesion: (A) Absent, (B) reticular, (C) reduced, and (D) reverse (polarized, DermLite DL3, 10×).

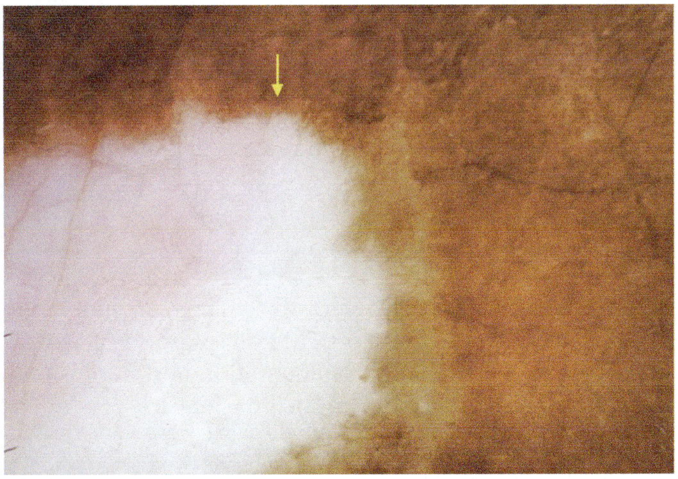

FIG. 5: Dermoscopic image of perilesional hyperpigmentation characteristic of stable lesion (polarized, DermLite DL3, 10×).

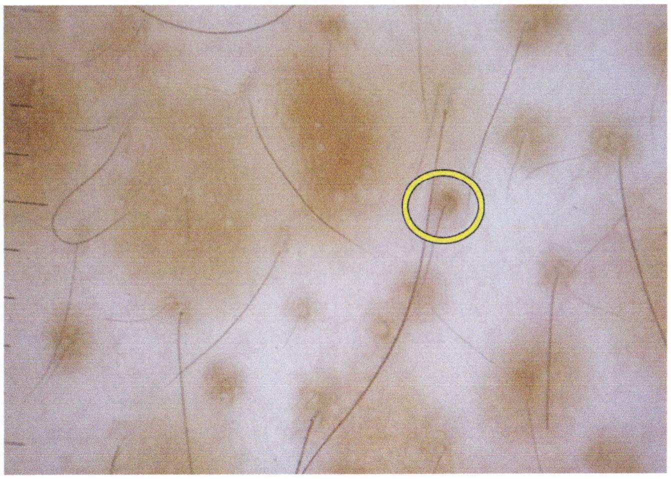

FIG. 6: Dermoscopic image of perifollicular pigmentation indicating stability (polarized, DermLite DL3, 10×).

Blue light dermatoscopy delineates sharp border in stable vitiligo better than white light dermatoscopy as blue light has a wavelength closer to the absorption peak of melanin (**Figs. 9A** and **B**).[5]

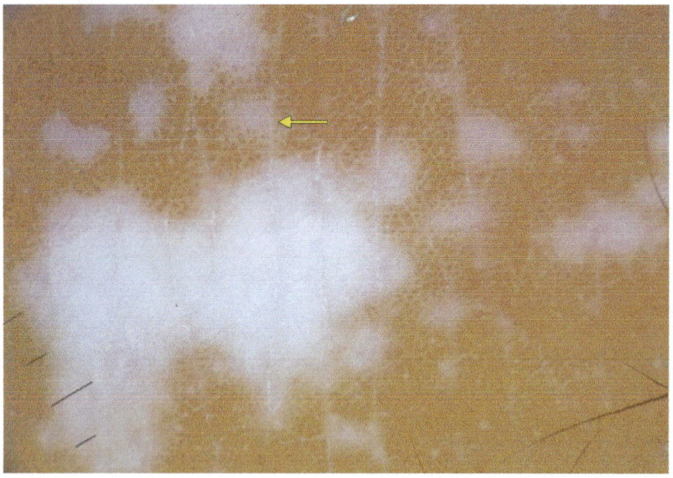

FIG. 7: Dermoscopic image of satellite lesions representing active vitiligo (polarized, DermLite DL3, 10×).

FIG. 8: Dermoscopic image of micro-Koebner phenomenon seen as "comet-tail" appearance indicating disease activity (polarized, DermLite DL3, 10×).

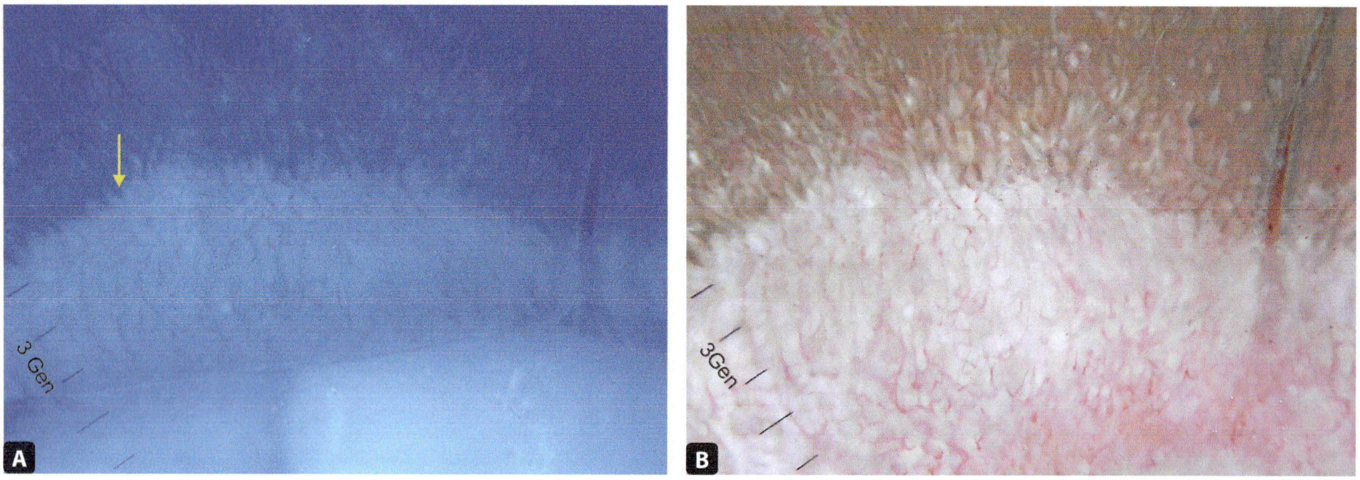

FIGS. 9A AND B: Dermoscopic image of stable vitiligo lesion: (A) Blue light (470 nm) delineates amelanotic vitiligo with the sharply demarcated border better than and (B) white-light dermoscopy (polarized, DermLite DL3, 10×).

Key Points

- *Stable vitiligo*: Sharp border, reticular/absent pigment network, perilesional hyperpigmentation, perifollicular pigmentation.
- *Unstable vitiligo*: Ill-defined/trichrome border, reduced/reverse pigment network, satellite lesions, micro-Koebner phenomenon.

NEVUS DEPIGMENTOSUS

Clinical Features

Nevus depigmentosus is a hypopigmented (unlike what the name would suggest!) macule with characteristic feathery or serrated margins. It is usually present since birth, and its size grows in proportion to body growth (**Fig. 10A**).

It may sometimes be confused with ash-leaf macule or vitiligo, and dermoscopy may help in the differential diagnosis.

Dermoscopic Features

White structureless areas with irregular extensions with a uniform faint brown reticulated pigment network (**Fig. 10B**).[6,7] Perifollicular pigmentation and perilesional pigmentation are other important features in nevus depigmentosus.

Key Points

- White structureless areas with irregular extensions with uniform faint reticular pigment network.

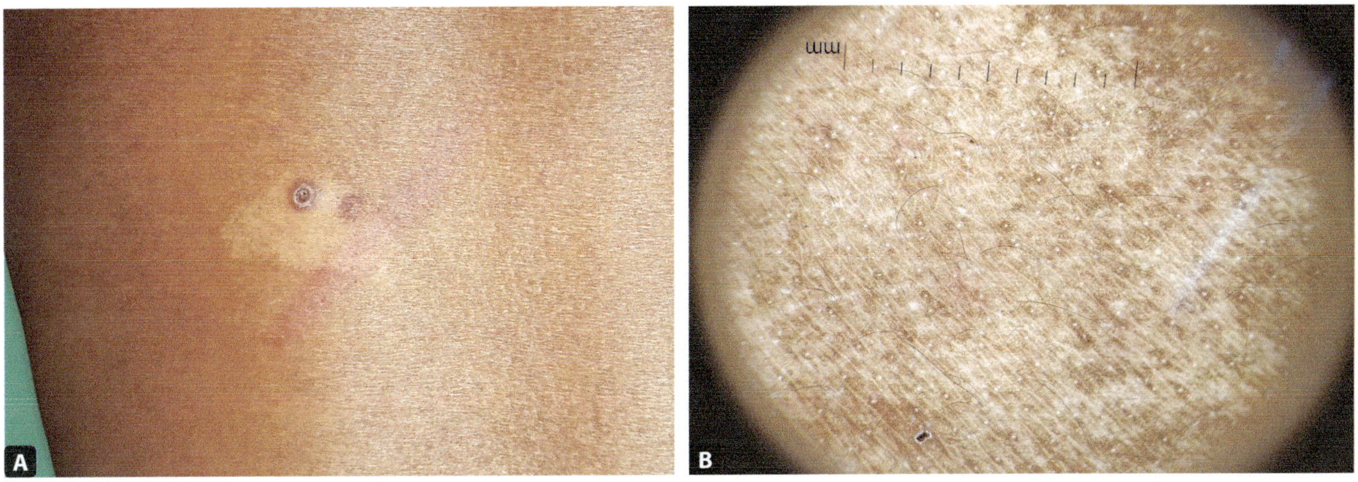

FIGS. 10A AND B: (A) Clinical image of nevus depigmentosus on the back; (B) Dermoscopy showing hypopigmented background with preserved faint pigment network (polarized, DermLite DL3, ×10).

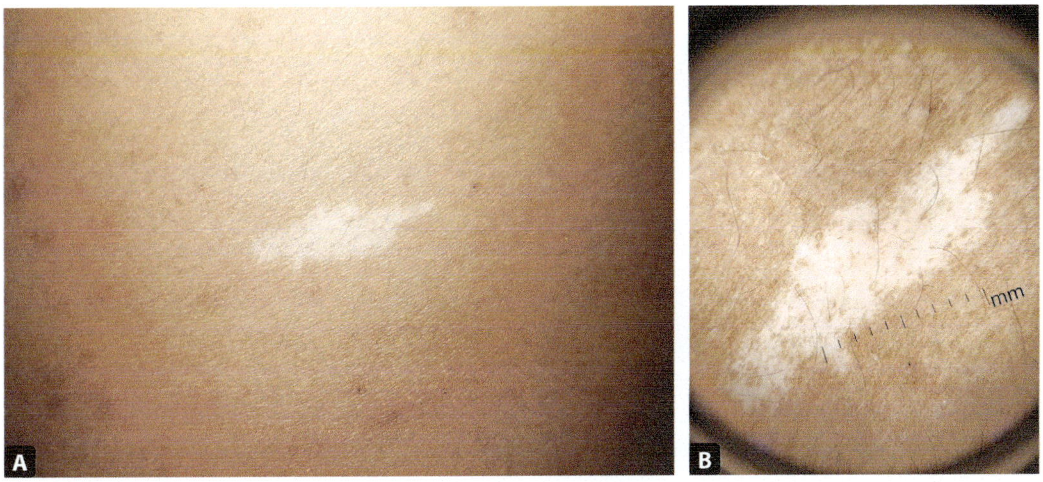

FIGS. 11A AND B: (A) Clinical image of ash-leaf macule on flank; (B) Dermoscopy shows hypopigmented background with absent pigment network, except for focal pigment network and focal areas of normal skin color (polarized, DermLite DL3, 10×).

ASH-LEAF MACULE

Clinical Features

Ash-leaf macules are one of the earliest manifestations of tuberous sclerosis complex, and clinically present as oblong hypopigmented macules usually on the trunk (**Fig. 11A**).

Dermoscopic Features

Faint whitish background and focally retained areas of pigmentation with pigment network. The pigment network is present focally and completely absent in other areas, and where present has a normal brown color (faint brown color in nevus depigmentosus) (**Fig. 11B**).[6] Though this dermoscopic pattern is highly suggestive of ash-leaf macule, it may rarely be seen in nevus depigmentosus (**Figs. 12A and B**). One of the authors (VG) has noted a similar pattern in some of the patients with pigmentary mosaicism of hypopigmented variety (personal observations) (**Figs. 13A and B**).

Key Points

- Faint whitish background with focal small areas of pigmentation and reticular network.

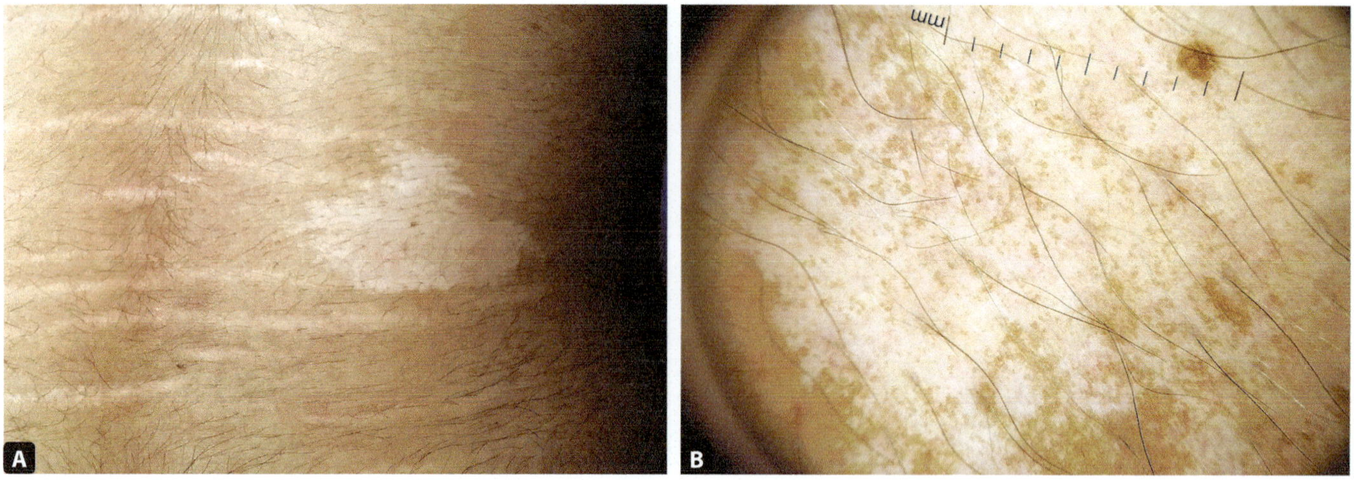

FIGS. 12A AND B: (A) Clinical image of nevus depigmentosus on the back; (B) Dermoscopy shows hypopigmented background with focal pigment network and focal areas of normal skin color; features similar to those described for ash-leaf macule (polarized, DermLite DL3, 10×).

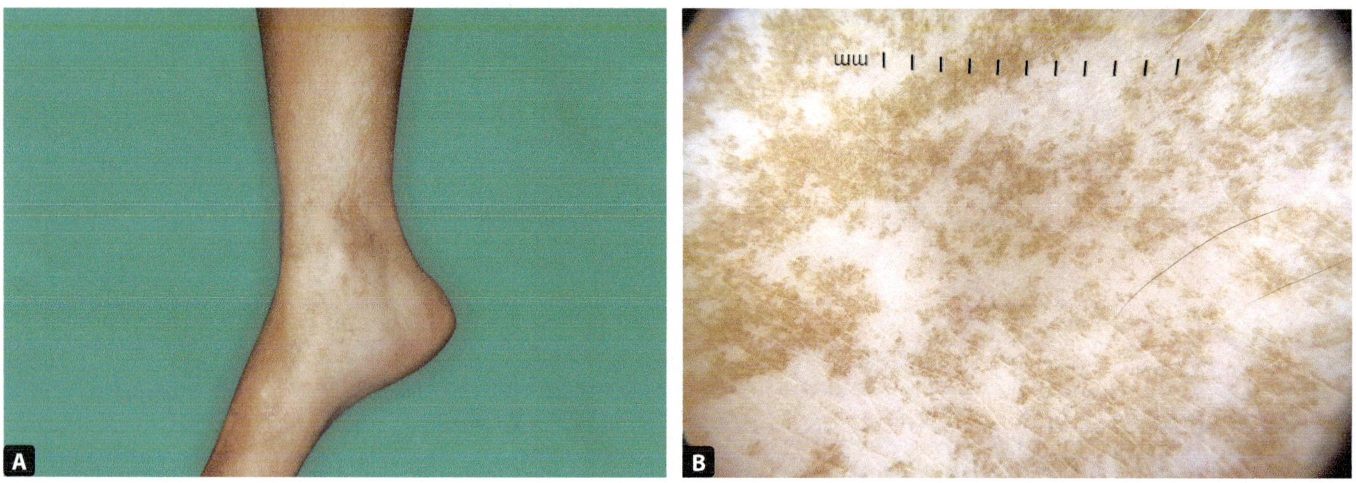

FIGS. 13A AND B: (A) Clinical image of pigmentary mosaicism of the hypopigmented type on the leg; (B) Dermoscopy shows hypopigmented background with islands of retained normal skin color and normal pigment network; features similar to those described for ash-leaf macule (polarized, DermLite DL3, 10×).

PIEBALDISM

Clinical Features

Piebaldism is a congenital depigmentary disorder that occurs due to a developmental defect in melanocytes as a result of mutation in *c-kit* proto-oncogene. It presents at birth as well-demarcated depigmented macules with irregular margins present over the central anterior trunk, mid-extremities, and central forehead (**Fig. 14A**).

Dermoscopic Features

There is little data on the dermoscopic features of piebaldism in the literature. One published report describes whitish areas with nonfollicular areas of normal or hyperpigmented skin (in vitiligo, such areas can be follicular in position). The pigment network is faint and present focally.[8] Additionally, author (VG) has observed perilesional hyperpigmentation and prominent leukotrichia on and outside the lesion (unpublished personal observations) (**Fig. 14B**).

Key Points

- Whitish area with nonfollicular areas of normal or hyperpigmented skin
- Focal faint pigment network
- *Other findings*: Leukotrichia and perilesional hyperpigmentation

IDIOPATHIC GUTTATE HYPOMELANOSIS

Clinical Features

Idiopathic guttate hypomelanosis (IGH) is an acquired leukoderma, commonly seen in elderly, presenting with discrete, round, or oval porcelain-white macules of approximately 2–5-mm diameter, which increase in number with aging.[9]

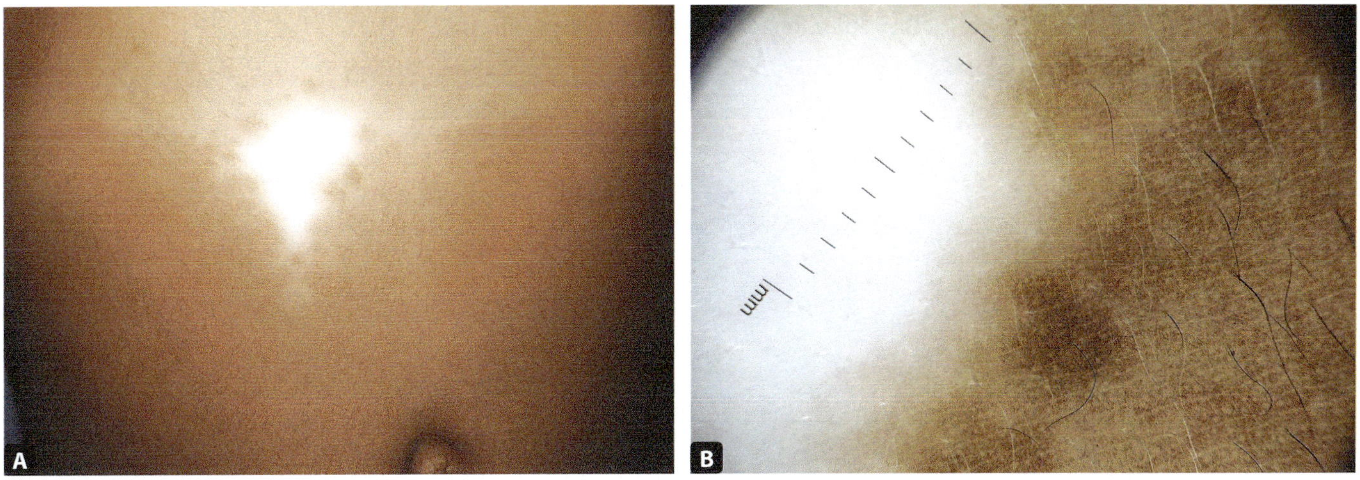

FIGS. 14A AND B: (A) Clinical image of piebaldism: Triangular depigmented macule on the right upper abdomen; (B) Dermoscopy shows depigmented white background with perilesional focal hyperpigmentation. Leukotrichia is present on the lesion as well as outside the depigmented lesion (polarized, DermLite DL3, 10×).

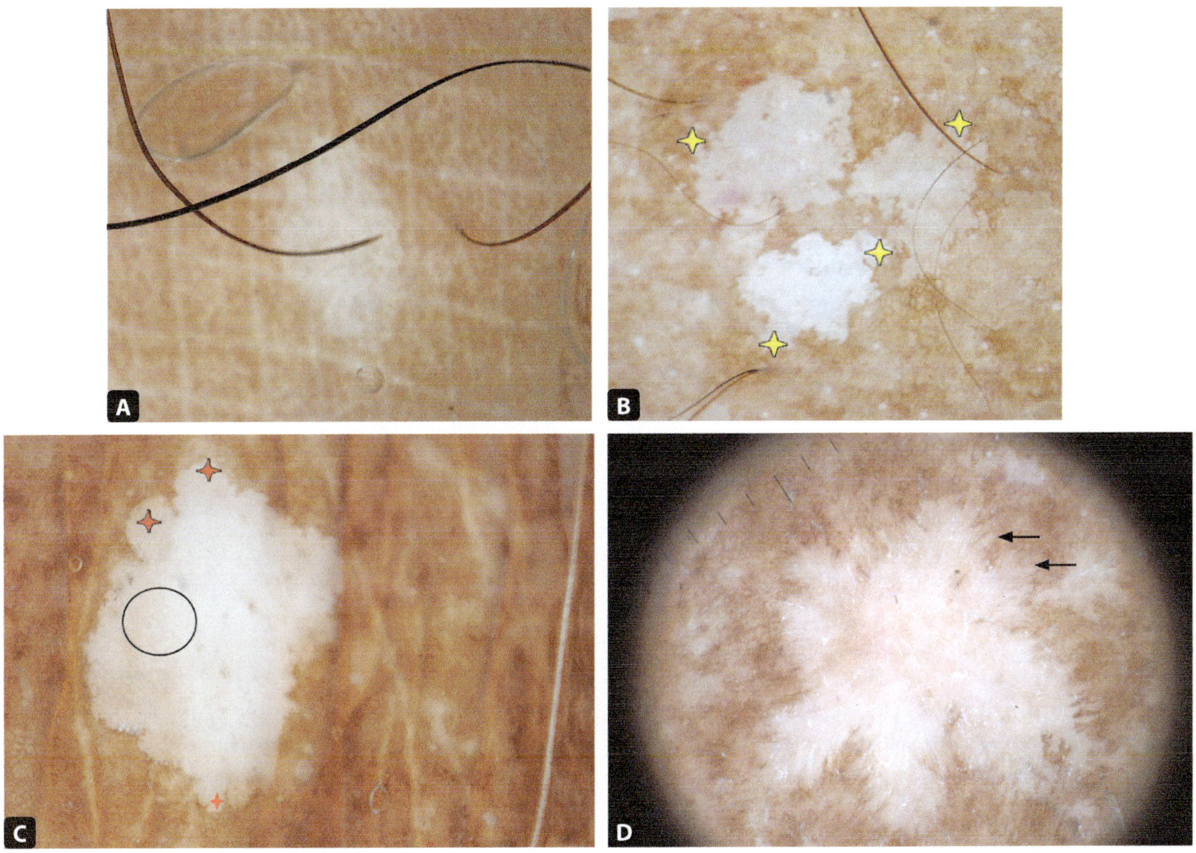

FIGS. 15A TO D: (A) Dermoscopy of idiopathic guttate hypomelanosis showing nebuloid pattern; (B) Dermoscopy of idiopathic guttate hypomelanosis showing homogeneous hypopigmentation with borders showing amoeba-like pseudopods (yellow stars) (polarized, DermLite DL3, 10×); (C) Dermoscopy of idiopathic guttate hypomelanosis showing homogeneous hypopigmented areas with borders extending like petals (red stars) and patchy reticular pigmentation seen (black circle) (polarized, DermLite DL3, 10×); (D) Dermoscopy of idiopathic guttate hypomelanosis showing homogeneous hypopigmentation with thin feathery borders (polarized, DermLite DL3, 10×).

Source (Figs. C and D): Reused with permission from Ankad BS, Beergouder SL. Dermoscopic evaluation of idiopathic guttate hypomelanosis: A preliminary observation. Indian Dermatol Online J. 2015;6:164-7.

Dermoscopic Features

Homogeneous white macules with well/ill-defined borders. Patchy hyperpigmented network can be observed in few lesions. Hair follicles in the lesion appear normal with no perifollicular hyperpigmentation.

Four patterns are appreciated on dermoscopy namely nebuloid, petaloid, feathery, and amoeboid (**Figs. 15A** to **D** and **Table 2**).[4] Different patterns can be seen in different lesions in same person.

TABLE 2: Description of dermoscopic patterns of idiopathic guttate hypomelanosis.

Dermoscopy patterns	Description
Nebuloid (**Fig. 15A**)	Ill-defined borders merging with normal skin
Petaloid (**Fig. 15C**)	Petal like well-defined borders
Feathery (**Fig. 15D**)	Thin feathery borders
Amoeboid (**Fig. 15B**)	Borders extending like pseudopods of amoeba

Key Points

- Homogenous white macules with well to ill-defined borders
- Arranged in nebuloid, petaloid, feathery, and amoeboid

POSTINFLAMMATORY HYPOPIGMENTATION

Clinical Features

Postinflammatory hypopigmentation (PIH) is an acquired partial or total loss of skin pigmentation occurring after cutaneous inflammation, occurs most commonly in dark-skinned people. It can be a result of cutaneous inflammation, injury, or dermatological treatment. Pityriasis lichenoides chronica, lichen striatus, and dermatological procedures tend to induce postinflammatory hypopigmentation rather than hyperpigmentation.

Dermoscopic Features

Dermoscopy reveals patterns that are similar to the original dermatosis with white structureless areas with pink background.[10,11] Dermoscopy of lichen simplex chronicus with chronic steroid abuse shows exaggerated skin markings, white structureless areas with red background (**Figs. 16A** and **B**), hypertrophic lichen planus after intralesional steroid injections shows white structureless areas with pink background and yellow follicular plugging (comedone-like openings) (**Figs. 16C** and **D**), depigmented lesion post-trauma shows white structureless areas in the area of trauma (**Figs. 16E** and **F**).[12,13]

Key Points

- White structureless areas, pink background with typical residual patterns of original dermatosis.

LICHEN SCLEROSIS ET ATROPHICUS

Clinical Features

Extragenital lichen sclerosis (LS) also known as white spot disease or guttate scleroderma is a rare chronic inflammatory dermatosis of unknown etiology. These lesions are usually asymptomatic and clinically lesions begin as polygonal, bluish-white, slightly elevated papules which coalesce into plaques and with time become increasingly atrophic and get a wrinkled surface (**Fig. 17A**).

Dermoscopic Features

White structureless areas, comedone-like openings (follicular plugging), and white crystalline structures (chrysalis-like structures) along with telangiectasias of various lengths and caliber.[14,15] Early lesions of LS are associated with dermoscopic findings of follicular plugging and white structureless areas, whereas in late cases, these features become less prominent (**Figs. 17B** and **C**). Peppering of brown and blue-gray dots is also a characteristic pattern.[16,17]

Key Points

- White structureless areas with comedone-like openings
- Telangiectasia
- White chrysalis structures
- Peppering

PITYRIASIS ALBA

Clinical Features

Pityriasis alba is a low-grade type of eczema or dermatitis seen in children and young adults. Hypopigmented, dry macules, or patches with mild scaling, more commonly seen over face in young children (**Fig. 18A**).

Dermoscopic Features

Fairly ill-demarcated white areas with fine scales distributed within and outside the area. Faint pigment network is observed at the background. Hairs within the lesion are normal (**Fig. 18B**).[13,18]

Key Points

- Ill-demarcated white areas with mild scaling on a faint pigment network.

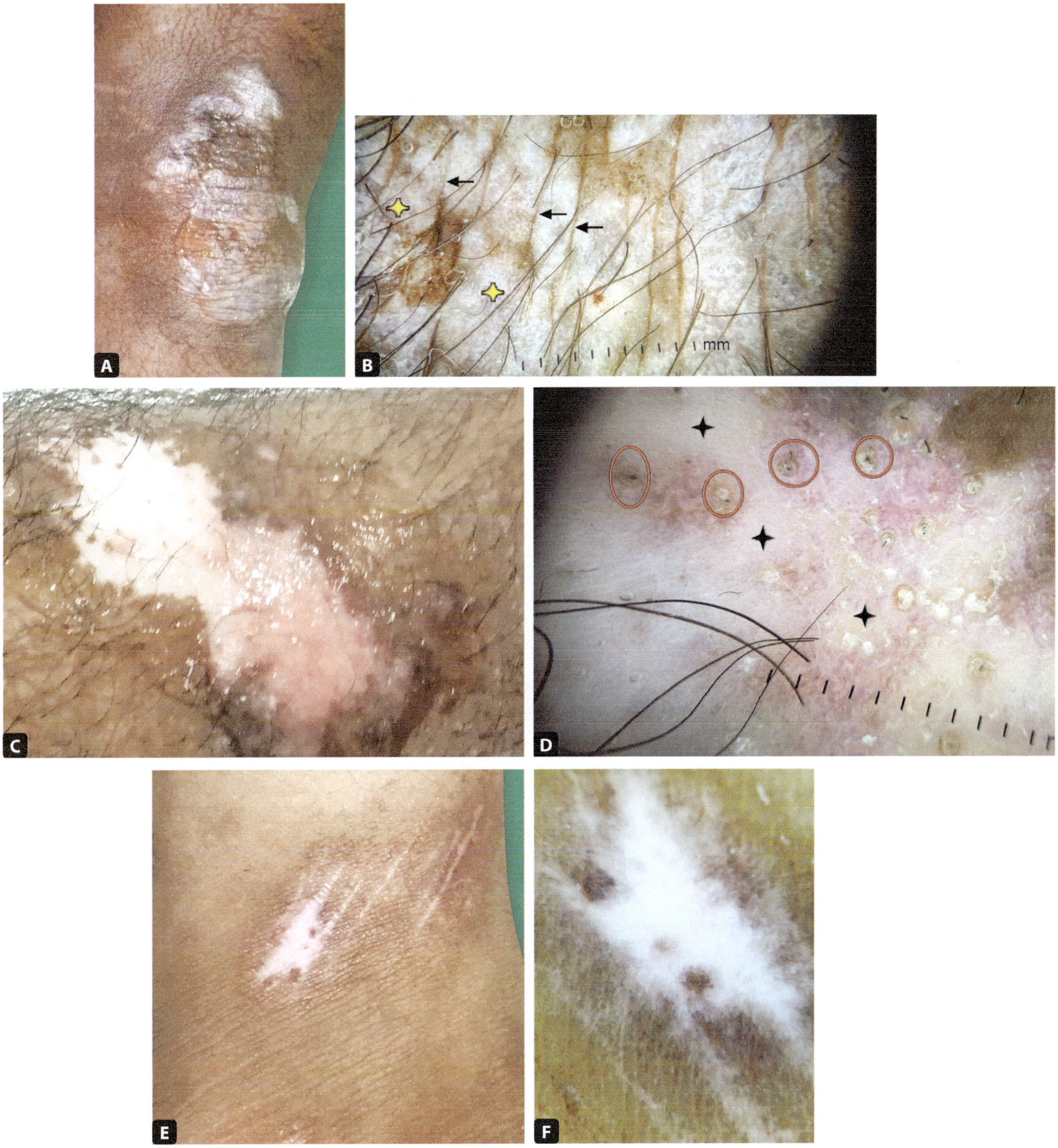

FIGS. 16A TO F: (A) Clinical picture of hypopigmented to depigmented plaque over the knee; (B) White structureless areas, exaggerated skin markings (black arrows) with dull red background (yellow stars) (polarized, DermLite DL3, 10×); (C) Clinical picture of depigmented erythematous plaque of hypertrophic lichen planus over shin; (D) Dermoscopy shows white structureless areas (black stars), pink background, and follicular plugging (red circles) (polarized, DermLite DL3, 10×); (E) Clinical picture of depigmented plaque over leg in the area of trauma; (F) Dermoscopy showing white structureless areas with pink background (polarized, DermLite DL3, 10×).

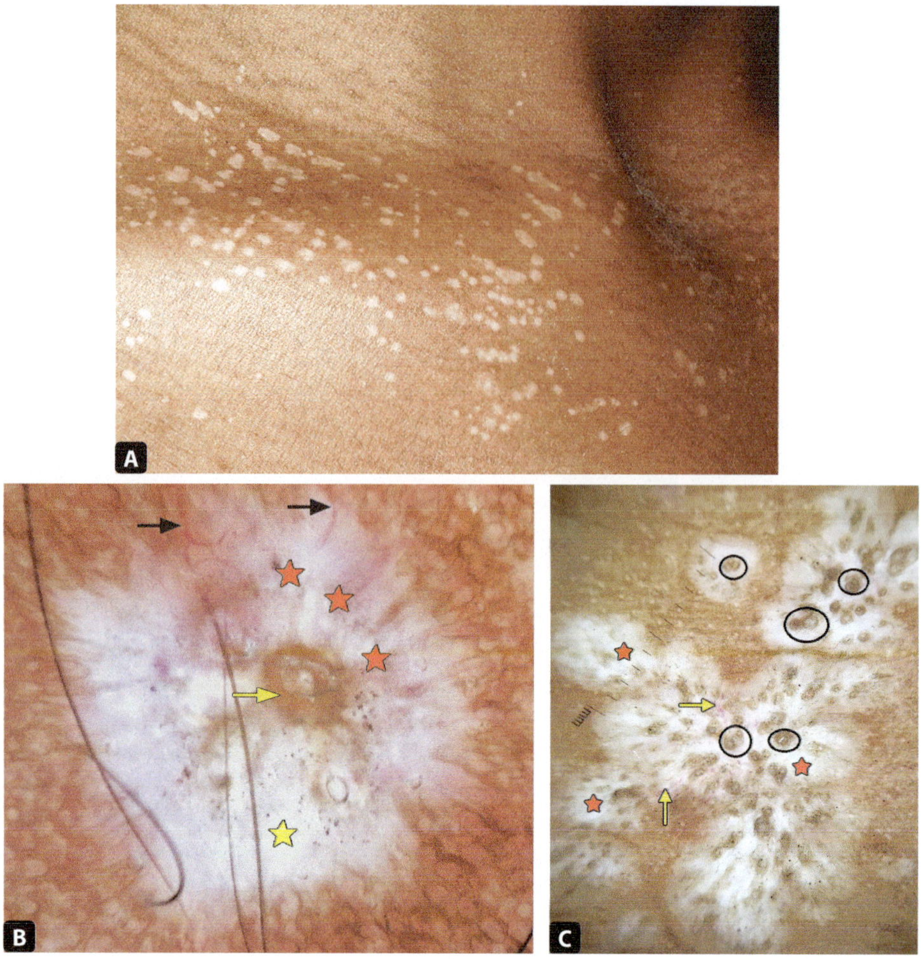

FIGS. 17A TO C: (A) Multiple depigmented macules, papules, and few plaques with mild atrophy in lichen sclerosus. Koebner phenomenon is seen; (B) Dermoscopy showing white structureless areas (yellow star) and comedone-like openings (yellow arrow) with telangiectasias of different lengths and calibers (black arrows) and white crystalline structures (white chrysalis) (red stars) (polarized, DermLite DL3, 10×); (C) White structureless areas (red stars), comedone-like openings (black circles), and telangiectasias of different lengths (yellow arrows) (polarized, DermLite DL3, 10×).

Source (Figs. A and B): Reused with permission from Ankad BS, Beergouder SL. Dermoscopic patterns in lichen sclerosus: A report of three cases. Indian Dermatol Online J. 2015;6(3):237-40.

Courtesy (Fig. C): Dr Chetan D Rajput, SBH Government Medical College, Dhule, Maharashtra, India.

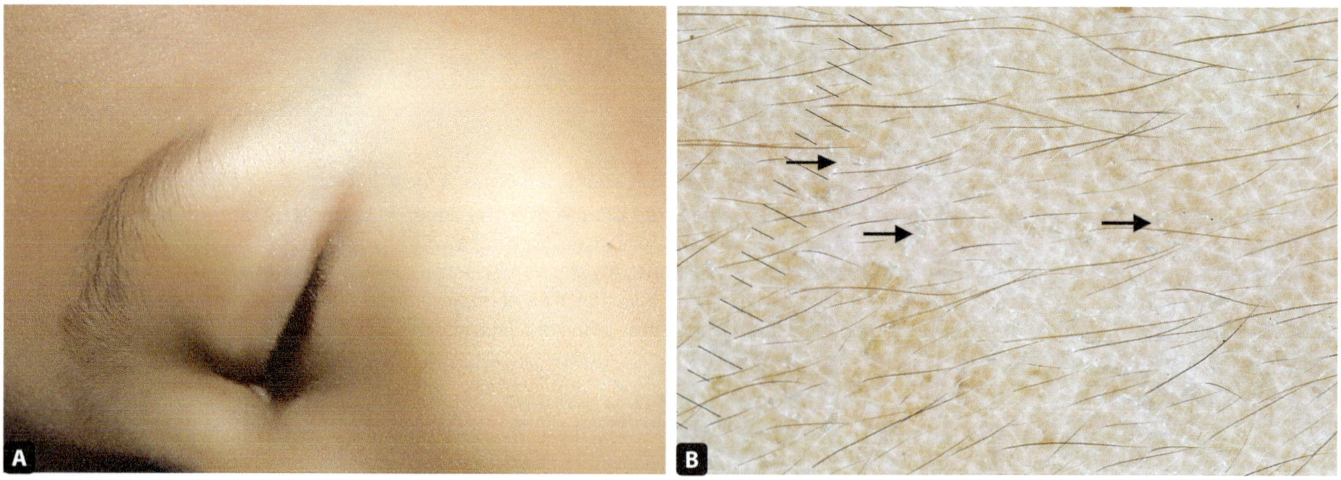

FIGS. 18A AND B: (A) Clinical picture of hypopigmented macule near eye; (B) Dermoscopy shows ill-defined hypopigmented area with mild scaling (black arrows) (polarized, DermLite DL3, 10×).

Courtesy (Fig. B): Dr Balachandra S Ankad, SN Medical College, Bagalkot, Karnataka, India.

PITYRIASIS VERSICOLOR

Clinical Features

Pityriasis versicolor (PV) is clinically characterized by hyperpigmented or hypopigmented or erythematous, round to oval lesions commonly found on the upper chest, back, upper part of arms, neck, and face. The surface of the patches may show mild scaling (**Fig. 19**).

Dermoscopic Features

Non uniform pigmentation, characterized by lighter and darker areas within the lesion (**Fig. 20**), faint brownish areas with increased reticular pigmentary network (**Fig. 21A**) and white structureless areas with faint pigment network are observed (**Fig. 21B**).[19,20]

Radial distribution of lesions from the hair follicle is noted. Marginal hyperpigmentation can be seen in hypopigmented lesions and marginal hypopigmentation in hyperpigmented lesions, the features being described as "contrast halo sign."[21]

Patchy scaling is reported in hypopigmented lesions. In hyperpigmented lesions, scaling in the furrows is more frequent (**Fig. 21C**), which may detach from the skin and break into two parts when the lesions are stretched, called as "double-edged" scales dermoscopically. Perilesional and perifollicular scaling can be observed. Folliculocentric scaling is a conspicuous feature (**Fig. 21C**).[20,21]

Inconspicuous ridges and furrows and varied vascular patterns are also reported. Hypopigmentation of the involved hair follicle as a result of follicular invasion of the yeast can be seen.[19,20]

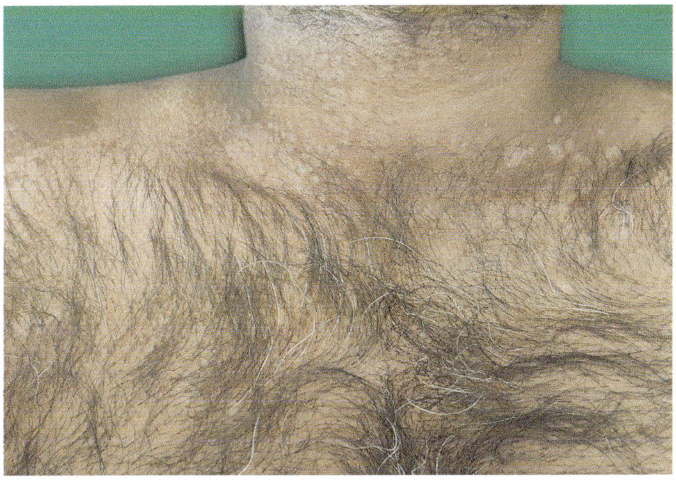

FIG. 19: Hypopigmented patches with mild scaling in pityriasis versicolor.

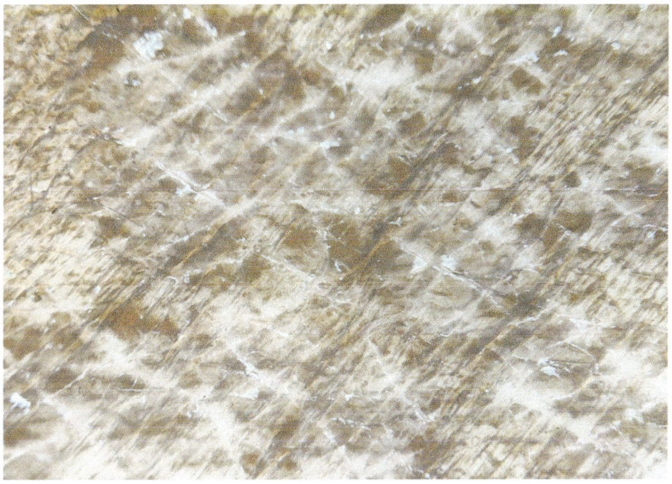

FIG. 20: Non uniform hyper- and hypopigmented areas (polarized, DermLite DL3, 10×).

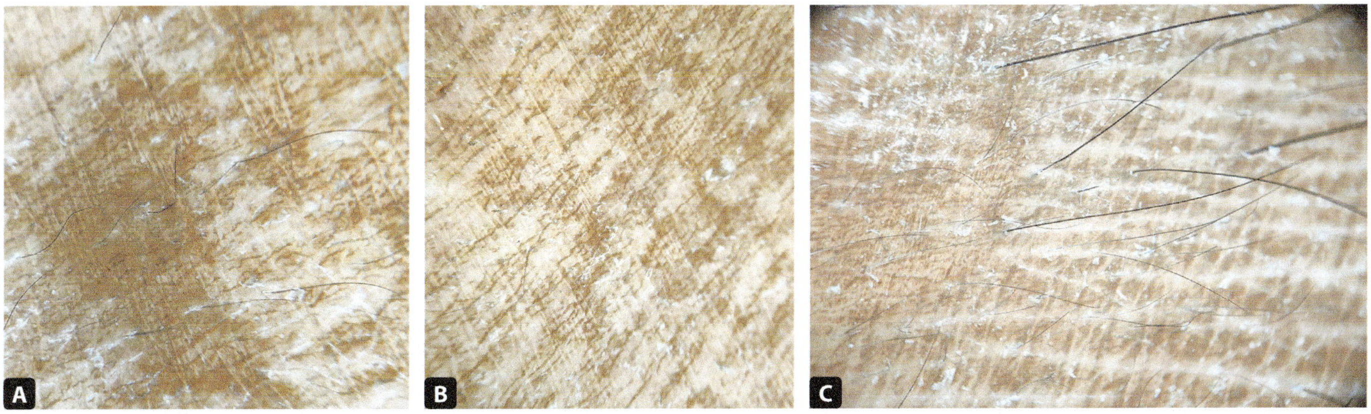

FIGS. 21A TO C: (A) Faint brown areas with increased reticular network (polarized, DermLite DL3, 10×); (B) White structureless areas in between brown pigment network (polarized, DermLite DL3, 10×); (C) Perifollicular scales and scaling in furrows appearing as white lines (polarized, DermLite DL3, 10×).

Key Points

- Folliculocentric scaling
- Scaling along furrows
- Increased reticular pigmentation in hyperpigmented patches
- White structureless areas with faint pigment network in hypopigmented lesions

LEPROSY

Clinical Features

Clinical presentation of cutaneous lesions vary from plaques (**Fig. 22**) patches (**Fig. 23**) to nodules, and ulcers depending on the spectrum of the disease.

Dermoscopic Features

Borderline tuberculoid leprosy shows white areas with sparse hair follicular openings as the most consistent pattern. Absence of skin appendages and white dots representing absent sweat glands is a characteristic feature (**Fig. 24**). Yellow globular structures represent granuloma.[22,23]

Lepromatous leprosy shows partial loss of hair follicles, dry xerotic skin, and white scaling (**Fig. 25**).

White areas noted in most lesions of leprosy, not in reaction, correspond to a decreased number of melanocytes in the affected patches of leprosy, differentiating it from other granulomatous infections.[22]

The dome-shaped nodules of histoid leprosy show crown vessels (linear branching vessels originating in the periphery which do not cross the center of the lesion), a central yellowish structureless area, shiny white structures, and peripheral hyperpigmentation.[24-26]

Type 1 lepra reaction shows characteristic diffuse erythematous background and blurry branching telangiectatic vessels along with sparse hair follicles and scaling, whereas erythema nodosum leprosum shows ill-defined branching blood vessels in the background of characteristic hyperpigmentation.[22] In conclusion, dermoscopic features such as linear blurry vessels within reddish or orangish areas could typify type 1 reaction.[27]

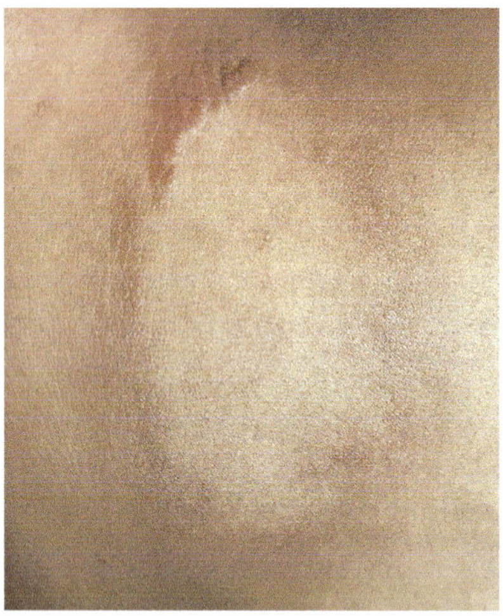

FIG. 22: Well-defined plaque of borderline tuberculoid leprosy.

FIG. 23: Ill-defined patch of lepromatous leprosy.

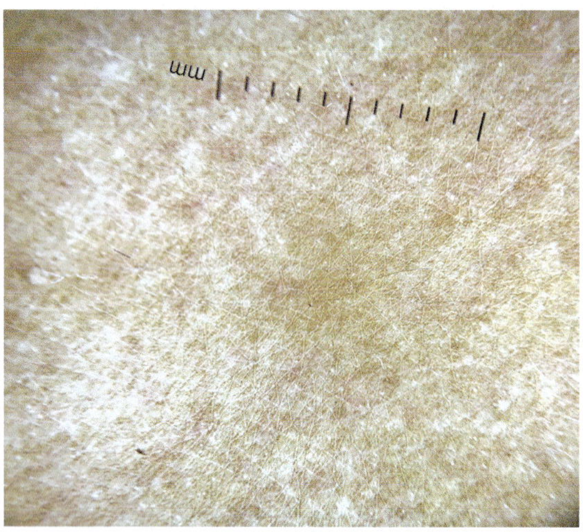

FIG. 24: Dermoscopy of borderline tuberculoid leprosy shows sparseness of follicular openings and hypopigmented areas (polarized, DermLite DL3, 10×).

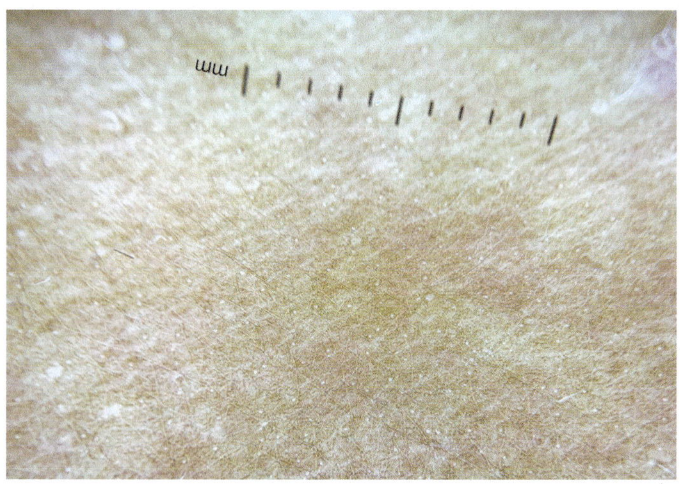

FIG. 25: Dermoscopy of lepromatous leprosy shows follicular openings seen with whitish areas (polarized, DermLite DL3, 10×).

Key Points

- Sparse follicular openings in tuberculoid spectrum
- White areas and dryness in lepromatous spectrum
- Vascular pattern in reactions

KEY POINTS

- Dermoscopy in hypopigmented lesions demonstrate definitive and specific features.
- Vitiligo and idiopathic guttate hypomelanosis do not reveal faint pigment network in fully developed lesions.
- Other conditions show faint pigment network at the background.
- Dermoscopy plays a significant role in the diagnosis and/or ruling out vitiligo, thus alleviating the apprehension.

CONCLUSION

Among the hypopigmentary disorders, dermoscopic findings of vitiligo have been studied in some detail. Apart from diagnosis, dermoscopic examination may also be helpful in assessing vitiligo disease activity and treatment response, though this needs further evaluation in large scale prospective studies. Dermoscopy can be potentially useful in distinguishing vitiligo from its clinical mimics. Dermoscopic findings of some diseases such as IGH, PV, and lichen sclerosus are well-characterized, while suggestive findings are being recognized for other hypopigmentary disorders as well.

REFERENCES

1. Nirmal B. Use of dermatoscope to monitor the repigmentation of various vitiligo surgical procedures. J Cutan Aesthet Surg. 2016;9(4):286-7.
2. Nirmal B, Antonisamy B, Dincy Peter CV, George L, George AA, Dinesh GM. Cross-sectional study of dermatoscopic findings in relation to activity in vitiligo: BPLeFoSK criteria for stability. J Cutan Aesthet Surg. 2019;12(1):36-41.
3. Thatte SS, Khopkar US. The utility of dermoscopy in the diagnosis of evolving lesions of vitiligo. Indian J Dermatol Venereol Leprol. 2014;80(6):505-8.
4. Vinay K, Ankad BS. Dermatoscopic features of pigmentary diseases in ethnic skin. Indian Dermatol Online J. 2021;12(1):24-33.
5. Nirmal B. Utility of blue light in dermoscopy for diagnosing stable lesions in vitiligo. Dermatol Pract Concept. 2021;11(1):e2021141.
6. Chatterjee M, Neema S. Dermoscopy of pigmentary disorders in brown skin. Dermatol Clin. 2018;36(4):473-85.
7. Oiso N, Kawada A. The diagnostic usefulness of dermoscopy for nevus depigmentosus. Eur J Dermatol. 2011;21(4):639-40.
8. Malakar S, Mukherjee SS, Malakar S. Looking through the dermoscope in a case of piebaldism. Our Dermatol Online. 2019;10:312-3.
9. Bambroo M, Pande S, Khopkar U. Dermoscopy in the differentiation of idiopathic guttate hypomelanosis (IGH) and Guttate vitiligo. In: Khopkar's Dermoscopy and Trichoscopy in diseases of the brown skin. Atlas and Short Text. 1st edition. New Delhi: Jaypee Brothers Medical Publishers (P) Ltd; 2012. p. 97-103.
10. Kittler H, Pehamberger H, Wolff K, Binder M. Diagnostic accuracy of dermoscopy. Lancet Oncol. 2002;3(3):159-65.
11. Vachiramon V, Thadanipon K. Postinflammatory hypopigmentation. Clinical and Experimental Dermatology. 2011;36(7):708-14.
12. Errichetti E, Stinco G. The practical usefulness of dermoscopy in general dermatology. G Ital Dermatol Venereol. 2015;150(5):533-46.
13. Errichetti E, Lallas A, Ioannides D. Hypopigmented dermatoses. In: Lallas A, Errichetti E, Ioannides D (Eds). Dermoscopy in General Dermatology. London: CRC Press; 2019. pp. 121-9.
14. Shim WH, Jwa SW, Song M, Kim HS, Ko HC, Kim MB, et al. Diagnostic usefulness of dermatoscopy in differentiating lichen sclerous et atrophicus from morphea. J Am Acad Dermatol. 2012;66(4):690-1.
15. Marghoob AA, Cowell L, Kopf AW, Scope A. Observation of chrysalis structures with polarized dermoscopy. Arch Dermatol. 2009;145(5):618.
16. Garrido-Ríos AA, Alvarez-Garrido H, Sanz-Muñoz C, Aragoneses-Fraile H, Manchado-López P, Miranda-Romero A. Dermoscopy of extra genital lichen sclerosus. Arch Dermatol. 2009;145(12):1468.
17. Tiodorovic-Zivkovic D, Argenziano G, Popovic D, Zalaudek I. Clinical and dermoscopic findings of a patient with co-existing lichen planus, lichen sclerosus and morphea. Eur J Dermatol. 2012;22(1):143-4.
18. Lapeere H, Boone B, Schepper SD, Verhaeghe E, Van Geel M, Ongenae K, et al. Hypomelanoses and hypermelanoses. In: Goldsmith LA, Katz MS, Gilchrest BA, Paller AS, Leffell DJ, Wolff K (Eds). Fitzpatrick's Dermatology in General Medicine, 8th edition. McGraw-Hill; 2012. p. 2049.
19. Mathur M, Acharya P, Karki A, KC N, Shah J. Dermoscopic pattern of pityriasis versicolor. Clin Cosmet Investig Dermatol. 2019;12:303-9.
20. Ankad BS, Koti VR. Dermoscopic approach to hypopigmentary or depigmentary lesions in skin of color. Clin Dermatol Rev. 2020;4:79-83.
21. Kaur I, Jakhar D, Singal A. Dermoscopy in the evaluation of pityriasis versicolor: A cross-sectional study. Indian Dermatol Online J. 2019;10(6):682-5.
22. Chopra A, Mitra D, Agarwal R, Saraswat N, Talukdar K, Solanki A. Correlation of dermoscopic and histopathologic patterns in leprosy: a pilot study. Indian Dermatol Online J. 2019;10(6):663-8.
23. Ankad BS, Sakhare PS. Dermoscopy of borderline tuberculoid leprosy. Int J Dermatol. 2018;57(1):74-6.
24. Abadías-Granado I, Navarro-Bielsa A, Gómez-Mateo MC, Bermúdez-Cameo R, Gilaberte Y. Crown vessels and shiny white structures in dermoscopy of histoid leprosy. JAAD Case Rep. 2020;6(11):1147-9.
25. Ankad BS, Sakhare PS. Dermoscopy of histoid leprosy: a case report. Dermatol Pract Concept. 2017;7(2):63-5.
26. Acharya P, Mathur MC. Clinicodermoscopic study of histoid leprosy: a case series. Intl J Dermatol. 2020;59(3):365-8.
27. Jha AK, Zeeshan MD, Tiwary P, Singh A, Roy PK, Chaudhary RKP. Dermoscopy of type 1 lepra reaction in skin of color. Dermatol Pract Concept. 2020;10(3):e2020083.

10 Facial Dermatoses

CHAPTER

Shagufta Rather, Mansi Kansal

INTRODUCTION

- Face is a common and many a times lone site of involvement for inflammatory and granulomatous skin disorders.
- Due to cosmetic concerns, face is always a nonpreferred anatomical site for an invasive procedure like biopsy and dermoscopic diagnosis can help overcome such diagnostic quandary.
- Different features on dermoscopy to be considered while evaluating these inflammatory disorders, include background color, vascular pattern, shape and distribution of vessels, color and distribution of the scales, follicular structures, and other additional findings.

Some of the disorders affecting face where dermoscopy can facilitate the noninvasive diagnosis are described.

ACNE AND ITS VARIANTS

Acne Vulgaris

Clinical Features

Lesions start as microcomedones present in the clinically normal appearing skin, mature into visible open or closed comedones. Inflammatory lesions such as erythematous papules and pustules appear as the disease progresses (**Figs. 1A** and **B**). There is background erythema, and in severe cases nodules and pseudocysts are seen. Scarring is the most common sequel.[1,2]

Dermoscopic Features

Features vary with the type of acne lesion present (**Figs. 1C** to **L**).[1,2] Nonpolarized dermoscopy of the comedones shows multiple, well-defined, structureless, homogeneous superficially placed circular areas, light to dark-brown, sometimes black in color, surrounding the keratin plugs. Open comedones typically show a hair follicle surrounded by central black ring while the ring is small with yellowish surroundings in white/closed comedones.

Polarized dermoscopy of papule shows background erythema, and a central yellowish-orange hue with some dotted vessels, a central vellus hair, folliculocentric pattern and surrounding erythema.

Pustular acne: Well to ill-defined dull white to yellowish-white raised central clod, with erythematous borders, surrounding erythema, folliculocentric nature.

Key Points

- Multiple, well-defined, structureless, homogeneous superficially placed circular areas, light to dark-brown, sometimes black in color, surrounding the keratin plugs.

Acne Keloidalis Nuchae

Clinical Features

Although it is a chronic inflammatory process affecting the nape of the neck and the occipital scalp, it is included here in view of its morphology, characterized by follicle-oriented papules and pustules (**Fig. 1M**).[3]

Dermoscopic Features

It reveals perifollicular pustules as white round structures and a vascular pattern composed of dotted and linear vessels. Tufted hairs and white chrysalis strands are also important features (**Fig. 1N**).[3]

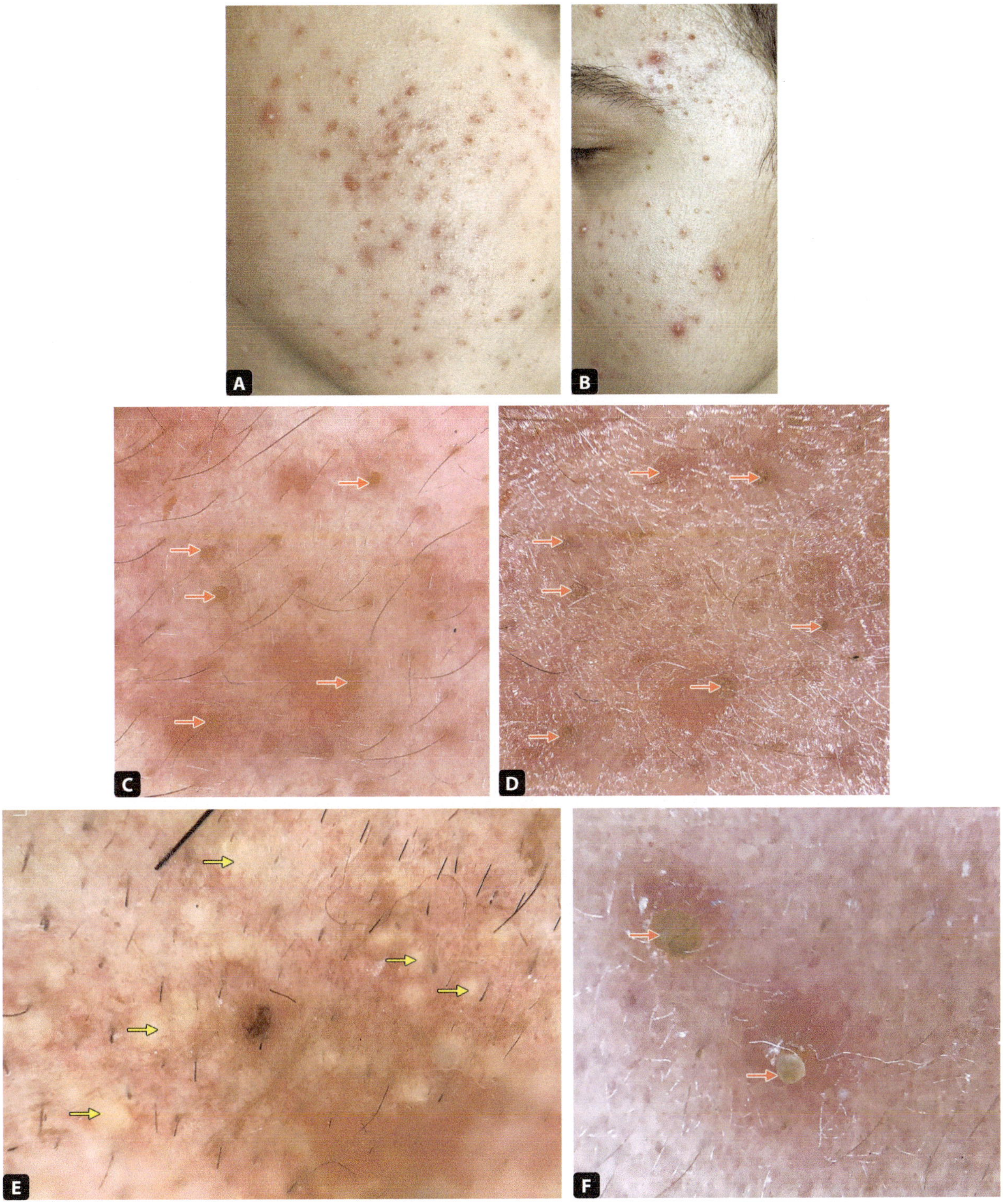

FIGS. 1A TO N: (*Continued*)

(*Continued***)**

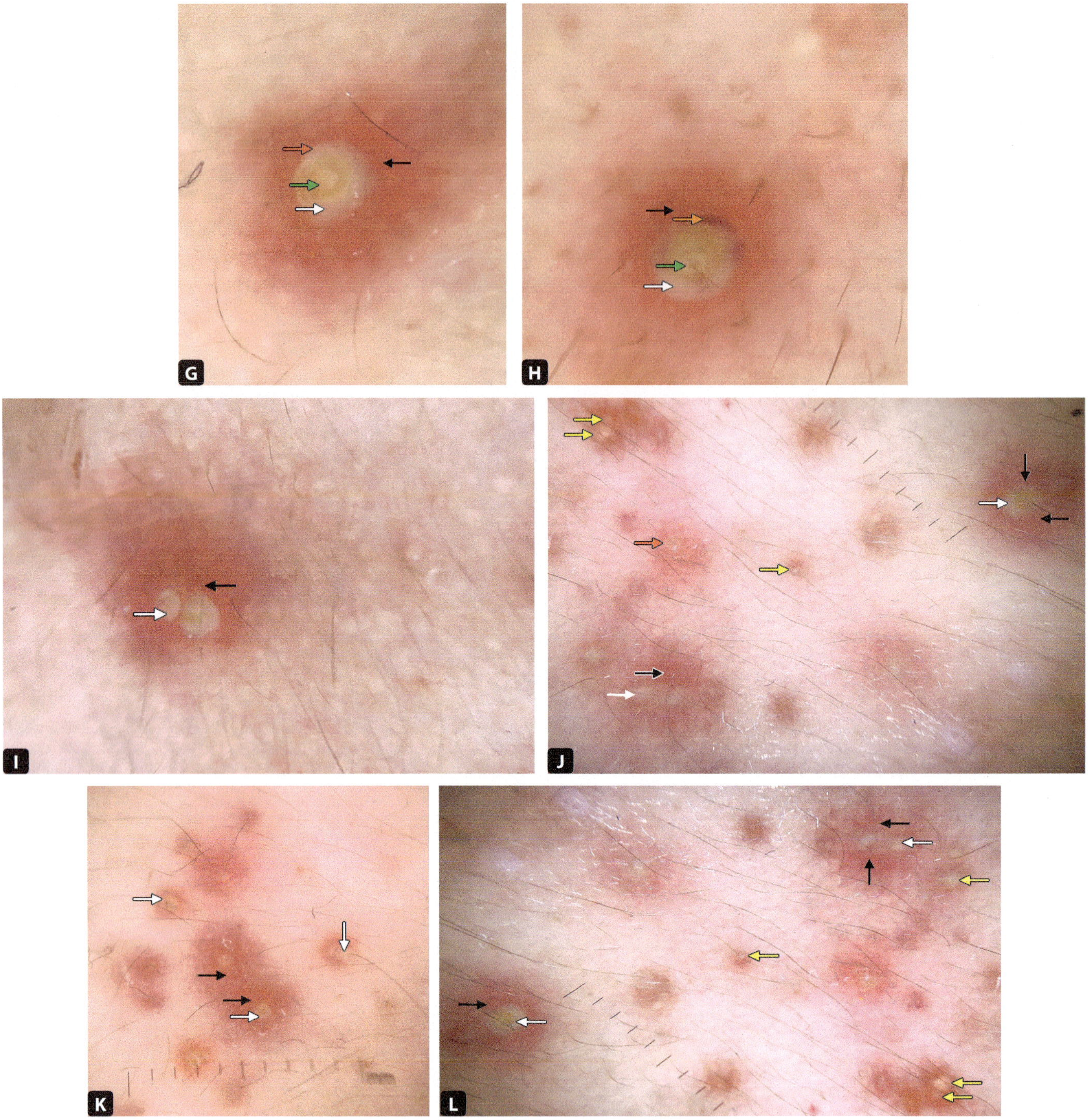

FIGS. 1A TO N: (*Continued*)

(*Continued*)

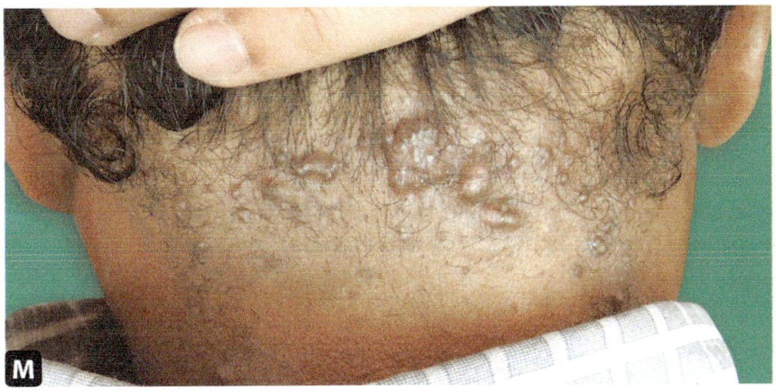

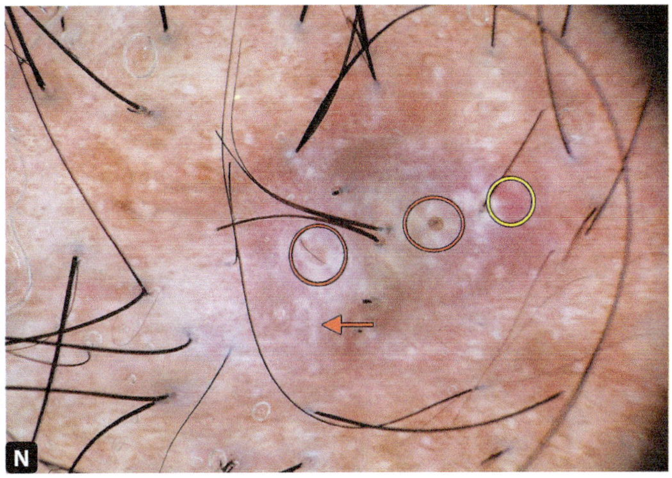

FIGS. 1A TO N: (A) Clinical image of acne vulgaris showing multiple comedones and papules on the face; (B) Clinical image of acne vulgaris showing multiple papules and pustules and few comedones on the face; (C) Dermoscopy of open comedones shows multiple, round dark brown globules with surrounding the keratin plugs (red arrows). Note that open comedones typically show a hair follicle surrounded by central black ring (polarized, DermLite DL4, 10×); (D) Dermoscopy of open comedones shows multiple, round dark brown globules with surrounding the keratin plugs (red arrows). Note that open comedones typically show a hair follicle surrounded by central black ring (nonpolarized, DermLite DL4, 10×); (E) Dermoscopy of closed comedones shows multiple, circular yellow globules (yellow arrows). Note that no keratin plugs or hair follicle is seen (polarized, DermLite DL4, 10×); (F) Dermoscopy of open comedones shows multiple round dark brown globules with surrounding the keratin plugs (red arrows) (polarized, DermLite DL4, 10×); (G) Dermoscopy of pustule shows central yellowish-brown zone (green arrow) surrounded by white areas (white arrow) with well-defined border (red arrow) and erythema at periphery (black arrow) (polarized, DermLite DL4, 10×); (H) Dermoscopy of pustule shows central yellowish-brown zone (green arrow) surrounded by white areas (white arrow) with well-defined border (red arrow) and erythema at periphery (black arrow) (polarized, DermLite DL4, 10×); (I) Dermoscopy of pustules shows white globules (white arrow) surrounded by erythema (black arrow) (polarized, DermLite DL4, 10×); (J) Dermoscopy of pustular lesions shows well- to ill-defined dull white to yellowish-white raised central clod (white arrows), with erythematous borders and surrounding erythema (black arrows). Few closed comedones present show small ring with yellowish-orange surrounding areas (yellow arrows) (polarized, DermLite DL4, 10×); (K) Dermoscopy of pustular lesions shows well- to ill-defined dull white to yellow-white raised central clod (white arrows), with erythematous borders and surrounding erythema (black arrows) (polarized, DermLite DL4, 10×); (L) Well- to ill-defined dull white to yellowish-white raised central clod (white arrows), with erythematous borders and surrounding erythema (black arrows). Few closed comedones present show small ring with yellowish-orange surrounding areas (yellow arrows) (polarized, DermLite DL4, 10×); (M) Clinical image of acne keloidalis nuchae shows papules and nodules in perifollicular and interfollicular areas with broken hairs on the nape of the neck; (N) Dermoscopy of acne keloidalis nuchae shows whitish round structures (red circles), white chrysalis strands (red arrow), and linear and dotted vessels (yellow circle) (polarized, DermLite DL3, 10×).

Courtesy (Figs. M and N): Dr BS Ankad, SN Medical College, Bagalkot, Karnataka, India.

Key Points

- Follicle-oriented white round globules with tuft of hairs and linear and dotted vessels

ROSACEA AND ITS VARIANTS

Clinical Features

Chronic inflammatory disorder that involves the facial pilo-sebaceous units and manifests clinically on the convexities of central face. It is most frequently observed in patients with fair skin, with onset at any time after 30 years. Females are predominantly affected, but rhinophyma occurs commonly in males.[4]

Clinical Subtype[5]

Erythematotelangiectatic type: It is characterized by persistent, fixed erythema, in a characteristic centrofacial pattern associated with burning and stinging sensation (**Fig. 2A**). There is roughness and scaling, "dry appearance" of skin, telangiectasia and facial edema, which may be persistent for few days.

Papulopustular rosacea: It is characterized by persistent central erythema, predominant dome-shaped red papules, accompanying pustules predominantly on the cheeks, chin, and forehead (**Fig. 2B**). There may be nodules also. Presence of comedones is not a part of rosacea process.

Phymatous rosacea: Characterized by persistent facial erythema along with skin thickening due to fibrosis and sebaceous gland hyperplasia. Most common is the rhinophyma but other phymas may occur. Thickened skin, patulous follicular orifices, and nodularities together impart the nose a bulbous appearance (**Figs. 2C** and **D**).

Dermoscopic Features

Linear reddish or purple vessels arranged in a polygonal network (polygonal vessels) are most sensitive and specific criterion for the diagnosis of rosacea and correspond to the dilatation of the vessels of the subpapillary plexus (**Fig. 2E**). Additional findings include follicular plugs (**Fig. 2F**), superficial white/yellow scales, rosettes, orange-white areas of pigmentation, and features related to the presence of *Demodex*, "*Demodex* tails", and whitish amorphic follicular material. Dilated follicles and follicular pustules are seen in papulopustular rosacea. Rhinophyma shows linear vessels and prominent follicular openings on reddish-background erythema (**Figs. 2G** and **H**). Dermoscopy can be quite useful in detection of telangiectasias, and erythema in patients with darker skin types (V and VI) where the initial stage is difficult to appreciate visually. Dermoscopy might help pick

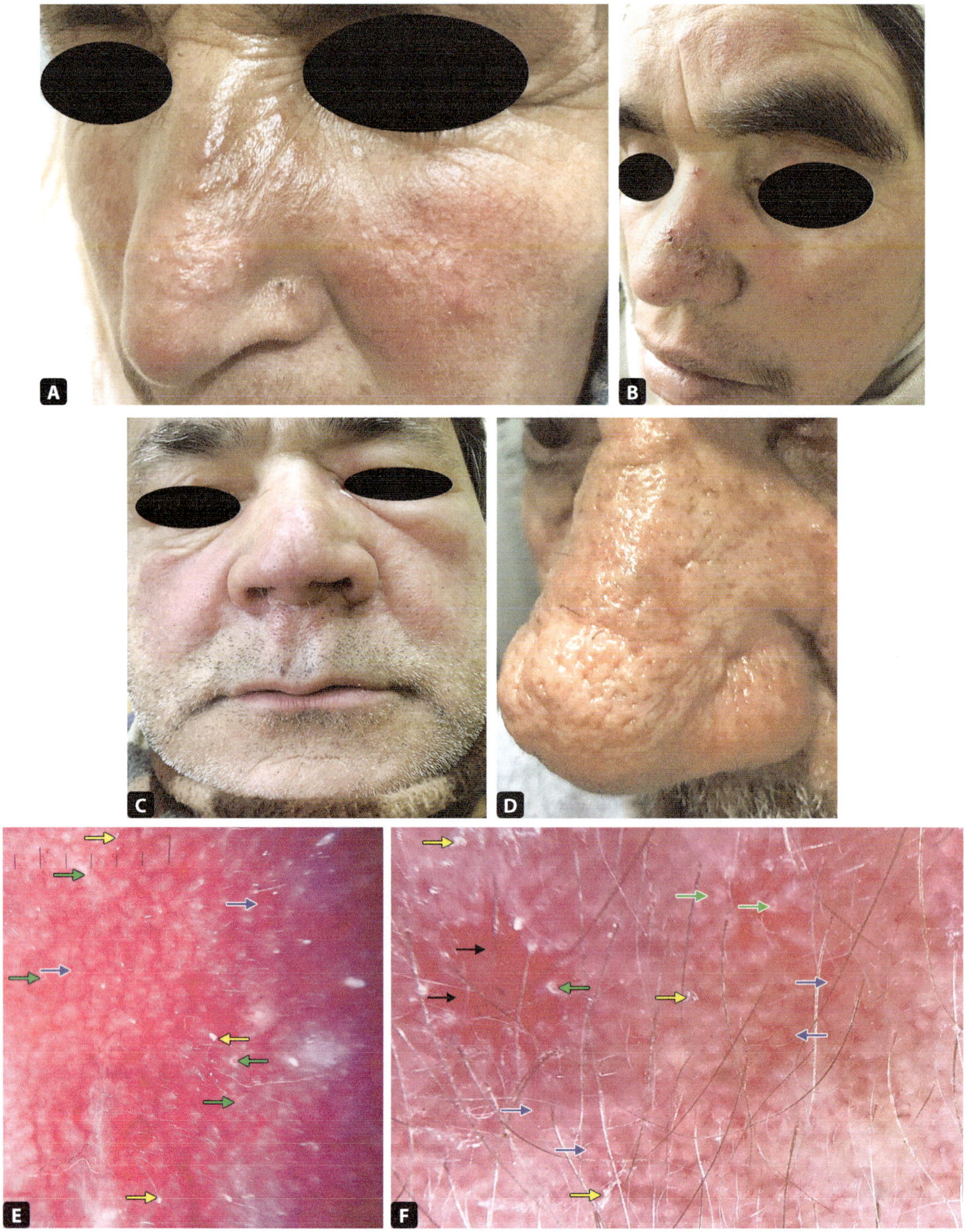

FIGS. 2A TO H: *(Continued)*

(*Continued*)

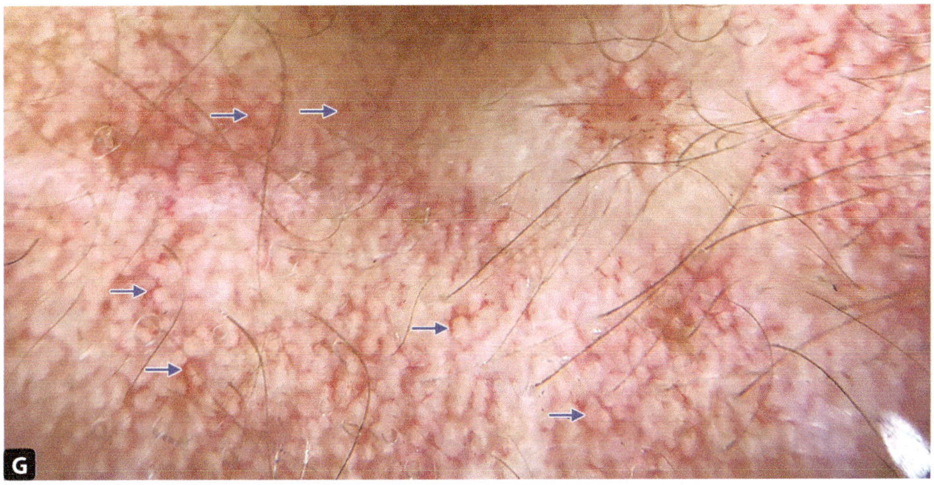

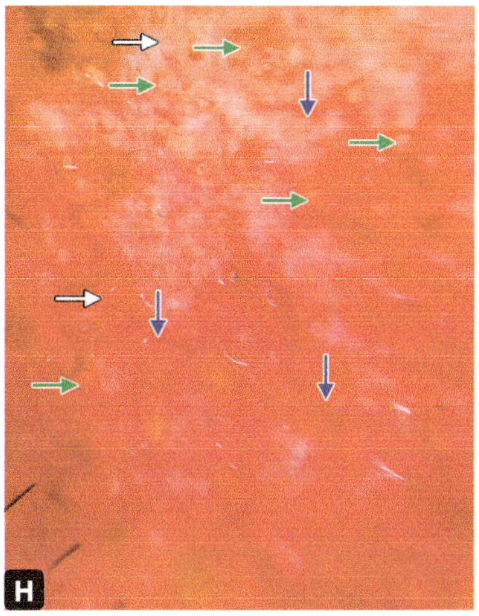

FIGS. 2A TO H: (A) Clinical image of rosacea shows erythema in a centrofacial pattern, accompanied by dome-shaped red papules, and pustules on the convexities of face; (B) Clinical image of rosacea shows erythema accompanied by dome-shaped crusted red papules, and pustules on the convexities of face in a characteristic distribution; (C) Clinical image of rhinophyma shows central facial erythema along with skin thickening on nose due to fibrosis and sebaceous gland hyperplasia; (D) Clinical image of rhinophyma shows thickened skin, patulous follicular orifices, and nodularities together impart nose a bulbous appearance; (E) Dermoscopy of rosacea shows reddish-background erythema, and linear reddish or purple vessels arranged in a polygonal network (polygonal vessels) (blue arrows), follicular plugs (green arrows), and superficial white/yellow scales (yellow arrows) (polarized, DermLite DL4, 10×); (F) Dermoscopy of rosacea shows red background (black arrows), and linear red or purple vessels arranged in a polygonal network (polygonal vessels) (blue arrows). Follicular plugs (green arrows) and white scales are noted (yellow arrows) (polarized, DermLite DL4, 10×); (G) Dermoscopy of rosacea/rhinophyma shows reddish-background erythema, and linear red or purple vessels arranged in a polygonal network (polygonal vessels) (blue arrows) (polarized, DermLite DL4, 10×); (H) Dermoscopy of rosacea/rhinophyma shows reddish-brown background (white arrows), prominent follicular openings (green arrows), and linear branching vessels (blue arrows) (polarized, DermLite DL4, 10×).

up the microcomedones and comedones to differentiate it from acne. Similarly, in papulopustular rosacea, clinically nonvisible pustules provide a useful dermoscopic clue for discrimination from lupus erythematosus.[4,5]

Key Points

- Vascular polygons are a highly sensitive and specific.
- Follicular plugs, superficial white/yellow scales, rosettes, orange-white areas, structures and features related to demodicosis.
- Dilated follicles and follicular pustules in papulopustular rosacea.

DEMODEX FOLLICULITIS (DEMODICOSIS)

Clinical Features

Demodex mite is an obligate parasite, inhabiting the pilosebaceous follicle. In older children and adults, it is mainly seen on the sebaceous areas of face and upper chest (**Fig. 3A**).[6] Inflammatory dermatoses associated with demodicosis seen are:

- *Pityriasis folliculorum* or *spinulate demodicosis* is characterized by presence of discrete, fine, whitish-yellow, isolated but grouped, follicular spicules, against diffuse facial erythema, giving it a sandpaper-like texture. The typical rough feel of skin helps to differentiate it from rosacea.[6]
- *Demodex* folliculitis, meaning inflammation of the follicle due to *Demodex* mites, can be morphologically divided into the following patterns: Papulopustular, nodulocystic, and conglobata demodicosis, which depicts abscess-like lesions.[7]
- *Rosacea-like (rosaceiform) demodicidosis*
- *Papulopustular demodicosis*: Perioral demodicosis, periorbital demodicosis, periauricular demodicosis.[7]

In addition, *Demodex* mite is implicated in seborrheic dermatitis, and steroid dermatitis along with other factors.

Dermascopic Features

Specific features in favor of *Demodex* infestation consist of "*Demodex* tails" or "*Demodex* follicular openings". "*Demodex* tails"—represented by nonfollicular and perifollicular gelatinous threads or filaments, 1–3 mm in length, protruding out of follicular openings, and account for the presence of the mite itself. Gray dots—"*Demodex* follicular openings" are identified as dilated follicular openings containing round, amorphic, gray/light brown plugs surrounded by an erythematous halo. Epidermal scale and red dots are other important dermoscopic findings in interfollicular areas of these patients. Reticular horizontal dilated blood vessels (arborizing red lines) can be seen in patients with an inflammatory variant of demodicidosis (**Figs. 3B** to **E**).[6-8]

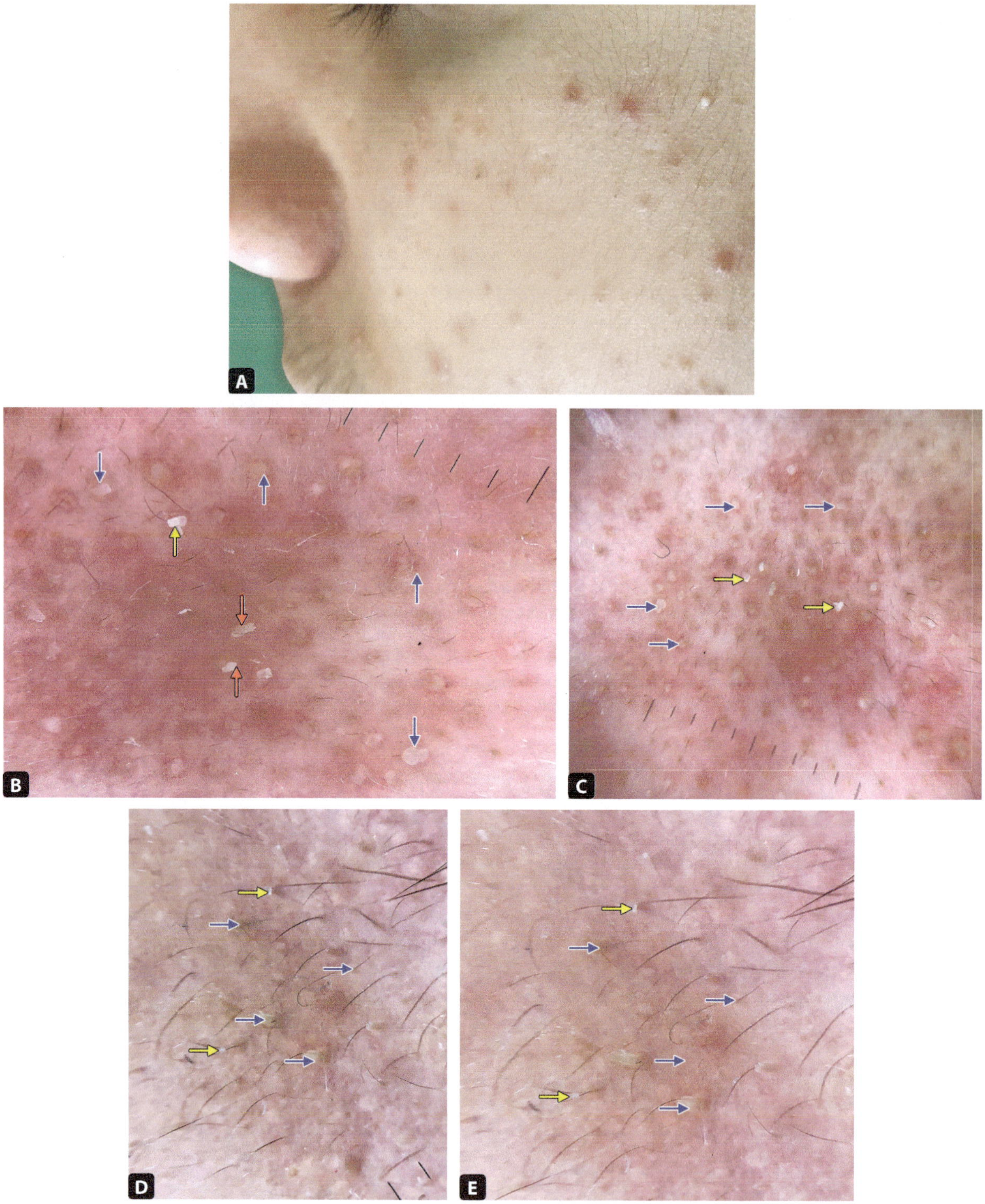

FIGS. 3A TO E: (A) Clinical image of demodicosis shows seborrhea and greasy skin in an adult male; (B) Dermoscopy of *Demodex* folliculitis shows dilated follicular openings containing round, amorphic, grayish/light brown plugs surrounded by an erythematous halo ("*Demodex* follicular openings") (blue arrows). Note the nonfollicular and perifollicular gelatinous threads or filaments, 1–3 mm in length, protruding out of follicular openings ("*Demodex* tails") (red arrows). Whitish scales are seen (yellow arrow) (polarized, DermLite DL4, 10×); (C) Dermoscopy of *Demodex* folliculitis. Dilated follicular openings containing round, amorphic, grayish/light brown plugs surrounded by an erythematous halo ("*Demodex* follicular openings") (blue arrows). Whitish scales are seen (yellow arrows) (polarized, DermLite DL4, 10×); (D) Dermoscopy of *Demodex* infestation. Dilated follicular openings containing round, amorphic, grayish/light brown plugs surrounded by an erythematous halo ("*Demodex* follicular openings") (blue arrows). Whitish scales are seen (yellow arrows) (polarized, DermLite DL4, 10×); (E) Dermoscopy of *Demodex* infestation. Dilated follicular openings containing round, amorphic, gray/light brown plugs surrounded by an erythematous halo ("*Demodex* follicular openings") (blue arrows). White scales are seen (yellow arrows) (polarized, DermLite DL4, 10×).

Key Points

- In addition to the diagnosis of various forms of demodicosis, dermoscopy helps to assess the response to treatment and follow-up.
- Specific features are "*Demodex* tails" or "*Demodex* follicular openings".
- Additional findings include epidermal scale and red dots and reticular horizontal dilated blood vessels.

LUPUS MILIARIS DISSEMINATUS FACIEI

Clinical Features

Clinically, it is characterized by discrete, multiple, asymptomatic, monomorphic, erythematous to reddish-brown, dome-shaped papules, involving central area of the face, particularly periorbital area, nasolabial folds, cheeks, and the perioral areas, in a symmetrical distribution (**Fig. 4A**).[9]

Dermoscopic Features

Dermoscopy shows reddish-brown background, multiple ill-defined, discrete, perifollicular, yellow to brown, structureless areas, which represent granulomas. White or yellow keratotic follicular plugs and perifollicular scales are seen. Keratotic follicular plugs on dermoscopy are secondary to the follicular hyperkeratosis and lateral pressure on follicles by the surrounding granulomas. Well-focused linear and branching vessels and white scar-like depigmented areas are present over reddish-brown background (**Figs. 4B** to **D**).[10,11]

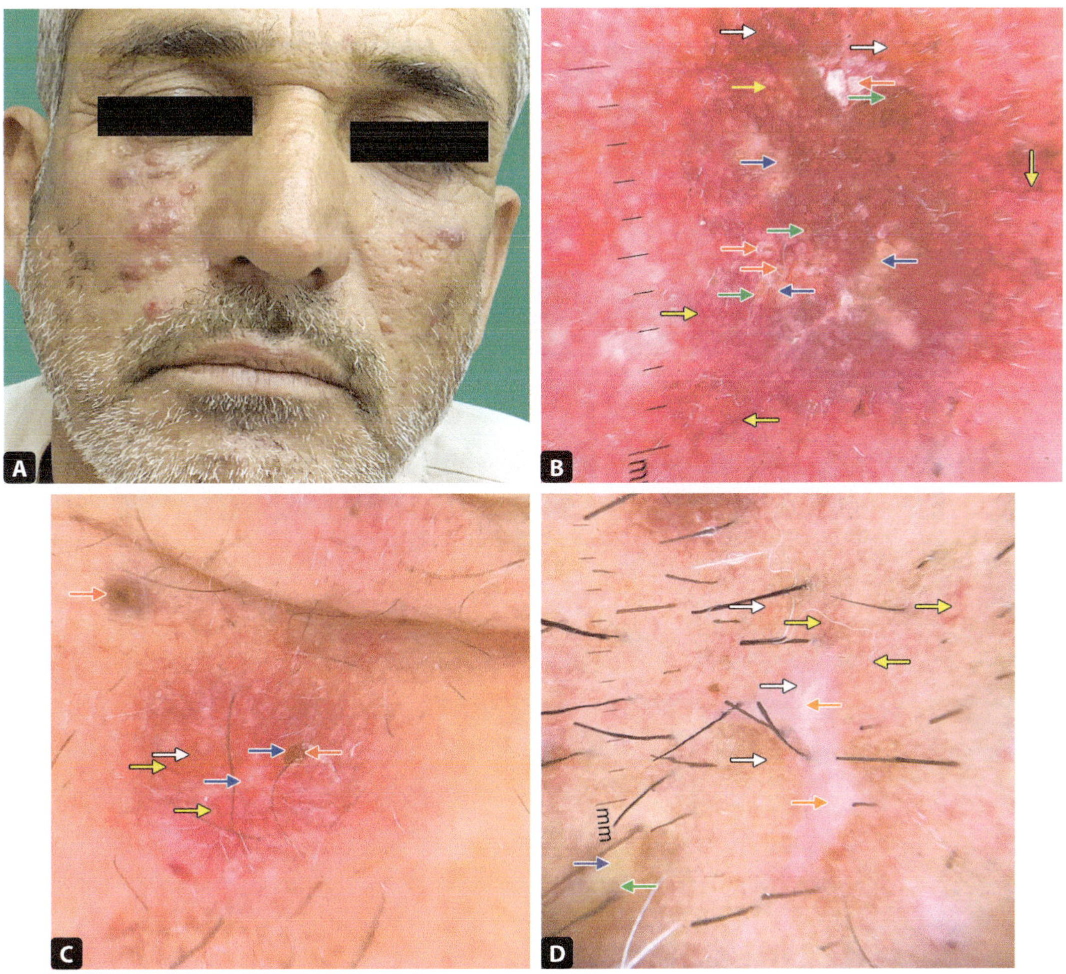

FIGS. 4A TO D: (A) Clinical image of lupus miliaris disseminatus faciei shows multiple, monomorphic, erythematous to reddish-brown, dome-shaped papules on the face, particularly on periorbital area, nasolabial folds, cheeks, and perioral areas; (B) Dermoscopy of lupus miliaris disseminatus faciei shows multiple, ill-defined, discrete, yellow to orange brown, structureless areas (blue arrows), arranged focally in perifollicular distribution. White or yellow keratotic follicular plugs (red arrows), perifollicular scales, well-focused linear and arborizing vessels (yellow arrows) present on over reddish-brown background (white arrows) (polarized, DermLite DL4, 10×); (C) Dermoscopy of lupus miliaris disseminatus faciei shows multiple, ill-defined, discrete, yellow to orangish brown, structureless areas (blue arrows), arranged focally around follicles. White or yellow keratotic follicular plugs (red arrows) perifollicular scales, well-focused linear and arborizing vessels (yellow arrows) seen over a reddish-brown background (white arrow) (polarized, DermLite DL4, 10×); (D) Dermoscopy of lupus miliaris disseminatus faciei shows white scar-like depigmented areas (orange arrows), structureless areas (blue arrow), short linear vessels (yellow arrows), and reddish-brown background (white arrows). Perifollicular pigmentation is also noted (green arrow) (polarized, DermLite DL4, polarized, 10×).

Key Points

- Multiple, ill-defined, discrete, perifollicular, yellow to brown, structureless areas, which represent granulomas.
- Whitish or yellow keratotic follicular plugs and perifollicular scales
- Well-focused linear and arborizing vessels are present.

GRANULOMA FACIALE

Clinical Features

Clinically, it is characterized by occurrence of asymptomatic, single or multiple, reddish-brown, papules, plaques or nodules, primarily on the sun-exposed areas, especially face (**Figs. 5A** and **B**). Lesions are usually soft, with prominent follicular openings, giving it a characteristic orange peel-like surface.[12]

Dermoscopic Features

It shows pink to reddish-brown background, with some areas of translucent white-gray color. Vascular inflammation, erythrocyte extravasation, and hemosiderin deposition may contribute to color of lesion. Whitish streaks in different directions, associated with fairly focused, linear branching vessels are commonly seen. Prominent follicular orifices or follicular accentuation giving it a "peau d'orange" appearance clinically, corresponding to the intense inflammatory infiltrate of lymphohistiocytes, neutrophils, and numerous eosinophils, in a micronodular arrangement with sparing of adnexal structures of skin. An amorphous yellowish or yellow-brown or brown area may be present in the center of lesion which has been correlated to the presence of abundance of hemosiderin deposition in these lesions on histopathology (**Figs. 5C** and **D**).[13,14]

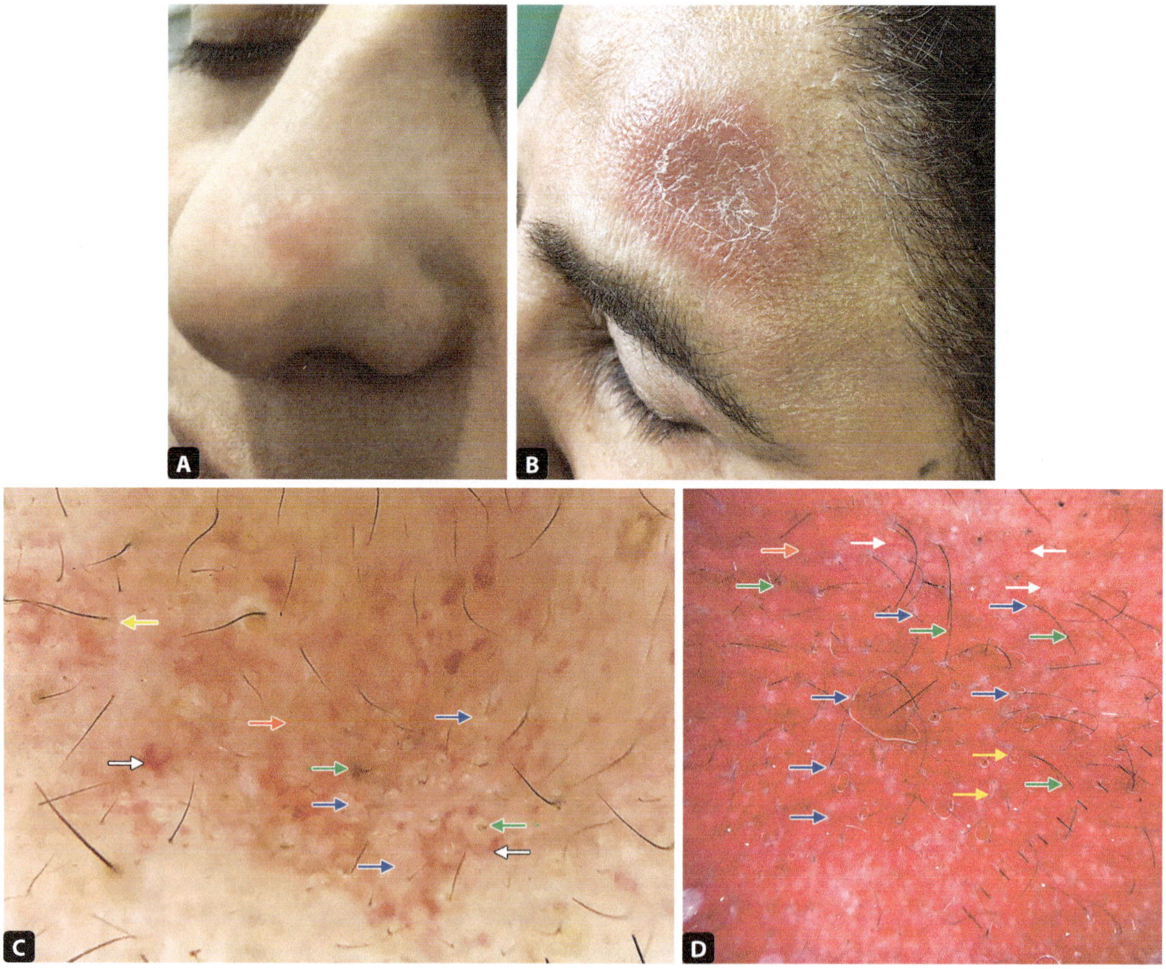

FIGS. 5A TO D: (A) Clinical image of granuloma faciale shows erythematous to violaceous plaque with prominent follicular openings on nose; (B) Clinical image of granuloma faciale shows erythematous to brownish plaque with scaling on the forehead; (C) Dermoscopy of granuloma faciale shows pink to reddish-brown background (red arrow), prominent follicular orifices (green arrows), areas of translucent white-gray color (blue arrows), few whitish streaks in different directions (yellow arrow), and fairly focused, linear branching vessels (white arrows) (polarized, DermLite DL4, 10×); (D) Dermoscopy of granuloma faciale shows reddish-brown background (red arrow), marked follicular accentuation (green arrows), areas of translucent white-gray color (blue arrows), and linear branching vessels (white arrows) (polarized, DermLite DL4, 10×).

Key Points

- Pink to reddish-brown background, with some areas of translucent white-gray color.
- Whitish streaks in different directions, associated with fairly focused, linear branching vessels
- Prominent follicular orifices or follicular accentuation giving it a "peau d'orange" appearance
- An amorphous yellowish or yellow-brown or brown area may be present in the center of lesion.

ERYTHROMELANOSIS FOLLICULARIS FACIEI ET COLLI

Clinical Features

A rare disorder described for the first time by Kitamura et al., has onset during early childhood and occurs predominantly in males. Clinically, it is characterized by presence of sharply demarcated erythema (with or without telangiectasia), reddish-brown patches of hyperpigmentation along with follicular papules present on face, mainly cheeks, preauricular and temporal areas, extending over to involve the submandibular areas of neck (**Figs. 6A** to **C**).[15]

Dermoscopic Features

It reveals whitish scales, numerous follicular keratotic plugs against a reddish-brown background and telangiectasias, which on histopathology correspond to presence of hyperkeratotic hair follicles, orthokeratosis, dilated infundibula with follicular plugging, and vasodilation and pigmentation of basal layer, respectively. Gray-blue dots and granules present in the perifollicular and interfollicular areas are seen, especially in subjects with longer duration of disease, and correlate with the presence of pigmentary incontinence and dermal melanophages, respectively (**Figs. 6D** and **E**). A coiled up or twisted hair retained inside a follicular prominence is usually observed, with an inflamed follicular papule overlying it. White shiny structures (rosettes) were observed in some patients under polarized light (**Fig. 6F**).[16-18]

TOPICAL STEROID-DEPENDENT FACE

It is common facial dermatosis due to the uncontrolled use of topical steroids in India.

Dermoscopic Features

Irregularly dilated, branching tortuous vessels almost interconnecting with each other are seen on dermoscopy, but between the larger interconnecting vessels, the smaller nonlinear vessels can be observed. In addition, red dots, white structureless areas and yellow areas, corresponding to epidermal and dermal atrophy, respectively, and coarse terminal areas are seen. Features like follicular plugs, follicular pustules, and rosettes are not seen (**Figs. 7A** and **B**).[19]

Key Points

- Vascular polygons are a highly sensitive and specific finding of rosacea.
- Follicular plugs, superficial white/yellow scales, rosettes, orange-white areas, structures and features related to demodicosis are additional findings.
- Dilated follicles and follicular pustules are seen in papulopustular rosacea.

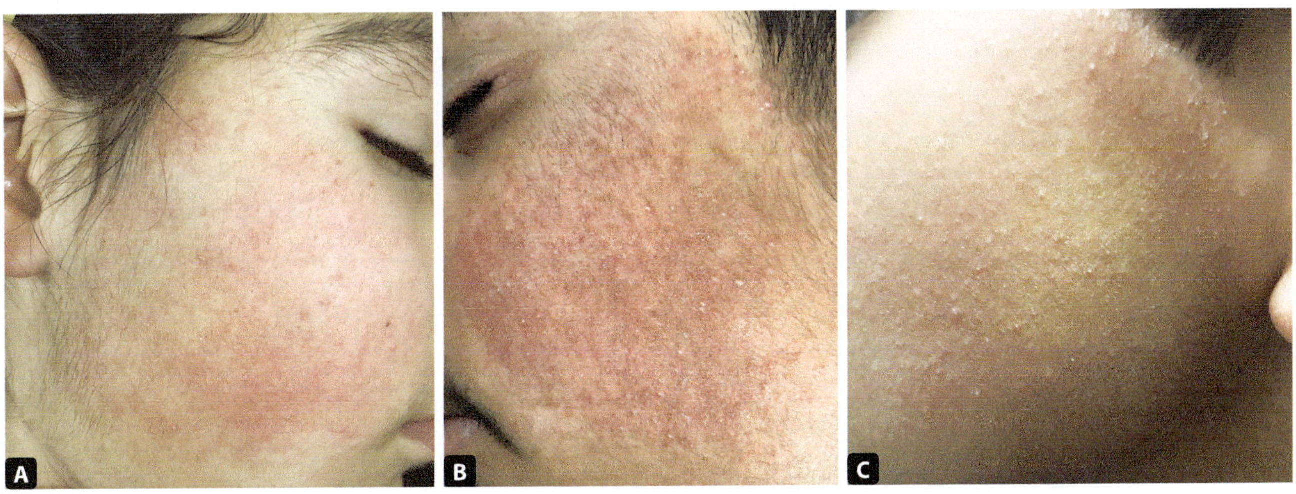

FIGS. 6A TO F: *(Continued)*

(*Continued*)

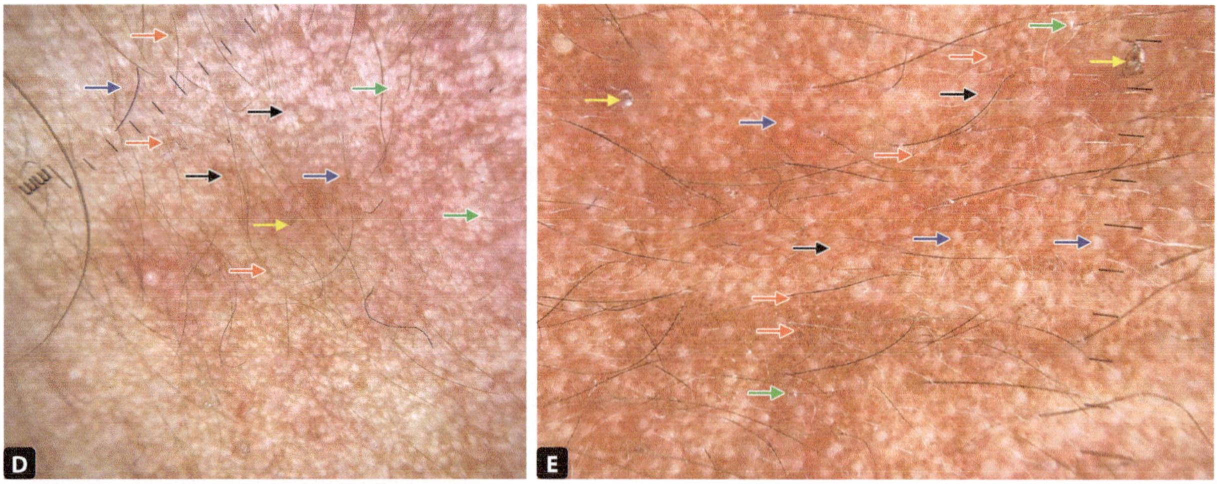

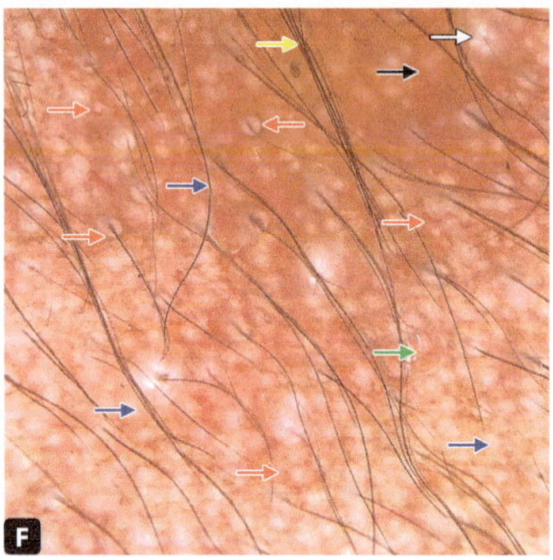

FIGS. 6A TO F: (A) Clinical image of erythromelanosis follicularis faciei et colli shows classical triad of erythema, hyperpigmentation, and follicular papules involving preauricular areas, cheeks, temporal areas, and side of nose; (B) Clinical image of erythromelanosis follicularis faciei et colli shows erythema, follicular papules, and hyperpigmentation in a classical distribution over preauricular areas, cheeks, and chin extending on to temples; (C) Erythromelanosis follicularis faciei et colli shows erythema, follicular papules, and hyperpigmentation in a classical distribution over preauricular area and cheek; (D) Dermoscopy of erythromelanosis follicularis faciei et colli shows white scales, mainly perifollicular in distribution (green arrows), numerous follicular keratotic plugs (blue arrows) against a reddish-brown background and telangiectasias (black arrows). Perifollicular and interfollicular gray-brown dots and granules (peppering) (red arrows). Twisted/coiled hairs (yellow arrow) are also seen (polarized, DermLite DL4, 10×); (E) Dermoscopy of erythromelanosis follicularis faciei et colli shows white scales (green arrows), numerous follicular keratotic plugs (blue arrows) against a red-brown background and telangiectasias (black arrows). Gray-blue dots and granules present in the perifollicular and interfollicular areas (red arrows). A coiled up or twisted hair retained inside a follicular prominence is observed, with an inflamed follicular papule overlying it (yellow arrows) (polarized, DermLite DL4, 10×); (F) Dermoscopy of erythromelanosis follicularis faciei et colli shows white scales (green arrow), numerous follicular keratotic plugs (blue arrows) against a reddish-brown background and telangiectasias (black arrow). Gray-blue dots and granules present in the perifollicular and interfollicular areas (red arrows). A coiled up or twisted hair (yellow arrows) and rosettes (white arrow) are noted (polarized, DermLite DL4, 10×).

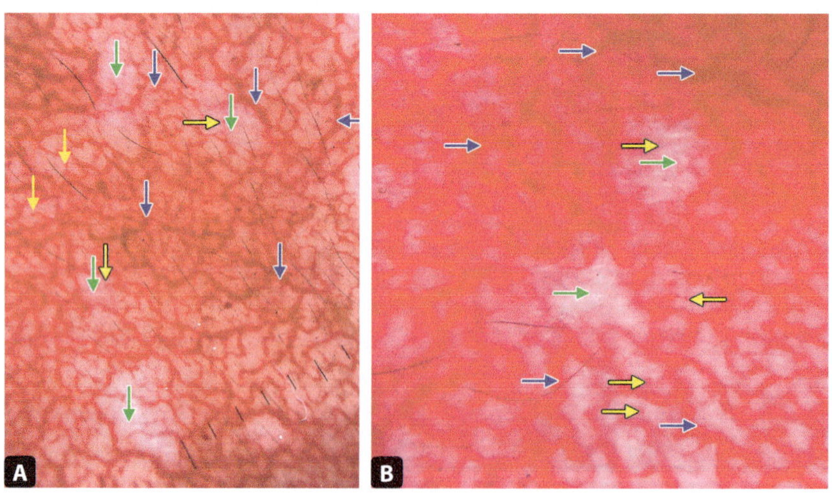

FIGS. 7A AND B: (A) Dermoscopy of topical steroid-dependent face shows irregularly dilated, branching tortuous vessels almost interconnecting with each other (blue arrows), along with white structureless areas (green arrows) and red dots (yellow arrows) (polarized, DermLite DL4, 10×); (B) Dermoscopy of topical steroid-dependent face shows irregularly dilated, branching tortuous vessels (blue arrows), white structureless areas (green arrows), and red dots (yellow arrows) (polarized, DermLite DL4, 10×).

KEY POINTS

- White scales, numerous follicular keratotic plugs against a reddish-brown background and telangiectasias
- Gray-blue dots and granules present in the perifollicular and interfollicular areas.
- A coiled up or twisted hair retained inside a follicular prominence, with an inflamed follicular papule overlying it.
- White shiny structures (rosettes) were observed in some patients under polarized light.

CONCLUSION

Dermoscopy can play a vital role in improving the diagnostic accuracy of various inflammatory facial dermatoses, evade the need for an invasive procedure like skin biopsy, bringing about a prompt resolution to clinicians confronted with diagnostic and therapeutic dilemmas in their routine practice.

REFERENCES

1. Alfaro-Castellon P, Mejia-Rodriguez SA, Valencia-Herrera A, Ramirez S, Mena-Cedillos C. Dermoscopy distinction of eruptive vellus hair cysts with molluscum contagiosum and acne lesions. Pediatr Dermatol. 2012;29:772-3.
2. Nayak SS, Mehta HH, Gajjar PC, Nimbark VN. Dermoscopy of general dermatological conditions in Indian population: a descriptive study. Clin Dermatol Rev. 2017;1:41-51.
3. Chouk C, Litaiem N, Jones M, Zeglaoui F. Acne keloidalis nuchae: clinical and dermoscopic features. BMJ Case Rep. 2017;2017:bcr2017222222.
4. Lallas A, Argenziano G, Longo C, Moscarella E, Apalla Z, Koteli C, et al. Polygonal vessels of rosacea are highlighted by dermoscopy. Int J dermatol. 2014;53:e325-7.
5. Kang IH, Seo JK, Shin MK. Useful dermoscopic findings for differentiating rosacea from seborrheic dermatitis. Indian J Dermatol. 2020;65:316-8.
6. Segal R, Mimouni D, Feuerman H, Pagovitz O, David M. Dermoscopy as a diagnostic tool in demodicidosis. Int J Dermatol. 2010;49:1018-23.
7. Donnelly A, Kenney A, DiCaudo D. Demodicosis: clinical, dermatoscopic, and microscopic correlation. J Am Acad Dermatol. 2013;68:117.
8. Friedman P, Sabban EC, Cabo H. Usefulness of dermoscopy in the diagnosis and monitoring treatment of demodicidosis. Dermatol Pract Concept. 2017;7:35-8.
9. Toda-Brito H, Aranha JM, Tavares ES. Lupus miliaris disseminatus faciei. An Bras Dermatol. 2017;92:851-3.
10. Ayhan E, Alabalik U, Avci Y. Dermoscopic evaluation of two patients with lupus miliaris disseminatus faciei. Clin Exp Dermatol. 2014;39:500-2.
11. Chauhan P, Jindal R, Shirazi N. Dermoscopy of lupus miliaris disseminatus faciei: a step closer to diagnosis. Dermatol Pract Concept. 2020;10(3):e2020055.
12. Marcoval J, Moreno A, Peyr J. Granuloma faciale: a clinicopathological study of 11 cases. J Am Acad Dermatol. 2004;51(2):269-73.
13. Teixeira DA, Estrozi B, Ianhez M. Granuloma faciale: a rare disease from a dermoscopy perspective. An Bras Dermatol. 2013;88(6 Suppl 1):97-100.
14. Lallas A, Sidiropoulos T, Lefaki I, Tzellos T, Sotiriou E, Apalla Z. Photoletter to the editor: dermoscopy of granuloma faciale. J Dermatol Case Rep. 2012;6:59-60.
15. Kitamura K, Kato H, Mishima Y, Sonoda S. Erythromelanosis follicularis faciei. Hautarzt. 1960;11:391-3.
16. Errichetti E, Pizzolitto S, Stinco G. Dermoscopy of erythromelanosis follicularis faciei et colli. Actas Dermosifiliogr. 2017;108(8):779-81.
17. Maouni S, EL Anzi O, Sqalli A, Znati K, Meziane M, Hassam B. Erythromelanosis follicularis faciei et colli: dermoscopy and dermatopathology correlates. JAAD Case Rep. 2019;5(6):535-6.
18. Rather S, Shah AA, Shah FY. Dermoscopy as a noninvasive diagnostic modality in erythromelanosis follicularis faciei et colli: a case series. Dermatol Pract Concept. 2021;11(2):e2021020.
19. Jakhar D, Kaur I. Dermoscopy of topical steroid damaged/dependent face. Indian Dermatol Online J. 2018;9:286-7.

11 CHAPTER

Connective Tissue Disorders

Kumudhini Subramanian, Shazia Jeelani

INTRODUCTION

Connective tissue disorders (CTDs) encompass a wide range of diseases caused by immune-mediated tissue injury and vascular inflammation. Dermoscopy being a reproducible, noninvasive and powerful diagnostic tool is imperative in the early diagnosis of CTD. Dermoscopic diagnosis of connective tissue diseases includes two important aspects.

1. Nailfold capillaroscopy (NFC)
2. Dermoscopy of the lesions

Nailfold capillaroscopy: Nailfold videocapillaroscopes (NVC) have been in use for performing NFC for >30 years but being heavy and difficult to carry, have been replaced now by dermoscopes. Both handheld and videodermoscopes are being used for NFC.

Nailfold capillaroscopy helps to predict the onset of complications, such as digital ulcers and internal organ involvement in connective tissue diseases such as systemic sclerosis by detecting the early microvascular changes. Morphology, diameter, architecture, and density (MDAD) is an approach to signify the proximal nailfold dermoscopic changes in a uniform, detailed manner.[1]

Dermoscopy of the lesions: Each CTD has some specific cutaneous rash with distinct dermoscopic findings.

SYSTEMIC LUPUS ERYTHEMATOSUS

Clinical Features

Acute cutaneous lupus is characterized clinically by lupus malar rash (**Fig. 1A**), maculopapular rash or toxic epidermal necrolysis variant of systemic lupus erythematosus (SLE). An important feature is nonerosive palatal, buccal, tongue or nasal ulcers. Nonscarring alopecia is noted with diffuse thinning or hair fragility with broken hairs.[2]

Dermoscopic Features

Characteristic dermoscopic findings of malar rash include reddish/salmon-colored follicular dots surrounded by white halos (**Fig. 1B**) ("inverse strawberry" pattern).[3] In SLE, histopathology may be nonspecific.

Hair: Trichoscopy shows decrease in hair shaft diameter and density, prominent blood vessels, brown-scattered pigmentation, black dots and blue-gray speckled pigmentation (**Fig. 1C**).[4]

Nailfold capillaroscopy shows mostly nonspecific pattern in the form of disorganized capillary architecture with dilated capillaries. Sometimes a normal NFC pattern or rarely a typical scleroderma pattern is also seen in case of SLE.

Key Points

- Malar rash on dermoscopy shows inverse strawberry pattern.
- NFC mostly shows a nonspecific pattern.
- Trichoscopy reveals decrease in hair shaft diameter and density with prominent vessels.

DISCOID LUPUS ERYTHEMATOSUS

Clinical Features

Discoid lupus erythematosus (DLE) on the scalp presents as scarring alopecia (**Fig. 2A**), erythema, areas of atrophy and scaling and dyspigmentation (**Fig. 2B**).[5] Chronic

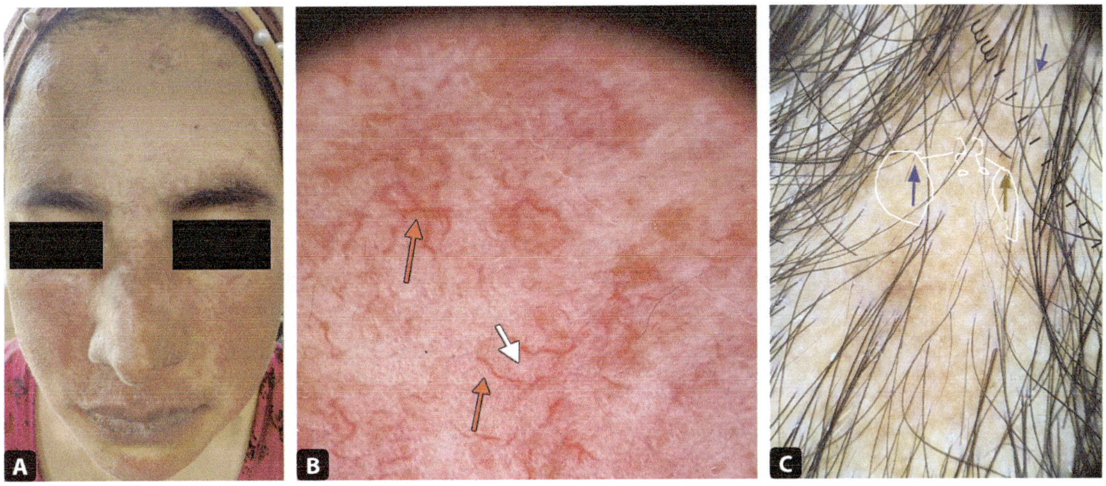

FIGS. 1A TO C: (A) Clinical image of a typical malar rash of systemic lupus erythematosus depicting erythema over the butterfly area of the face sparing the nasolabial folds; (B) Dermoscopic image of malar rash of systemic lupus erythematosus shows the classic "inverse strawberry" pattern where reddish follicular dots (red arrows) are surrounded by white halos (white arrow) (polarized, Dermlite DL4, 10×); (C) Dermoscopic image of scalp of systemic lupus erythematosus patient. Note the decrease in number and diameter of hair shaft (blue arrow) and brown scattered pigmentation (brown arrow) (polarized, DermLite DL4,10×).

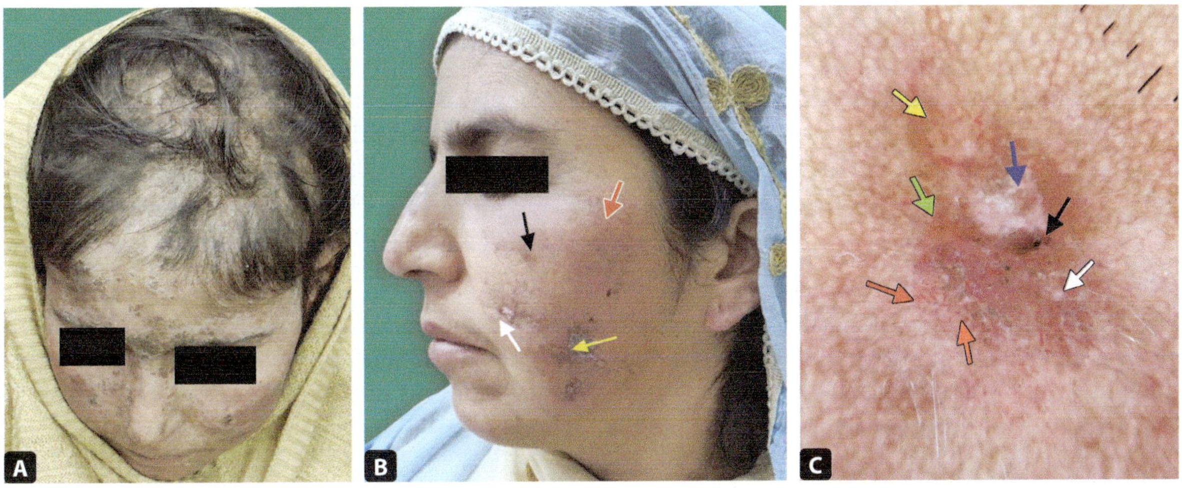

FIGS. 2A TO C: Clinical photograph of scalp of discoid lupus erythematosus with erythematous to hyperpigmented crusted plaque with atrophy and scarring over the scalp and face; (B) Clinical photograph of discoid lupus erythematosus on the left cheek. Note the follicular plugging (yellow arrow), erythema (red arrow), pigmentation (black arrow), and areas of atrophy (white arrow); (C) Dermoscopic image of discoid lupus erythematosus. Take note of the follicular keratotic plugs (black arrow), perifollicular whitish halo (white arrow), linear vessels (yellow arrow) as well as branching vessels (red arrow), rosettes (orange arrow), and structureless white areas (blue arrow), and structureless brown areas (green arrow) (polarized, DermLite DL4, 10×).

cutaneous lupus may also present as classic discoid rash, hypertrophic (verrucous) lupus, lupus panniculitis (profundus), mucosal lupus, lupus erythematosus tumidus, chilblain lupus or discoid lupus/lichen planus overlap.

Dermoscopic Features

Active DLE lesions show follicular red dots corresponding to dilated vessels and extravasated erythrocytes in perifollicular distribution on histopathology and large, yellow-brown dots corresponding to keratotic plugs in the dilated follicular ostia. Follicular red dots are characteristic of scalp DLE and not so much in facial or body lesions of DLE. White rosettes appear in early stages due to the optical effect of the polarized light and its interaction with adnexal openings that are narrowed or filled with keratin; larger rosettes are due to concentric perifollicular fibrosis.[6]

Inactive or long-standing lesions show absence of follicular openings, cicatricial milky red or white patches and structureless white and brown areas; brown areas corresponding to pigment incontinence and white areas to fibrosis. Patterns noted in late DLE include "red spider in a yellow dot" (large yellow dots with thin arborizing vessels at the periphery), and a "red stardust pattern" (telangiectasia, epidermal hyperplasia, and underlying dermal fibrosis) (**Fig. 2C**).[7]

Discoid lupus erythematosus in dark skin includes loss of pinpoint white dots, blue-gray dots in a speckled pattern, and a peripheral pigmented network. A blue-white veil with "ground-glass" hue, corresponding to the hyperkeratosis overlying interface changes at the dermal-epidermal junction, with melanophages in the papillary dermis can be seen.[8]

The dermoscopy of mucosal DLE differs from cutaneous DLE in lacking follicular plugs, perifollicular halo, and reduced number of follicular ostia. Mucosal DLE shows grayish-black to brown pigment dots, whitish-yellow scales, white structureless areas, and pink background with dilated vessels.[9]

Key Points

- Acute DLE shows follicular keratotic plugging, telangiectasia, perifollicular red dots, perifollicular white halo, and white scales.
- Late DLE reveals white structureless areas, telangiectasia, dotted vessels, and blue-gray globules or honeycomb pigmentation.
- DLE in dark skin shows an additional blue-white veil with ground-glass hue.
- Mucosal DLE shows gray-black pigment dots, white structureless areas with dilated vessels with absent follicular plugs.

DERMATOMYOSITIS

Clinical Features

Dermatomyositis (DM) is an idiopathic inflammatory myopathy with characteristic skin changes and proximal skeletal muscle weakness. Gottron's papules, pathognomonic cutaneous feature, are flat-topped, erythematous to violaceous papules and plaques over bony prominences (**Fig. 3A**).

Dermoscopic Features

Nailfold capillaroscopy: Nailfold capillary changes are as prevalent and as prominent in DM as in scleroderma. NVC patterns are referred to as a "scleroderma-like pattern" or "sclerodermoid" if the pattern is found in disorders other than scleroderma.

Proximal NFC shows capillary loss, altered capillary architecture, and presence of capillary hemorrhage with characteristic bushy capillaries or giant capillaries (**Fig. 3B**).

Dermoscopy of lesions: Dermoscopic findings of Gottron's sign are not specific. Irregular arrangement of venules and scales are found on a light red background. The punctate hemorrhage may reflect vascular injury (**Fig. 3C**).[10] The dermoscopy of poikiloderma skin lesions in DM shows enlarged linear irregular vessels with mixed pigmentation and depigmentation. Though poikiloderma is not specific for DM, the confirmation using dermoscopy may be useful to distinguish poikiloderma from other skin lesions.

The scalp of DM patients often shows elongated and tortuous vessels with persistence of follicular openings and irregularly enlarged, giant vessels with root-like appearance and thick arborizing vessels even when there is no clinical evidence of scalp involvement.[11]

Key Points

- NFC shows capillary loss, altered capillary architecture, capillary hemorrhage with bushy capillaries.
- Gottron's papules show irregular arrangement of venules and scales found on a light red background.

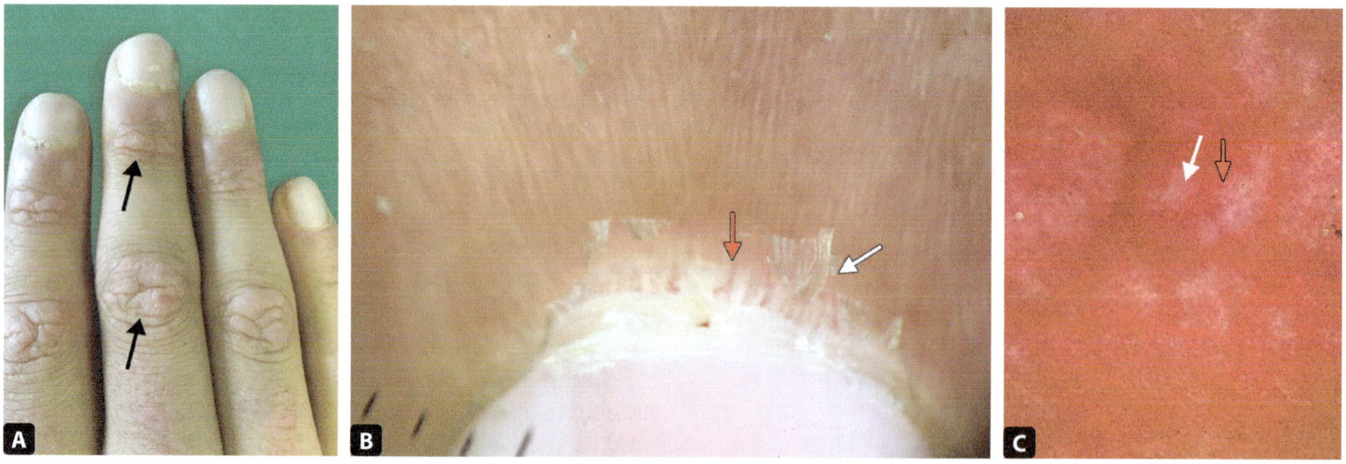

FIGS. 3A TO C: (A) Clinical picture of Gottron's papule showing flat topped, erythematous to violaceous papules and plaques over the metacarpophalangeal joints (black arrows); (B) Nailfold capillaroscopy (NFC) in case of dermatomyositis showing classical bushy appearance of the capillaries (red arrow). Note the scaling of the periungual fold (white arrow) (polarized, DermLite DL4, 10×); (C) Dermoscopic image of Gottron's papule showing central whitish area (white arrow) indicating underlying mucin deposition with peripheral dotted vessels (red arrow) (polarized, DermLite DL4, 10×).

Courtesy (A and C): Dr Yasmeen J Bhat, Associate Professor, Dermatology, Venereology and Leprosy, Government Medical College, Srinagar, Jammu and Kashmir, India.

- Poikiloderma lesions show enlarged linear irregular vessels with mixed pigmentation and depigmentation.
- Scalp shows elongated and tortuous vessels, persistence of follicular openings and irregularly enlarged, giant vessels.

MIXED CONNECTIVE TISSUE DISEASE

Clinical Features

Mixed connective tissue disease (MCTD) may clinically present as Raynaud's phenomenon, arthritis, puffy hands, patchy hypopigmentation, calcinosis, sclerodactyly (**Fig. 4A**), hypomotility of esophagus, interstitial lung disease, pulmonary artery hypertension, pleurisy, pericarditis, facial erythema, lymphadenopathy, neurological involvement, myositis, nephritis.[12]

Dermoscopic Features of Proximal Nailfold Capillaries

A sclerodermiform pattern is visible in the proximal nailfold with tortuous vessels, hemorrhages, avascular zones, rarefaction of capillaries and megacapillaries (**Fig. 4B**).[13]

Sclerodermiform pattern is present in 70% scleroderma patients, 50% in MCTD, and 45% in DM.

Key Points

- Sclerodermiform pattern of NFC.

SCLERODERMA

Clinical Features

Systemic sclerosis or scleroderma is a complex autoimmune connective tissue disease where inflammation, fibrosis, and vasculopathy lead to cutaneous and internal organ damage. It can be limited cutaneous systemic sclerosis or diffuse cutaneous systemic sclerosis. Salt-and-pepper pigmentation (**Fig. 5A**), sclerodactyly or skin thickening of fingers and toes with vasculopathy leads to digital pitted scars, matted telangiectasias (**Fig. 5B**), proximal NVC changes have characteristic dermoscopic findings.

Dermoscopic Features

Dermoscopy of proximal NFC: According to Cutolo et al., three patterns have been described: normal pattern, nonspecific pattern, and sclerodermoid pattern.[14]

Normal NFC shows homogeneously aligned hairpin arrangement of the capillary plexus with mean linear density of 6–14/mm or 30/5 mm, with no morphological alterations, no hemorrhages and no evidence of neovascularization (**Fig. 5C**). In nonspecific pattern, the changes observed on NFC do not have the complete sclerodermoid pattern.

In systemic sclerosis, three patterns have been described by Maricq et al.[15] and Bergman et al.[16]

Early scleroderma pattern shows looped morphology, regularly enlarged diameter, organized architecture, and normal density capillaries (**Fig. 5D**).

Active scleroderma pattern shows looped morphology, regularly enlarged diameter, slightly disorganized architecture with few capillary dropouts with frequent giant capillaries, capillary hemorrhages, and mild reduction of density (**Figs. 5E** and **F**). Capillary microhemorrhage due to the recurrent bleeding episodes forms a characteristic "fumarole-like" image. This pattern, although not pathognomonic, is strongly suggestive of secondary Raynaud's phenomenon due to autoimmune diseases.

Late scleroderma pattern shows capillaries with looped and branched morphology, regularly enlarged diameter, severe capillary disorganization and severe reduction of density with numerous capillary dropouts depicting large avascular areas, fewer giant capillaries, and hemorrhages.

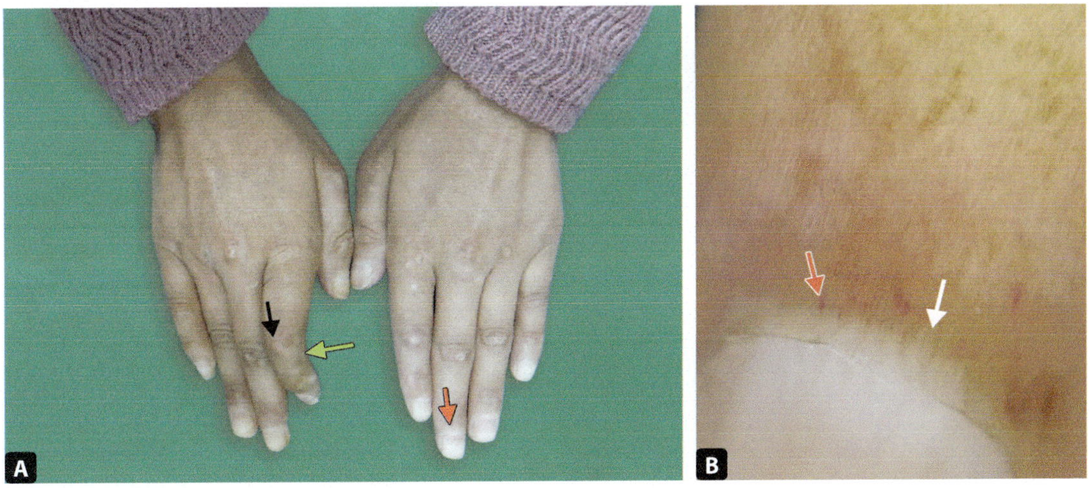

FIGS. 4A AND B: (A) Clinical photograph of mixed connective tissue disease patient showing sclerodactyly (green arrow), patchy hypopigmentation, cutaneous calcinosis (black arrow), and tapering of fingers (red arrow); (B) Proximal nailfold capillaroscopy of mixed connective tissue disease patient showing enlarged capillaries (red arrow), large avascular areas (white arrow), and rarefaction of capillaries demonstrating a late sclerodemoid pattern (polarized, DermLite DL4, 10×).

There is evidence of neovascularization in the form of markedly ramified or bushy capillaries (**Fig. 5G**).

Dermoscopy is used to differentiate a primary Raynaud's from a secondary one, to make an early diagnosis of scleroderma and it also helps to classify the activity of scleroderma.[17] NFC may show changes even before the antibody detection in some cases. Dermoscopy detects "late scleroderma" NVC pattern (the horizontal plexus alteration aka reticular dermoscopy pattern) better than NVC.[18]

Dermoscopy of lesions:

Skin telangiectasias: For telangiectasia in systemic sclerosis, two patterns are recognized:[10]

1. Matted lesions with well-circumscribed dense telangiectasia in patients with anticentromere antibodies (**Fig. 5H**)
2. Stellate lesions with poorly marginated light telangiectasia in patients with antitopoisomerase antibodies

Salt-and-pepper pigmentation: Salt-and-pepper pigmentation presents as irregular white homogeneous areas with perifollicular pigment (**Fig. 5I**). It can be differentiated from vitiligo by the absence of leukotrichia, and sometimes polka dot appearance.

Whitish perifollicular halo may be an important dermoscopic clue for diagnosis of systemic and pulmonary fibrosis in systemic sclerosis.[19]

Digital scars: Dermoscopically, keratotic plugs within an irregular shaped pitted scar is noticed in digital pitted scars (**Fig. 5J**).

Key Points

- Capillary architecture is well preserved in early and slightly disorganized in active scleroderma.
- Severe capillary disorganization is seen in late scleroderma pattern.
- Salt-and-pepper pigmentation presents as irregular white homogeneous areas with perifollicular pigment.
- Keratotic plugs within an irregular shaped pitted scar are noticed in digital pitted scars.

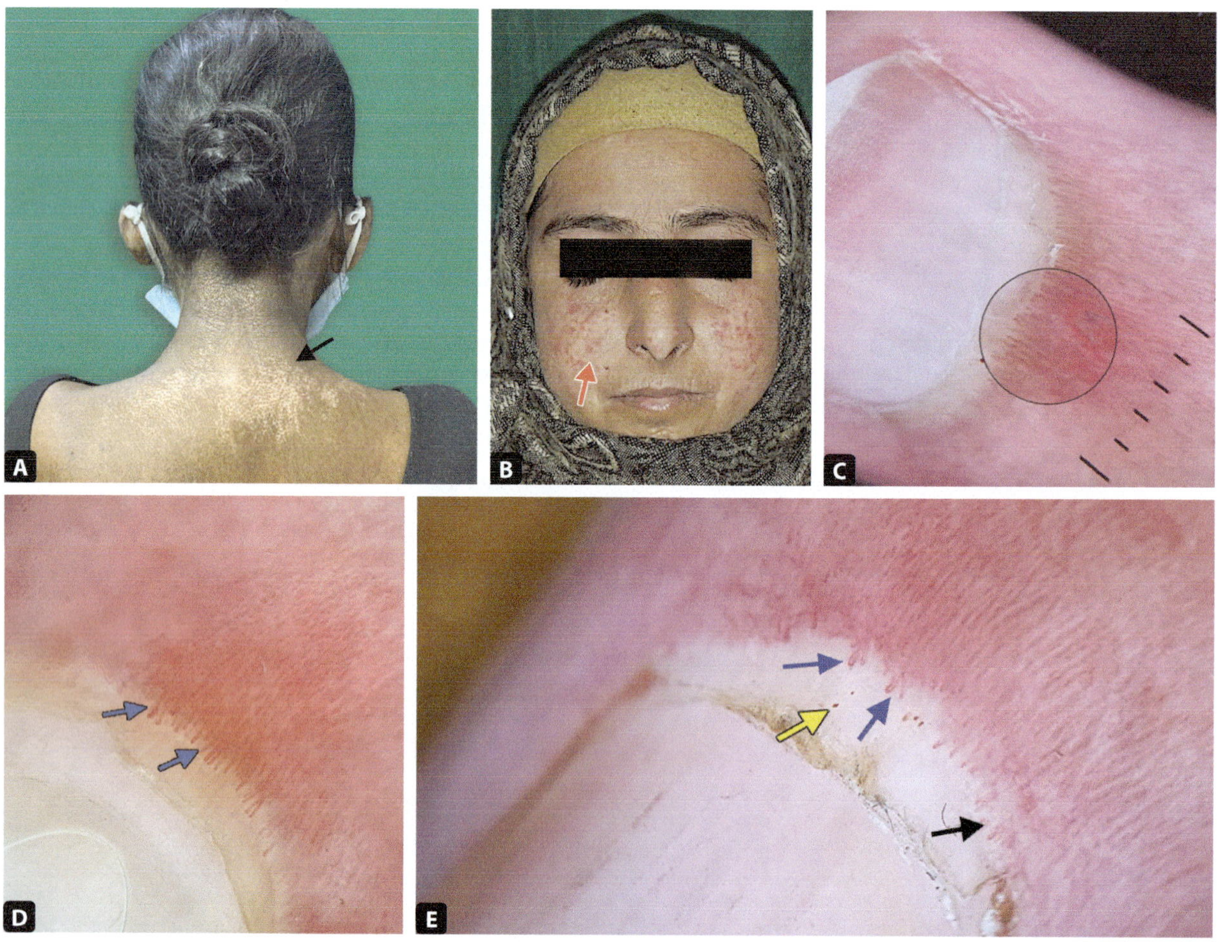

FIGS. 5A TO J: *(Continued)*

(*Continued*)

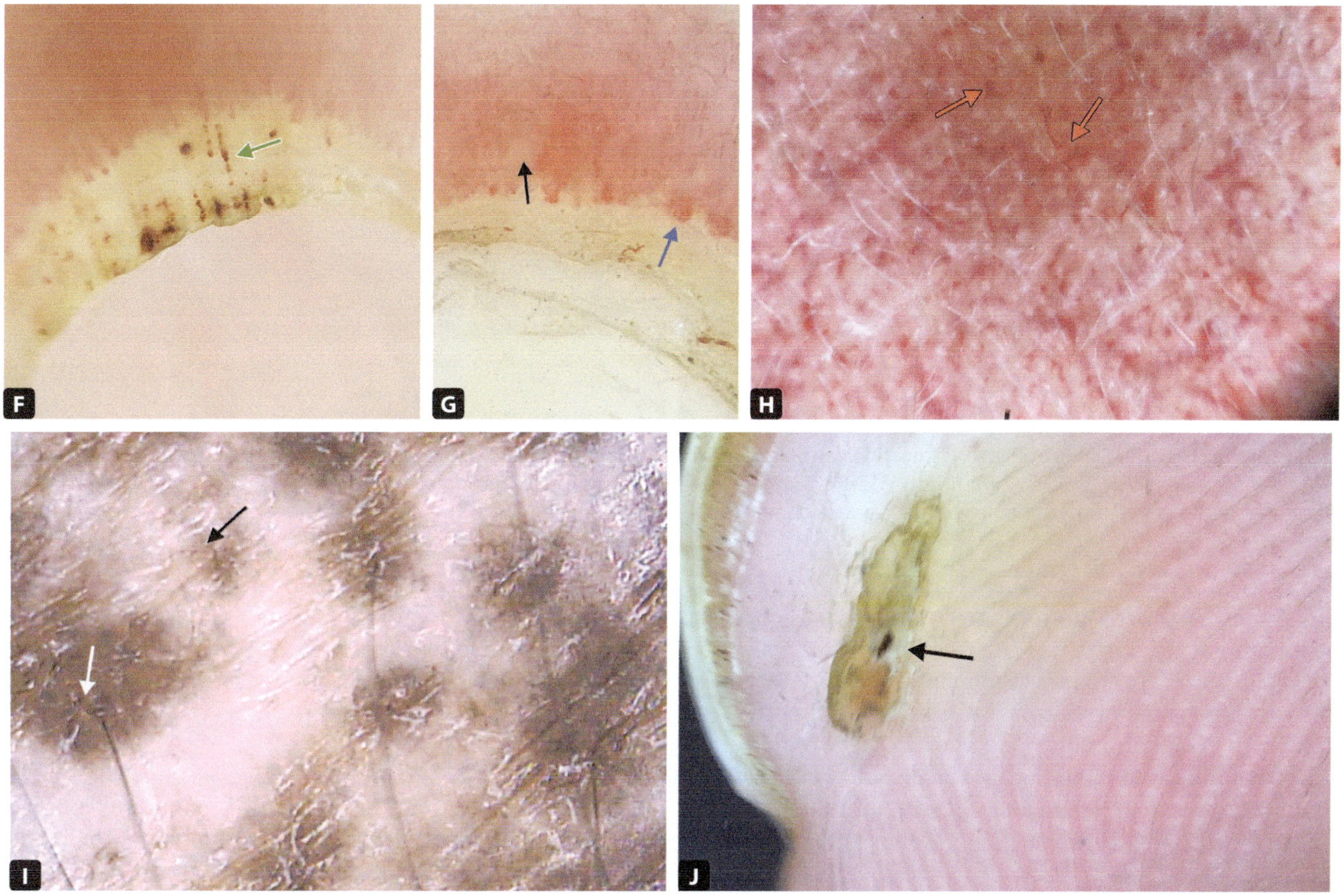

FIGS. 5A TO J: (A) Clinical photograph of salt-and-pepper pigmentation on the upper back (black arrow); (B) Clinical image of widespread mat-like telangiectasia (red arrow) in the cheeks of a scleroderma patient; (C) Proximal nailfold of left hand ring finger depicting normal nailfold capillaries showing looped morphology, regularly enlarged diameter, organized architecture, and normal density of capillaries at 30 capillaries/5 mm (black circle) (polarized, DermLite DL4, 10×); (D) Dermoscopic image of proximal nailfold of ring finger showing early scleroderma pattern. Note the looped morphology, regularly enlarged diameter capillaries, relatively well-organized capillary architecture with no evident loss of capillaries, few giant capillaries (blue arrows), few capillary hemorrhages and normal density (polarized, DermLite DL4, 10×); (E) Dermoscopic image of proximal nailfold of middle finger showing active scleroderma pattern with looped and branched morphology, regularly enlarged diameter, mild disorganization of capillary architecture with frequent giant capillaries (blue arrows) and frequent capillary hemorrhages (yellow arrow), moderate loss of capillaries (black arrow), and mild reduction in density (polarized, DermLite DL4, 10×); (F) Dermoscopic image of proximal nailfold of ring finger showing presence of microhemorrhage in a fumarole pattern (green arrow) suggesting repeated microhemorrhages in an active scleroderma pattern on NFC (polarized, DermLite DL4, 10×); (G) Dermoscopic image of proximal nailfold of ring finger showing late scleroderma pattern with looped and branched morphology, regularly enlarged diameter, severe capillary architecture disorganization with extensive avascular areas/"capillary dropouts" (black arrow) and neovascularization with ramified/bushy capillaries (blue arrow) leading to severe reduction of density (polarized, DermLite DL4, 10×); (H) Dermoscopic image of matted telangiectasia of face showing mat-like and linear telangiectasia (red arrows) (polarized, DermLite DL4, 10×); (I) Dermoscopic image of irregular white homogeneous areas (white arrow) with perifollicular pigment (black arrow) (polarized, DermaIndia videodermoscope, 40×); (J) Dermoscopic image of a digital scar showing irregular pitted scar with keratotic plug (black arrow) (polarized, DermLite DL4, 10×).

MORPHEA

Clinical Features

Morphea or localized scleroderma is a fibrosing disorder that presents with erythema on a localized area followed by tightening of skin with surface and pigmentary changes followed by atrophy at a later stage (**Fig. 6A**). The characteristic histopathological features include an atrophic epidermis with a thickened, hyalinized dermis. Dermoscopy plays a major role in identifying the active stage of morphea.

Dermoscopic Features

On polarized light dermoscopic examination, morphea classically presents with white fibrotic beams (white clouds) interspersed with linear to irregular telangiectatic vessels crossing them (**Fig. 6B**).[20,21] The fibrotic beams

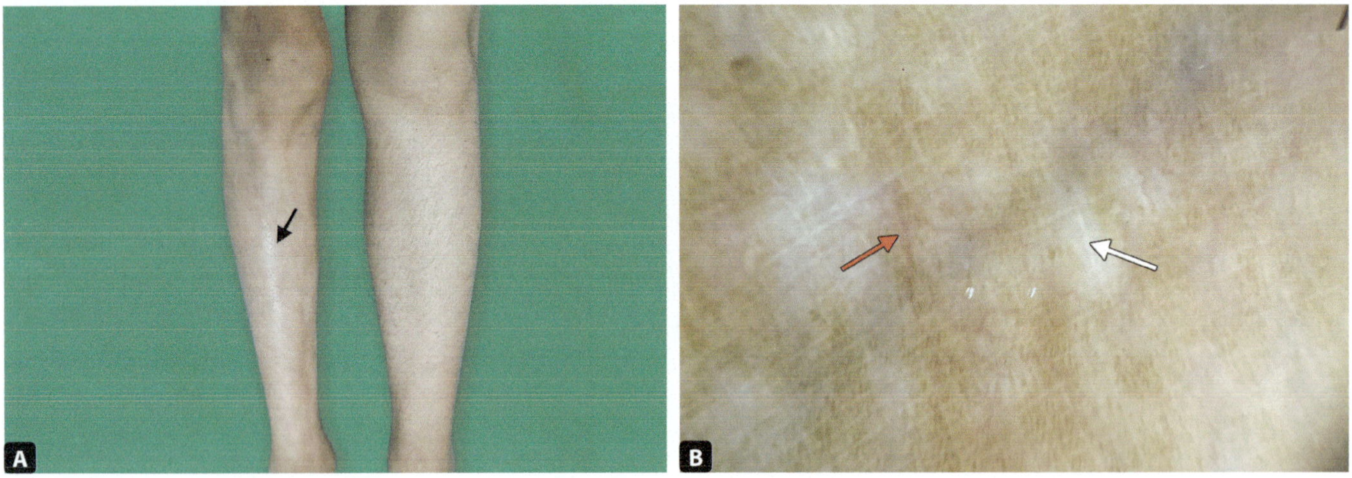

FIGS. 6A AND B: (A) Clinical picture of morphea shows a sclerotic yellowish patch in the right anterior aspect of leg (black arrow); (B) Dermoscopic image shows white fibrotic beams (white arrow) traversed by longitudinal branching vessels which are interspersed with telangiectasia (red arrow) and absent follicular openings (polarized, DermLite DL4, 10×).

observed in morphea indicate sclerotic dermis on histopathology.[22]

White fibrotic beams are seen in inflammatory, sclerotic, and atrophic stage of morphea. Crystalline structures are noticed in the inflammatory and sclerotic stage of morphea whereas unfocused large purple vessels and yellow structureless areas can be seen in late stage of morphea.[23]

Key Points

- Accentuated white fibrotic beams crossed by spreading telangiectasia is characteristic.

KEY POINTS

- Connective tissue disorders encompass a wide range of disorders.
- Dermoscopy using a hand held dermoscope helps in early detection of microvascular changes in the nail fold capillaries in cases of connective tissue disorders, especially systemic sclerosis and dermatomyositis.
- Dermoscopy of various lesions associated with these disorders helps to detect the skin changes and differentiate from other common diseases.

CONCLUSION

Dermoscopy shows definitive features in various connective tissue diseases. It plays an important role in the analysis of nailfold capillaries whereby it can predict the stage of the condition and also assists in the treatment monitoring.

ACKNOWLEDGMENT

A special credit and thanks for the figures goes to all the team of [Professor Iffat Hassan Shah (Professor and head), Dr Shazia Jeelani, Dr Subreen Kour, Dr Yakzata Bashir, Dr. Sumaya Zeerak] of 'Connective Tissue Disease Special Clinic", Department of Dermatology, Venereology and Leprosy, Government Medical College, Srinagar, Jammu and Kashmir, India.

REFERENCES

1. Rennie D. Nailfold dermatoscopy in general practice. Aust Fam Physician. 2015;44:809-12.
2. Goodfield M, Dutz J, McCourt C. Lupus erythematosus. In: Griffiths C, Barker J, Bleiker T, Chalmers R, Creamer D. Rook's Textbook of Dermatology, 9th edition. Chichester, West Sussex: John Wiley and Sons Ltd; 2016. pp. 51.15-24.
3. Errichetti E, Lallas A, De Marchi G, Apalla Z, Zabotti A, De Vita S, et al. Dermoscopy in the differential diagnosis between malar rash of systemic lupus erythematosus and erythematotelangiectatic rosacea: an observational study. Lupus. 2019;28:1583-8.
4. Suchonwanit P, Udompanich S, Thadanipon K, Chanprapaph K. Trichoscopic signs in systemic lupus erythematosus: a comparative study with 109 patients and 305 healthy controls. J Eur Acad Dermatol Venereol. 2019;33:774-80.
5. Jha AK, Sonthalia S, Sarkar R. Dermoscopy of discoid lupus erythematosus. Indian Dermatol Online J. 2016;7:458.
6. Ankad BS, Shah SD, Adya KA. White rosettes in discoid lupus erythematosus: a new dermoscopic observation. Dermatol Pract Concept. 2017;7:9-11.
7. Malakar S, Pal A, Pradhan P. 'Red starburst' pattern: a new dermoscopic indicator in discoid lupus erythematosus. Our Dermatol Online. 2019;10: 103-5.
8. Cervantes J, Hafeez F, Miteva M. Blue-white veil as novel dermatoscopic feature in discoid lupus erythematosus in 2 African-American patients. Skin Appendage Disord. 2017;3:211-4.
9. Chandela M, Misri R, Jakhar D. Mucoscopy of discoid lupus erythematosus on lower lip. Indian Dermatol Online J. 2020;11:296-7.
10. Hasegawa M. Use of dermoscopy in the evaluation of connective tissue diseases. Dermatol Clin Res. 2015;1:41-8.
11. Jasso-Olivares JC, Tosti A, Miteva M, Domínguez-Cherit J, Díaz-González JM. Clinical and dermoscopic features of the scalp in 31 patients with dermatomyositis. Skin Appendage Disord. 2017;3:119-24.
12. Alves MR, Isenberg DA. "Mixed connective tissue disease": a condition in search of an identity. Clin Exp Med. 2020;20:159-66.

13. Barbach Y, Chaouche M, Cherif AD, Elloudi S, Baybay H, Mernissi FZ. Dermoscopy of nail fold capillaries in connective tissue diseases. Madridge J Case Rep Stud. 2019;3:130-1.
14. Cutolo M, Sulli A, Pizzorni C, Accardo S. Nailfold videocapillaroscopy assessment of microvascular damage in systemic sclerosis. J Rheumatol. 2000;27:155-60.
15. Maricq HR, Harper FE, Khan MM, Tan EM, LeRoy EC. Microvascular abnormalities as possible predictors of disease subsets in Raynaud's phenomenon and early connective tissue disease. Clin Exp Rheumatol. 1983;1:195-205.
16. Bergman R, Sharony L, Schapira D, Nahir MA, Balbir-Gurman A. The handheld dermatoscope as a nail-fold capillaroscopic instrument. Arch Dermatol. 2003;139:1027-30.
17. Nirmal B. Checklist for nailfold capillaroscopy findings in systemic sclerosis: ABCDEGH. Int J Dermoscop. 2017;1:54-5.
18. Gianpetruzzi A, Bono R, Mondino C, Facchiano A, Didona B, Puddu P, et al. AB1286 Dermoscopic images of telangiectasias and nailfold videocapillaroscopic patterns in systemic sclerosis patients. Ann Rheum Dis. 2013;71:711.
19. Singh A, Ambujam S, Varghese A, Vishranth SP, Sadanandan N. Salt-and-pepper appearance: a cutaneous clue for the diagnosis of systemic sclerosis. Indian J Dermatol. 2012;57:412-3.
20. Bhat YJ, Akhtar S, Hassan I. Dermoscopy of morphea. Indian Dermatol Online J. 2019;10:92-3.
21. Tiodorovic-Zivkovic D, Argenziano G, Popovic D, Zalaudek I. Clinical and dermoscopic findings of a patient with co-existing lichen planus, lichen sclerosus and morphea. Eur J Dermatol. 2012;22:143-4.
22. Campione E, Paterno EJ, Diluvio L, Orlandi A, Bianchi L, Chimenti S. Localized morphea treated with imiquimod 5% and dermoscopic assessment of effectiveness. J Dermatolog Treat. 2009;20:10-3.
23. Errichetti E, Lallas A, Apalla Z, Di Stefani A, Stinco G. Dermoscopy of morphea and cutaneous lichen sclerosus: clinicopathological correlation study and comparative analysis. Dermatology. 2017;233(6):462-70.

12 Erythemas

CHAPTER

Malcom Noronha, Dilip Kumar NR

INTRODUCTION

Dermoscopy of erythematous plaque or patch shows dotted/linear vessels depending on the level of blood vessels. Type of scaling helps in indicating the diagnosis. Conditions with erythematous macules usually show network of erythematous blood vessels. In this chapter, we will discuss dermoscopic features of few conditions which show erythema as their predominant clinical feature.

ERYTHEMA MULTIFORME

Clinical Features

Characteristic lesion is target or "iris" lesion, described as a round lesion with three concentric rings and a well-defined border. The peripheral ring is erythematous, middle zone is pale, edematous, and the center is erythematous, covered with a blister (**Fig. 1**). Lesions are commonly located over acral areas (palms, soles, dorsal aspect of hands and feet) and might involve mucous membrane (oral, ocular, or genital).[1]

Dermoscopic Features

Central dusky zone shows clods of different color—red, blue, purple, black which correspond histologically to presence of intraepidermal or subepidermal blister with apoptotic cells in epidermis. Middle pale zone reveals pale structureless area and the peripheral zone shows erythema (**Fig. 2**). Few linear vessels are noted occasionally.[2]

Key Points

- Target lesions, characterized by three zones of clods, pale areas, and erythema from center to periphery.

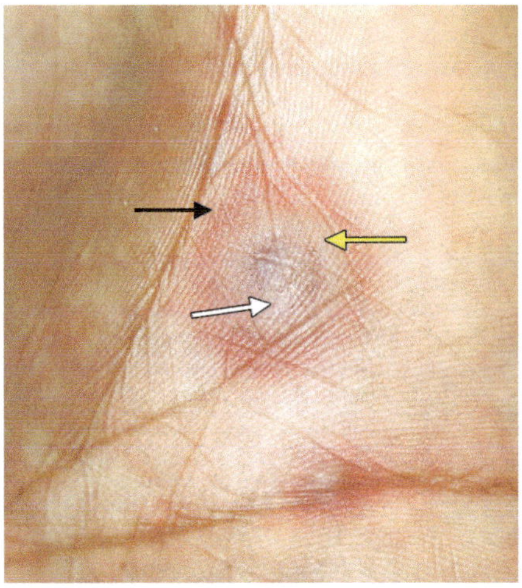

FIG. 1: Clinical image of typical target lesion in erythema multiforme on palm showing dusky erythema (white arrow), pale zone (yellow arrow) surrounded by erythema (black arrow).

Source: Kaliyadan F. Dermoscopy of erythema multiforme. Indian Dermatol Online J. 2017;8(1):75.

ERYTHEMA ANNULARE CENTRIFUGUM

Clinical Features

It is characterized by asymptomatic, annular, or polycyclic lesions which grow slowly, developing central clearance, rarely reaching > 10 cm in diameter. Trailing scale is seen at the inner border of the annular erythema (**Fig. 3**).[3]

Dermoscopic Features

Homogeneous collar-like scales are seen, which are fine and fragile. Scaling edge appears irregular, thinner with no distinct direction of peeling when observed on dermoscopy (**Fig. 4**).[3]

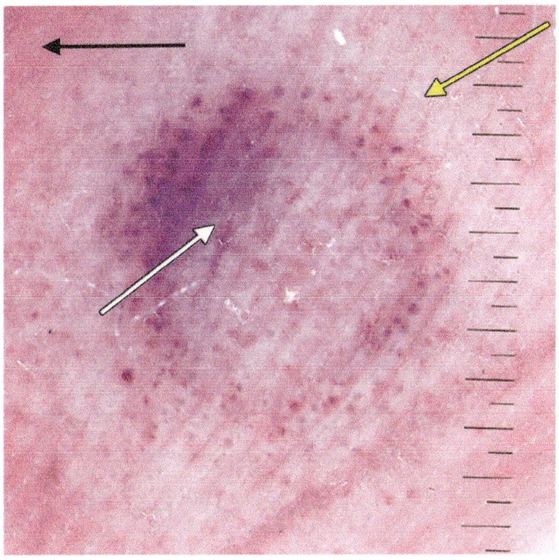

FIG. 2: Dermoscopy of typical lesion in erythema multiforme shows white arrow—central dusky zone showing clods of different colors—red, blue, purple, and black. Yellow arrow shows a plain featureless area corresponding to the pale edematous zone, and black arrow shows homogeneous erythema corresponding to outer ring. A few short linear vessels also seen (polarized, DermLite Foto II Pro, 10×).

Source: Kaliyadan F. Dermoscopy of erythema multiforme. Indian Dermatol Online J. 2017;8(1):75.

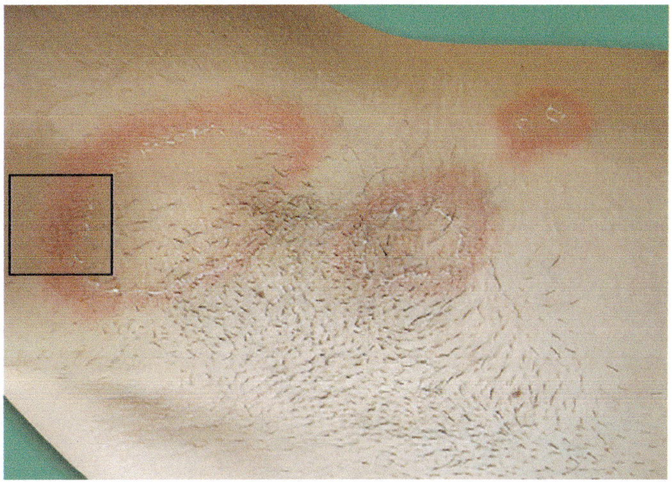

FIG. 3: Clinical image of erythema annulare centrifugum in axillae of a 63-year-old male.

Source: Tognetti L, Sbano P, Fimiani M, Rubegni P. Dermoscopy of Biett's sign and differential diagnosis with annular maculo-papular rashes with scaling. Indian J Dermatol Venereol Leprol. 2017;83:270-3.

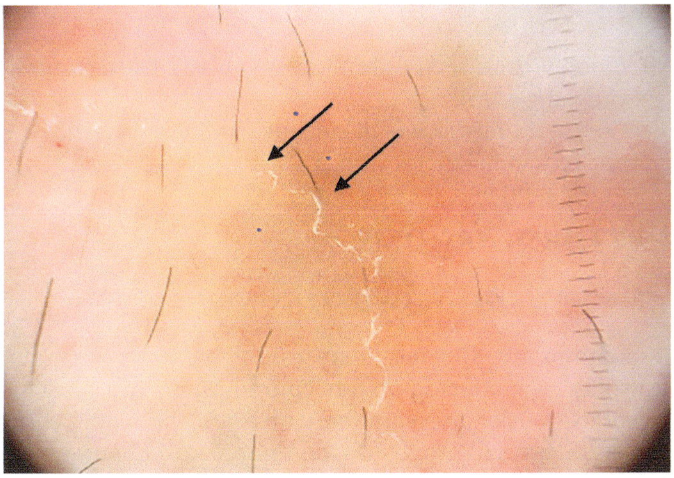

FIG. 4: Dermoscopy image showing thin scaling with irregular edge (black arrows) and unclear direction of peeling (polarized, DermLite Foto II Pro, 10×).

Source: Tognetti L, Sbano P, Fimiani M, Rubegni P. Dermoscopy of Biett's sign and differential diagnosis with annular maculo-papular rashes with scaling. Indian J Dermatol Venereol Leprol. 2017;83:270-3.

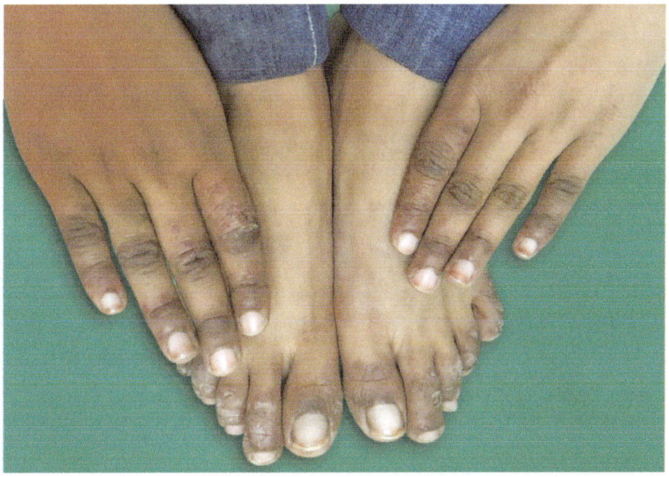

FIG. 5: Clinical image of perniosis or chilblain showing erythematous and hemorrhagic patches with scaling.

Courtesy: Dr Payal Chauhan, Assistant Professor, AIIMS, Bilaspur, Himachal Pradesh, India.

Key Points

- Trailing scale sign is seen.
- Irregular peripheral scales with no distinct direction of peeling.

CHILBLAINS

Clinical Features

It is an inflammatory skin condition typically presenting as red or blue, tender, pruritic lesions located symmetrically over dorsal aspect of toes, ears, and nose. The lesions usually start after 12–24 hours of cold exposure and resolve within 1–3 weeks.[4] There has been a significant association of chilblain-like lesions (two types—erythematous-edematous type and blistering type) with coronavirus disease 2019 (COVID-19) infection without any exposure to cold or underlying autoimmune or hematologic disorder (**Fig. 5**).[5,6]

Dermoscopic Features

Background color varies from coppery to red in color. Erythema appears to be blanching in initial but becomes nonblanching in long-standing lesions with red-purple

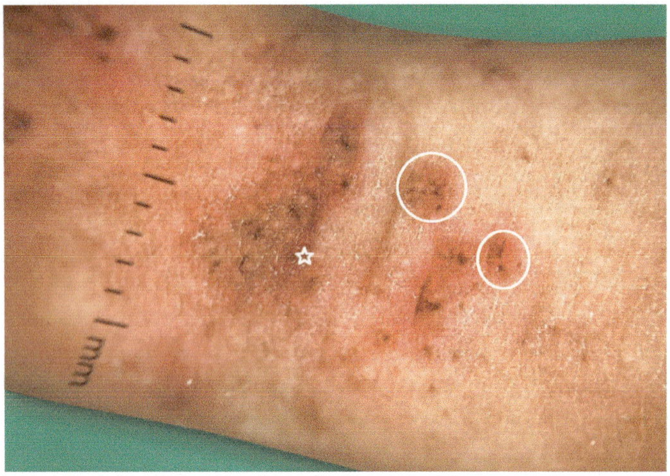

FIG. 6: Dermoscopy findings of a classical erythematous-edematous lesion of the dorsal aspect of the toe showing a predominant coppery red background (star) associated with dotted vessels and hemorrhagic spots (circles) (polarized, DermLite DL4, 10×).

Courtesy: Dr Payal Chauhan, Assistant Professor, AIIMS, Bilaspur, Himachal Pradesh, India.

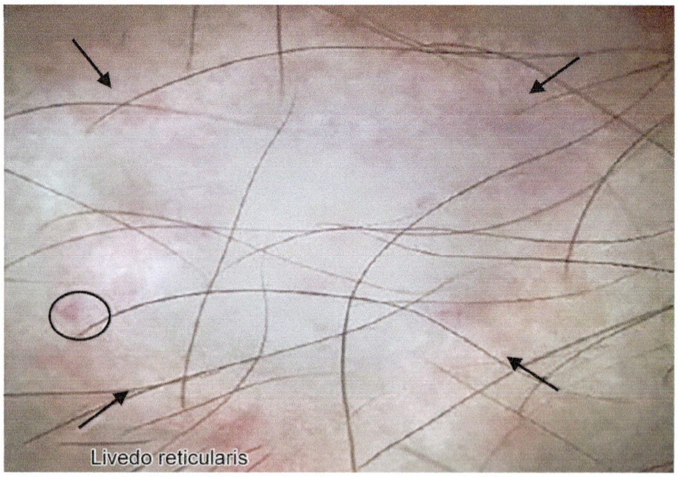

FIG. 7: Image shows presence of erythematous ring (arrow), comma-shaped vessels (circle) (polarized, DermLite II, 10×).

Source: Nayak SS, Mehta HH, Gajjar PC, Nimbark VN. Dermoscopy of general dermatological conditions in Indian population: a descriptive study. Clin Dermatol Rev. 2017;1(2):41-51.

lesions. In the plantar area, erythema mostly involves the ridges. Blood vessels are seen in all cases which might look like hemorrhagic dots (most common), blanching blurred dots, linear, glomerular, or irregular in shape (**Fig. 6**).[5,6]

Key Points

- Coppery red background
- Blood vessels appear as red dots, blanching blurred dots, linear, or glomerular.

LIVEDO RETICULARIS

Clinical Features

Typically, livedo reticularis (LR) presents as a complete network-like reddish-violet discoloration of the limbs, which reduces on limb elevation or warming of skin. In contrast to this, when there is an incomplete and broken network appearing like branching configuration, the term livedo racemosa is used.[7,8]

Dermoscopic Features

It shows homogeneous red lines, comma vessels and regular, complete network-like pattern of purple vessels (erythematous ring) and sparse-dotted vessels which correspond to dilated subpapillary vessels and papillary vessels, respectively.[9] In contrast, livedo racemosa shows broken network-like and blurry vessels; linear-irregular blurry vessels and diffuse-dotted vessels (**Fig. 7**).[9]

Key Points

- Blood vessels seen as homogeneous red lines, comma-shaped vessels.
- Complete formation of network in LR versus broken network in livedo racemosa.

ERYTHROCYANOSIS

Clinical Presentation

The commonly affected areas are thighs, lower legs, and buttocks. The affected area is cold to touch and presents as diffuse dusky discoloration which may be blanched by pressure, which Krogh has compared to subcutaneous lake of ink.[10] Angiokeratomas, keratosis pilaris, and telangiectasias may be seen along with the lesions. Long-standing cases may present with edema, fibrosis, and nodular perniotic lesions.[8]

Dermoscopic Features

Characteristic dermoscopic features are coarse network-like, reddish-purple vessels and less commonly sparsely distributed vessels of dotted or linear-irregular morphology. These network-like vessels and dotted vessels histologically correspond to subpapillary vessels and papillary vessels, respectively.[9]

Key Points

- Red to purple color dot to linear vessels.

RAYNAUD'S PHENOMENON

Clinical Presentation

The typical appearance of white (pallor), blue (cyanosis), and red (rubor) color changes in sequence was first described by Maurice Raynaud. These triphasic color changes represent the ischemic phase, deoxygenation phase, and reperfusion phase, respectively.[11] The episodes usually last for a few minutes and resolves without sequelae but can be of prolonged duration in secondary Raynaud's phenomenon and may be associated with telangiectasia of nail fold, nail changes, etc.[8]

Dermoscopic Features

The nail fold capillaroscopic findings of secondary Raynaud's phenomenon are: architectural disorganization, reduction of capillary density, giant capillaries, enlarged loops, avascular areas, microhemorrhages, and angiogenesis.[9,12] Primary Raynaud's phenomenon on the other hand usually shows a normal capillaroscopic architectural pattern or slight vessel dilation (**Figs. 8A** to **C**).[9]

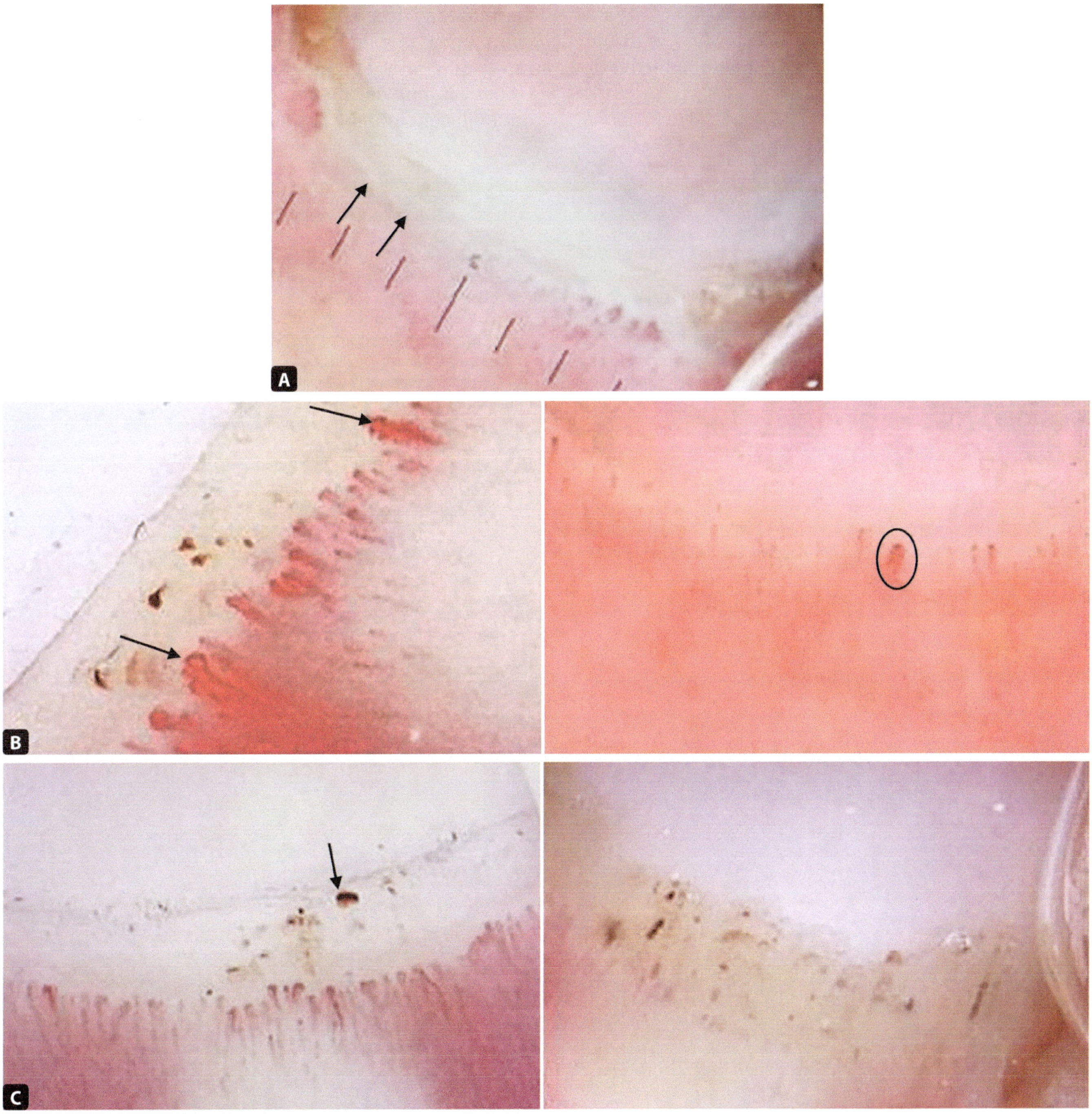

FIGS. 8A TO C: Dermoscopy of nail fold capillaries showing (A) reduction of capillary density (arrows), (B) giant capillaries, and (C) microhemorrhages (marked in black arrows and circle in respective images) (polarized, DermLite DL4, 10×).

Source: Moreau J, Dupond AS, Dan N, Untereiner T, Vidal C, Aubin F. Comparative evaluation of dermoscopy and capillaroscopy in Raynaud's phenomenon. Ann Dermatol Venereol. 2017;144(5):333-40.

Key Points

- Loss of blood vessel architecture and morphology
- Giant capillaries → microhemorrhages→ reduced capillary density → avascular areas

KEY POINTS

- Erythema multiforme is characterized by target lesions, which shows three zones—characterized by three zones of clods, pale areas, and erythema from centre to periphery.
- Erythema annulare centrifugum—scaling is seen on the inner edge of the annular erythema.
- Chilblains show coppery red background with blood vessels appearing as red dots, blanching blurred dots, linear, or glomerular.
- Livedo reticularis shows network of blood vessels which appears as homogeneous red lines and comma shaped vessels.
- Erythrocyanosis commonly appears as dusky erythema over lower limbs, shows red to purple dots to linear vessels on dermoscopy.
- Raynaud's phenomenon shows—Giant capillaries → microhemorrhages → reduced capillary density → avascular areas as sequential changes on dermoscopy of affected area.

CONCLUSION

Dermoscopy acts as a useful tool to differentiate between common erythematous scaly lesions and helps in providing rapid diagnosis and might avoid biopsy in most cases. Understanding dermoscopy in such conditions provides a better insight into the pathology of the condition.

REFERENCES

1. Kaliyadan F. Dermoscopy of erythema multiforme. Indian Dermatol Online J. 2017;8(1):75.
2. Vázquez-López F, Kreusch J, Marghoob AA. Dermoscopic semiology: further insights into vascular features by screening a large spectrum of nontumoral skin lesions. Br J Dermatol. 2004;150:226-31.
3. Tognetti L, Sbano P, Fimiani M, Rubegni P. Dermoscopy of Biett's sign and differential diagnosis with annular maculo-papular rashes with scaling. Indian J Dermatol Venereol Leprol. 2017;83:270-3.
4. Vano-Galvan S, Martorell A. Chilblains. CMAJ. 2012;184(1):67.
5. Piccolo V, Neri I, Filippeschi C, Argenziano G, Battarra VC, Berti S, et al. Chilblain-like lesions during COVID-19 epidemic: a preliminary study on 63 patients. J Eur Acad Dermatol Venereol. 2020;34(7):e291-3.
6. Piccolo V, Bassi A, Argenziano G, Mazzatenta C, Guglielmo A, Patrizi A, et al. Dermoscopy of chilblain-like lesions during the COVID-19 outbreak: a multicenter study on 10 patients. J Am Acad Dermatol. 2020;83(6):1749-51.
7. Sajjan VV, Lunge S, Swamy MB, Pandit AM. Livedo reticularis: a review of the literature. Indian Dermatol Online J. 2015;6(5):315-21.
8. Bashir SJ, Chew A. Cutaneous reactions to cold and heat. In: Griffiths CE, Barker J, Bleiker T, Chalmers R, Creamer D (Eds). Rook's Textbook of Dermatology, 9th edition. Oxford: Wiley-Blackwell; 2016. pp. 125.1-13.
9. Meo ND, Corneli P, Zalaudek I. Erythemas. In: Lallas A, Errichetti E, Ioannides D (Eds). Dermoscopy in General Dermatology. Boca Raton, FL: CRC Press; 2019. pp. 97-105.
10. Telford ED, Simmons HT. Erythrocyanosis. Br Med J. 1936;1(3925):629-30.
11. Temprano KK. A review of Raynaud's disease. Mo Med. 2016;113(2):123-6.
12. Moreau J, Dupond AS, Dan N, Untereiner T, Vidal C, Aubin F. Comparative evaluation of dermoscopy and capillaroscopy in Raynaud's phenomenon. Ann Dermatol Venereol. 2017;144(5):333-40.

13 CHAPTER Benign Tumors

Balachandra S Ankad, Tejinder Kaur, Priyanka Jaju

INTRODUCTION

Dermoscopy is a noninvasive tool which helps in the diagnosis of benign tumors of the skin by recognizing the peculiar dermoscopic patterns and pigment distribution patterns. It helps in the differentiation of benign from malignant skin lesions. This chapter covers the dermoscopic findings of benign skin tumors.

SEBORRHEIC KERATOSIS

Clinical Features

They are common, benign epidermal tumors developing after middle age. They involve any part of the body, mainly the face and trunk with sparing of the palms and soles. They are usually multiple and begin as sharply defined brown macules, that develop into slightly raised, brown to black, oval papules, or into polypoidal lesions. The surface is uneven, verrucous, and dull, with multiple plugged follicles (**Fig. 1A**). The lesions have a characteristic "stuck-on" appearance (**Fig. 1B**).[1]

Dermoscopic Features

- Milia-like cysts are small, whitish or yellowish round structures, corresponding to intraepidermal keratin-filled cysts resembling milia (**Fig. 1C**). They are mainly seen in seborrheic keratoses but some small milia-like cysts can also be seen in congenital melanocytic nevi and rarely in other melanocytic tumors. They are better visible under nonpolarized dermoscopy.
- Comedo-like openings are round, brown to black-colored structures (**Fig. 1D**) which correspond to keratin-filled invaginations of the epidermis.[2]
- Fissures and ridges (cerebriform pattern) are irregular linear keratin-filled structures giving a "gyri and sulci" of brain or "mountain and valley pattern" appearance. Hypo- or hyperpigmented gyri (ridges) that have thicker width are known as "fat fingers" (**Fig. 1E**).
- Fingerprint-like structures are thin, brown, parallel lines resembling fingerprints (**Fig. 1C**). Although they can be seen in some flat seborrheic keratosis, they are predominant features of solar lentigo.
- Moth-eaten border is a sharply demarcated and irregularly concave border that gives a moth-eaten appearance to the lesion (**Fig. 1C**). This is typically seen in some flat seborrheic keratosis on the face.
- Hairpin vessels are elongated capillary vessels folded in a loop that resembles a hairpin. They are typically found at the periphery of the lesions. Mostly, hairpin blood vessels are grouped together, and each of them is surrounded by a hypopigmented halo. Atypical hairpin blood vessels may be seen in melanomas.
- *Network-like structures*: This reticulation resembling pigment network is larger than the classic pigment network (**Fig. 1F**) and does not correspond to melanin pigment but appears to be due to keratin-filled structures.
- *Sharp demarcation*: An abrupt interruption of the pigmented edge at the border of the lesion is often present in seborrheic keratosis (**Fig. 1G**).
- *Wobble test*: This dynamic test is performed using a contact dermoscopy device. Once the contact plate of the dermoscope is firmly pressed down (pressure in vertical direction) against the lesion, it is then moved slightly back and forth in the horizontal plane (parallel to the skin surface). In, Seborrheic keratoses, the superficial part of the lesion "stays stuck" to the dermoscope and move en bloc with the movement of the dermoscopic face plate. In contrast, nevi will not move en bloc but, rather roll back and forth. In other words, intradermal nevi will wobble. This sign reflects the consistency of the lesion, which is rather stiff and rigid (in seborrheic keratosis) compared to dermal nevi.[3,4]

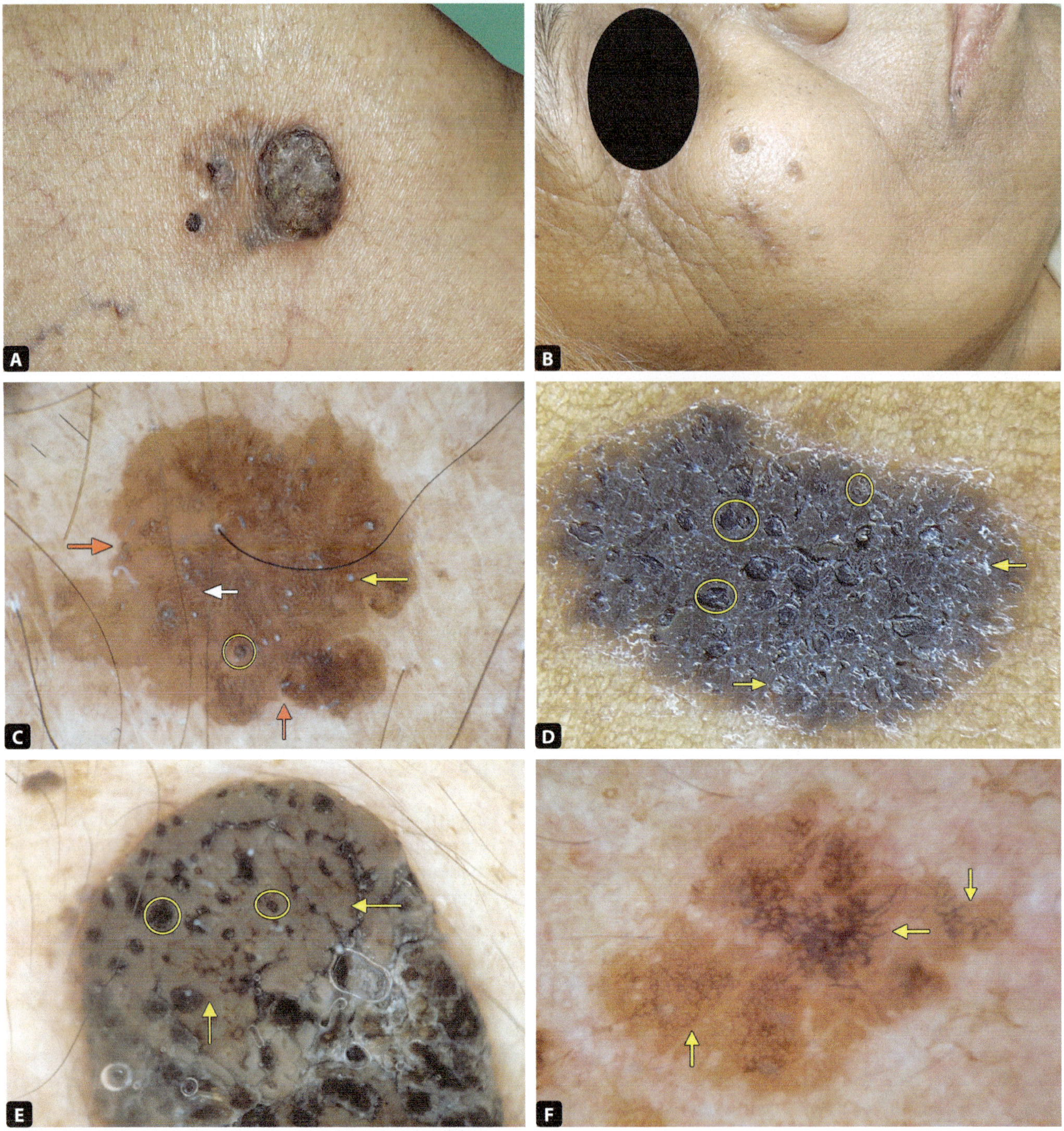

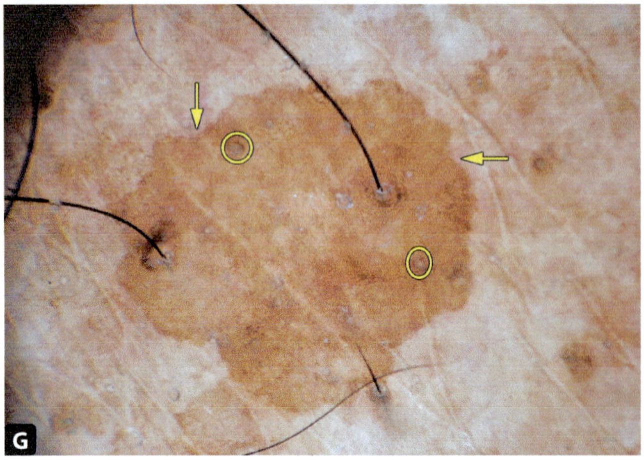

FIGS. 1A TO G: (A) Clinical image of seborrheic keratosis showing well-defined plaque with verrucous surface with follicular plugs; (B) Clinical image of seborrheic keratosis showing well-defined plaques with stuck-on appearance; (C) Dermoscopy of seborrheic keratosis shows milia-like cysts (yellow arrow), moth-eaten borders (red arrows), and fingerprint-like structures (white arrow) with comedo-like openings (yellow circle) (polarized, DermLite DL3, 10×); (D) Dermoscopy of seborrheic keratosis shows multiple comedo-like openings (circles) with surface scales (arrows) (nonpolarized, DermLite DL3, 10×); (E) Dermoscopy of seborrheic keratosis shows fissure and ridges in cerebriform pattern with multiple comedo-like openings (circles) and fat finger-like structures (arrows) (polarized, DermLite DL4, 10×); (F) Dermoscopy of seborrheic keratosis shows network-like structures (arrows) and well-demarcated borders (polarized, DermLite DL3, 10×); (G) Dermoscopy of seborrheic keratosis shows sharp borders (arrows) and comedo-like openings (circles) (polarized, DermLite DL3, 10×).

Source (Figs. C and G): Ankad BS, Sakhare PS, Prabhu MH. Dermoscopy of non-melanocytic and pink tumors in brown skin: a descriptive study. Indian J Dermatopathol Diagn Dermatol. 2017;4:41-51.

Key Points

- In global view characteristic cerebriform pattern is observed with moth-eaten borders.
- Local view reveals comedo-like openings, milia-like cysts with other definitive features such as fat finger-like and fingerprint-like structures, hairpin-like vessels.

DERMATOSIS PAPULOSA NIGRA

Clinical Features

They present as multiple black to brownish smooth, firm papules on face (**Fig. 2A**), neck and even chest, and back.[5]

Dermoscopic Features

It is characterized by fissures and ridges that give cerebriform pattern (**Fig. 2B**). Broad ridges appear as fat finger-like structures (**Fig. 2C**).[6] Comedo-like openings are noted especially with higher magnification.

Key Points

- Ridges and fissures in cerebriform pattern and comedo-like openings are definitive patterns.

SKIN TAGS

Clinical Features

Skin tags, also known as fibroepithelial polyps, are seen in individuals as they become older. They are found in neck, axillae, and groin areas. Obese and diabetics are common predisposing factors. They are asymptomatic and present as skin or dark brown color, sessile or pedunculated papules (**Fig. 3A**). They result from irritation of skin folds or insulin resistance and human papillomavirus is also attributed.[7]

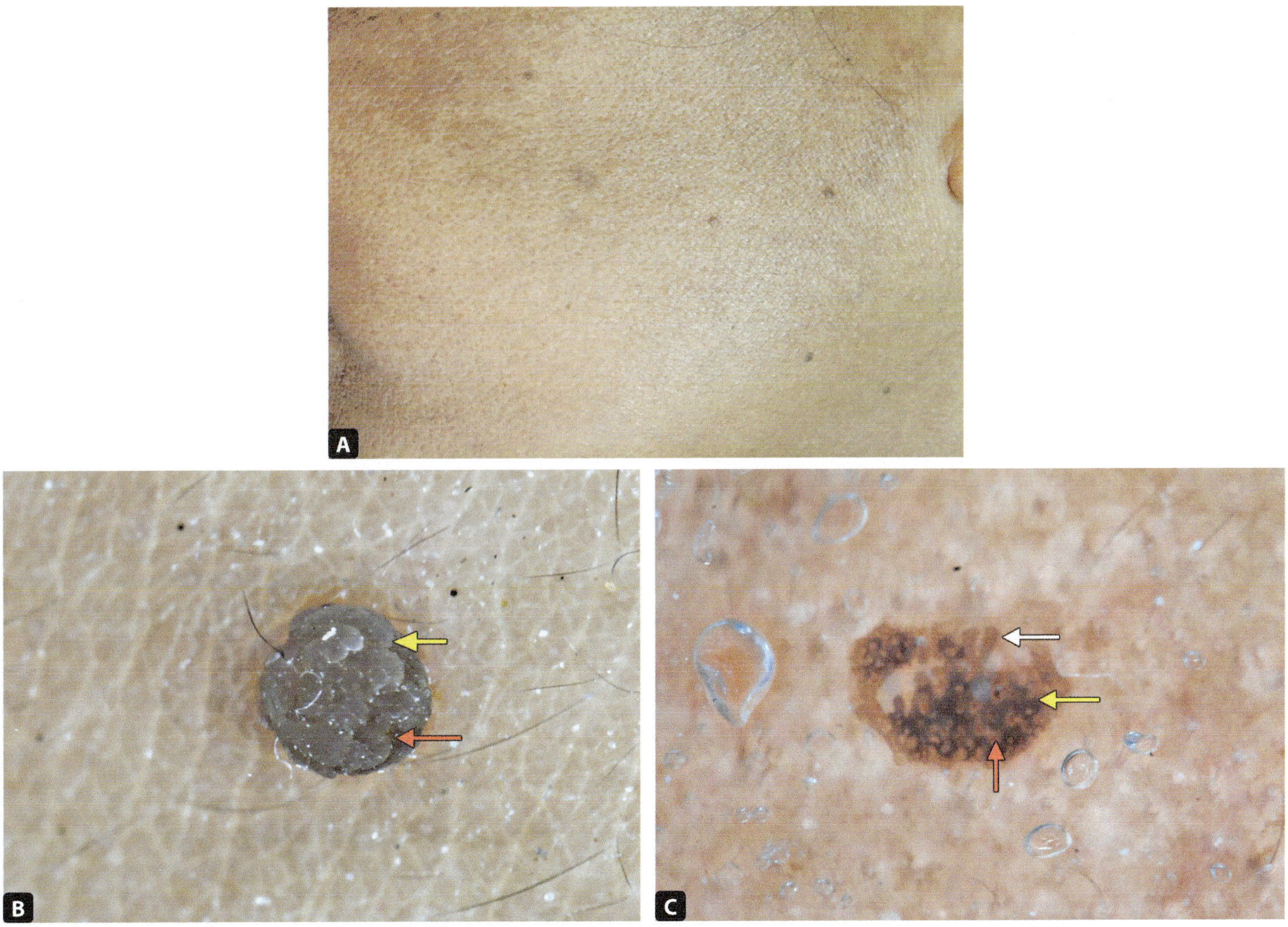

FIGS. 2A TO C: (A) Clinical image of dermatosis papulosa nigra showing brown papules on the check; (B) Dermoscopy of dermatosis papulosa nigra shows fissures (red arrow) and ridges (yellow arrow) giving a cerebriform pattern (polarized, DermLite Foto II Pro Plus, 10×); (C) Dermoscopy of dermatosis papulosa nigra shows fissures (red arrow) and ridges (yellow arrow) giving a cerebriform pattern. Note the fat finger-like structures (white arrow) (polarized, DermLite DL3, 10×).

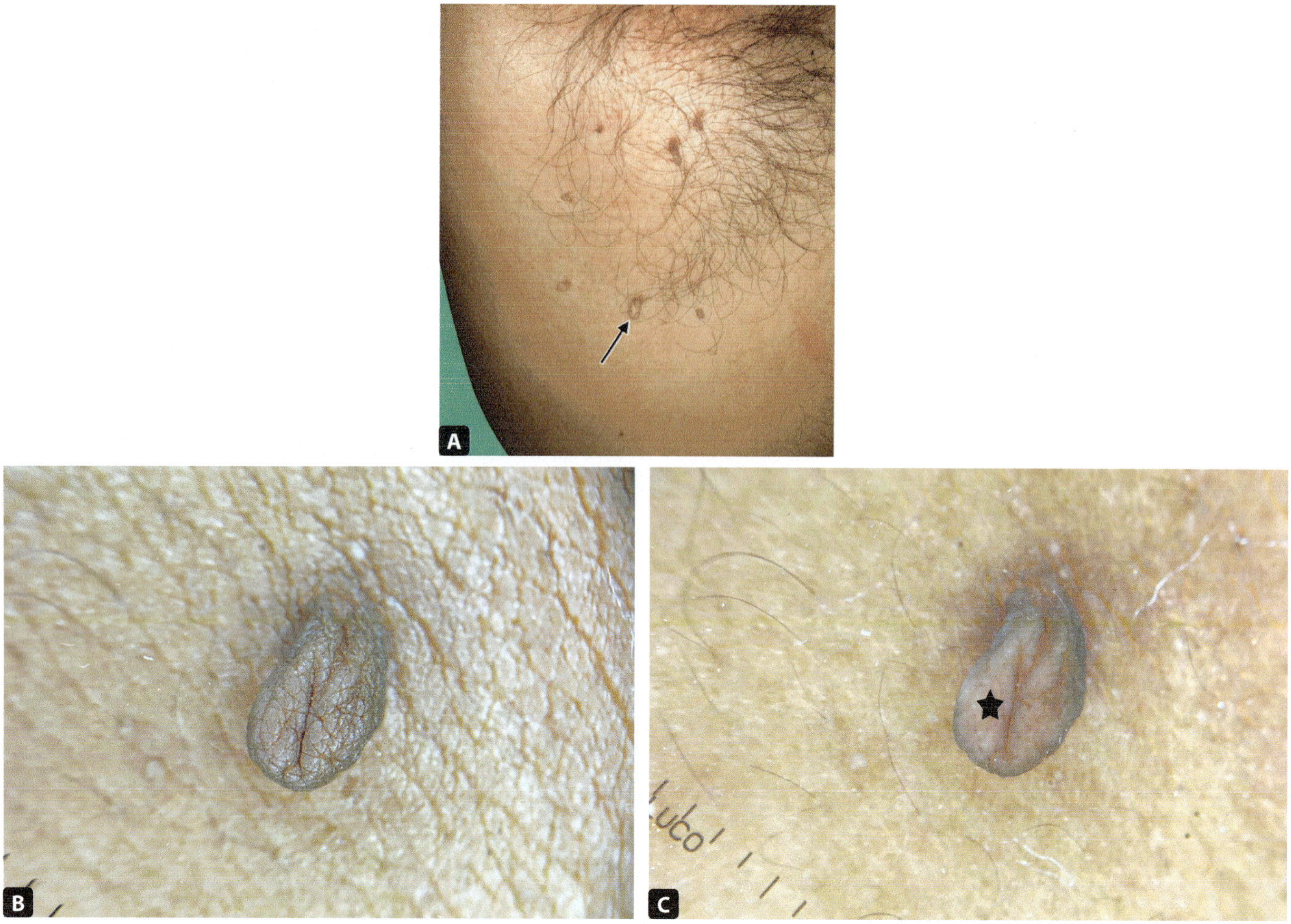

FIGS. 3A TO C: (A) Clinical image of skin tag showing brown pedunculated papules in the axillae; (B) Dermoscopy of skin tag shows verrucous and irregular surface (nonpolarized, Illuco IDS 1100, 10×); (C) Dermoscopy of skin tag shows brownish structureless area (black star). Note the absence of vascular elements (polarized, Illuco IDS 1100, 10×).

Dermoscopic Features

It shows verrucous surface in nonpolarized mode (**Fig. 3B**) and brown to grayish structureless area without vascular elements (**Fig. 3C**).

Key Points

- Brown or gray structureless area without vascular elements is characteristic of skin tag.

LICHEN PLANUS-LIKE KERATOSIS

Clinical Features

It is also called benign lichenoid keratosis, presents as a solitary, flat hyperkeratotic papule with irregular border (**Fig. 4A**). It is usually seen on the sun-exposed skin of middle-aged to elderly individuals. It is considered as an intermediate inflammatory stage of a regressing solar lentigo or seborrheic keratosis that has some histological features similar to lichen planus.[8,9]

Dermoscopic Features

Dermoscopic features include uniform-pigmented areas with granular pattern consisting of multiple blue-gray dots (**Fig. 4B**). This granular pattern can be localized or diffuse and these granules are coarse and show various shades of gray. Reticulate grayish lines on a pink background are also noted.[9] Occasionally, surface white scales are noted. Its dermoscopy features are believed to change with lesion progression and regression.

Key Points

- Blue-gray pigment granules that are coarse with different shades of gray color and uniform-pigmented areas are found.

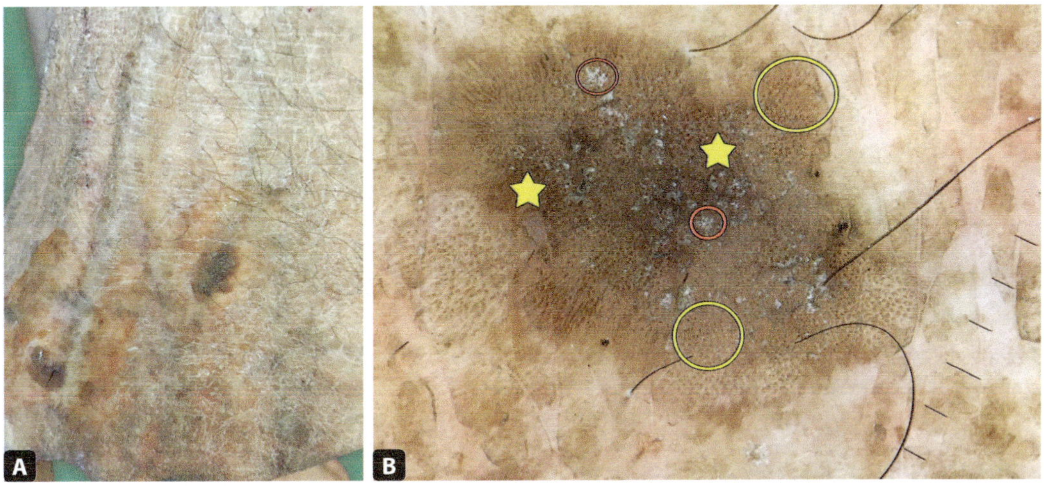

FIGS. 4A AND B: (A) Clinical image of lichen planus-like keratosis showing well-demarcated plaque on the forearm; (B) Dermoscopy of lichen planus-like keratosis shows brown to grayish coarse (yellow circles) granules with brown-pigmented areas (yellow stars). White surface scales are well-appreciated (red circles) (polarized, DermLite DL3, 10×).

Courtesy: Dr Yasmeen J Bhat, Government Medical College, Srinagar, Jammu and Kashmir, India.

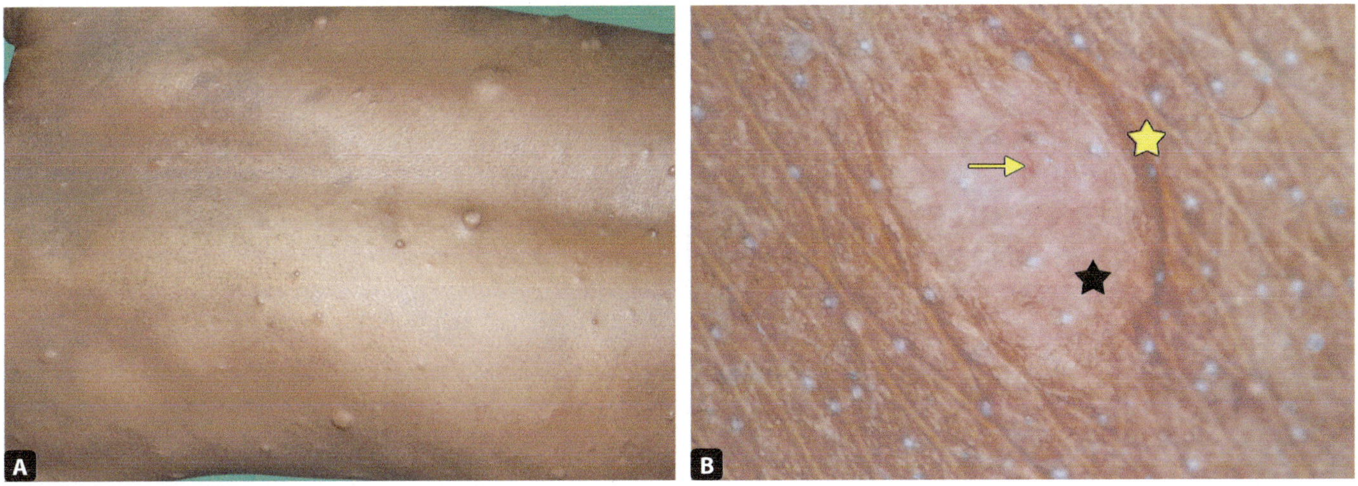

FIGS. 5A AND B: (A) Clinical image of neurofibromas in neurofibromatosis type 1 showing multiple soft to firm subcutaneous papules and nodules; (B) Dermoscopy of neurofibroma shows pinkish-red area (black star) with brown rim at the periphery (yellow star). Note the short linear vessels (yellow arrow) and white dots of eccrine openings (polarized, DermLite DL3, 10×).

NEUROFIBROMA

Clinical Features

Neurofibroma develops from nerve sheath. It is characteristic of neurofibromatosis type 1 and easy to diagnose.[10] Difficulty arises when solitary lesion is present. Clinically, soft to firm papule and nodule is noted (**Fig. 5A**). It demonstrates classical "buttonhole" sign.

Dermoscopic Features

Dermoscopy shows homogeneous pink-red area with peripheral brown pigmentation (**Fig. 5B**). Scar-like white areas and fingerprint-like lines are also noted.[10,11] Vascular elements include linear and dotted vessels. White dots of eccrine openings are noted.

Key Points

- Homogeneous pink-red area with peripheral brown pigmentation
- Scar-like white areas and fingerprint-like lines

ECCRINE SPIRADENOMA

Clinical Features

Spiradenoma presents as a solitary, pink, gray, or blue, dermal nodule located on the face, scalp and upper trunk in young to middle-aged adults (**Fig. 6A**). Rarely, multiple, painful nodules of varying sizes may present in a segmental pattern.

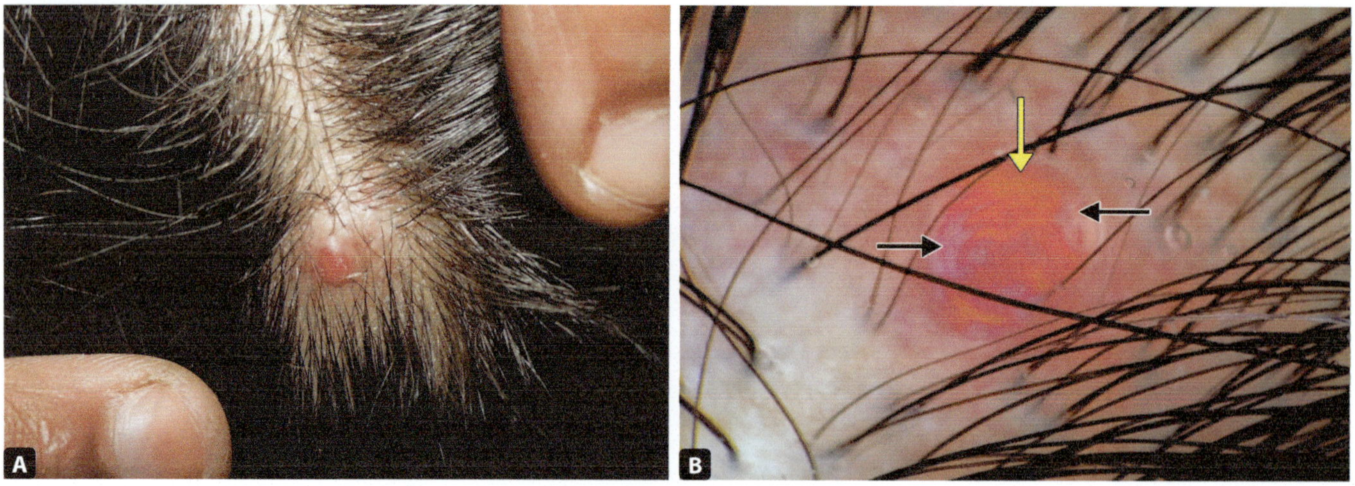

FIGS. 6A AND B: (A) Clinical image of eccrine spiradenoma presenting as erythematous nodule on the scalp (nonpolarized, DermLite DL3, 10×); (B) Trichoscopy of eccrine spiradenoma showing "serpentine-like" linear reddish structure (yellow arrow) surrounded by whitish areas (black arrows) (polarized, DermLite DL3, 10×).

Source: Ankad BS, Beergouder SL, Domble V, Sujana L. A serpentine inside eccrine spiradenoma: a new trichoscopic sign. Int J Trichology. 2015;7(1):38-40.

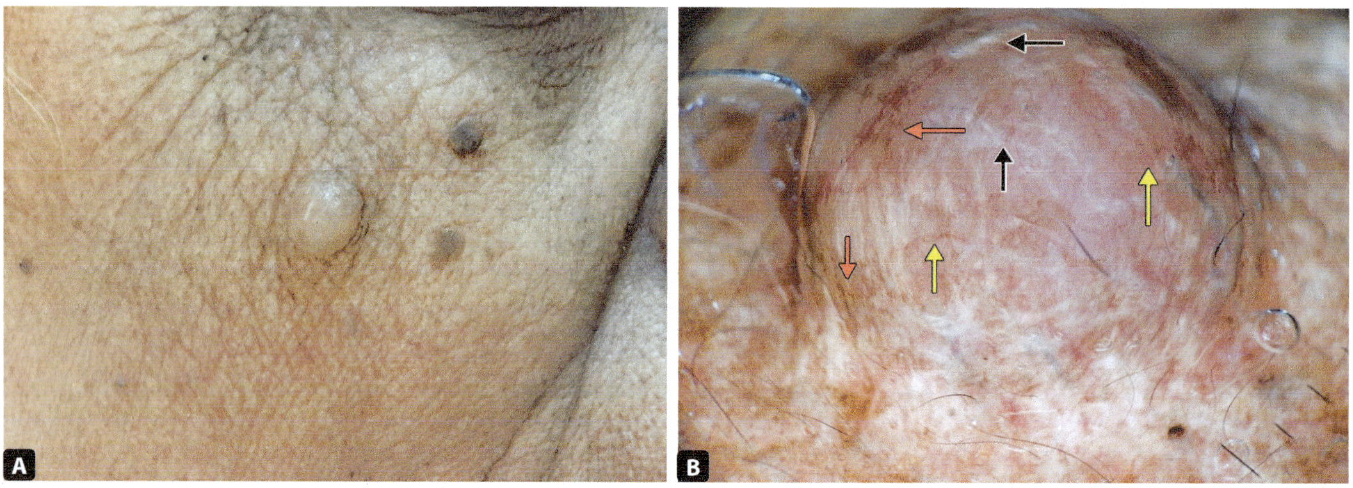

FIGS. 7A AND B: (A) Clinical image of apocrine hidrocystoma showing skin-colored translucent tumor on the right cheek; (B) Dermoscopy of apocrine hidrocystoma showing brown pigment globules (red arrows), telangiectasia (yellow arrows) and whitish strands (black arrows) (polarized, DermLite DL3, 10×).

Source: Ankad BS, Domble V, Sujana L. Dermoscopy of apocrine hydrocystoma: a first case report. Our Dermatol Online J. 2015;6(3):334-6.

Dermoscopic Features

Dermoscopically, faint grayish-blue clods with white structureless areas have been reported.[12] Linear serpiginous vessels are found occasionally (**Fig. 6B**).[13] The presence of blue clods with serpentine, branched vessels are also found in basal cell carcinoma (BCC). However, the blue clods in BCC represent nests of pigmented tumor cells, on the contrary the blue clods in spiradenoma correspond to hemorrhages.[13] Linear serpiginous vessels are found occasionally (**Fig. 6B**).[14]

Key Points

- Faint grayish-blue clods with white structureless areas
- Linear serpiginous vessels are noted.

APOCRINE HIDROCYSTOMA

Clinical Features

Apocrine hidrocystomas are benign cystic dilatation of apocrine glands. They are found on the head, neck, and eyelids. Typically, a solitary dome-shaped lesion containing a clear or bluish fluid is noted (**Fig. 7A**).[15] It mimics BCC, blue nevus, amelanotic melanoma requiring histopathological confirmation.[16]

Dermoscopic Features

It is characterized by skin-colored, pink, yellow or blue homogeneous area occupying the whole lesion with whitish areas and arborizing vessels on dermoscopy.[15,17] In skin of color, brown pigment globules, arborizing telangiectasia and whitish structures are found (**Fig. 7B**).

Key Points

- Yellow to blue homogeneous areas and arborizing vessels are found.
- Brown pigment globules are prominently observed in skin of color.

SYRINGOMA

Clinical Features

Syringomas are benign sweat duct tumors typically seen in adolescent and young, adult females. They are often present as multiple, 1–3 mm, skin-colored, dome-shaped or flat papules. They are commonly found on the face in a periorbital distribution (**Fig. 8A**).[18] They can be confused with xanthoma, hidrocystoma, milia, trichoepithelioma.

Dermoscopic Features

Dermoscopy of syringoma shows homogeneous light brown pseudonetwork with multifocal and glittering white dots and globules (**Fig. 8B**), and occasionally linear vessels (**Fig. 8C**). White dots correspond to eccrine duct openings. Size of white dots is bigger in lesional skin as compared to uninvolved skin.[10]

Key Points

- Multiple homogeneous light brown areas of pseudonetwork with irregular borders
- Multifocal glittering white dots and globules

SYRINGOCYSTADENOMA PAPILLIFERUM

Clinical Features

Syringocystadenoma papilliferum is a rare, benign neoplasm that is seen in children and young adults. Single or multiple, grouped, brown to red papules are noted. They are typically seen on areas of the head and neck (**Fig. 9A**). It gradually increases in size forming a plaque with a cerebriform surface at puberty.[19]

Dermoscopic Features

It demonstrates exophytic milky-red projections with microulceration, polymorphous vascular pattern consisting of hairpin-like, dotted and comma vessels (**Fig. 9B**), and arborizing vessels (**Fig. 9C**). Bright pinkish-white background is noted. Occasionally, perivascular whitish halo and yellowish areas within the ulceration may be present.[20,21]

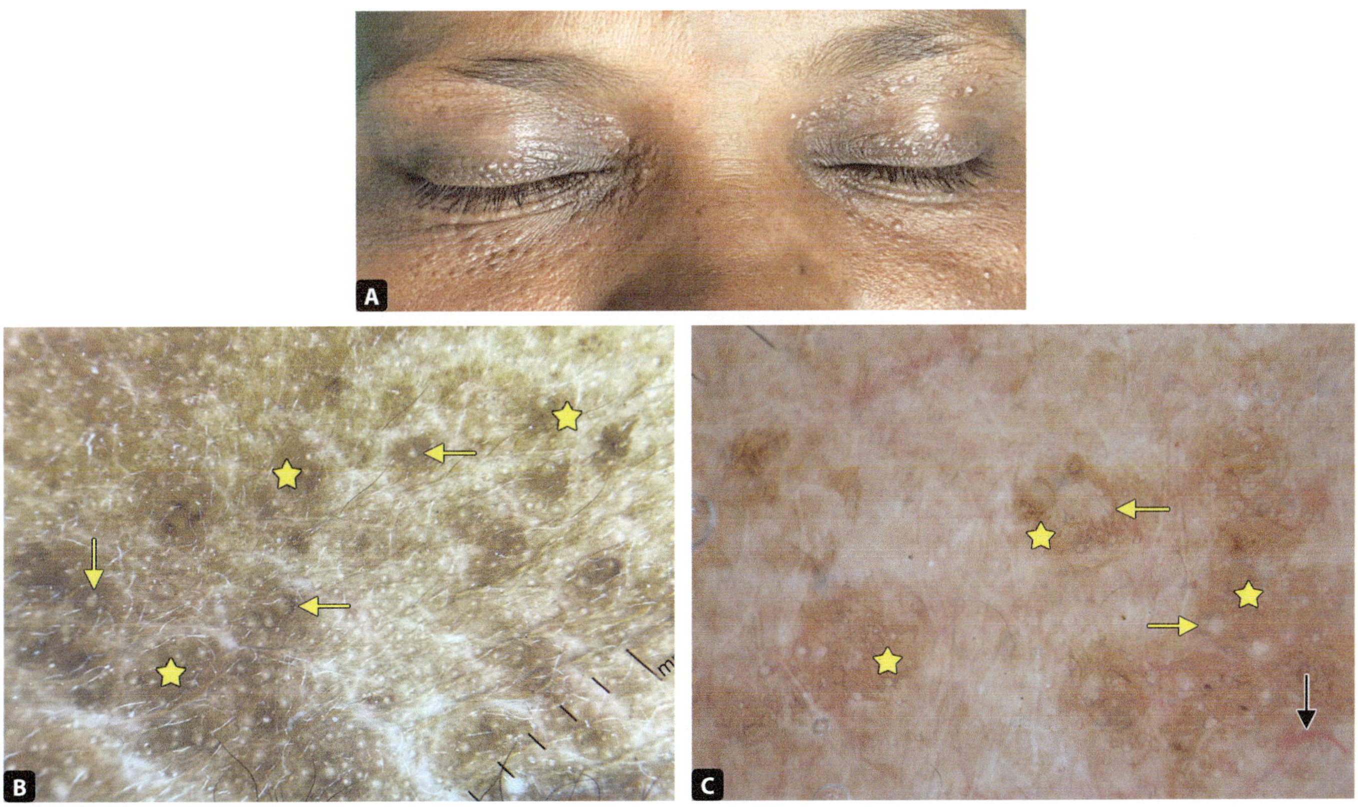

FIGS. 8A TO C: (A) Clinical image of syringoma showing skin-colored papules around the eyes in a symmetrical pattern; (B) Dermoscopy of syringoma showing glittering white dots and globules (yellow arrows) and pseudopigment network (yellow stars) (polarized, Illuco IDS 1100, 10×); (C) Dermoscopy of syringoma showing glittering white dots and globules (yellow arrows) and pseudopigment network (yellow stars). Note the short linear vessels (black arrow) (polarized, DermLite DL3, 10×).

Source (Fig. C): Ankad BS, Sakhare PS, Prabhu MH. Dermoscopy of non-melanocytic and pink tumors in brown skin: a descriptive study. Indian J Dermatopathol Diagn Dermatol. 2017;4:41-51.

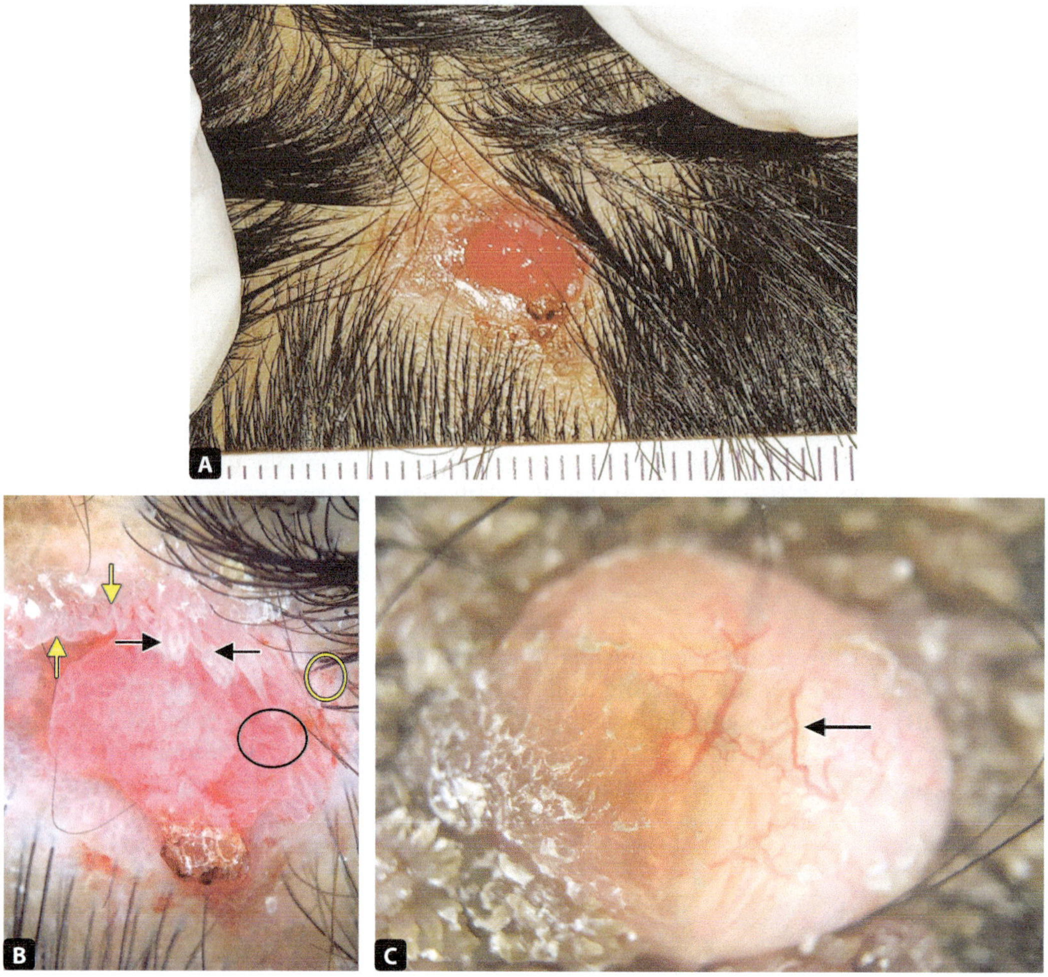

FIGS. 9A TO C: (A) Clinical image of syringocystadenoma papilliferum showing erythematous plaque on the scalp; (B) Dermoscopy of syringocystadenoma papilliferum showing exophytic milky-red projections (yellow arrows) with vascular structures such as hairpin-like (black circle) and dotted vessels (yellow circle). Note the white halo (black arrows) and pinkish-white background (polarized, DermLite DL4, 10×); (C) Dermoscopy of syringocystadenoma papilliferum showing arborizing vessels (black arrow) with whitish-yellow background (polarized, DermLite DL4, 10×).

Courtesy: Dr Keshav Adya, Associate Professor, Vijayapura, Karnataka, India.

Key Points

- Polymorphous vascular elements consisting of dotted, comma and linear vessels
- Exophytic projections with white halo and microulceration

TRICHOEPITHELIOMA

Clinical Features

Trichoepithelioma is a benign neoplasm arising from hair germ. It affects middle-aged adults. Trichoepithelioma presents as flesh-colored, 5–7 mm, firm papules in the nasolabial folds and cheeks (**Fig. 10A**). Three distinct subtypes are recognized; solitary, multiple, and desmoplastic trichoepithelioma.[22] Desmoplastic trichoepithelioma presents as a single, white to yellow, firm papule or plaque with a central depression.

Dermoscopic Features

It reveals white globular structures, small and fine arborizing telangiectasias with white background (**Figs. 10B** and **C**).[23,24] In skin of color, background is brownish-white. Desmoplastic trichoepithelioma shows arborizing telangiectasias, focal shiny, bright white areas, orthogonally oriented linear streaks, also known as "crystalline or chrysalis structures" and ivory-white color of the entire lesion.[25]

Key Points

- White globular structures with fine arborizing telangiectasias on bright white background are characteristically seen.

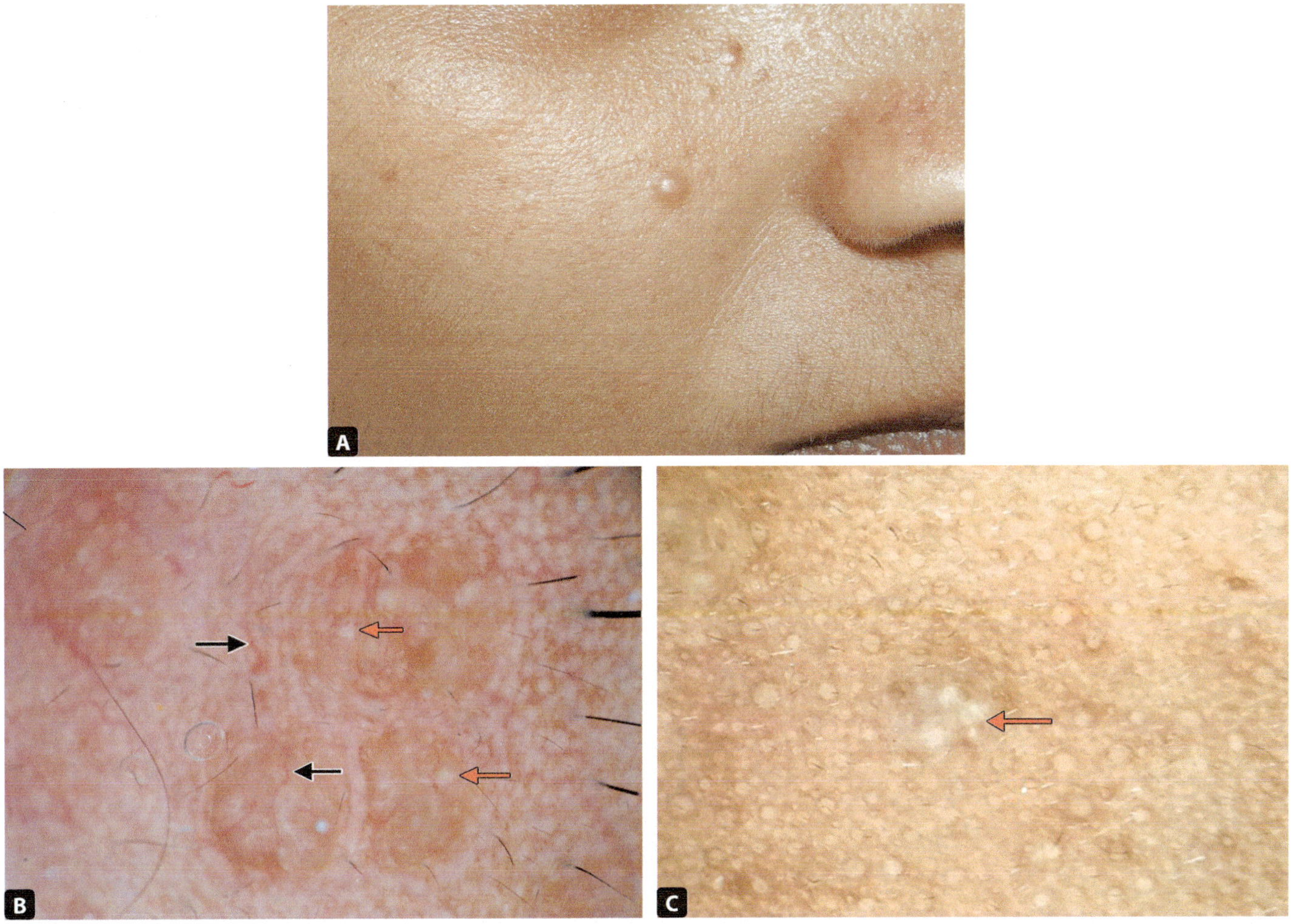

FIGS. 10A TO C: (A) Clinical image of trichoepithelioma showing flesh-colored papule on the cheek; (B) Dermoscopy of trichoepithelioma showing white globular structures (red arrows) with fine arborizing vessels (black arrows). Note the brownish-white background (polarized, DermLite DL3, 10×); (C) Dermoscopy of trichoepithelioma showing white globular structures (red arrow) with brownish-white background (polarized, DermLite DL3, 10×).

DILATED PORE OF WINER

Clinical Features

Dilated pore of Winer presents as a benign tumor of the infundibulum. It manifests as a single, enlarged pore with a keratin plug with normal surrounding skin. It occurs most frequently on the head and neck (**Fig. 11A**).[26]

Dermoscopic Features

Central bluish-black homogeneous structureless area surrounded by translucent grayish-whitish halo and a peripheral rim of pigment network (**Fig. 11B**). The central homogeneous bluish-black material corresponds to large, open comedones noted clinically. The translucent grayish-white margin corresponds to scaling due to epidermal hyperplasia around the follicular infundibulum.[27]

Key Points

- Central bluish-black homogeneous structureless area surrounded by translucent grayish-white halo and a peripheral rim of pigment network.

SEBACEOUS HYPERPLASIA

Clinical Features

It presents as yellow or white papules with central umbilication (**Fig. 12A**). Incidence of sebaceous hyperplasia increases with age and most commonly found on the face.[28]

Dermoscopic Features

Dermoscopy of sebaceous hyperplasia shows aggregates of white to yellow clods (**Fig. 12B**). This is seen due to increased

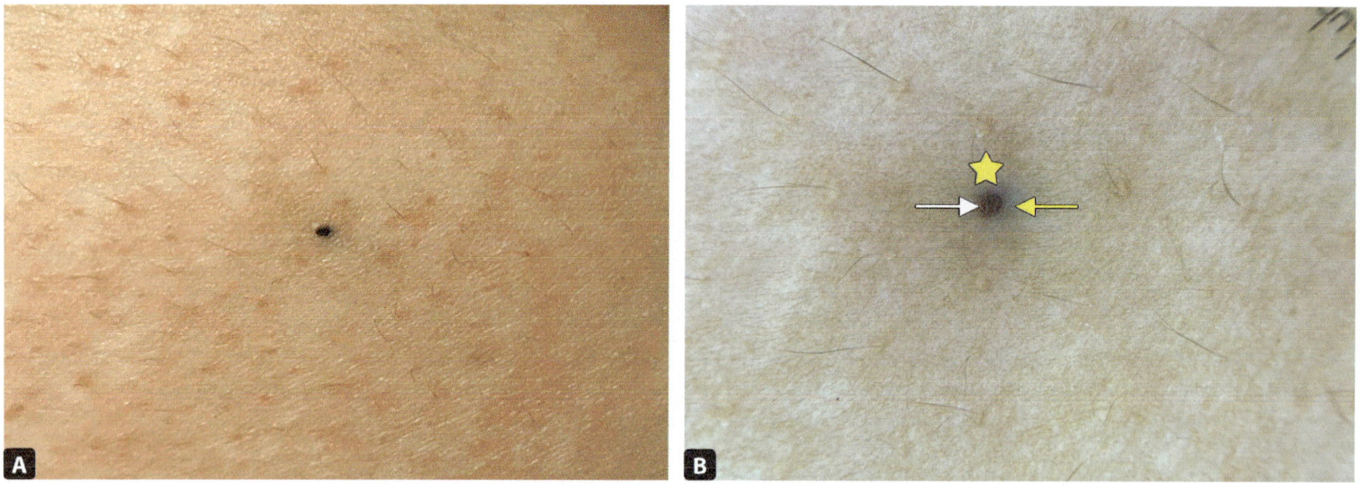

FIGS. 11A AND B: (A) Clinical image of dilated pore of Winer showing flesh-colored papule on the cheek; (B) Dermoscopy of dilated pore of Winer shows bluish-black area in the center (white arrow) and grayish-white translucent area (yellow arrow) with perilesional pigment network (yellow star) (polarized, Illuco IDS 1100, 10×).

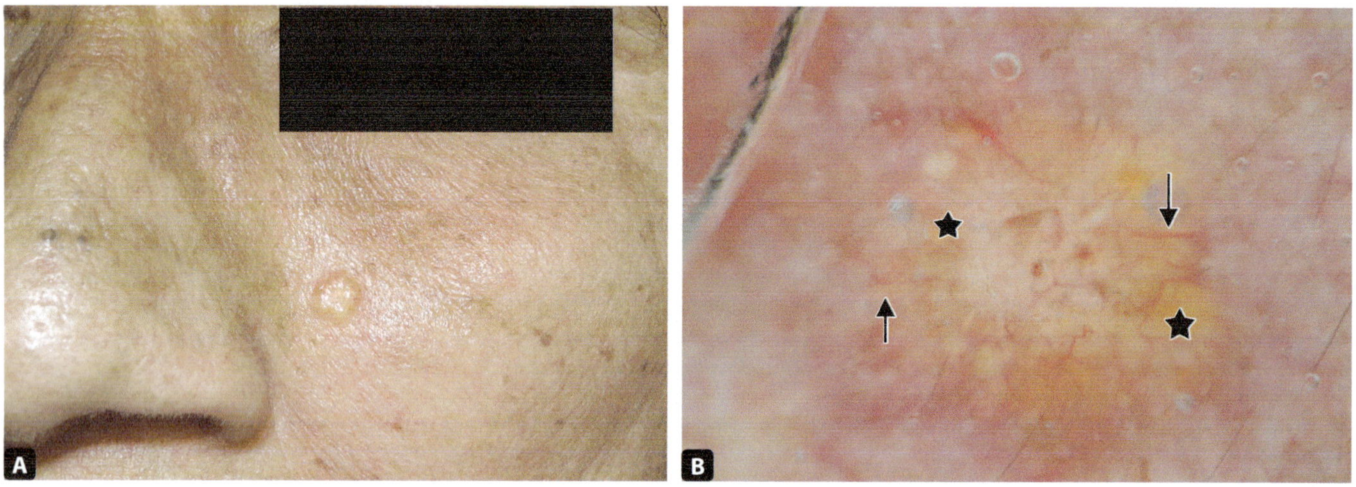

FIGS. 12A AND B: (A) Clinical image of sebaceous hyperplasia showing flesh-colored papule on the cheek; (B) Dermoscopy of sebaceous hyperplasia shows yellowish globular structures (black stars) with linear and branching vessels (black arrows). These are referred to as crown vessels (polarized, DermLite DL3, 10×).

Source: Ankad BS, Sakhare PS, Prabhu MH. Dermoscopy of non-melanocytic and pink tumors in brown skin: a descriptive study. Indian J Dermatopathol Diagn Dermatol. 2017;4:41-51.

sebum production and is referred to as "cumulus sign". Vessels around the lesion are arranged at the periphery which may extend into the lesion but characteristically do not cross midline. They are termed as "crown vessels".[29] Central umbilication is referred to as "bonbon toffee" sign.[28-30]

Key Points

- White to yellow clods which are traversed by crown vessels, and central umbilication are classically found.

STEATOCYSTOMA MULTIPLEX

Clinical Features

Steatocystoma multiplex consists of benign tumor arising from pilosebaceous unit. They are characterized by multiple; skin-colored nonpruritic papules and nodules of size of varying sizes over face, neck, and chest (**Fig. 13A**).[10]

Dermoscopic Features

Dermoscopy shows homogeneous pale or bright yellowish area that occupies the entire lesion (**Fig. 13B**).[31] Peripheral rim of brownish pigment is characteristically seen in skin of color (**Fig. 13C**). Many times, brown-pigmented area is noted on the yellowish area. Linear vessels are also found running from the periphery of the lesion (**Fig. 13D**). White dots of eccrine openings are preserved on the lesion.[10]

Key Points

- Homogeneous yellow area with brownish rim
- Brown pigmentation and linear vessels

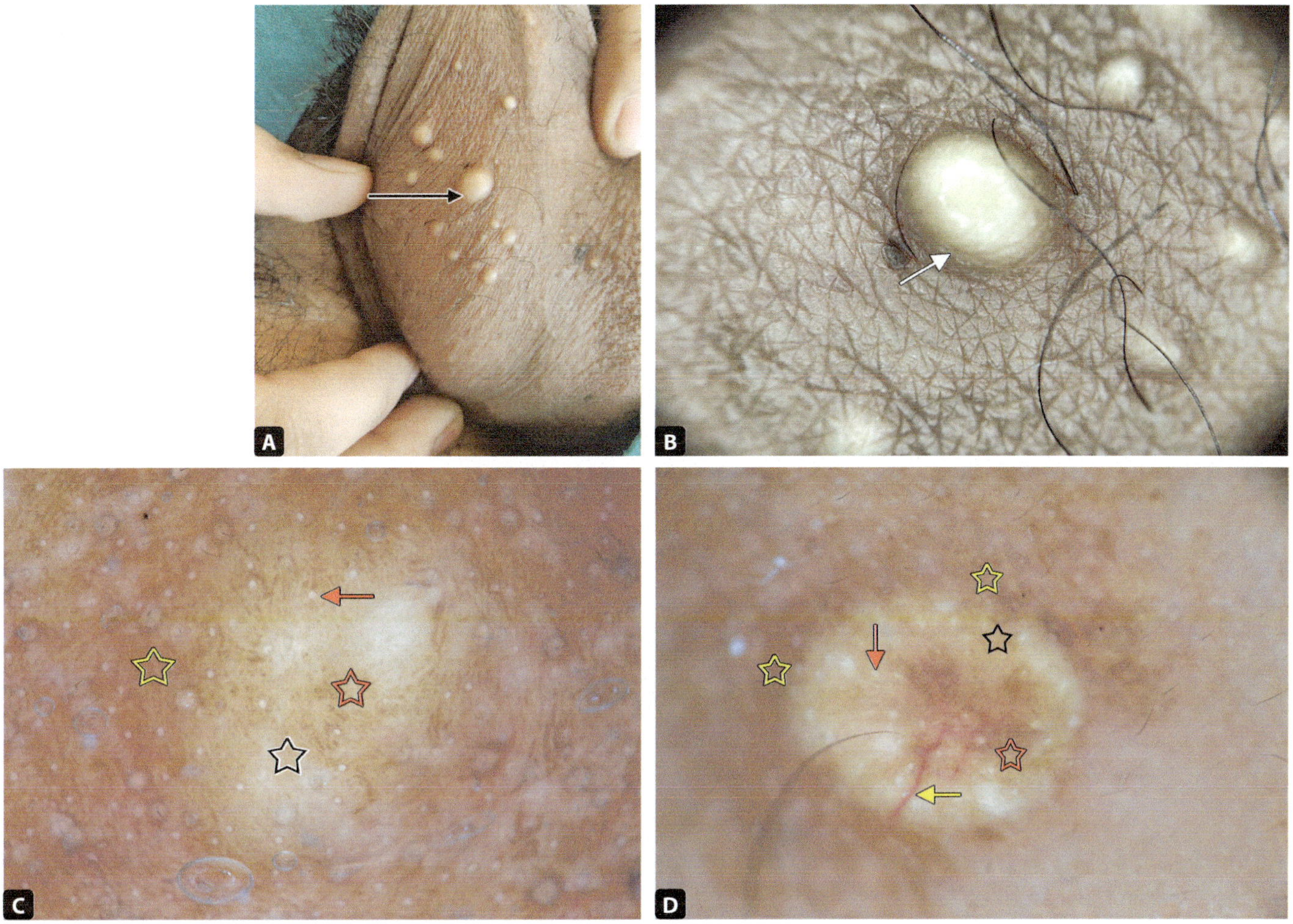

FIGS. 13A TO D: (A) Clinical image of steatocystoma multiplex showing multiple yellow-colored papules and nodules; (B) Dermoscopy of steatocystoma multiplex shows yellow area (white arrow) occupying the entire lesion (nonpolarized, DermLite DL2, 10×); (C) Dermoscopy of steatocystoma multiplex shows pale yellow homogeneous area (black star), brown-pigmented area (red star) and brown rim at the periphery (yellow star). Note the preservation of white dots of eccrine openings (red arrow) (polarized, DermLite DL3, 10×); (D) Dermoscopy of steatocystoma multiplex shows pale yellow homogeneous area (black star), brown-pigmented area (red star) and brown rim at the periphery (yellow stars). Note the preservation of white dots of eccrine openings (red arrow). Linear vessels running from the periphery are well-appreciated (yellow arrow) (polarized, DermLite DL3, 10×).

MILIA

Clinical Features

Milia are the epidermal inclusion cysts usually present on the face. They can be single or multiple (**Fig. 14A**). They are typified by tiny whitish papules with rubbery feel.[12]

Dermoscopic Features

Dermoscopy classically demonstrates whitish or yellowish homogeneous area that covers entire lesions. Brown rim at the periphery is typically observed in skin of color (**Fig. 14B**).[10] Larger lesions show arborizing vessels that traverse the entire lesion (**Fig. 14C**).[32]

Key Points

- White or yellow homogeneous area with brown pigmented rim at the periphery
- Large and chronic lesions reveal arborizing vessels.

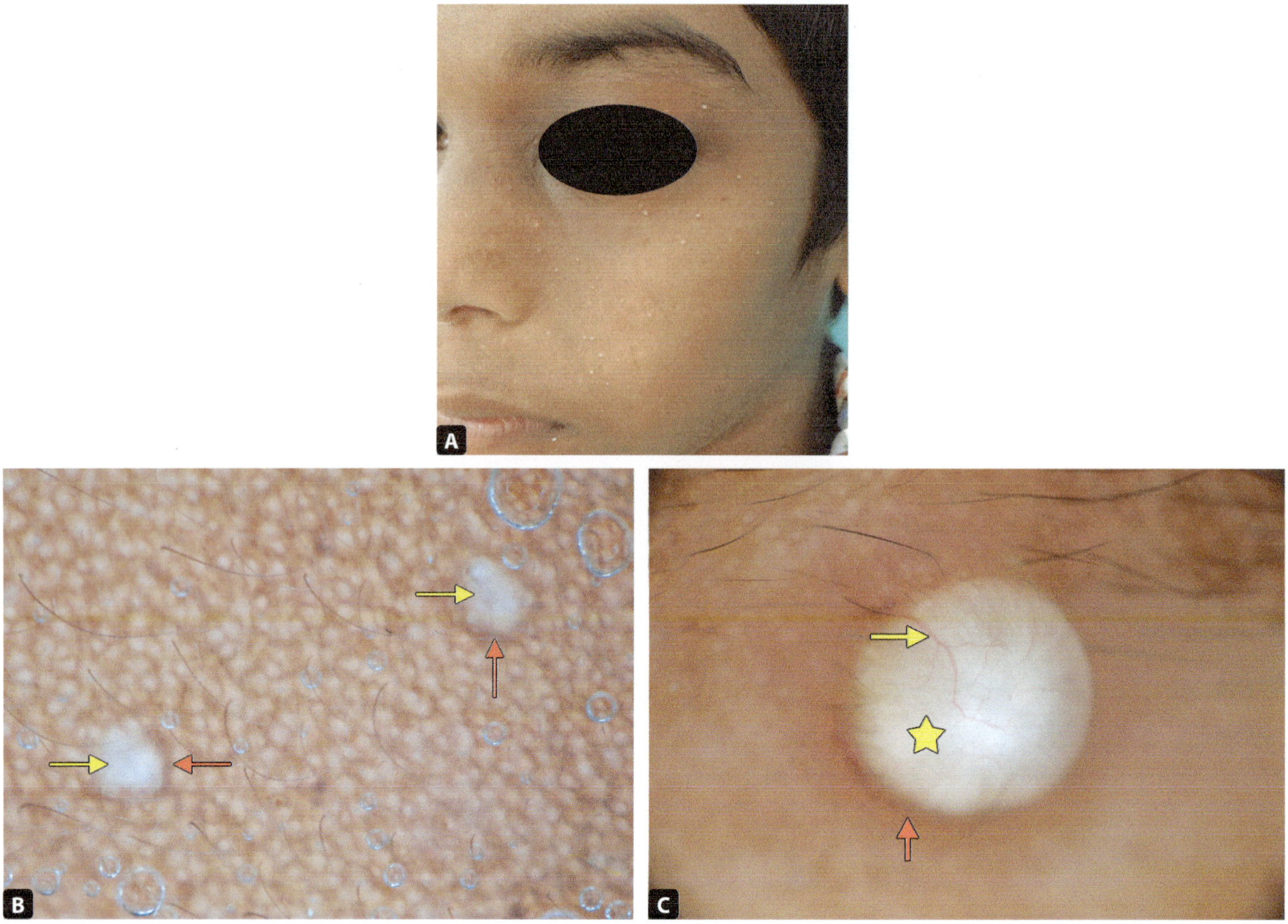

FIGS. 14A TO C: (A) Clinical image of milia showing multiple tiny white papules on the face; (B) Dermoscopy of milia shows white homogeneous area in the center (yellow arrows) and brownish rim at periphery (red arrows) (polarized, DermLite DL3, 10×); (C) Dermoscopy of larger and chronic lesion of milia shows white homogeneous area in the center (yellow star) and brownish rim at periphery (red arrow). Note the arborizing vessels traversing the lesion (yellow arrow) (polarized, DermLite DL3, 10×).

DERMATOFIBROMA

Clinical Features

It presents as single or multiple, firm nodules with smooth surface found on lower extremities (**Fig. 15A**). Characteristically, the lateral compression of lesion produces a dimple-like depression, referred to as dimple or Fitzpatrick's sign.[33]

Dermoscopic Features

Classical dermoscopic patterns: Delicate pigment network that is typified by fine light-to-medium brown pigment network located at the periphery, gradually fading into surrounding skin (**Fig. 15B**). Irregularly outlined and sharply demarcated central scar-like white patch (**Fig. 15C**).[34]

Atypical dermoscopic patterns: White lines surrounding small islands of brown pigment or surrounding globule-like, i.e., ring-like structures. Irregular folds with pseudofollicular openings (**Fig. 15D**) and homogeneous brownish pigmentation (**Fig. 15E**) are other dermoscopic patterns. Vascular structures include erythema, dotted vessels, hairpin vessels and comma vessels more commonly.[35]

Key Points

- Classical dermoscopic features include delicate pigment network.
- Irregularly outlined and sharply demarcated central scar-like white area.

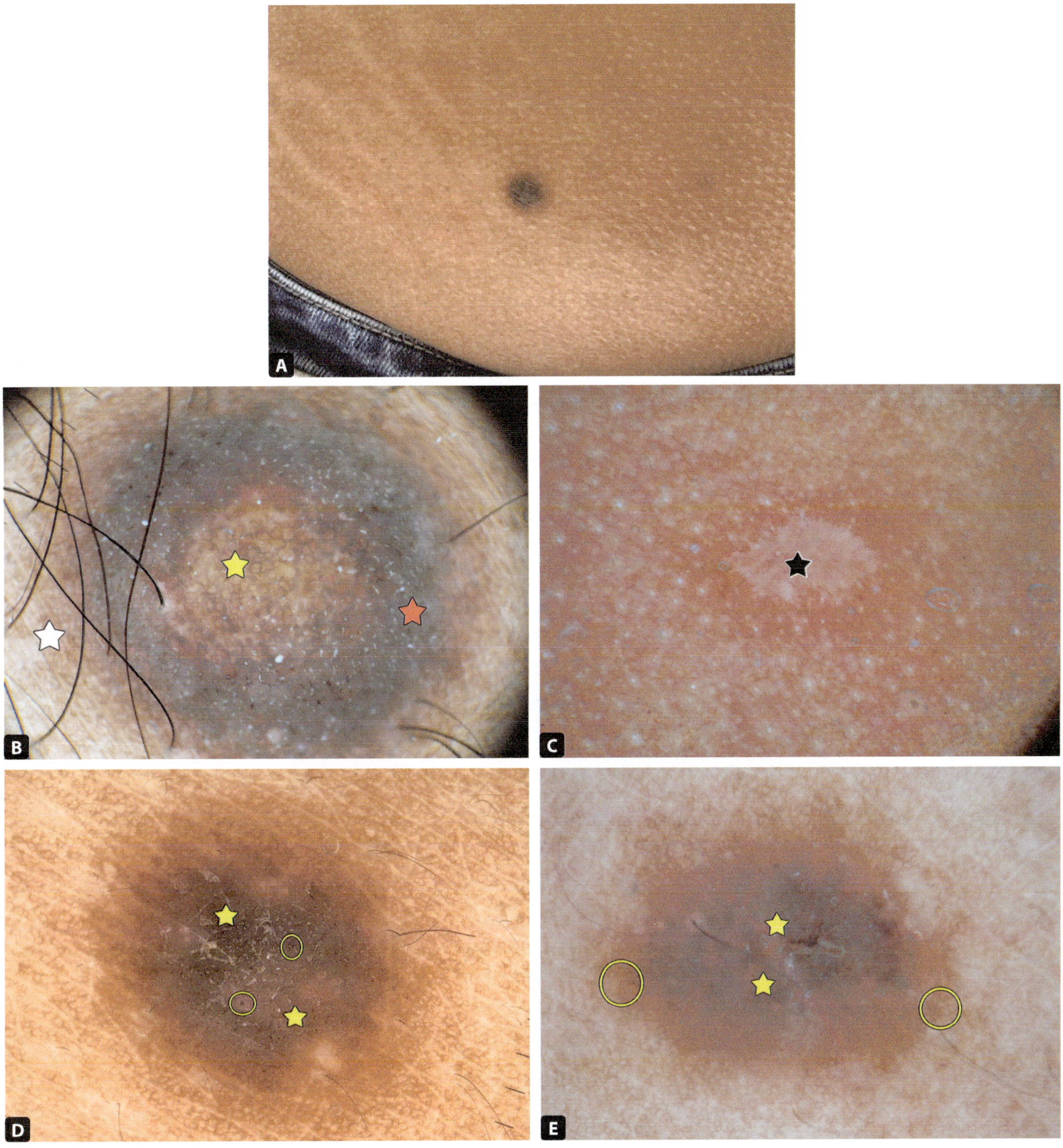

FIGS. 15A TO E: (A) Clinical image of dermatofibroma showing hyperpigmented plaque on the gluteal area; (B) Dermoscopy of dermatofibroma shows yellowish scar-like area in the center (yellow star) surrounded by heavily pigmented pigment network (red star) which is fading away in the normal skin (white star) (polarized, DermLite DL3, 10×); (C) Dermoscopy of dermatofibroma shows whitish scar-like area occupying the entire lesions with irregular outline (black star). Note the brown pigmentation in the periphery (polarized, DermLite DL3, 10×); (D) Dermoscopy of dermatofibroma shows papillomatous blackish-brown-pigmented area in the center (stars). Note the pseudofollicular openings (circles) (polarized, DermLite DL4, 10×); (E) Dermoscopy of dermatofibroma shows brownish-pigmented area in the center (stars) with delicate pigment network in the periphery (circles) (polarized, DermLite DL3, 10×).

Courtesy (Figs. A and D): Dr Nitin Barde, Consultant Dermatosurgeon, Radiance Skin, Antiaging, Hair Transplant Clinic, Nagpur, Maharashtra, India.

Source (Fig. B): Ankad BS, Sakhare PS, Prabhu MH. Dermoscopy of non-melanocytic and pink tumors in brown skin: a descriptive study. Indian J Dermatopathol Diagn Dermatol. 2017;4:41-51.

FIBROKERATOMA

Clinical Features

Fibrokeratoma is a benign tumor that consists of keratin and fibrous tissue. It manifests as solitary, asymptomatic skin-colored or brownish nodule (**Fig. 16A**). It mimics neurofibroma.[36]

Dermoscopic Features

Dermoscopy shows rosy white areas with brownish linear lines that traverse the lesion (**Fig. 16B**).[10] Mostly a homogeneous white area occupying the whole lesion is observed. Dotted vessels are also described in the literature. Red lacunae can be found especially in digital fibrokeratoma.[37]

Key Points

- Rosy white area and homogeneous white area which are traversed by brownish linear structures.
- Red lacunae are noted in instance of trauma.

PYOGENIC GRANULOMA

Clinical Features

It is a common vascular skin tumor and manifests as a solitary, red-colored nodule that tends to ulcerate and bleed (**Fig. 17A**). It looks similar to amelanotic melanoma and poroma. Hence, accurate diagnosis is of prime importance.[38]

Dermoscopic Features

It is characterized by reddish-white homogeneous structureless area with ring-shaped or arcuate white collarette at the periphery (**Figs. 17B** and **C**).[39] White rails are found intersecting the lesion. Vascular structures such as dotted, linear irregular, hairpin-like and polymorphous vessels are also seen. Sometimes, microulceration may be seen (**Fig. 17B**).[10,38]

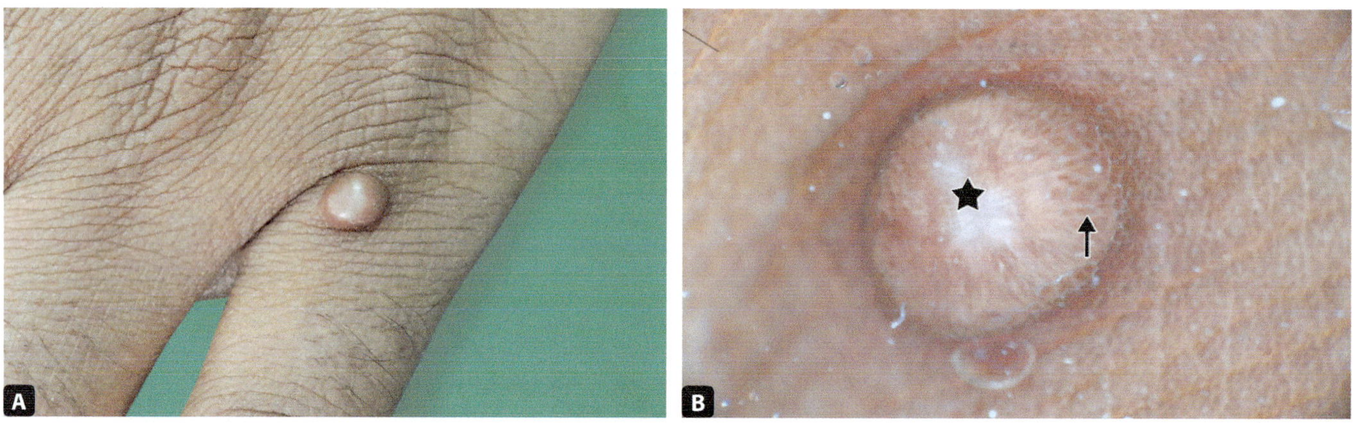

FIGS. 16A AND B: (A) Clinical image of fibrokeratoma showing solitary brown nodule; (B) Dermoscopy of fibrokeratoma shows rosy white area (star) with brownish linear structures (arrow) (polarized, DermLite DL3, 10×).

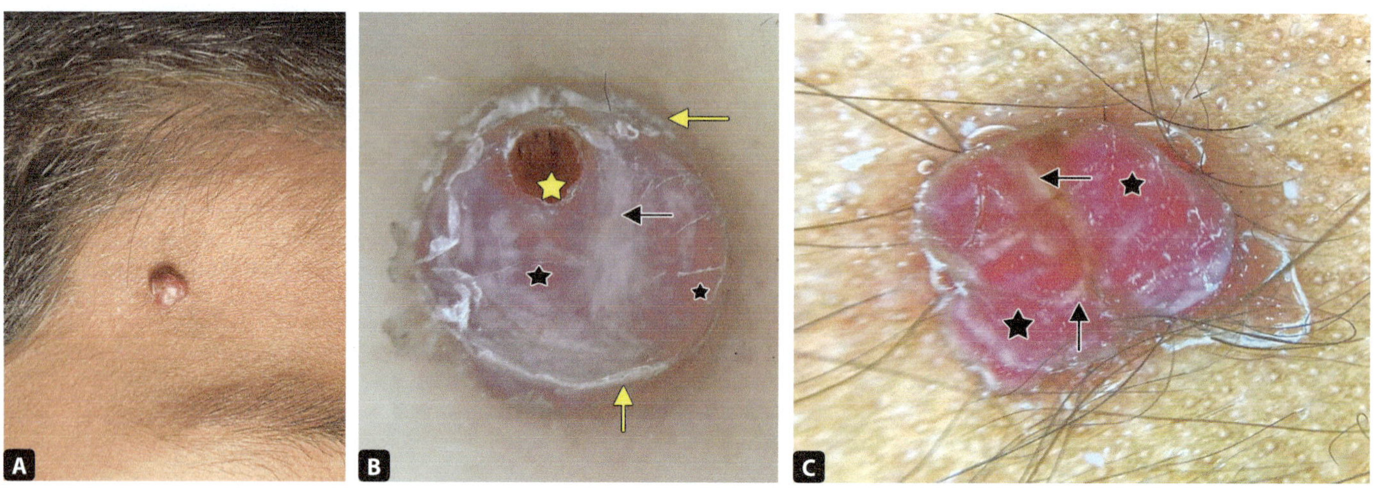

FIGS. 17A TO C: (A) Clinical image of pyogenic granuloma showing reddish nodule on the forehead; (B) Dermoscopy of pyogenic granuloma shows reddish homogeneous areas (black stars), white rail lines (black arrow) and white collarette (yellow arrows). Microulceration is well-appreciated (yellow star) (polarized, DermLite DL4, 10×); (C) Dermoscopy of pyogenic granuloma shows reddish homogeneous areas (black stars) and white rail lines (black arrows).

Courtesy (Fig. B): Dr Raghunatha S, Professor, ESIC Medical College and PGIMSR, Bengaluru, Karnataka, India.

Key Points

- Reddish-white homogeneous structureless area surrounded by a white collarette.
- White rails are seen separating the homogeneous areas.

CHERRY ANGIOMA

Clinical Features

Cherry angiomas develop from postcapillary venules and are commonly seen in older individuals.[10] They are asymptomatic. They are either pinpoint macules (**Fig. 18A**) or dome-shaped papules (**Fig. 18B**). They appear blackish when vessels are thrombosed.

Dermoscopic Features

Dermoscopy of cherry angioma reveals numerous reddish lacunae separated by septae. Lacunae are round to oval in shape and color may vary from red to purple (**Fig. 18C**).[40] Chronic lesions typically show bluish-white veil on the surface (**Fig. 18D**). Peripheral brown pigmentation is strikingly observed in skin of color.[10]

Key Points

- Reddish lacunae separated by septae and brown pigmentation at periphery.

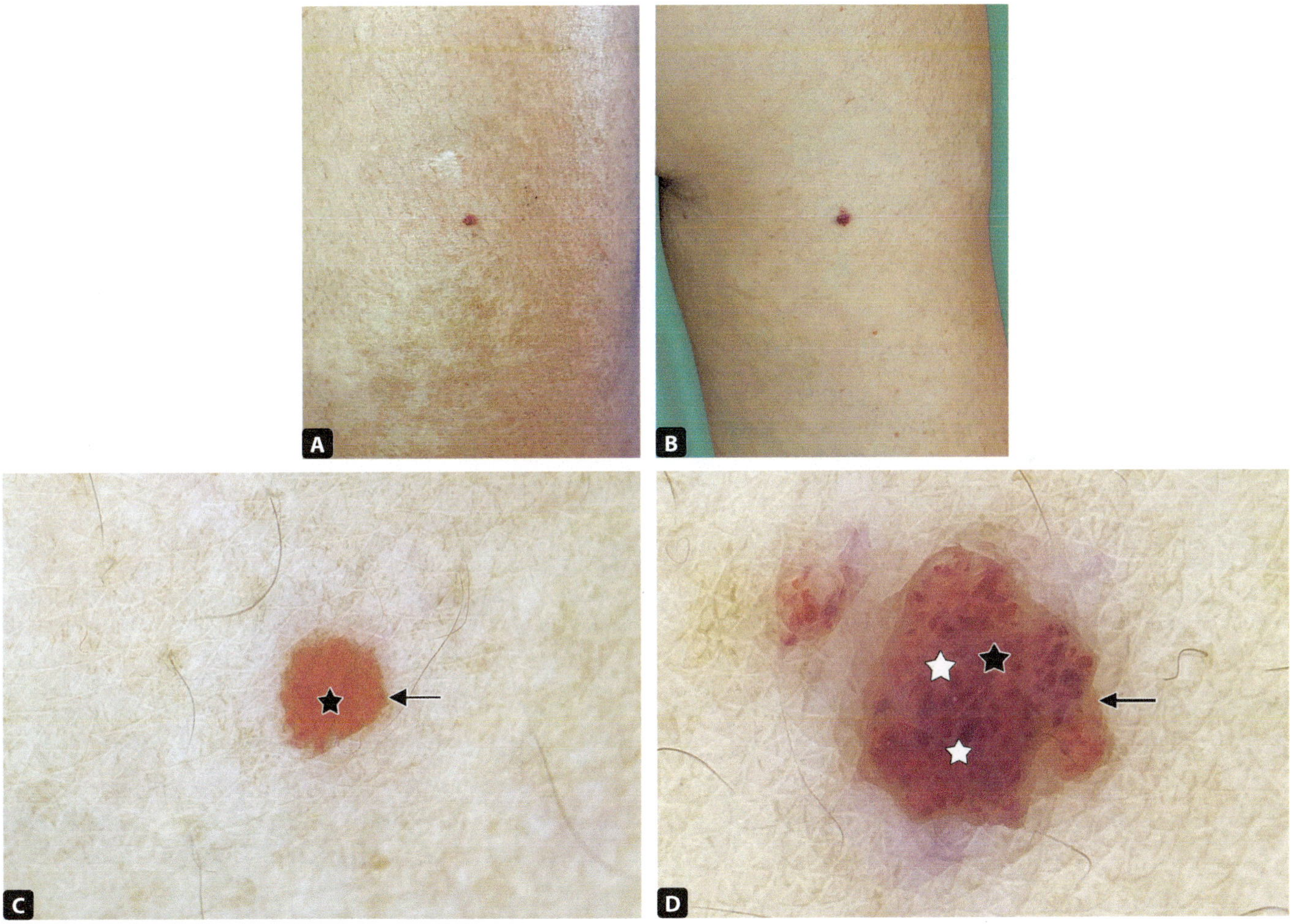

FIGS. 18A TO D: (A) Clinical image of cherry angioma showing pinpoint macule on the arm; (B) Clinical image of cherry angioma showing dome-shaped papule; (C) Dermoscopy of cherry angioma shows reddish to purplish lacunae (star) that are separated by septae. Note the brown pigmentation at the periphery (arrow) (polarized, FotoFinder Handyscope, 20×); (D) Dermoscopy of chronic cherry angioma shows reddish to purplish lacunae (black star) that are separated by septae. Note the brown pigmentation at the periphery (black arrow). Bluish-white veil is well-appreciated (white stars) (polarized, FotoFinder Handyscope, 20×).

ANGIOFIBROMA

Clinical Features

Angiofibroma manifest as multiple, skin-colored to erythematous papules of variable size over face, neck, and genitalia. The lesions on the male genitalia are called pearly penile papules (**Fig. 19A**) whereas the lesions on the face in tuberous sclerosis are misnamed as adenoma sebaceum.[10] Differentials are melanocytic nevi and BCC.

Dermoscopic Features

Dermoscopy demonstrates white globules on the whitish-red or pinkish background.[41] The other characteristic patterns include bluish-white lacunae, red dots, and white globules.[10] Pearly penile papules of longer duration reveal linear and looped linear (hairpin-like) vessels with white globules (**Fig. 19B**). Histopathologically, white globules are seen due to fibrosis and bluish-white lacunae correspond to proliferative vessels.

Key Points

- White globules with linear and looped linear vessels on a whitish-red background.

ANGIOMA SERPIGINOSUM

Clinical Features

It manifests with multiple, minute, erythematous macules coalescing into patches that are arranged in serpiginous or gyrate pattern (**Fig. 20A**). The color of the macules varies from purple to red.[42]

Dermoscopic Features

Multiple, relatively well-demarcated, round to oval red lacunae are characteristic. The arrangement of lacunae is described as "school of red fish in a pond" appearance. It should be noted that linear vessels are not seen (**Fig. 20B**).[43]

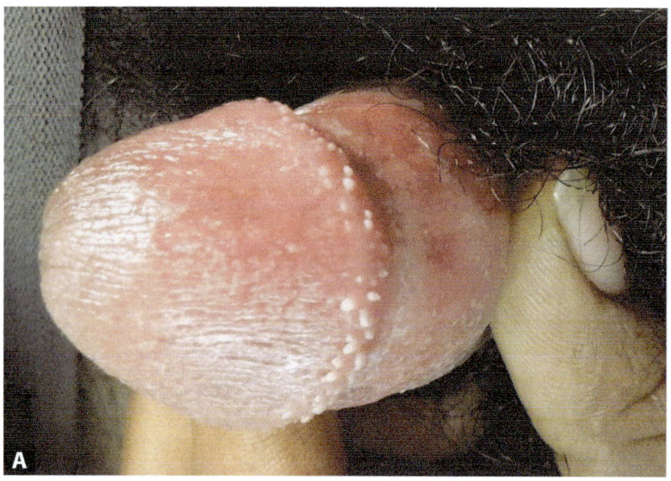

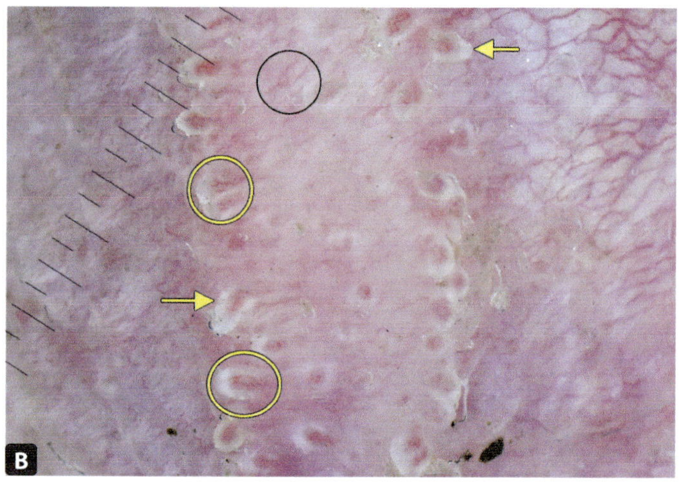

FIGS. 19A AND B: (A) Clinical image of angiofibroma (pearly penile papule) showing multiple papules in circumferential arrangement in front of corona sulcus; (B) Dermoscopy of angiofibroma (pearly penile papule) shows white globules (yellow arrows) on the whitish-red background. Linear (black circle) and hairpin-like (yellow circles) vessels are well-appreciated (polarized, DermLite Foto II Pro Plus, 10×).

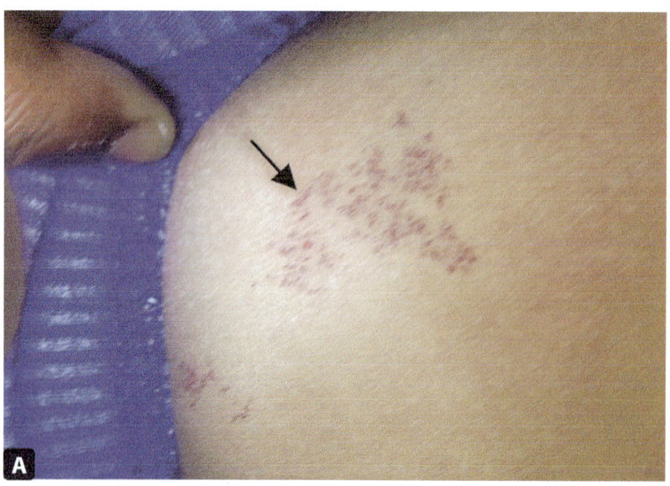

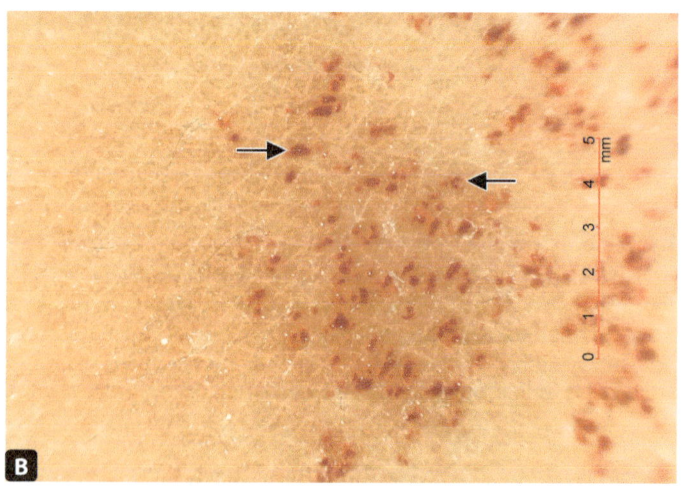

FIGS. 20A AND B: (A) Clinical image of angioma serpiginosum showing erythematous patches arranged in serpiginous pattern; (B) Dermoscopy of angioma serpiginosum shows round to oval red lacunae (black arrows) in a "school of red fish in a pond" pattern (polarized, Handyscope, 10×).

Key Points

- Multiple round to oval lacunae in a “school of red fish in a pond” pattern.

ANGIOKERATOMA

Clinical Features

Angiokeratoma is a benign vascular tumor that results from the pressure in the proximal area of the lesions. It presents as shiny, soft, dark red to violaceous, 2–10 mm papules which may develop a blue-violaceous to black color and a surface scale (**Fig. 21A**).[44]

Dermoscopic Features

Dermoscopy shows multiple lacunae or lagoons of different colors. Color varies from dark red to purple to bluish-red. They are sharply demarcated and ovoid structures. Bluish-white veil is classically seen as confluent bluish pigmentation overlying the lesion. Peripheral erythema (red area) is also characteristic (**Fig. 21B**).[10,44] Ulceration and surface scale may be seen. Rarely, rainbow pattern may be seen.

Key Points

- Multiple lacunae or lagoons of different colors that vary from red to purple to bluish-red, bluish-white veil and peripheral red area.

LYMPHANGIOMA CIRCUMSCRIPTUM

Clinical Features

Lymphangioma circumscriptum is present at birth and increases in size. Axillae, proximal portion of limbs (**Fig. 22A**), and gluteal area are common sites. Clinically, fluid-filled translucent vesicles are found. The color of the vesicles varies from skin color to yellowish which is imparted from the lymph fluid. Blood inside the vesicle gives red or bluish-black color.[10]

Dermoscopic Features

Dermoscopy reveals pale yellow lacunae that are surrounded by gray septae (**Fig. 22B**). Occasionally, pale pink lacunae are noted. Hemorrhage inside the vesicles results in reddish lacunae. Many times, blood settles down at the bottom of the lacunae giving characteristic “hypopyon” sign (**Fig. 22C**).[45] Chronic lesions show white scale at the surface.[10]

Key Points

- Pale yellow or pale pink lacunae separated by gray septae.
- Blood in the lacunae is seen as hypopyon and white scales are especially in chronic lesions.

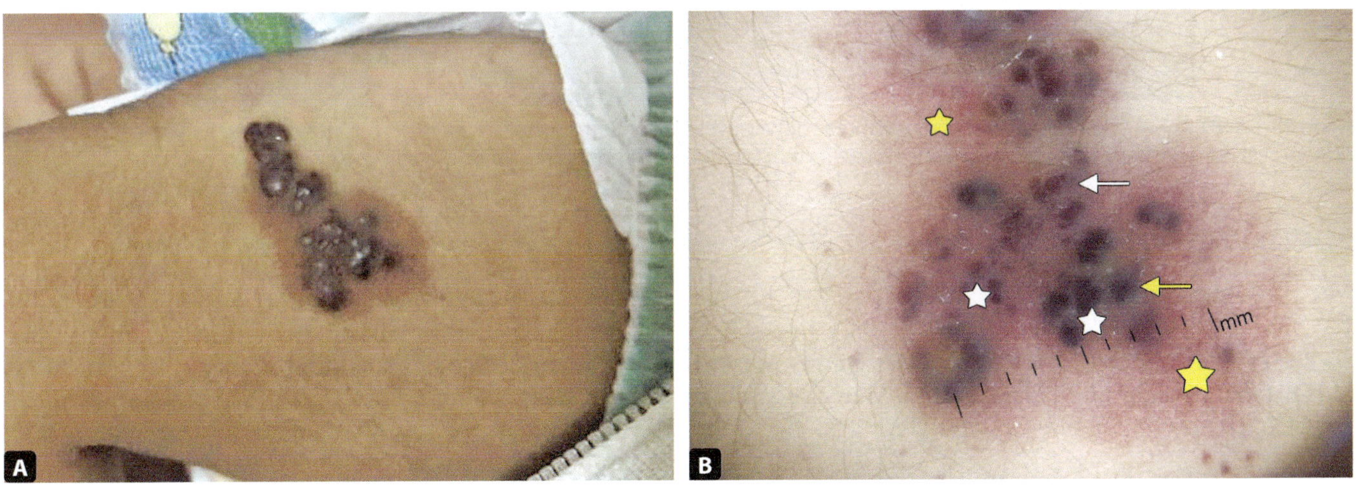

FIGS. 21A AND B: (A) Clinical image of angiokeratoma showing dark red to violaceous papules; (B) Dermoscopy of angiokeratoma shows dark blue (yellow arrow) and dark red (white arrow) lacunae with peripheral erythema (yellow stars). Note the bluish-white veil overlying the lesions (white stars) (polarized, DermLite DL3, 10×).

Courtesy: Dr Samipa Mukherjee, Pediatric Dermatologist, Cloudnine Hospital, Bengaluru, Karnataka, India.

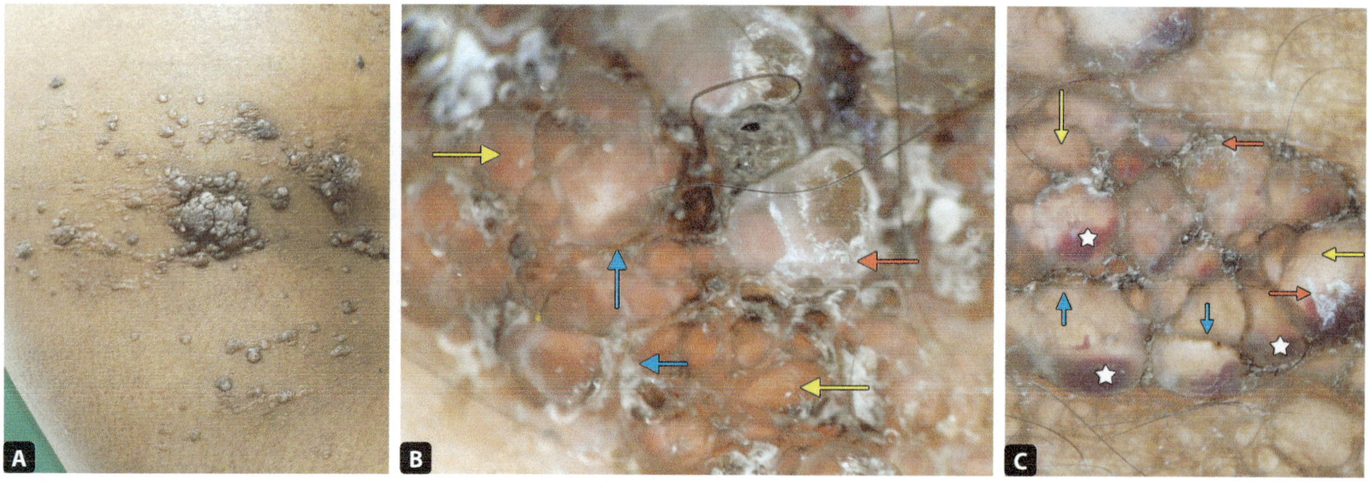

FIGS. 22A TO C: (A) Clinical image of lymphangioma circumscriptum showing fluid-filled vesicles on the proximal portion of the lower limb; (B) Dermoscopy of lymphangioma circumscriptum showspale yellow lacunae (yellow arrows), gray septae (blue arrows) and white scales on the surface (red arrow) (polarized, DermLite DL3, 10×); (C) Dermoscopy of lymphangioma circumscriptum shows pale yellow lacunae (yellow arrows), gray septae (blue arrows) and white scales on the surface (red arrows). Note the characteristic "hypopyon" sign representing blood at the bottom of lacunae (white stars) (polarized, DermLite DL3, 10×).

Source (Fig. C): Ankad BS, Sakhare PS, Prabhu MH. Dermoscopy of non-melanocytic and pink tumors in brown skin: a descriptive study. Indian J Dermatopathol Diagn Dermatol. 2017;4:41-51.

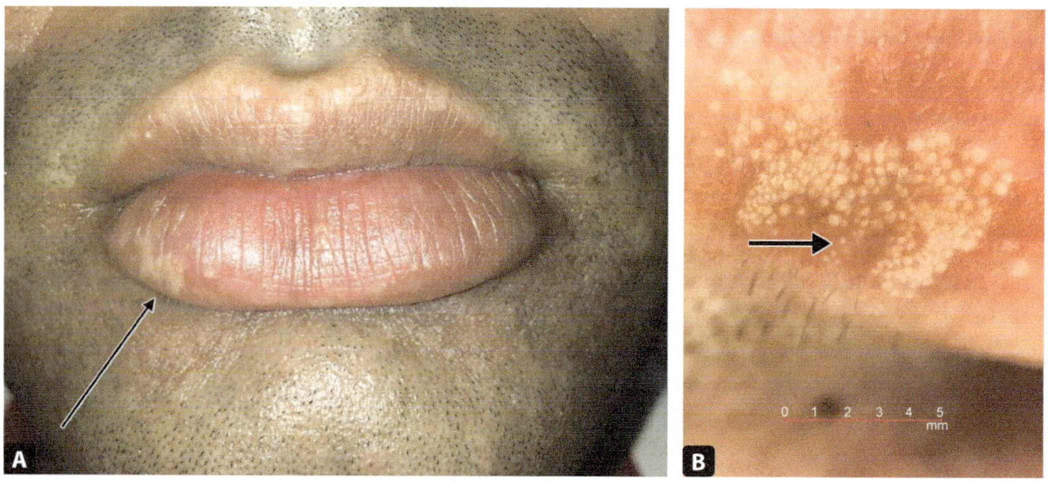

FIGS. 23A AND B: (A) Clinical image of Fordyce spots showing yellowish plaque on the lower lip; (B) Dermoscopy of Fordyce spots shows white dots and whitish to yellowish ovoid structures (arrow) (polarized, Handyscope, 10×).

FORDYCE SPOTS

Clinical Features

Fordyce spots (FS) are ectopic sebaceous glands present with distinct papules and plaques on the mucosal surface and glabrous skin of lips and genitalia (**Fig. 23A**).[46]

Dermoscopic Features

Dermoscopy shows bright white dots and whitish ovoid structures (**Fig. 23B**). Linear and branching vessels are noted. Occasionally, hair can be present in the white dot.[47]

Key Points

- Bright white dots and whitish or yellowish ovoid structures with vessels are definitive pattern of FS.

KEY POINTS

- Dermoscopy of benign tumors demonstrate characteristic patterns which vary from white, yellow, brown to blue and red color depending on the presence of keratin and hemoglobin.
- Presence of predominant polymorphic vascular pattern in malignant tumors helps in differentiating them from benign tumors on dermoscopy.
- Recognition of distinctive keratin and vascular pattern is of great help in diagnosis of benign tumors.

CONCLUSION

Dermoscopic patterns and structures of various benign cutaneous lesions are easy to identify. Dermoscopy is a valuable aid for the diagnosis of the benign skin tumors and their differentiation from malignant tumors.

REFERENCES

1. Madan V, Lear JT. Benign keratinocytic acanthomas and proliferations. In: Griffiths C, Barker J, Bleiker T, Chalmers R, Creamer D (Eds). Rook's Textbook of Dermatology, 9th edition. United Kingdom: Wiley-Blackwell Publishing; 2016. pp. 133.1-3.
2. Minagawa A. Dermoscopy-pathology relationship in seborrheic keratosis. J Dermatol. 2017;44(5):518-24.
3. Malvehy J, Puig S, Argenziano G, et al. Principles of Dermoscopy. Barcelona: GEDE; 2002.
4. Argenziano G, Soyer HP, Chimenti S, Talamini R, Corona R, Sera F, et al. Dermoscopy of pigmented skin lesions: results of a consensus meeting via the internet. J Am Acad Dermatol. 2003;48(5):679-93.
5. Grimes PE, Arora S, Minus HR, Kenney JA. Dermatosis papulosa nigra. Cutis. 1983;32:385-6.
6. Bhat RM, Patrao N, Monteiro R, Sukumar D. A clinical, dermoscopic, and histopathological study of dermatosis papulosa nigra (DPN): an Indian perspective. Int J Dermatol. 2017;56(9):957-60.
7. Dianzani C, Paolini F, Conforti C, Silvestre M, Flagiello F, Venuti A. Human papillomavirus in skin tags: a case series. Dermatol Pract Concept. 2018;8(4):295-6.
8. Zaballos P, Martí E, Cuéllar F, Puig S, Malvehy J. Dermoscopy of lichenoid regressing seborrheic keratosis. Arch Dermatol. 2006;142(3):410.
9. Mhatre A, Nadkarni N, Patil S, Agarwal S. A case of benign lichenoid keratosis. Indian J Dermatopathol Diagn Dermatol. 2015;2:49-51.
10. Ankad BS, Sakhare PS, Prabhu MH. Dermoscopy of non-melanocytic and pink tumors in brown skin: a descriptive study. Indian J Dermatopathol Diagn Dermatol. 2017;4:41-51.
11. Duman N, Elmas M. Dermoscopy of cutaneous neurofibromas associated with neurofibromatosis type 1. J Am Acad Dermatol. 2015;73:529-31.
12. Lallas A, Moscarella E, Argenziano G, Longo C, Apalla Z, Ferrara G, et al. Dermoscopy of uncommon skin tumours. Australas J Dermatol. 2014;55(1):53-62.
13. Ankad BS, Beergouder SL, Domble V, Sujana L. A serpentine inside eccrine spiradenoma: a new trichoscopic sign. Int J Trichology. 2015;7(1):38-40.
14. Tschandl P. Dermatoscopic pattern of a spiradenoma. Dermatol Pract Concept. 2012;2(4):204-9.
15. Zaballos P, Bañuls J, Medina C, Salsench E, Serrano P, Guionnet N. Dermoscopy of apocrine hidrocystomas: a morphological study. J Eur Acad Dermatol Venereol. 2014;28:378-81.
16. Calonje E. Tumours of the skin appendages. In: Griffiths C, Barker J, Bleiker T, Chalmers R, Creamer D (Eds). Rook's Textbook of Dermatology, 9th edition. United Kingdom: Wiley-Blackwell Publishing; 2016. pp. 138.19-20.
17. Ankad BS, Domble V, Sujana L. Dermoscopy of apocrine hydrocystoma: a first case report. Our Dermatol Online J. 2015;6(3):334-6.
18. Patrizi A, Neri I, Marzaduri S, Varotti E, Passarini B. Syringoma: a review of twenty-nine cases. Acta Derm Venereol. 1998;78:460-2.
19. Karg E, Korom I, Varga E, Ban G, Turi S. Congenital syringocystadenoma papilliferum. Pediatr Dermatol. 2008;25(1):132-3.
20. Duman N, Ersoy-Evans S, Erkin Özaygen G, Gököz Ö. Syringocystadenoma papilliferum arising on naevus sebaceus: a 6-year-old child case described with dermoscopic features. Australas J Dermatol. 2015;56(2):53-4.
21. Bruno CB, Cordeiro FN, do Soares FE, Takano GH, Mendes LS. Dermoscopic aspects of syringocystadenoma papilliferum associated with nevus sebaceus. An Bras Dermatol. 2011;86(6):1213-6.
22. Brownstein MH, Starink TM. Desmoplastic trichoepithelioma and intradermal nevus: a combined malformation. J Am Acad Dermatol. 1987;17:489-92.
23. Navarrete-Dechent C, Bajaj S, Marghoob AA, González S, Muñoz D. Multiple familial trichoepithelioma: confirmation via dermoscopy. Dermatol Pract Concept. 2016;6(3):51-4.
24. Sharma S, Chauhan P, Kansal NK. Dermoscopy of trichoepithelioma: a clue to diagnosis. Indian Dermatol Online J. 2018;9:222-3.
25. Khelifa E, Masouyé I, Kaya G, Le Gal FA. Dermoscopy of desmoplastic trichoepithelioma reveals other criteria to distinguish it from basal cell carcinoma. Dermatology. 2013;226(2):101-4.
26. Winer LH. The dilated pore, a tricho-epithelioma. J Invest Dermatol. 1954;23(3):181-8.
27. Adya KA, Inamadar AC, Palit A. Dermoscopic characterization of dilated pore of Winer: report of two cases. Clin Dermatol Rev. 2019;3:96-8.
28. Zaballos P, Ara M, Puig S, Malvehy J. Dermoscopy of sebaceous hyperplasia. Arch Dermatol. 2005;141(6):808.
29. Zalaudek I, Kreusch J, Giacomel J, Ferrara G, Catricalà C, Argenziano G. How to diagnose nonpigmented skin tumors: a review of vascular structures seen with dermoscopy: part II. Nonmelanocytic skin tumors. J Am Acad Dermatol. 2010;63(3):377-86; quiz 387-8.
30. Bryden AM, Dawe RS, Fleming C. Dermatoscopic features of benign sebaceous proliferation. Clin Exp Dermatol. 2004;29(6):676-7.
31. Bañuls J, Arribas P, Berbegal L, DeLeón FJ, Francés L, Zaballos P. Yellow and orange in cutaneous lesions: clinical and dermoscopic data. J Eur Acad Dermatol Venereol. 2015;29:2317-25.
32. Malakar S, Mukherjee SS. Vascular pattern of milia on dermatoscopy. Our Dermatol Online. 2017;8(4):497-8.
33. Camara MF, Pinheiro PM, Jales RD, da Trindade Neto PB, Costa JB, de Sousa VL. Multiple dermatofibromas: dermoscopic patterns. Indian J Dermatol. 2013;58(3):243.
34. Zaballos P, Puig S, Llambrich A, Malvehy J. Dermoscopy of dermatofibromas: a prospective morphological study of 412 cases. Arch Dermatol. 2008;144:75-83.
35. Ferrari A, Argenziano G, Buccini P, Cota C, Sperduti I, De Simone P, et al. Typical and atypical dermoscopic presentations of dermatofibroma. J Eur Acad Dermatol Venereol. 2013;27:1375-80.
36. Ali M, Mbah CA, Alwadiya A, Nur MM, Sunderamoorthy D. Giant fibrokeratoma, a rare soft tissue tumor presenting like an accessory digit, a case report and review of literature. Int J Surg Case Rep. 2015;10:187-90.
37. Rubegni P, Poggiali S, Lamberti A, Chiantini A, De Paola M, Peccianti C, et al. Dermoscopy of acquired digital fibrokeratoma. Australas J Dermatol. 2012;53:47-8.
38. Zaballos P, Carulla M, Ozdemir F, Zalaudek I, Banuls J, Llambrich, et al. Dermoscopy of pyogenic granuloma: a morphological study. Br J Dermatol. 2010;163(6):1229-37.
39. Ankad BS, Beergouder SL, Shaik MA. Pink nodule with a peculiar pattern on trichoscopy. Int J Trichol. 2013;5:161-2.
40. Piccolo V, Russo T, Moscarella E, Brancaccio G, Alfano R, Argenziano G. Dermatoscopy of vascular lesions. Dermatol Clin. 2018;36(4):389-95.
41. Ozeki M, Saito R, Tanaka M. Dermoscopic features of pearly penile papules. Dermatology. 2008;217:21-2.
42. Ohnishi T, Nagayama T, Morita T, Miyazaki T, Okada H, Ohara K, et al. Angioma serpiginosum: a report of 2 cases identified using epiluminescence microscopy. Arch Dermatol. 1999;135:1366-8.
43. Ankad BS, Arora P, Sardana K, Bhardwaj M. Differentiation of acquired port wine stain and angioma serpiginosum: a dermoscopic perspective. Int J Dermatol. 2019;58(3):e62-4.
44. Zaballos P, Daufı C, Puig S, Argenziano G, Moreno-Ramıxrez G, Cabo H, et al. Dermoscopy of solitary angiokeratomas: a morphological study. Arch Dermatol. 2007;143:318-25.
45. Abhijeet KJ, Lallas A, Sonthalia S. Dermoscopy of cutaneous lymphangioma circumscriptum. Dermatol Pract Concept. 2017;7(2):37-8.
46. Hay RJ, Jones MR, Jemec GB. Other acquired disorders of the pilosebaceous unit. In: Griffiths C, Barker J, Bleiker T, Chalmers R, Creamer D (Eds). Rook's Textbook of Dermatology, 9th edition. United Kingdom: Wiley-Blackwell Publishing; 2016. pp. 93.10-2.
47. Jakhar D, Kaur I. Mucoscopy of Fordyce's spots on lips. Indian Dermatol Online J. 2019;10(4):498-9.

14 CHAPTER

Premalignant and Malignant Tumors

Yasmeen J Bhat, Usha N Khemani, Dincy Peter CV

INTRODUCTION

Dermoscopy is a noninvasive tool which helps in the early diagnosis of premalignant and malignant tumors and to differentiate them from benign tumors of the skin.

PREMALIGNANT LESIONS OF THE SKIN

Actinic Keratosis

Clinical Features

Actinic keratosis (AK) is an ultraviolet light induced most common premalignant lesion, 0.1–10% may subsequently progress to cutaneous squamous cell carcinoma.[1] Clinically, AK appears as erythematous, skin-colored or pigmented, scaly lesions with a rough, sandpaper-like texture, often easier to feel than to see (**Fig. 1A, Fig. 2A**, and **Fig. 3A**).

Dermoscopic Features

The features of nonpigmented AKs are graded as I–IV: I—red pseudonetwork; II—strawberry pattern; III—structureless, white to yellow areas, keratotic follicular openings; and IV—structureless, white to yellow keratotic areas.[2] The "strawberry pattern" is characterized by background erythema with unfocused, large, straight or wavy vessels located between hair follicles associated with prominent follicular openings surrounded by a white halo (**Figs. 1B** and **C**).[3] In skin of color, the vessels may not be prominent hence the typical strawberry pattern cannot be seen. Pigmented AKs demonstrate slate gray to brown dots and globules around follicular ostia, annular granular

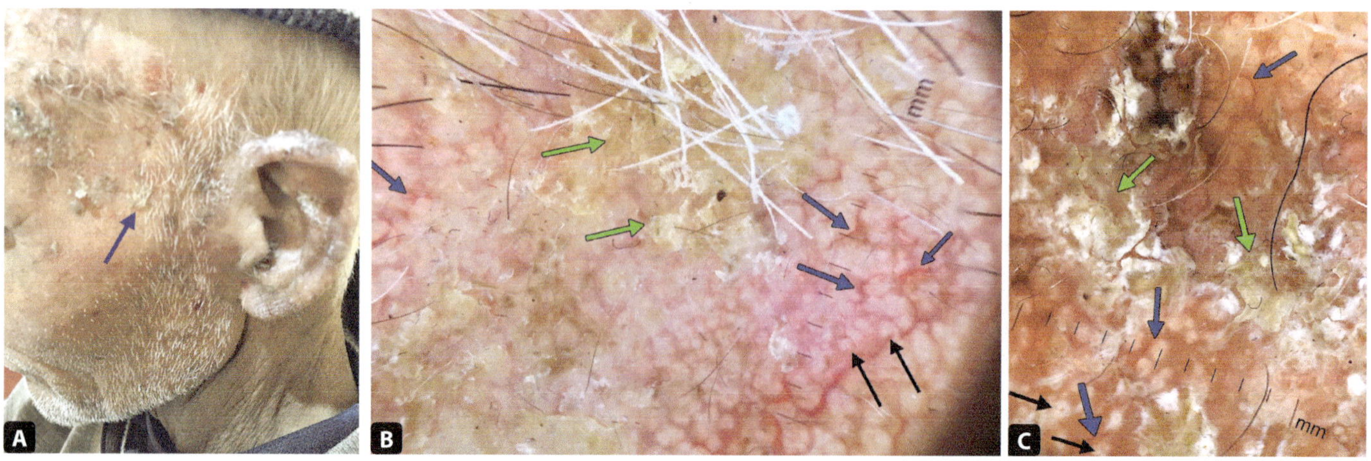

FIGS. 1A TO C: (A) Clinical image of actinic keratosis (blue arrow) on the face; (B and C) Dermoscopy showing scales and crusts on the surface (green arrows), rosettes and white circles (black arrows), perifollicular dilated unfocused vessels (blue arrows) (polarized, DermLite DL3N, 10×).

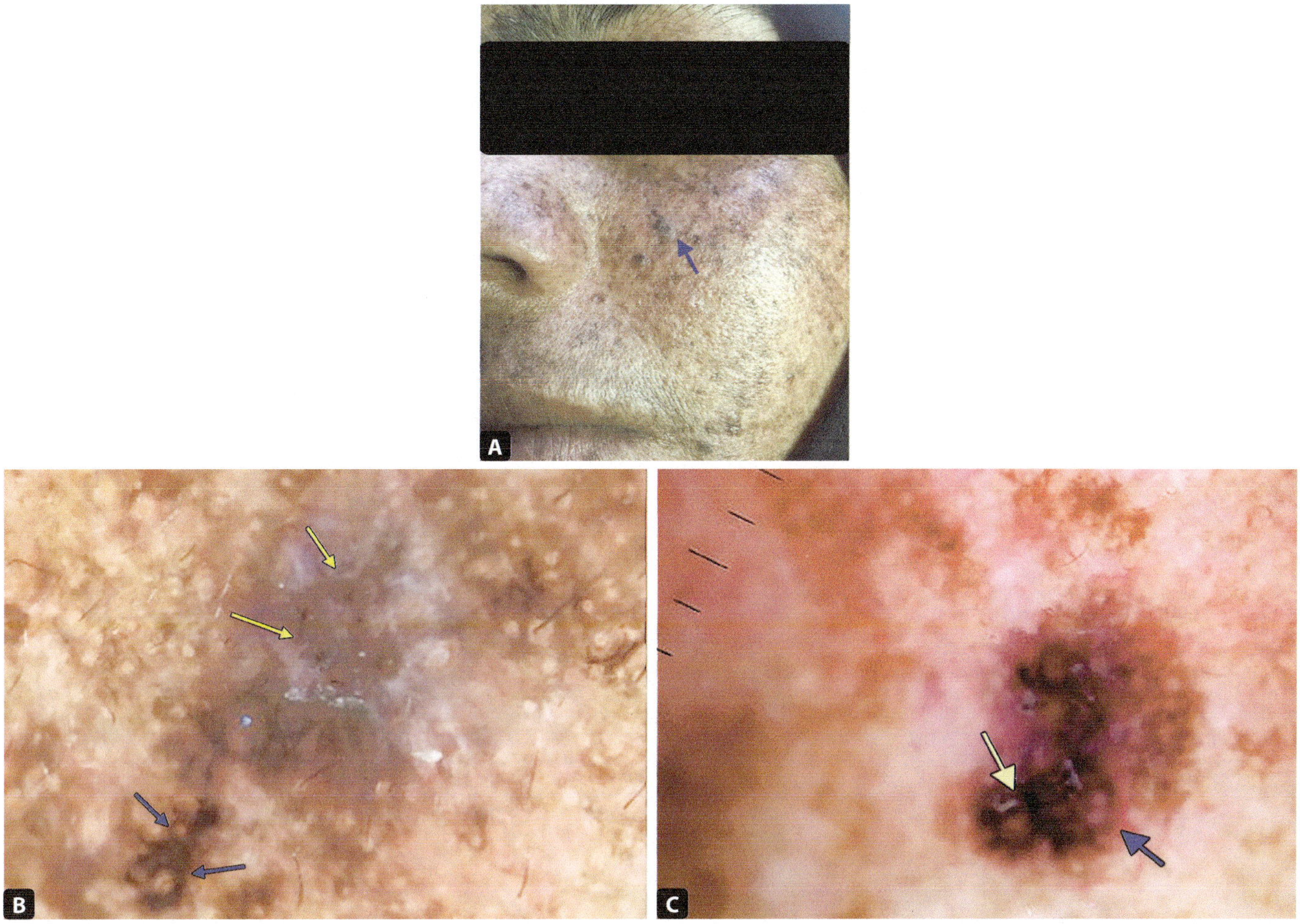

FIGS. 2A TO C: (A) Clinical image of actinic keratosis showing diffuse freckling with multiple erythematous to hyperpigmented macules over face. Blue arrow shows the lesion scoped; (B) Discrete whitish veil (yellow arrows), pigmented pseudonetwork with asymmetric dots and faint coiled vessels around the dilated follicles (blue arrows) (polarized, DermLite DL3N, 10×); (C) Pigmented pseudonetwork with asymmetric pigmented clods around dilated hair follicles (yellow arrow) with vessels surrounding them (blue arrow). Erythematous background intermingled with white to yellow, keratotic, and enlarged follicular openings giving strawberry appearance (polarized, DermLite DL3N, 10×).

and rhomboid structures, jelly sign, star-like appearance in periphery (**Figs. 2B** and **C**).[4] The follicles may have inner gray halo, white circle sign, rosettes, double white clods, dermoscopic horn (**Figs. 3B** to **E**).[5]

Key Points

- Strawberry pattern
- Rosettes
- Slate gray to brown dots and globules around follicular ostia

Bowen's Disease

Clinical Features

Bowen's disease (BD), a squamous cell carcinoma in situ with a 3–5% risk of developing into invasive squamous cell carcinoma, presents clinically as asymptomatic, slowly enlarging, erythematous, scaly plaques which may become hyperkeratotic, crusted, or ulcerated (**Fig. 4A, Fig. 5A**, and **Fig. 6A**).

Dermoscopic Features

It typically demonstrates glomerular and dot vessels grouped in clusters, surrounded by a white halo (sign of keratinization) and surface scales.[6] Pigmented BD shows brown globules or linear array of black dots regularly packed in a patchy distribution (melanophages in the dermoepidermal junction) and also gray to brown homogeneous pigmentation or brown structureless areas (acanthosis), white rosettes, double edge sign (two parallel pigmented edges at the periphery) (**Figs. 4B** and **C, Fig. 5B**, and **Figs. 6B** and **C**).[7,8]

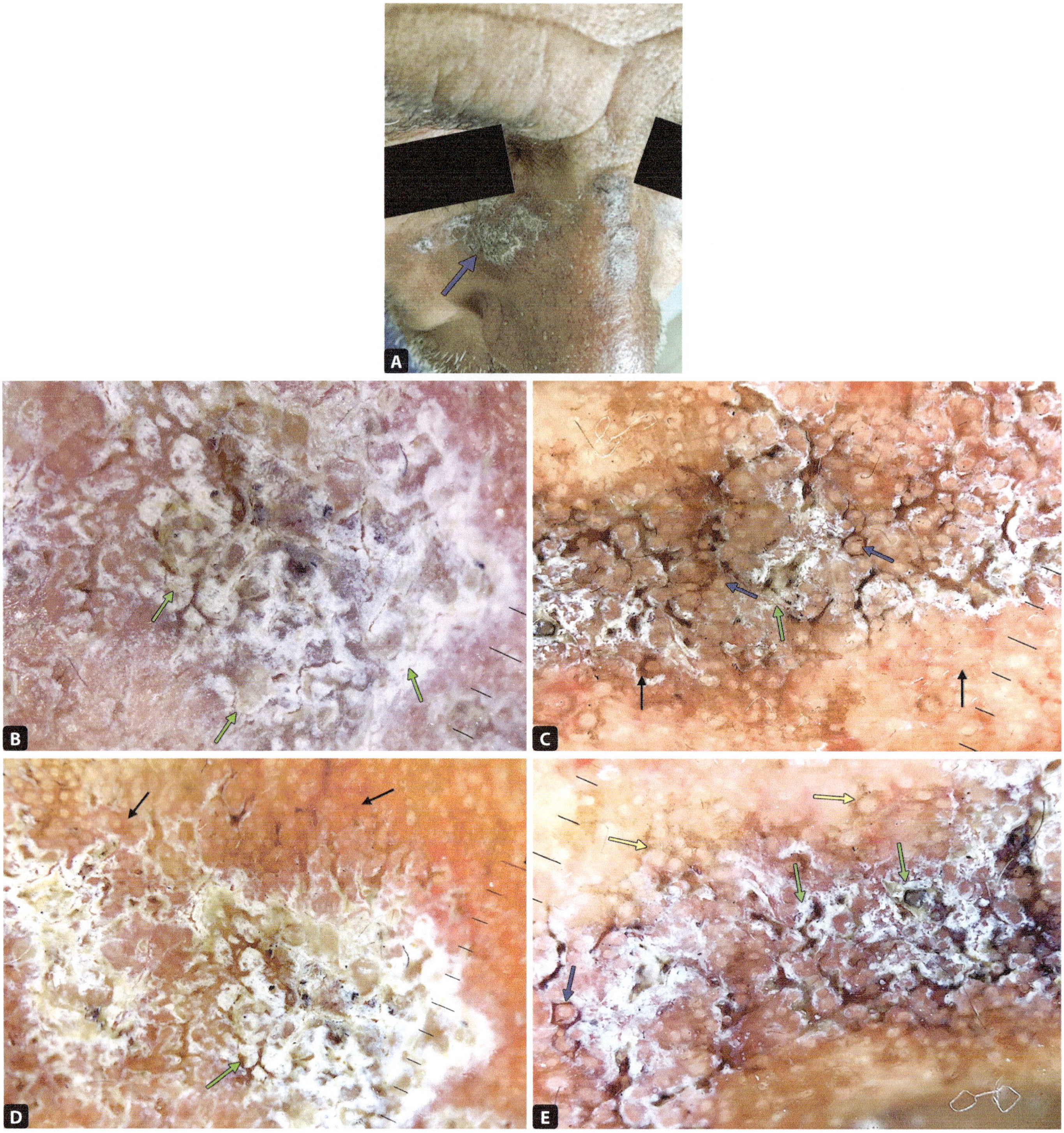

FIGS. 3A TO E: (A) Actinic keratosis on face (blue arrow); (B to E) Scales and crusts on the surface (green arrows), rosettes and white circles (blue arrows), perifollicular dilated unfocused vessels (black arrows), annular granular dots (yellow arrows) (polarized, DermLite DL3N, 10×).

Key Points

- Glomerular and dot vessels grouped in clusters
- White halo (sign of keratinization) and surface scales
- White rosettes
- Gray to brown homogeneous pigmentation or brown structureless areas

Keratoacanthoma

Clinical Features

Keratoacanthoma (KA) is a cutaneous squamoproliferative tumor with the potential for spontaneous resolution and needs to be treated due to its resemblance to cutaneous squamous cell carcinoma (**Fig. 7A** and **Fig. 8A**).

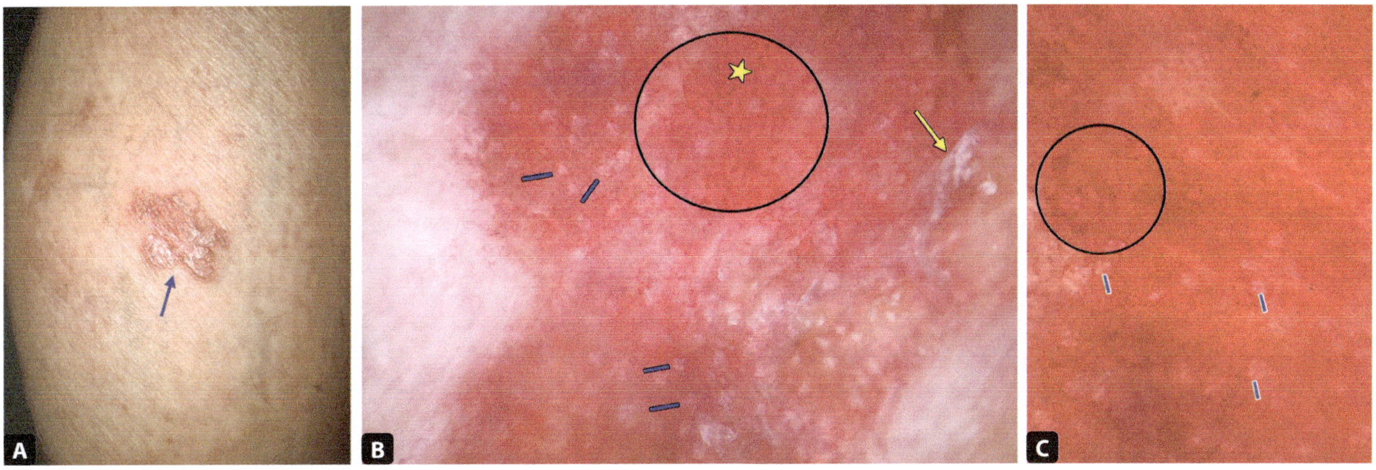

FIGS. 4A TO C: (A) Clinical image of Bowen's disease on leg; (B and C) Clusters of red dots and glomerular capillaries (black circle, yellow star), white rosettes (blue lines), white surface scales (yellow arrow) (polarized, DermLite DL3N, 10×).

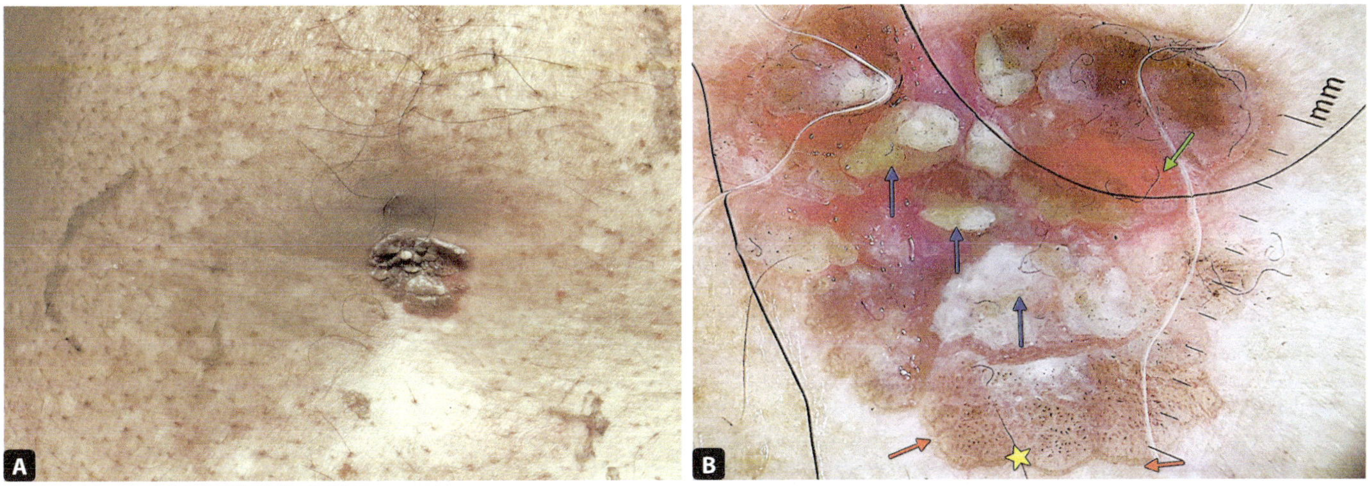

FIGS. 5A AND B: (A) Pigmented Bowen's disease on the abdomen; (B) Pigmented dots (yellow star), two parallel pigmented edges at the periphery (red arrows), whitish-brown structureless areas (blue arrows), and adherent fabric sign (green arrow) (polarized, DermLite DL3N, 10×).

Dermoscopic Features

It reveals concentric circles of central crater with blood spots, an ivory whitish area, adjacent peripheral vessels, dotted vessels, most outer circle of whitish halo. Surface scales and white structureless zones can be seen.[9,10] Keratin and white circles differ from other amelanotic tumors like amelanotic melanoma, AK, and BD. White circles are due to acanthosis and hypergranulosis of infundibular epidermis (**Figs. 7B** and **C**, and **Fig. 8B**).

Key Points

- Central crater with blood spots
- Surface scales with white structureless zones
- Whitish halos
- Peripheral vessels—short linear, curved, or dotted

MALIGNANT LESIONS OF THE SKIN

Squamous Cell Carcinoma

Clinical Features

Cutaneous squamous cell carcinoma is a common type of keratinocytic or nonmelanoma skin cancer with cumulative ultraviolet ray exposure being the main risk factor, involving face, neck, dorsum of hands, lower lip, and extremities. The typical lesion is an indurated, firm, papulonodular, plaque-like, papillomatous or exophytic growth with ulceration (**Fig. 9A, Fig. 10A**, and **Fig. 11A**).

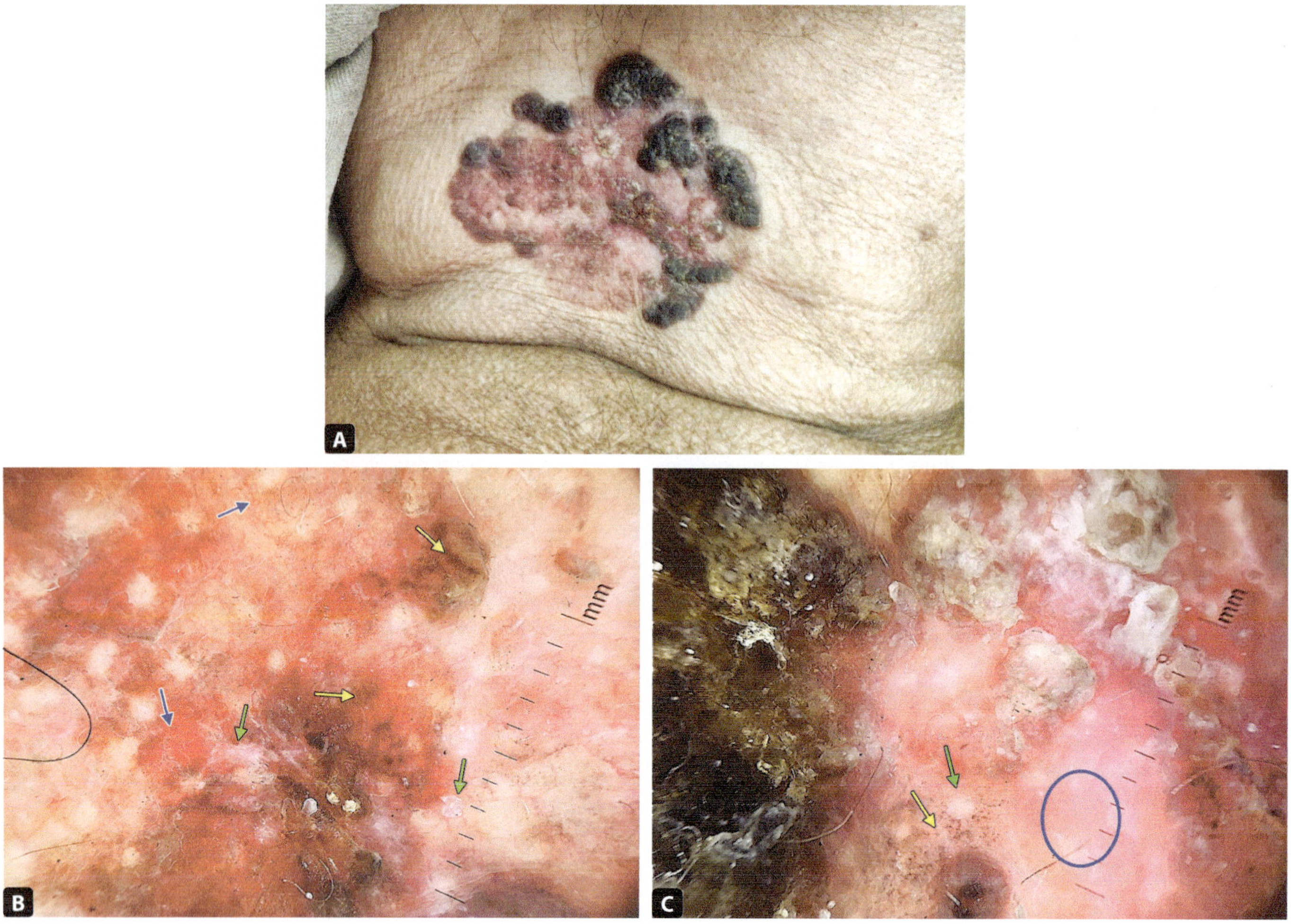

FIGS. 6A TO C: (A) Pigmented Bowen's disease on the chest; (B) Brown structureless areas (yellow arrows), clusters of glomerular capillaries (blue arrows), white scales (green arrows) (polarized, DermLite DL3N, 10×); (C) Reddish-white structureless areas (blue circle), pigmented dots (yellow arrow), nonpigmented follicles (green arrow) (polarized, DermLite DL3N, 10×).

Dermoscopic Features

Nonpigmented invasive squamous cell carcinoma frequently reveals linear, serpentine, irregular, hairpin, or dotted vessels, or combination of these vascular elements which is called as polymorphous or atypical vascular pattern. Typically, these vessels are surrounded by a whitish halo, which is a dermoscopic hallmark of all keratinizing tumors.

Pigmented invasive squamous cell carcinoma shows scales, keratin crust, keratin masses, white circles, and white structureless areas, diffuse or homogeneous blue pigmentation and/or irregularly distributed, blue-gray granular structures. A four-clover leaf pattern—"rosettes" with four bright white clods or dots arranged in two by two pattern may be seen. If ulcerated, dark-brown to black blood spots are visible. Due to pigmentation, vessels may not be appreciated, and if present are polymorphous vessels (serpentine, dotted or linear or looped, irregular or hairpin-like) with perivascular white halos.[11-14]

The dermoscopic structures differ among the clinical variants reflecting the different grades of differentiation (well differentiated, moderately differentiated or low differentiation) (**Fig. 9B, Figs. 10B** to **D**, and **Figs. 11B** and **C**).[15,16]

Key Points

- Keratin crusts or masses
- White circles/clods
- White structureless areas
- Perivascular white halos
- Polymorphous vessels

Basal Cell Carcinoma

Clinical Features

Basal cell carcinoma (BCC) is a nonmelanoma slow growing skin cancer and locally invasive. Clinical types—nodular, superficial, pigmented, morpheaform, fibroepithelioma of Pinkus, giant BCC, and subcutaneous (**Fig. 12A, Fig. 13A,** and **Fig. 14A**).[17]

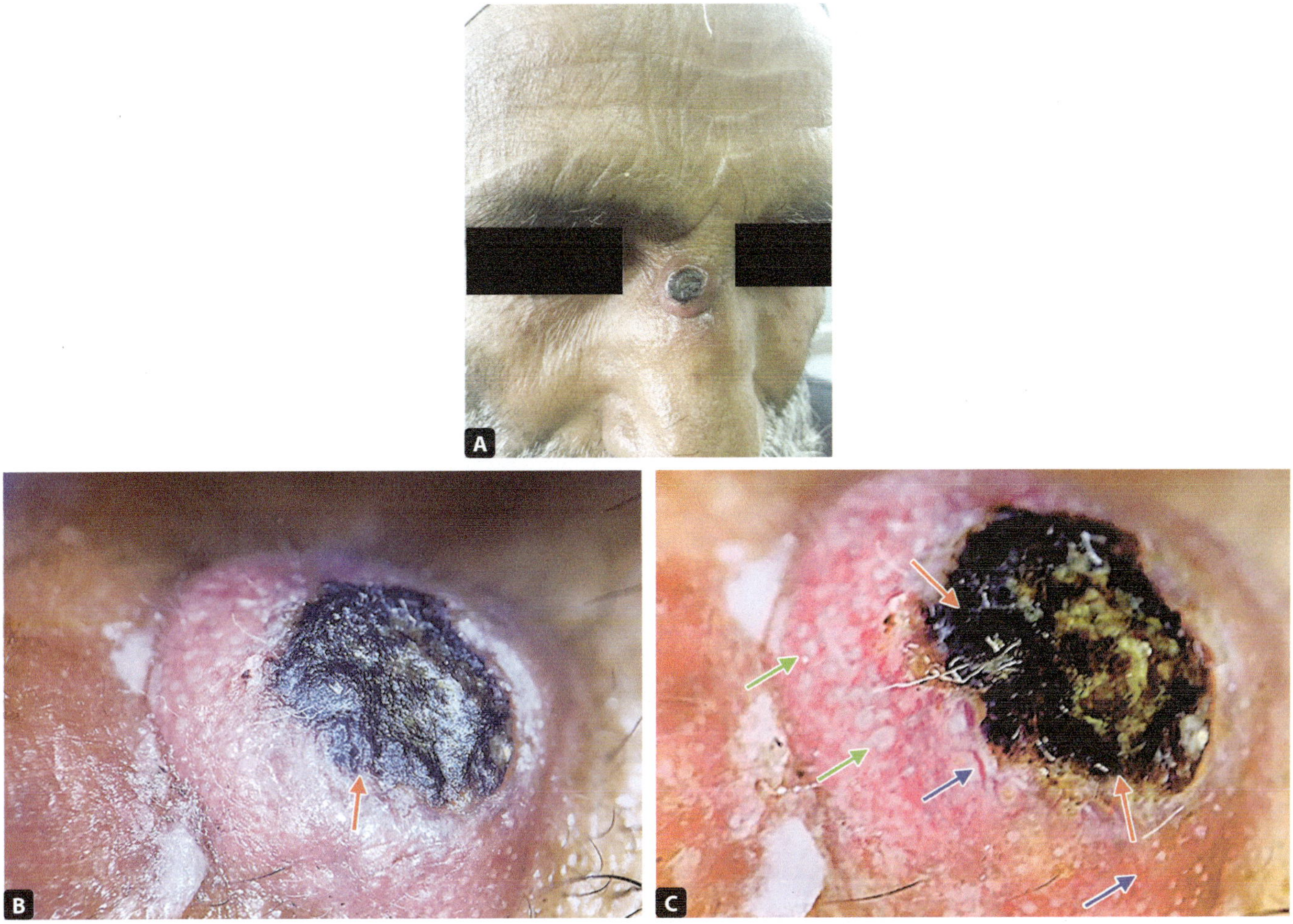

FIGS. 7A TO C: (A) Clinical image of keratoacanthoma on face; (B) Central crater with blackish areas (hemorrhage) (red arrow) (nonpolarized, DermLite DL3N, 10×); (C) Central crater with blackish areas (hemorrhage) (red arrows), whitish circles (green arrows), short linear and curved vessels (blue arrows) (polarized, DermLite DL3N, 10×).

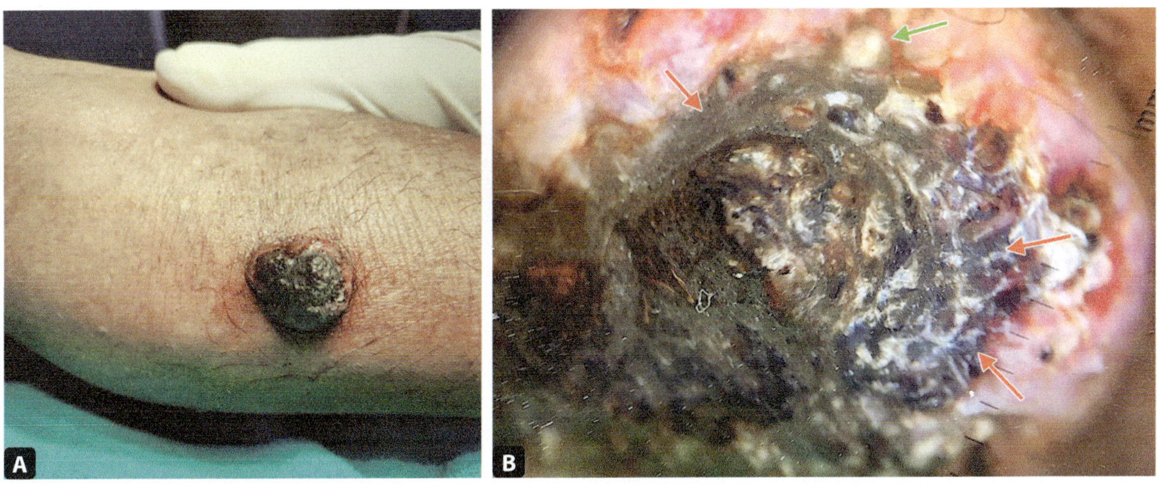

FIGS. 8A AND B: (A) Clinical image of keratoacanthoma on leg; (B) Central crater with blackish areas (hemorrhage) (red arrows), whitish circles (green arrow) (polarized, DermLite DL3N, 10×).

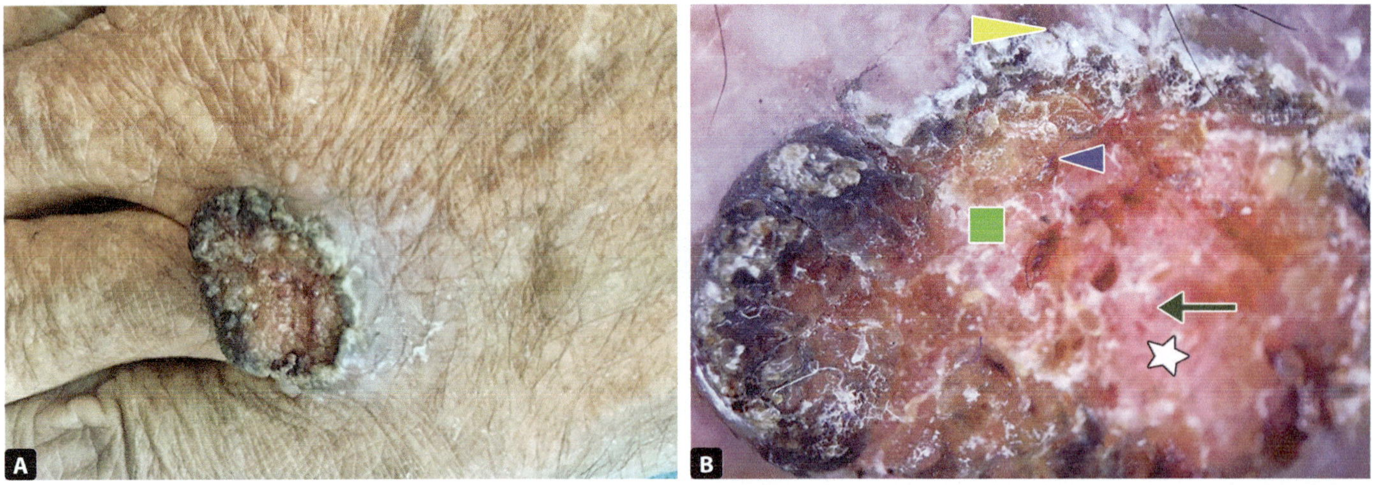

FIGS. 9A AND B: (A) Clinical image of ulcerated squamous cell carcinoma on the dorsum of the hand on photodamaged skin; (B) Dermoscopy showing keratin masses as white scales (yellow arrowhead), blood spots on keratin scale (blue arrowhead), fine white scales (green square), milky-red areas (white star) and polymorphous vessels such as coiled and glomerular (dark green arrow) (polarized, DermLite DL3N, 10×).

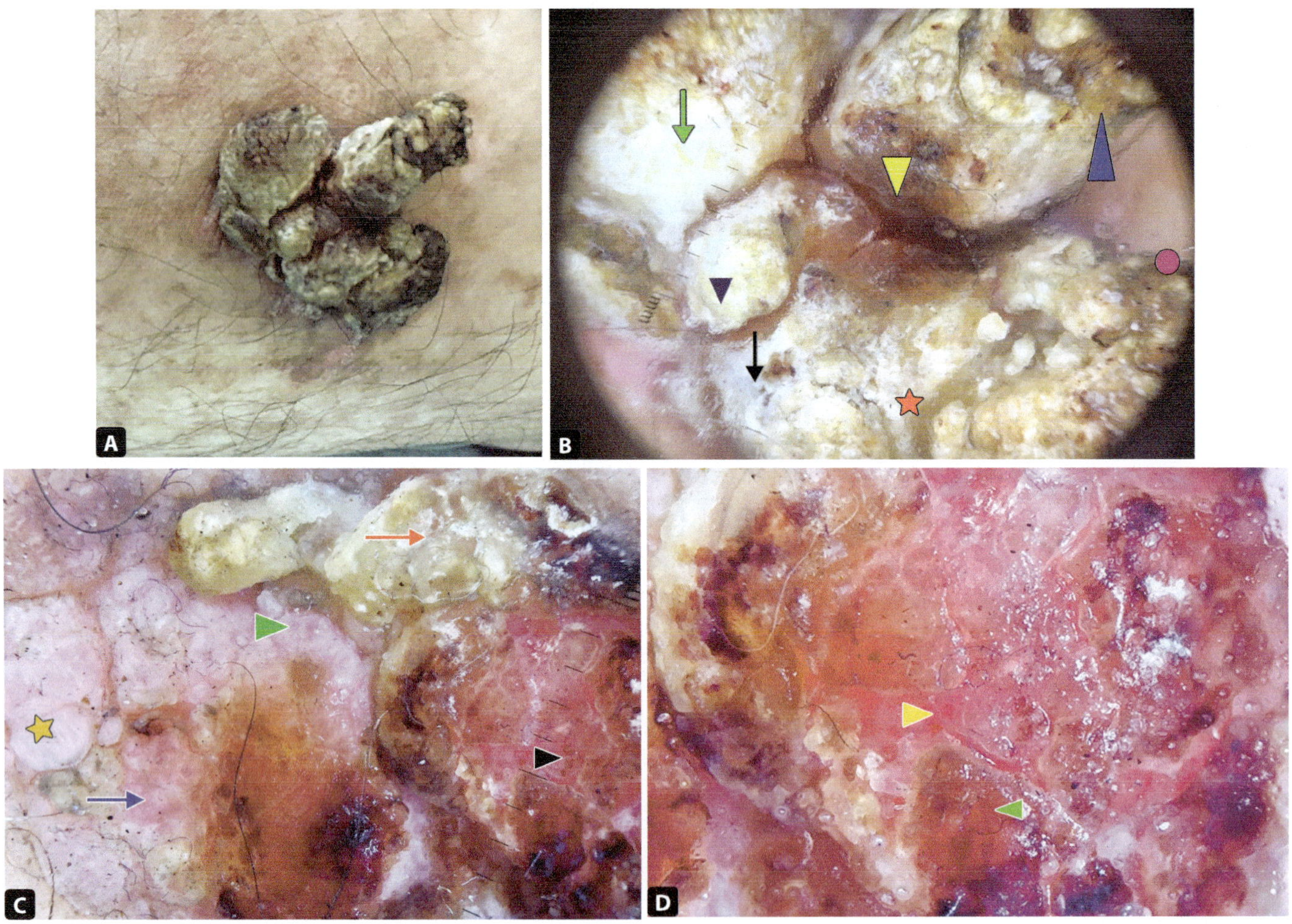

FIGS. 10A TO D: (A) Clinical image showing an exophytic squamous cell carcinoma with cutaneous horn with actinic keratosis at a distant site; (B) Dermoscopy displaying a combination color white being predominant color, white scales (green arrow), yellowish keratin with blood spots (blue arrowhead) and central hemorrhage (yellow arrowhead), white circles (purple arrowhead) and clod (red star) and brownish (pink circle) and white structureless areas (black arrow) (polarized, DermLite DL3N, 10×); (C) Dermoscopy showing yellowish keratin masses (red arrow), white circle with yellowish center (green arrowhead), perivascular white halo around vessels (blue arrow), white clod (yellow star), and polymorphous vessels (coiled, hair pin, dotted) (black arrowhead) (polarized, DermLite DL3N, 10×); (D) Dermoscopy showing polymorphous vessels coiled and glomerular (yellow and green arrowhead) (polarized, DermLite DL3N, 10×).

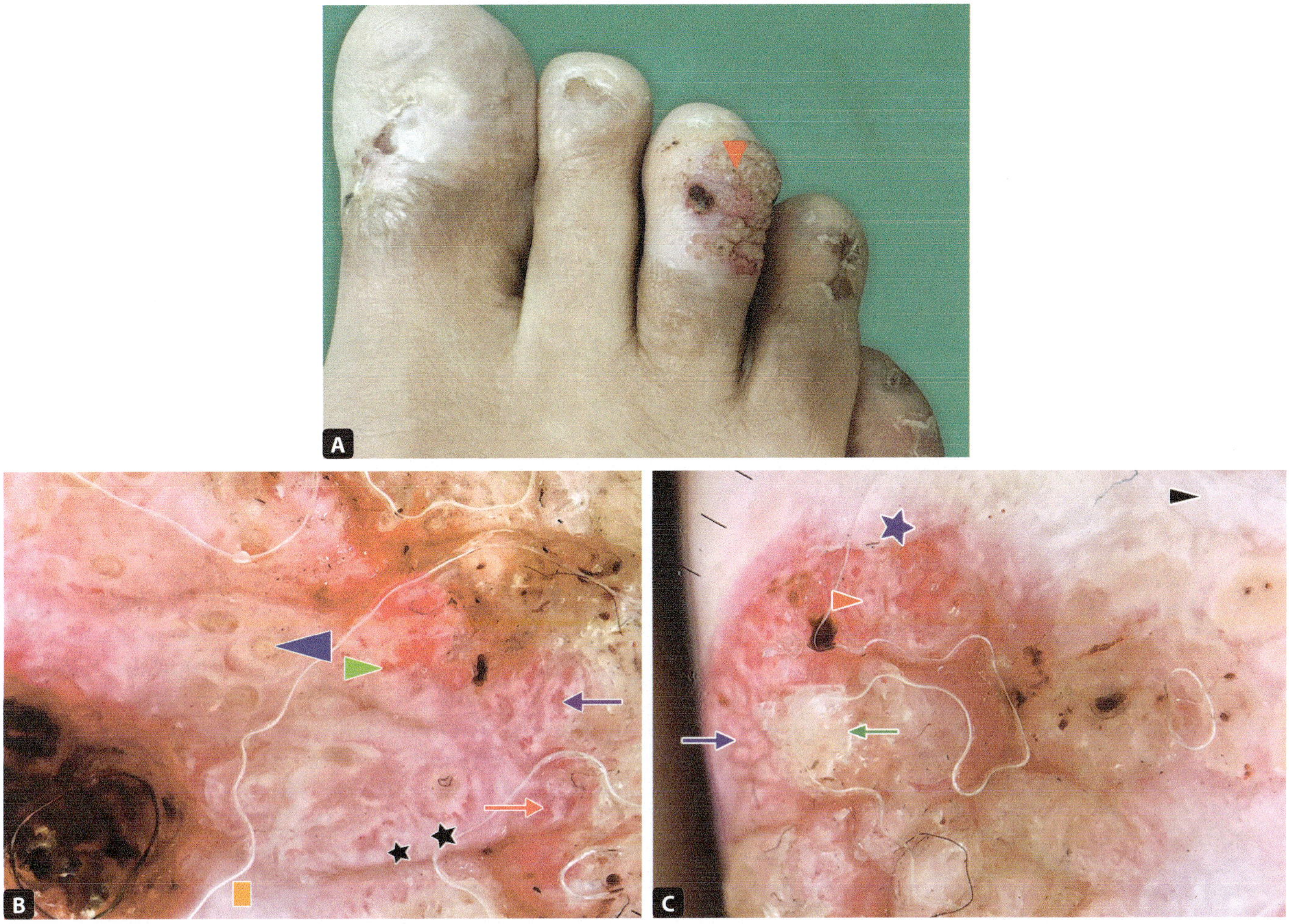

FIGS. 11A TO C: (A) Clinical image showing fungating mass verrucous squamous cell carcinoma (red arrowhead) overlying the middle toe of right foot with mitten toes and anonychia; (B) Dermoscopy showing white color predominantly with polymorphous vessels such as coiled (red arrow), dotted (purple arrow) and glomerular (green arrowhead) with a perivascular white halo (black stars), white circles with center yellowish plug (blue arrowhead) and rosettes, white structureless area (orange rectangle) with hemorrhage (polarized, DermLite DL3N, 10×); (C) Dermoscopy showing polymorphous vessels (blue star) with perivascular white halo around them (red arrowhead) white clods (purple arrow), amorphous white structures (green arrow) and white structureless areas at periphery (black arrowhead) (polarized, DermLite DL3N, 10×).

Dermoscopic Features

It helps as a screening technique in doubtful lesions and in the management of the tumor, since it provides valuable diagnostic information about it and the expansion of the tumor beyond clinically visible margins.[18,19]

The concept of the signature pattern of BCC as introduced by Zalaudek et al. indicates that multiple BCCs in an individual usually display a repetitive dermatoscopic pattern (**Tables 1** and **2**).[20-23] According to the degree of dermoscopic pigmentation, lesions are categorized as:[19]

- Nonpigmented BCCs—only red and/or white structureless areas
- Lightly pigmented BCCs—pigmented areas <30% of lesion
- Pigmented BCCs—pigmented areas 30–70% of lesion
- Heavily pigmented BCCs—presence of pigmentation >70%

TABLE 1: Dermoscopic features of basal cell carcinoma.[23]

Vascular structures	Pigmented structures	Nonvascular, nonpigmented structures
Arborizing vessels Thin arborizing Short fine telangiectasias	Globules	Milky-red area
Other vessels	Blue-gray ovoid nests	Ulceration
Serpentine	Dots	Crusts
Helical	Maple leaf	Scale
Polymorphous	Spoke wheel	Erosions
Linear	Concentric globules	Blue-white veil
Looped		Shiny white structures

Source: Wozniak-Rito A, Zalaudek I, Rudnicka L. Dermoscopy of basal cell carcinoma. Clin Exp Dermatol. 2018;43:241-7.

TABLE 2: Dermoscopic criteria of basal cell carcinoma according to subtype.

Dermoscopic pattern	Definition
Superficial pigmented	• Superficial fine telangiectasia, no ovoid nests • Multiple small erosions • Shiny white-red structureless areas • Maple leaf-like areas • Spoke-wheel areas • Concentric structures • Multiple blue-gray dots • In-focus dots
Nodular pigmented	• Arborizing vessels • Ulceration • Short white streaks on polarized dermoscopy • Blue-gray ovoid nests • Multiple blue-gray dots • Maple leaf-like areas* • Spoke-wheel areas* • Concentric structures*
Morpheaform pigmented	• Arborizing vessels finer, few branches • Ulceration • Whitish background • Blue-gray ovoid nests • Multiple blue-gray dots • In-focus dots
Infiltrative pigmented	• Arborizing vessels few branches • Ulceration • White-red structureless areas • Blue-gray ovoid nests • Multiple blue-gray dots • In-focus dots
Fibroepithelioma of Pinkus	• White-pinkish background • Fine arborizing vessels in center • Dotted vessels at periphery
Basosquamous carcinoma pigmented	• Arborizing vessels • Keratin masses, scale, may show blood spots • White structureless areas • Ulceration/blood crusts • Blue-gray ovoid nests • Multiple blue-gray dots

*Typically at peripheral, superficial parts of the lesion.

Source: Lallas A, Apalla Z, Argenziano G, Longo C, Moscarella E, Specchio F, et al. The dermatoscopic universe of basal cell carcinoma. Dermatol Pract Concept. 2014;4:11-24.

Classic BCC patterns—lack of pigment network, ulceration, multiple blue/gray globules, leaf-like areas, large blue/gray ovoid nests, spoke-wheel areas, and arborizing telangiectasia

Nonclassic BCC patterns—short fine superficial telangiectasia, multiple small erosions, concentric structures, multiple in-focus blue/gray dots (**Fig. 12B, Fig. 13B**, and **Fig. 14B**).[20]

Key Points

- Arborizing telangiectasias, short fine telangiectasias
- Bluish-gray ovoid nests, blue-gray globules
- Maple leaf-like areas, spoke-wheel areas, concentric structures
- Ulceration, erosions, white red structureless areas, chrysalis

Melanoma

Clinical Features

Melanoma is an aggressive and highly metastatic disease. Metastatic melanoma is a fatal disease with a rapid systemic dissemination. Cutaneous melanoma is classified as melanoma in situ when confined within the epidermis, or invasive when atypical melanocytes progressively invade into the dermis. Subtypes of invasive melanoma are superficial spreading melanoma (SSM) (41%) (**Fig. 15A**), lentigo maligna melanoma (LMM) (2.7–14%) (**Fig. 16A**), nodular melanoma (16%) (**Fig. 17A**), and acral lentiginous melanoma (ALM) (1–5%) (**Fig. 18A**).[24,25]

Dermoscopic Features

Using dermoscopic scoring systems, such as asymmetry, border irregularity, color variegation, diameter >6 (ABCD) rule, pattern analysis, Menzies method, 7-point checklist, modified asymmetry, border irregularity, color variegation (ABC)-point list and CASH (color, architecture, symmetry, and homogeneity) helps to identify whether the melanocytic lesion is benign, suspicious or frankly malignant.[26] Characteristic features for the diagnosis of melanoma, also called melanoma-specific criteria, include:

- An atypical pigment network
- Irregular brown-black dots/globules and streaks
- Pigmentation with multiple colors asymmetrically distributed.
- Additional criteria, e.g., blue-whitish veil and polymorphic vessels are common in invasive melanoma.
- A parallel ridge pattern and irregular diffuse pigmentation are the main dermoscopic features of early and invasive acral melanoma, respectively.[27]
- Atypical vascular structures (including polymorphic vessels, milky-red areas, and homogeneous red areas) and the simultaneous presence of blue and black areas (seen as dots, globules, blotches, or ulceration) involving at least 10% of the lesion surface are significantly associated with nodular melanomas.

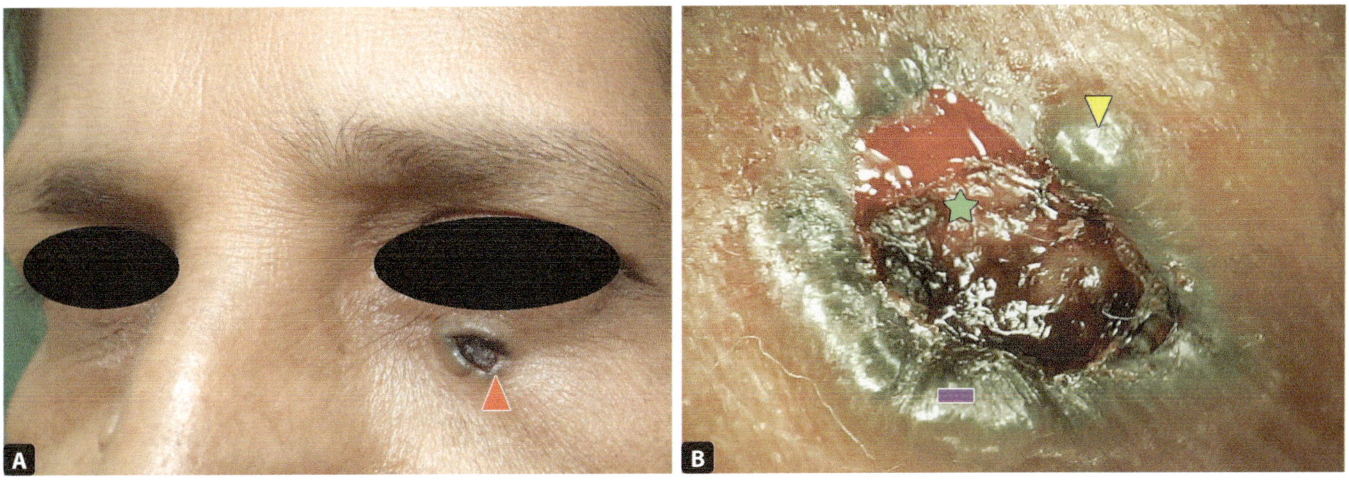

FIGS. 12A AND B: (A) Clinical photograph showing classical pigmented noduloulcerative basal cell carcinoma below the left lower eyelid with rolled out everted border (red arrowhead); (B) Dermoscopic image showing multiple confluent grayish-blue ovoid nests (lilac rectangle), single ovoid nest (yellow arrowhead), with central hemorrhagic crust (green star) (polarized, Dino-Lite, 10×).

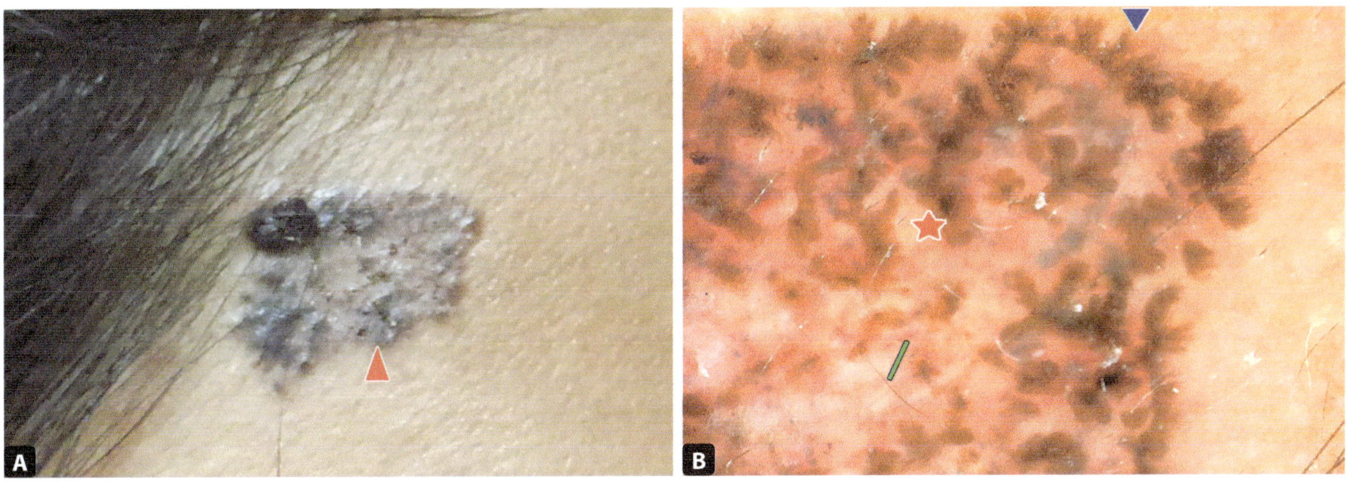

FIGS. 13A AND B: (A) Clinical photograph of superficial spreading basal cell carcinoma on the left forehead (red arrowhead); (B) Dermoscopic image showing maple leaf-like areas (blue arrowhead), with concentric structures (red star) and brown dots (green line) (polarized, Dino-Lite, 10×).

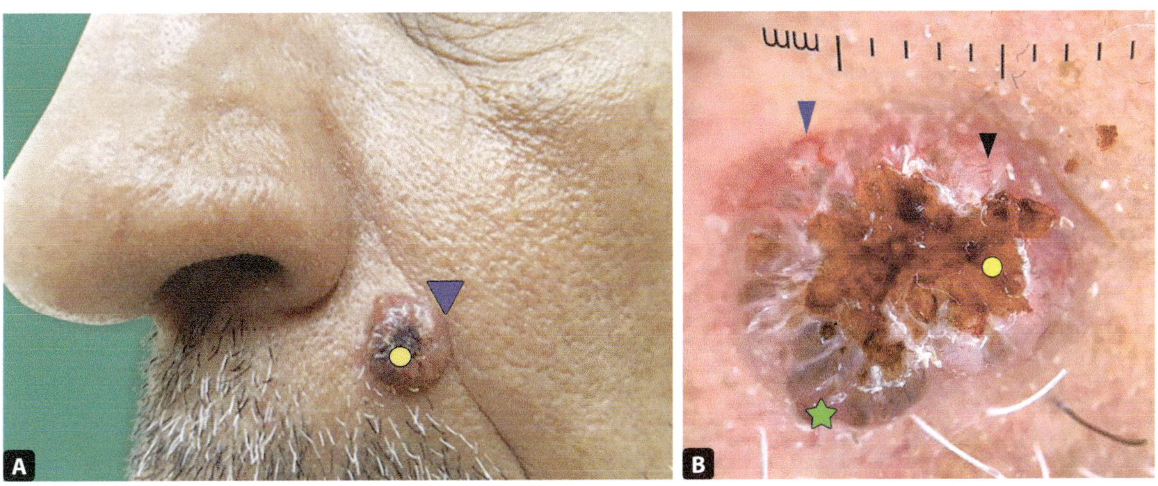

FIGS. 14A AND B: (A) Clinical photograph showing nonpigmented nodular variant of basal cell carcinoma (blue arrowhead) with central erosion and crust (yellow circle); (B) Dermoscopic image showing arborizing telangiectasias (blue arrowhead), with short fine telangiectasias (black arrowhead), grayish ovoid nests (green star) and hemorrhagic crust (yellow circle) (polarized, DermLite DL4, 10×).

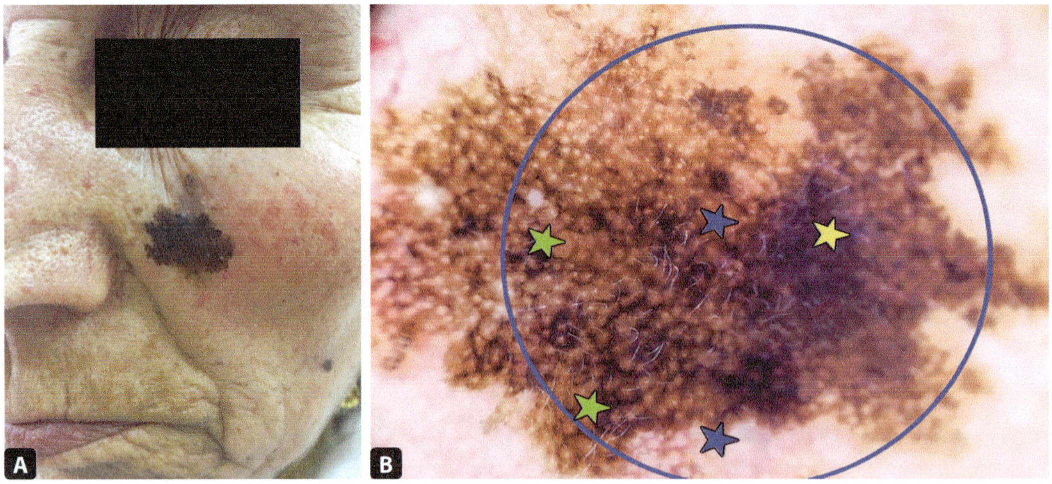

FIGS. 15A AND B: (A) Pigmented plaque on left cheek with color variegation; (B) Dermoscopy shows irregular pseudonetwork (blue circle), blue-white veil (yellow star), angulated lines (blue stars), and irregular thick lines (green stars) (polarized, DermLite DL3N, 10×).

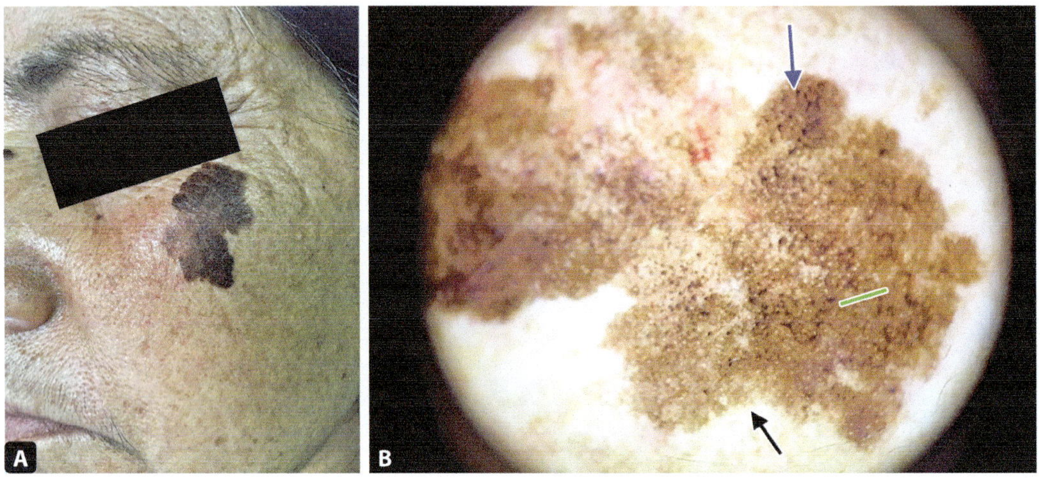

FIGS. 16A AND B: (A) Pigmented plaque on left cheek; (B) Dermoscopy showing multiple brown dots, peripheral black dots/globules (blue arrow), multiple colors, broad network (green line), focal sharply cut-off border (black arrow), irregular vascularity (polarized, DermLite DL3N, 10×).

Facial melanoma is typified by a pseudonetwork background, gray circles (asymmetric pigmented follicular openings), circle within the circle-isobar sign (gray dots in the follicular openings), granular-annular structures (fine gray dots, globules, and streaks around the follicles), rhomboidal structures (thick pigmented lines around appendageal openings due to melanocytes that surround or completely obliterate the follicular openings), black/gray blotches (diffuse brown-black pigmentation that obscures the recognition of other dermoscopic features). Other melanomas difficult to diagnose are those of special locations including mucosal, acral, and nail apparatus melanoma.[28]

Key Points

- Superficial spreading melanoma—blue-whitish veil, pseudopods, radial streaming, scar-like depigmentation, peripheral black dots/globules, multiple (5–6) colors, broad network, focal sharply cut-off border, negative network, irregular vascularity (**Fig. 15B**)
- Lentigo maligna melanoma—a pseudonetwork background, circle within the circle, granular-annular structures, and rhomboidal structures (**Fig. 16B**).
- Nodular melanoma—atypical vascular structures and the simultaneous presence of blue and black areas (**Fig. 17B**)
- Acral lentiginous melanoma—a parallel ridge pattern and irregular diffuse pigmentation, ulceration (**Fig. 18B**)
- Amelanotic melanoma—absence of pigment network, ulceration, polymorphic vessels

Appendageal Tumors

Leiomyosarcoma

Clinical Features

Leiomyosarcoma is a rare smooth muscle neoplasm of the skin. Clinically, it presents as skin-colored nodules. The

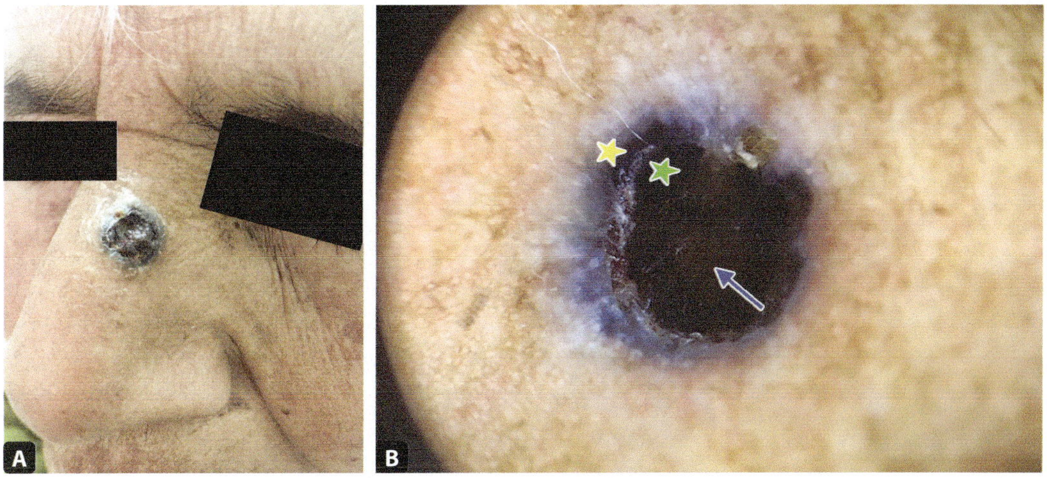

FIGS. 17A AND B: (A) Pigmented nodule on left side of nose; (B) Dermoscopy shows blue-black veil (yellow star), ulceration with black pigmentation (green star) and irregular vessels (blue arrow) (polarized, DermLite DL3N, 10×).

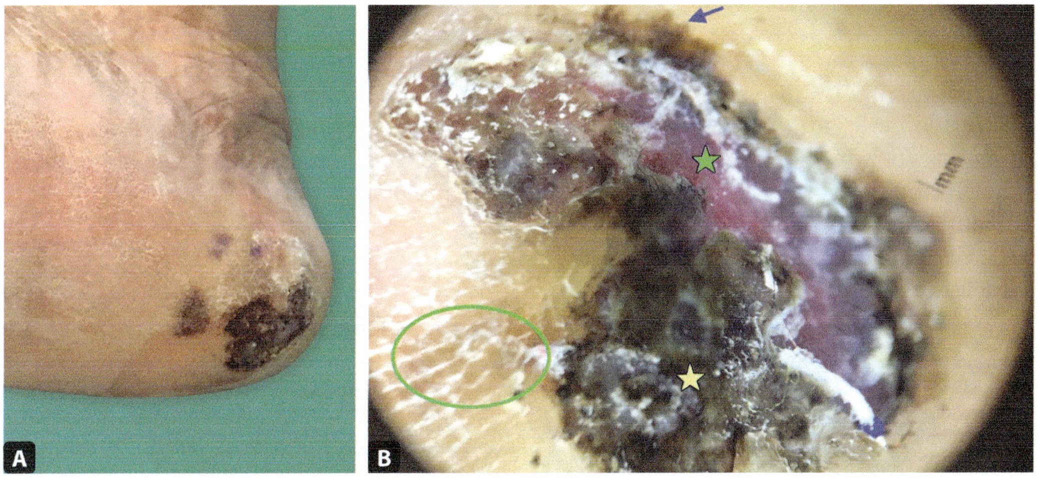

FIGS. 18A AND B: (A) Clinical image of acral lentiginous melanoma; (B) Dermoscopy showing bluish veil (yellow star), ulceration (green star), parallel ridge pattern (green circle), and irregular pigmented streaks (blue arrow) (polarized, DermLite DL3N, 10×).

most common sites of involvement include head and neck and extremities especially the legs (**Fig. 19A**).[29]

Dermoscopic Features

It include asymmetry, ulceration, multilobulation, atypical pigment network, multifocal lesions, polymorphic vessels with linear, irregular and atypical vessels, milky-red areas, and white structures including chrysalis (**Fig. 19B**).[29] The dermoscopic differentials include malignant tumors such as melanoma, Merkel cell carcinoma, angiosarcoma, dermatofibrosarcoma protuberans, porocarcinoma, and B-cell lymphomas. De Giorgi et al. reported the presence of arborizing vessels and telangiectasias on a background of whitish area on dermoscopy of a cutaneous nodule of leiomyosarcoma.[30] Atypical pigmentary lesion with a peripheral brownish network and central white roundish globules with scar-like features on dermoscopy have been described in a case of clear cell variant of cutaneous leiomyosarcoma.[31]

Key Points

- Asymmetry
- Ulceration
- Multilobulation
- Atypical pigment network
- Polymorphic atypical vessels

Dermatofibrosarcoma Protuberans

Clinical Features

Dermatofibrosarcoma protuberans is a rare, low-grade malignant skin tumor. It is considered the cutaneous equivalent of malignant extracutaneous soft tissue fibrous histiocytoma. The tumor has a high tendency to recur after incomplete surgical excision. Clinically, it may be confused with dermatofibroma or keloid (**Fig. 20A**).

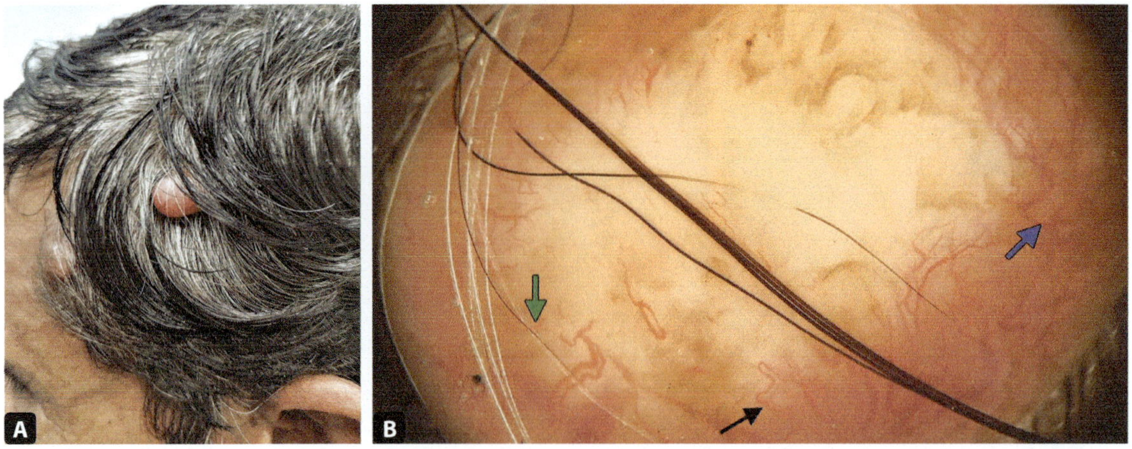

FIGS. 19A AND B: (A) Clinical photograph showing erythematous nodule over scalp. Histopathology was consistent with leiomyosarcoma; (B) Dermoscopic image showing central homogeneous yellowish structureless area with polymorphous vessels with thick arborizing (blue arrow), thin arborizing, linear (green arrow) and serpentine vessels (black arrow) at the periphery (nonpolarized, FotoFinder Systems, 20×).
Courtesy: Department of Dermatology, CMC, Vellore, Tamil Nadu, India.

Dermoscopic Features

The reported dermoscopic findings in 15 dermatofibrosarcoma protuberans include delicate pigmented network (87%), vessels (80%), structureless light brown areas (73%), shiny white streaks (67%), pink background coloration (67%), and structureless hypo- or depigmented areas (60%). Arborizing vessels represented the most frequent vascular feature (**Figs. 20B** and **C**).[32]

Key Points

- Arborizing vessels
- Delicate pigment network

Merkel Cell Carcinoma

Clinical Features

Merkel cell carcinoma is a rare neuroendocrine carcinoma of skin. It presents as an asymptomatic, rapidly growing nonpigmented erythematous or violaceous nodule (**Fig. 21A**). The clinical differential diagnoses include cutaneous lymphoma, atypical fibroxanthoma, porocarcinoma, achromic melanoma, angiosarcoma, and hemangioma or skin metastasis from internal malignancy.

Dermoscopic Features

The dermoscopic patterns described in Merkel cell carcinoma include polymorphous vessels, milky pink areas, architectural disorder, and structureless areas.[33-36] The most common dermoscopic pattern includes milky-red areas with vascular pattern.[34] The vascular patterns described include dotted vessels, linear irregular vessels, arborizing vessels, and glomerular vessels (**Fig. 21B**). The combination of both sharply focused and poorly focused vessels in the one dermoscopic field is a useful diagnostic feature and shiny white areas are seen with both polarized and nonpolarized dermoscopy.[35] Blue-gray veil and pigmented structure are conspicuously absent.

Key Points

- A polymorphous vascular pattern is a characteristic finding in Merkel cell carcinoma.
- Milky-red areas are characteristic dermoscopic finding in Merkel cell carcinoma.

Mycosis Fungoides

Clinical Features

Mycosis fungoides (MF) is the most common variant of primary cutaneous T-cell lymphoma and has an indolent course. It is characterized by polymorphic patches and plaques usually involving trunk, extremities, the breast, and especially the buttock area. Patients can occasionally present with nodules and erythroderma. Clinically, early MF can mimic chronic dermatitis or plaque psoriasis (**Fig. 22A, Fig. 23A**, and **Fig. 24A**). A diagnosis of MF is made by the characteristic histopathology and immunohistochemistry.

Dermoscopic Features

The various dermoscopic patterns described in MF include white scales, orange-yellow patches, white structureless areas, linear and spermatozoa-like vessels. The characteristic dermoscopic pattern consists of fine short linear vessels, vascular structure resembling spermatozoa, and orange-yellowish patchy areas.[37,38] The term "spermatozoa-like structure" refers to a specific vascular structure composed of a dotted and a short curved linear vessel, giving an overall shape similar to a spermatozoon.[37] White scales (80%) with a patchy distribution pattern (36.6%) and dotted and linear vessel type (80%) were prominent in a study by Bilgic et al.[39] In terms of background color, Lallas et al. reported yellow-orange (90.6%), Xu et al. reported dull red (83.9%), and Bilgic et al. reported dull red (45%) and yellow-orange (35%) as the most prominent background colors.

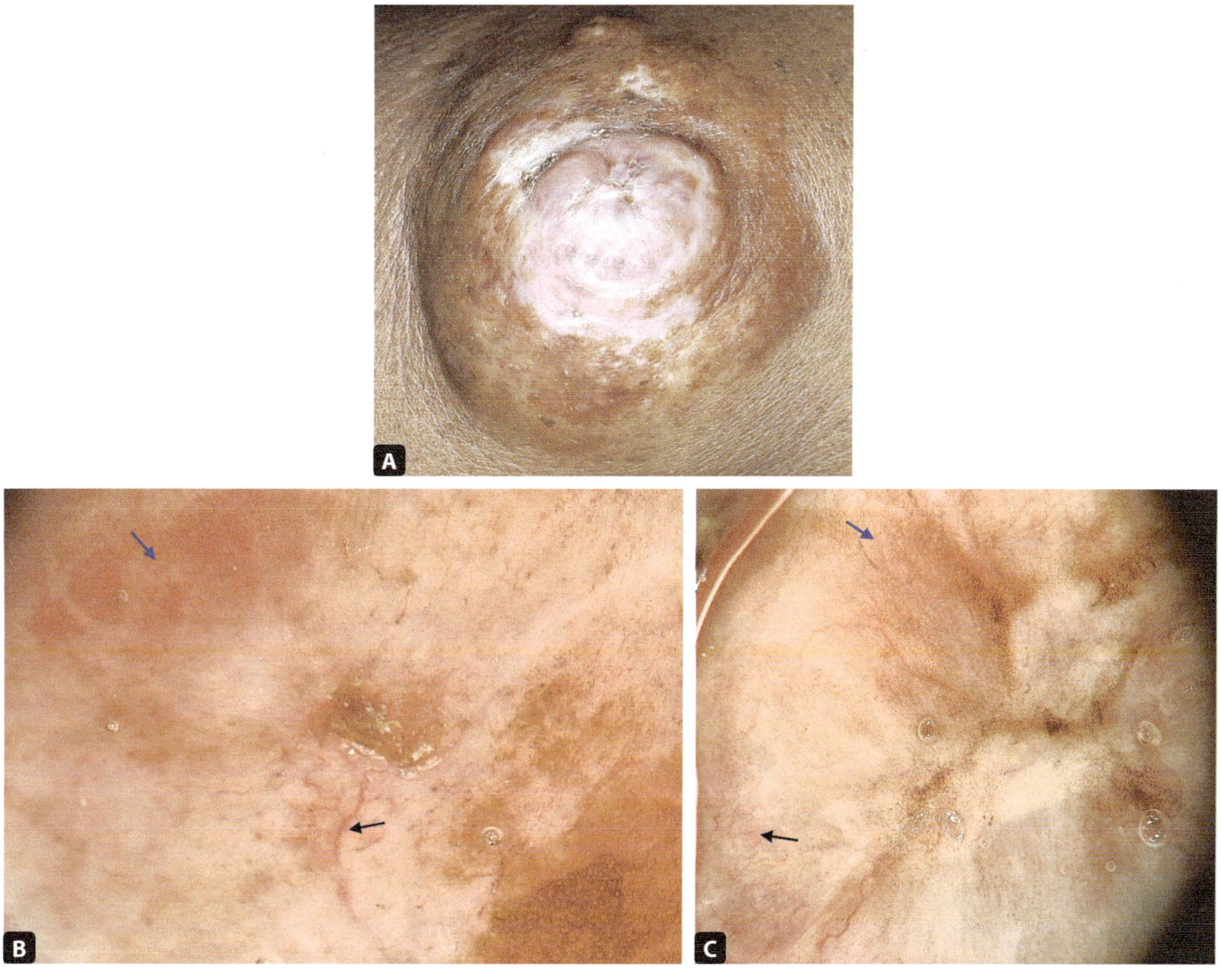

FIGS. 20A TO C: (A) Clinical photograph showing skin-colored nodule with central depigmentation over the arm. Histopathology was consistent with dermatofibrosarcoma protuberans; (B) Dermoscopic image showing central white structureless area with milky-red areas (blue arrow) with brown pigment network and an arborizing vessel (black arrow) from the periphery (nonpolarized, FotoFinder Systems, 20×); (C) Dermoscopic image showing central white structureless area with milky-red areas (blue arrow) with brown dots and brown pigment network with unfocused thin arborizing vessel (black arrow) at the periphery (nonpolarized, FotoFinder Systems, 20×).

Courtesy: Department of Dermatology, CMC, Vellore, Tamil Nadu, India.

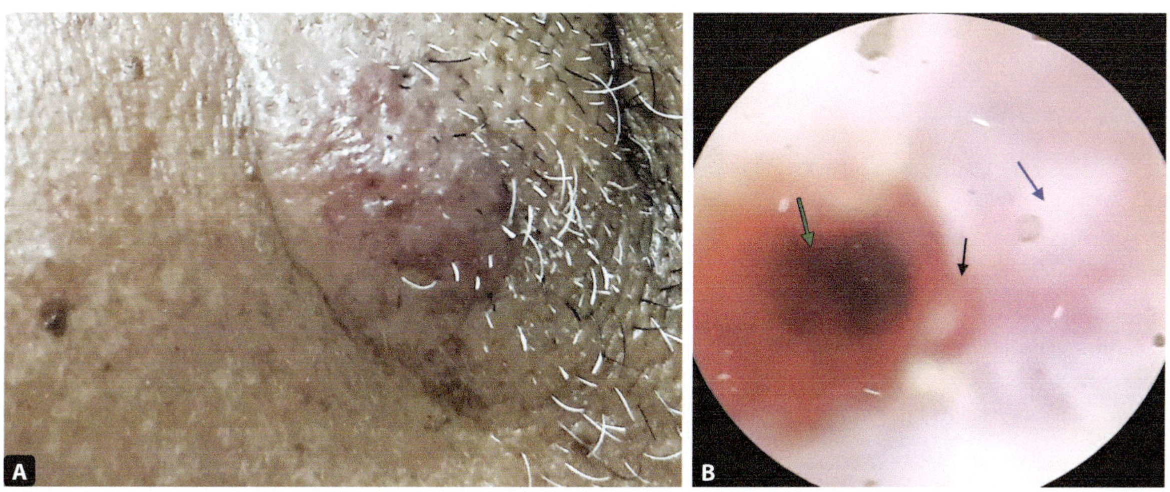

FIGS. 21A AND B: (A) Clinical photograph of erythematous nodules over right upper lip below the nasolabial fold, histopathology was consistent with Merkel cell carcinoma; (B) Dermoscopic image of Merkel cell carcinoma showing ulceration, nonfocused vessels (black arrow), red ulceration (green arrow), milky-red areas and structureless white areas (blue arrow) (nonpolarized, Heine Delta 20T, 10×).

In a study by Ghahramani et al., MF was characterized by interconnected white structureless patches encircling small fine linear vessels, yielding an overall trabeculated to fenestrated pattern under dermoscopy (**Figs. 22B** and **C, Fig. 23B**, and **Fig. 24B**).[40]

Key Points

- Fine short linear vessels
- Spermatozoa-like vessels
- White scales

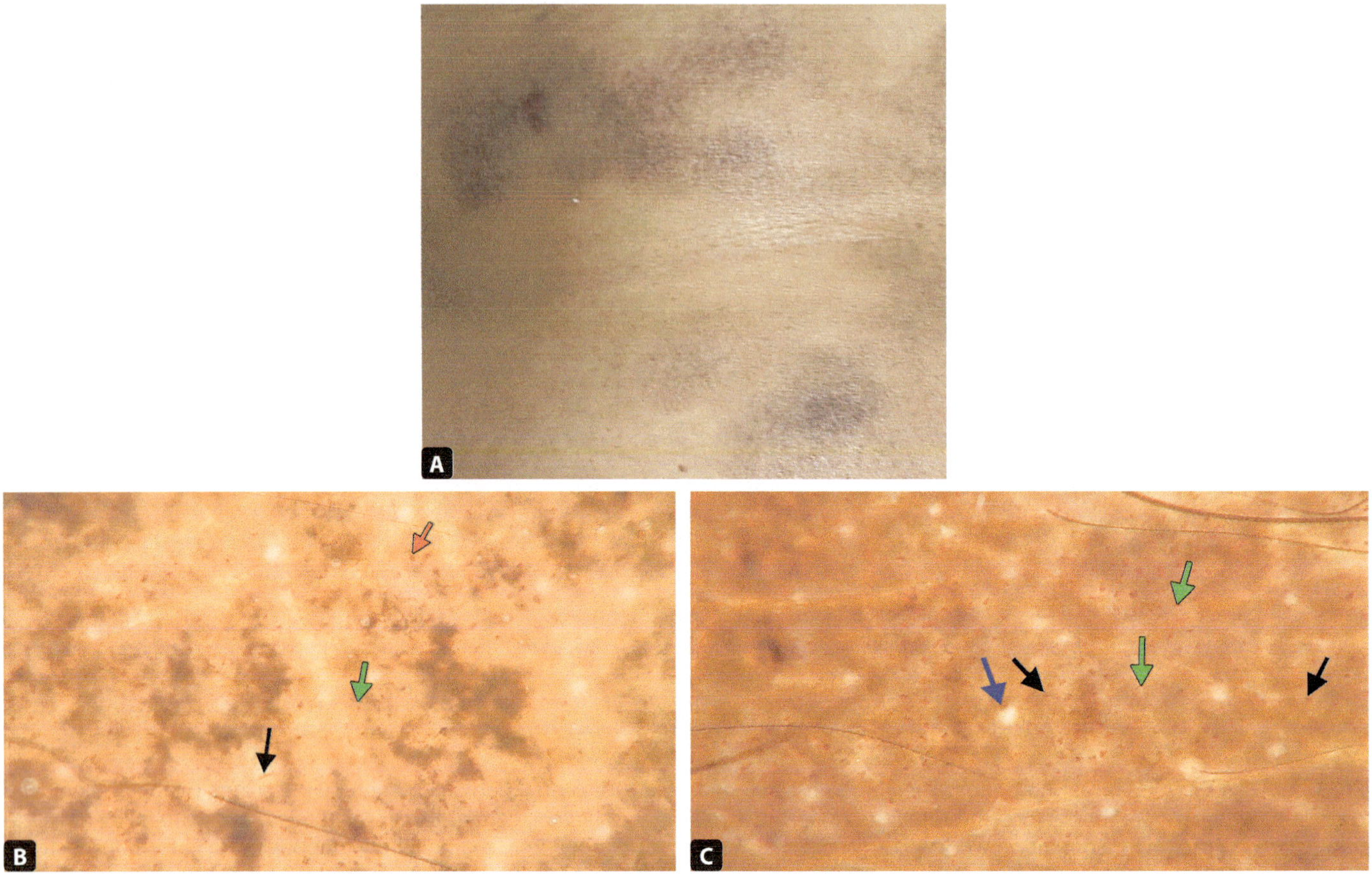

FIGS. 22A TO C: (A) Clinical photograph showing mycosis fungoides with dull erythematous xerotic macules over abdomen. Histopathology was suggestive of CD8+; (B) Dermoscopic image showing scattered red dots (green arrow), occasional spermatozoa-like vessels (red arrow) and linear vessels (black arrow) on an orange-yellow background with bluish-gray globules and structureless white areas (nonpolarized, FotoFinder Systems, 20×); (C) Dermoscopic image showing predominant red dots (black arrows), occasional linear vessels (green arrows) with white globules (blue arrow) on an orange-yellow background (nonpolarized, FotoFinder Systems, 20×).

Courtesy: Department of Dermatology, CMC, Vellore, Tamil Nadu, India.

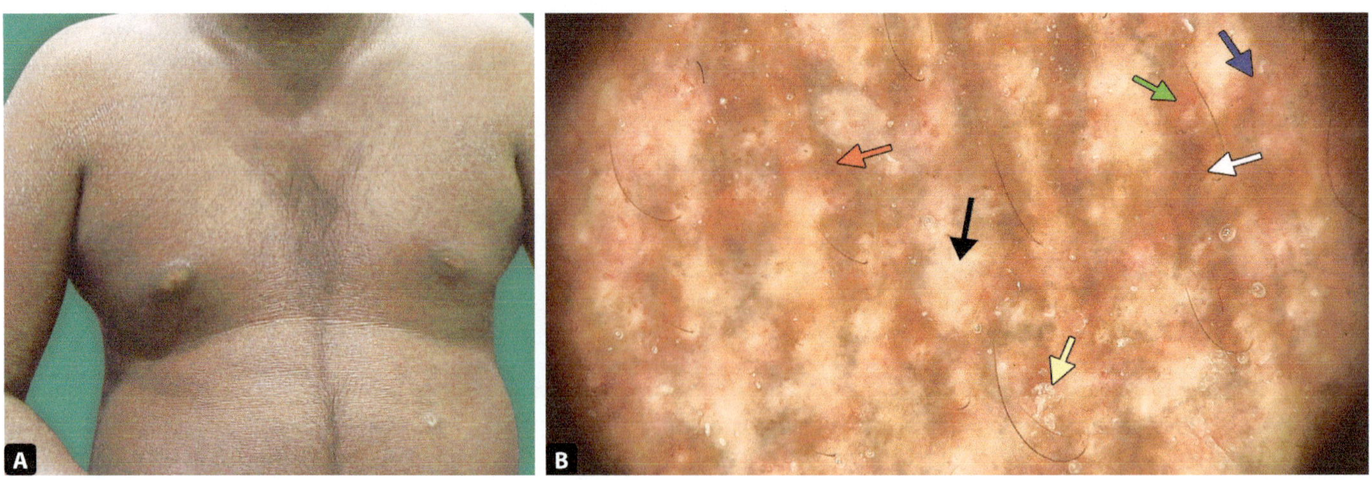

FIGS. 23A AND B: (A) Clinical photograph of an erythrodermic mycosis fungoides; (B) Dermoscopic image showing dotted (red arrow), linear vessels (light green arrow), and occasional spermatozoa-like structures (white arrow), structureless white areas (black arrow), few white scales (yellow arrow) and milky-red areas (blue arrow) (nonpolarized, FotoFinder Systems, 20×).

Courtesy: Department of Dermatology, CMC, Vellore, Tamil Nadu, India.

Cutaneous Metastasis

Clinical Features

Cutaneous metastasis may develop rarely in patients with solid tumor. Skin metastases may represent the first sign of extranodal disease in 7.6% of patients with a primary oncologic diagnosis.[41] The clinical presentation of cutaneous metastases could be skin-colored or erythematous solitary or multiple nodules, plaques, ulcers (**Fig. 25A** and **Fig. 26A**). The common differential diagnoses include cysts, lipoma, fibroma, or appendageal tumors.

Dermoscopic Features

The most common dermoscopic finding seen with cutaneous metastasis is a vascular pattern. Discrete vessels were observed in 88%, most frequent subtype being serpentine (or linear irregular vessels), seen in 77%, followed by arborizing vessels in 53%, dotted vessels and comma-shaped vessels.[42] The presence of pigmented metastases, in the absence of a history of melanoma, may suggest a primary breast carcinoma.[42] Dermoscopy showing vascular structures within a cutaneous nodule in patients with a known cancer diagnosis should raise suspicion for cutaneous metastasis (**Fig. 25B,** and **Figs. 26B** and **C**).[42]

Key Points

- A vascular pattern is a characteristic finding in cutaneous metastasis.

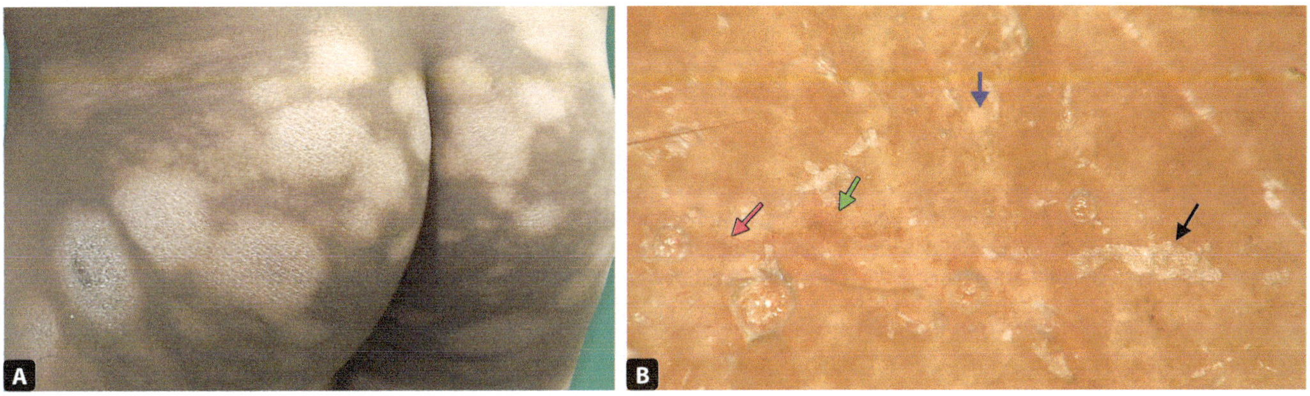

FIGS. 24A AND B: (A) Clinical photograph showing hypopigmented xerotic patches of mycosis fungoides over low back and gluteal region. Histopathology was suggestive of CD8⁺; (B) Dermoscopic image showing white scales (black arrow), linear vessels (pink arrow) and occasional dotted vessels (green arrow), white globules (blue arrow) over an orange-yellow background (nonpolarized, FotoFinder Systems, 20×).

Courtesy: Department of Dermatology, CMC, Vellore, Tamil Nadu, India.

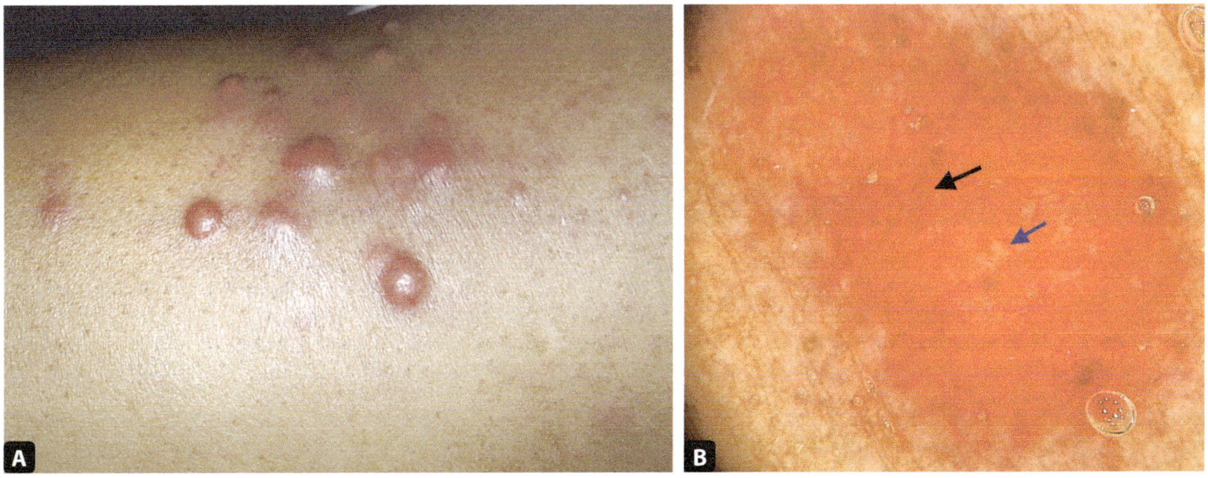

FIGS. 25A AND B: (A) Clinical photograph of metastatic breast carcinoma with erythematous nodules over forearm; (B) Dermoscopic image of metastatic breast carcinoma showing arborizing vessels (black arrow) in the periphery and linear irregular vessels (blue arrow) at the center over a bright red background (nonpolarized, FotoFinder Systems, 20×).

Courtesy: Department of Dermatology, CMC, Vellore, Tamil Nadu, India.

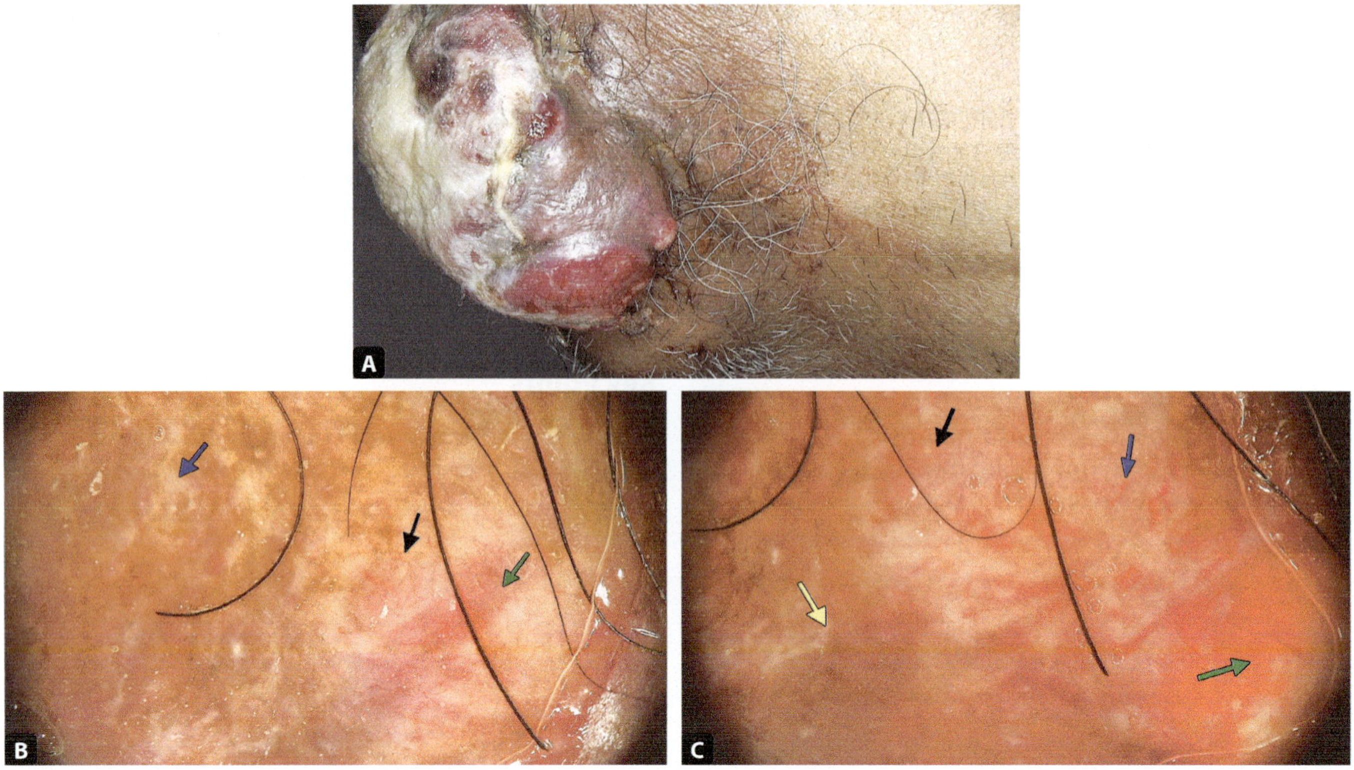

FIGS. 26A TO C: (A) Clinical photograph of salivary duct carcinoma with ulcerated nodule over left parotid region; (B) Dermoscopic image of salivary duct carcinoma showing thin arborizing vessels (black arrow), milky-red areas (green arrow), and white structureless areas (blue arrow) (nonpolarized, FotoFinder Systems, 20×); (C) Dermoscopic image of salivary duct carcinoma showing unfocused linear serpentine vessels (blue arrow) and thin arborizing (black arrow) vessels over a milky-red background with white structureless areas (yellow arrow) and ulceration (green arrow) (nonpolarized, FotoFinder Systems, 20×).

Courtesy: Department of Dermatology, CMC, Vellore, Tamil Nadu, India.

KEY POINTS

- Dermoscopy, being non-invasive acts as a quick adjunctive diagnostic tool. Specific and definitive patterns are observed in majority of premalignant and malignant tumors.
- Dermoscopy guided biopsy would yield accurate histopathological findings. Accurate grading of lesions cannot be done.

CONCLUSION

Dermoscopy is a valuable tool for the early diagnosis of several premalignant and malignant lesions. It also serves as a guide to select an appropriate area for performing skin biopsy.

REFERENCES

1. Glogau RG. The risk of progression to invasive disease. J Am Acad Dermatol. 2000;42:23-4.
2. Zalaudek I, Argenziano G. Dermoscopy of actinic keratosis, intraepidermal carcinoma and squamous cell carcinoma. Curr Probl Dermatol. 2015;46:70-6.
3. Peris K, Micantonio T, Piccolo D, Concetta M. Dermoscopic features of actinic keratosis. J Dtsch Dermatol Ges. 2007;5:970-6.
4. Akay BN, Kocyigit P, Heper AO, Erdem C. Dermatoscopy of flat facial lesions: diagnostic challenge between pigmented actinic keratosis and lentigo maligna. Br J Dermatol. 2010;163:1212-7.
5. Kelati A, Baybay H, Moscarella E, Argenziano G, Gallouj S, Mernissi FZ. Dermoscopy of pigmented actinic keratosis of the face: a study of 232 cases. Actas Dermosifiliogr. 2017;108:844-51.
6. Bhat YJ, Bashir S, Wani R, Hassan I. Dermoscopy of Bowen's disease. Indian J Dermatopathol Diagn Dermatol. 2019;6:60-1.
7. Zalaudek I, Argenziano G, Leinweber B, Citarella L, Hofmann-Wellenhof R, Malvehy J, et al. Dermoscopy of Bowen's disease. Br J Dermatol. 2004;150: 1112-6.
8. Yang Y, Lin J, Fang S, Han S, Song Z. What's new in dermoscopy of Bowen's disease: two new dermoscopic signs and its differential diagnosis. Int J Dermatol. 2017;56:1022-5.
9. Rosendahl C, Cameron A, Argenziano G, Zalaudek I, Tschandl P, Kittler H. Dermoscopy of squamous cell carcinoma and keratoacanthoma. Arch Dermatol. 2012;148(12):1386-92.
10. Kwiek B, Schwartz RA. Keratoacanthoma (KA): an update and review. J Am Acad Dermatol. 2016;74:1220-33.
11. Zalaudek I, Giacomel J, Schmid K, Bondino S, Rosendahl C, Cavicchini S, et al. Dermatoscopy of facial actinic keratosis, intraepidermal carcinoma, and invasive squamous cell carcinoma: a progression model. J Am Acad Dermatol. 2012;66:589-97.
12. Chandrashekhar L, Behera B. Dermoscopy of malignant cutaneous tumors. In: Chatterjee M, Neema S, Malakar S (Eds). Dermoscopy in Darker Skin. New Delhi: Jaypee Brothers Medical Publishers (P) Ltd; 2017. pp. 81-5.

13. Hanan MS, Manal MM, Azza EM. Dermoscopic criteria of squamous cell carcinoma in relation to clinical variant and histopathologic differentiation grade. J Egypt Womens Dermatol Soc. 2020;17:83-90.
14. Ankad BS, Sakhare PS, Prabhu MH. Dermoscopy of non-melanocytic and pink tumors in brown skin: a descriptive study. Indian J Dermatopathol Diagn Dermatol. 2017;4:41-51.
15. Fania L, Didona D, Di Pietro FR, Verkhovskaia S, Morese R, Paolino G, et al. Cutaneous squamous cell carcinoma: from pathophysiology to novel therapeutic approaches. Biomedicines. 2021;9:171.
16. Lallas A, Pyne J, Kyrgidis A, Andreani S, Argenziano G, Cavaller A, et al. The clinical and dermoscopic features of invasive cutaneous squamous cell carcinoma depend on the histopathological grade of differentiation. Br J Dermatol. 2015;172:1308-15.
17. Popadic M. Dermoscopic features in different morphologic types of basal cell carcinoma. Dermatol Surg. 2014;40:725-32.
18. Lallas A, Apalla Z, Argenziano G, Longo C, Moscarella E, Specchio F, et al. The dermatoscopic universe of basal cell carcinoma. Dermatol Pract Concept. 2014;4:11-24.
19. Menzies SW, Westerhoff K, Rabinovitz H, Kopf AW, McCarthy WH, Katz B, et al. Surface microscopy of pigmented basal cell carcinoma. Arch Dermatol. 2000;136:1012-6.
20. Altamura D, Menzies SW, Argenziano G, Zalaudek I, Soyer HP, Sera F, et al. Dermatoscopy of basal cell carcinoma: morphologic variability of global and local features and accuracy of diagnosis. J Am Acad Dermatol. 2010;62: 67-75.
21. Rosendahl C, Tschandl P, Cameron A, Kittler H. Diagnostic accuracy of dermatoscopy for melanocytic and nonmelanocytic pigmented lesions. J Am Acad Dermatol. 2011;64:1068-73.
22. Zalaudek I, Moscarella E, Longo C, Pace BD, Argenziano G. The 'signature' pattern of multiple basal cell carcinomas. Arch Dermatol. 2012;148:1106-7.
23. Wozniak-Rito A, Zalaudek I, Rudnicka L. Dermoscopy of basal cell carcinoma. Clin Exp Dermatol. 2018;43:241-7.
24. Matas-Nadal C, Malvehy J, Ferreres JR, Boada A, Bodet D, Segura S, et al. Increasing incidence of lentigo maligna and lentigo maligna melanoma in Catalonia. Int J Dermatol. 2019;58:577-81.
25. Teramoto Y, Keim U, Gesierich A, Schuler G, Fiedler E, Tuting T, et al. Acral lentiginous melanoma: a skin cancer with unfavorable prognostic features. A study of the German central malignant melanoma registry (CMMR) in 2050 patients. Br J Dermatol. 2018;178:443-51.
26. Goodson AG, Grossman D. Strategies for early melanoma detection: approaches to the patient with nevi. J Am Acad Dermatol. 2009;60:719-38.
27. Garbe C, Amaral T, Peris K, Hauschild A, Arenberger P, Bastholt L, et al. European consensus-based interdisciplinary guideline for melanoma. Part 1: Diagnostics - Update 2019. Eur J Cancer. 2020;126:141-58.
28. Russo T, Piccolo V, Lallas A, Jacomel J, Moscarella E, Alfano R, et al. Dermoscopy of malignant skin tumours: what's new?" Dermatology. 2017;233:64-73.
29. Zaballos P, Del Pozo LJ, Argenziano G, Medina C, Lacarrubba F, Ferrer B, et al. Dermoscopy of cutaneous smooth muscle neoplasms: a morphological study of 136 cases. J Eur Acad Dermatol Venereol. 2019;33:693-9.
30. De Giorgi V, Scarfi F, Silvestri F, Maida P, Gori A, Trane L, et al. Cutaneous leiomyosarcoma: a clinical, dermoscopic, pathologic case study. Exp Oncol. 2019;41:80-1.
31. Atzori L, Pilloni L, Zanniello R, Ferreli C, Rongioletti F. Clear-cell variant of superficial cutaneous leiomyosarcoma associated with RB1 mutation: clinical, dermoscopic, and histopathological characteristics. J Cutan Pathol. 2020;47:571-5.
32. Bernard J, Poulalhon N, Argenziano G, Debarbieux S, Dalle S, Thomas L. Dermoscopy of dermatofibrosarcoma protuberans: a study of 15 cases. Br J Dermatol. 2013;169:85-90.
33. Harting MS, Ludgate MW, Fullen DR, Johnson TM, Bichakjian CK. Dermatoscopic vascular patterns in cutaneous Merkel cell carcinoma. J Am Acad Dermatol. 2012;66:923-7.
34. Dalle S, Parmentier L, Moscarella E, Phan A, Argenziano G, Thomas L. Dermoscopy of Merkel cell carcinoma. Dermatology. 2012;224:140-4.
35. Jalilian C, Chamberlain AJ, Haskett M, Rosendahl C, Goh M, Beck H, et al. Clinical and dermoscopic characteristics of Merkel cell carcinoma. Br J Dermatol. 2013;169:294-7.
36. Suarez AL, Louis P, Kitts J, Busam K, Myskowski PL, Wong RJ, et al. Clinical and dermoscopic features of combined cutaneous squamous cell carcinoma (SCC)/neuroendocrine [Merkel cell] carcinoma (MCC). J Am Acad Dermatol. 2015;73:968-75.
37. Lallas A, Apalla Z, Lefaki I, Tzellos T, Karatolias A, Sotiriou E, et al. Dermoscopy of early stage mycosis fungoides. J Eur Acad Dermatol Venereol. 2013;27: 617-21.
38. Xu C, Liu J, Wang T, Luo Y, Liu Y. Dermoscopic patterns of early-stage mycosis fungoides in a Chinese population. Clin Exp Dermatol. 2019;44(2):169-75.
39. Bilgic SA, Cicek D, Demir B. Dermoscopy in differential diagnosis of inflammatory dermatoses and mycosis fungoides. Int J Dermatol. 2020;59(7):843-50.
40. Ghahramani GK, Goetz KE, Liu V. Dermoscopic characterization of cutaneous lymphomas: a pilot survey. Int J Dermatol. 2018;57(3):339-43.
41. Lookingbill DP, Spangler N, Helm KF. Cutaneous metastases in patients with metastatic carcinoma: a retrospective study of 4020 patients. J Am Acad Dermatol. 1993;29:228-36.
42. Chernoff KA, Marghoob AA, Lacouture ME, Deng L, Busam KJ, Myskowski PL. Dermoscopic findings in cutaneous metastases. JAMA Dermatol. 2014;150(4):429-33.

15 CHAPTER

Nevi and Nevoid Disorders

Kinjal D Rambhia, Balachandra S Ankad, Yasmeen J Bhat

INTRODUCTION

Dermoscopy is a noninvasive technique for visualization of subsurface structures. It is a valuable aid in the diagnosis of keratinocytic and melanocytic nevi. It is a noninvasive, painless, quick tool to aid the clinician in diagnosis of nevi and may prove useful to avoid biopsies.

KERATINOCYTIC NEVI

Epidermal Nevus

Verrucous Epidermal Nevus

Clinical Features

Verrucous epidermal nevus (VEN) is a benign cutaneous hamartoma usually present at birth. Clinically, VEN is characterized by well-defined skin-colored to brown papules coalescing to plaques (**Figs. 1A** and **2A**).

Dermoscopic Features

The common dermoscopic features are large thick brown circles on a brownish background, thick brown-branched lines, and terminal hair.[1] The large brown circles correlate with the dermal papillae. Other findings include brown globules, brown dots forming lines, serpiginous brown dots, white and brown exophytic papillary structures, fine scale, thick adherent scale, and cerebriform structures (**Figs. 1B** and **C**, and **Fig. 2B**). Dotted vessels are the most common vascular finding.

Key Points

- Large thick brown circles on a brownish background
- Thick brown branched lines

Inflammatory Linear Verrucous Epidermal Nevus

Clinical Features

Inflammatory linear verrucous epidermal nevus (ILVEN) is an uncommon variant of keratinocytic epidermal nevus that clinically presents as linear erythematous and verrucous papules and plaques (**Fig. 3A**).

Dermoscopic Features

Dermoscopic features of ILVEN are alternating red and brown glomerular-type structures over a white background (**Figs. 3B** and **C**).[2]

Key Points

- Alternating red and brown glomerular type structures over a white background.

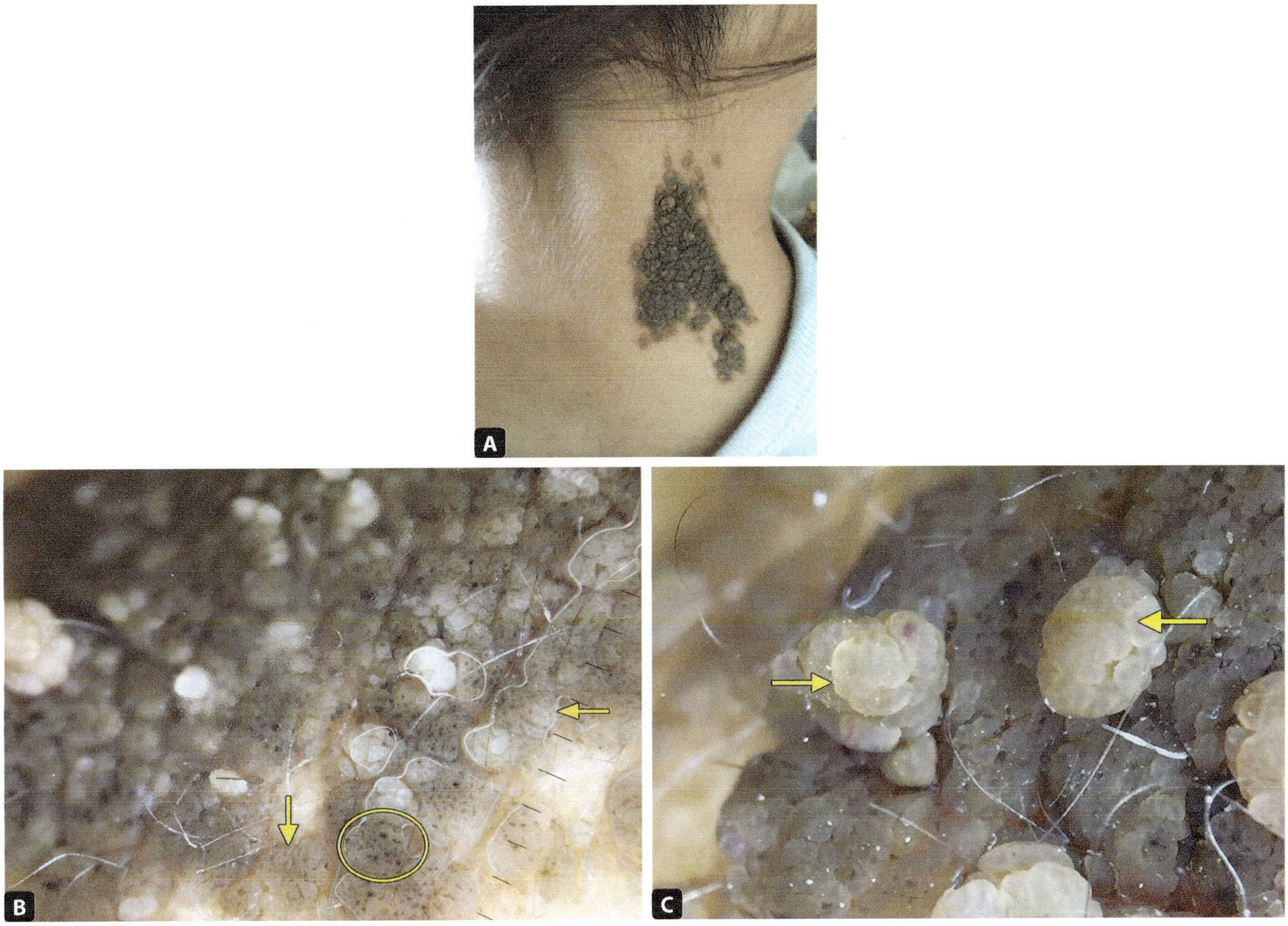

FIGS. 1A TO C: (A) Clinical image of verrucous epidermal nevus showing hyperpigmented verrucous papules coalescing to form plaques; (B) Dermoscopy showing large thick brown circles (arrows) on a brownish background, thick brown-branched lines, and brown globules (circle) (polarized, DermLite DL3N, 10×); (C) Dermoscopy showing white and brown exophytic papillary structures (arrows) and terminal hair (polarized, DermLite DL3N, 10×).

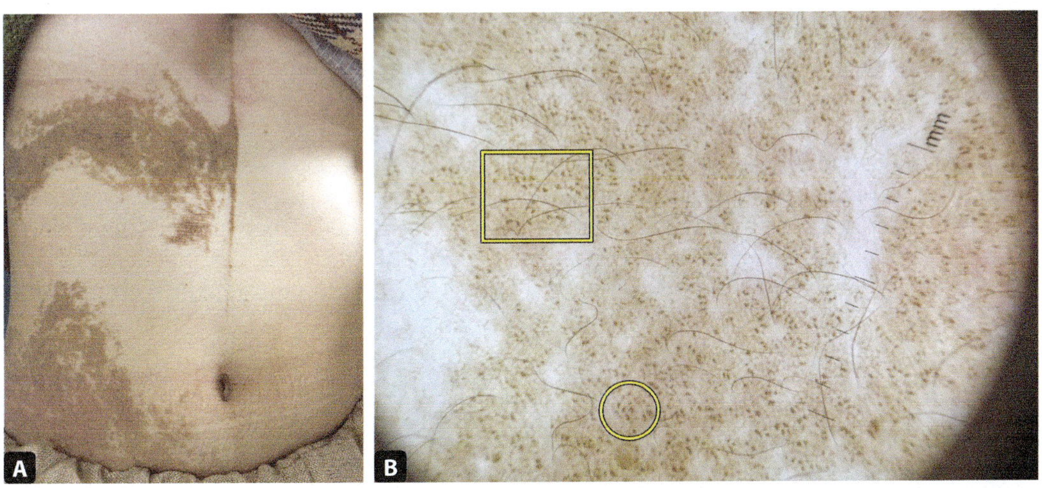

FIGS. 2A AND B: (A) Clinical image of verrucous epidermal nevus showing hyperpigmented verrucous papules coalescing to form plaques in Blaschkoid pattern; (B) Dermoscopy showing scattered brown globules and dots (circle) and few of them are forming lines, serpiginous tracks (box) on a faint brownish background (polarized, DermLite DL3N, 10×).

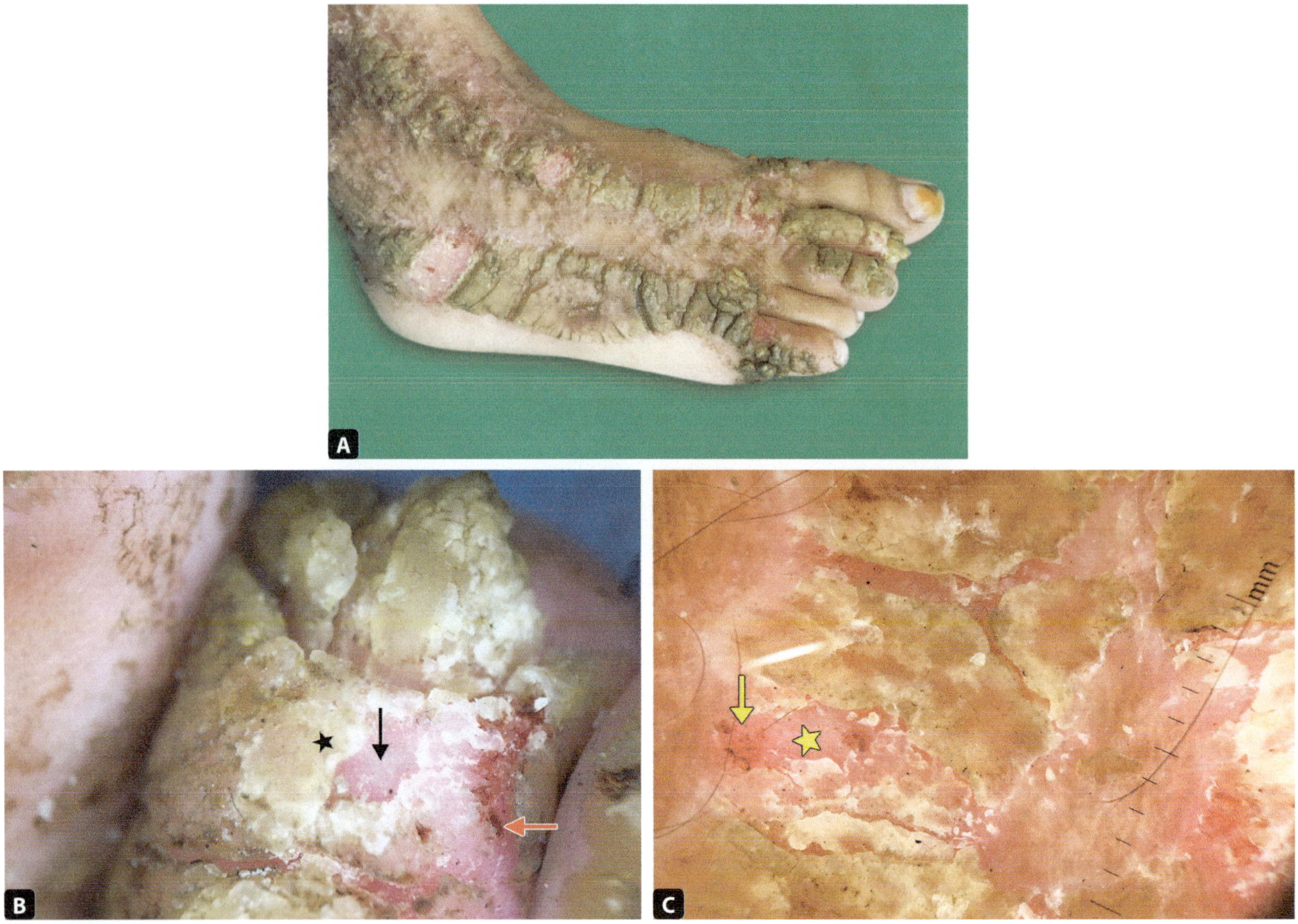

FIGS. 3A TO C: (A) Clinical image of inflammatory linear verrucous epidermal nevus showing linear erythematous papules and plaques on the foot; (B) Dermoscopy of inflammatory linear verrucous epidermal nevus showing alternating red and brown glomerular-type structures (red arrow) over a whitish pink background (black arrow) with whitish keratotic structures (black star) (polarized, DermLite DL3N, 10×); (C) Dermoscopy of inflammatory linear verrucous epidermal nevus showing alternating red and brown glomerular-type structures (arrow) over a whitish pink background (star) (polarized, DermLite DL3N, 10×).

Nevus Sebaceous

Clinical Features

Nevus Sebaceous (NS) of Jadassohn is a benign asymptomatic hamartomatous lesion present since birth. In infantile stage, it presents as smooth yellowish alopecic plaque, becomes verrucous or mamillated at puberty and in the final stage it is characterized by nodular or tumoral appearance with peripheral telangiectasias (**Fig. 4A**).[3]

Dermoscopic Features

Infantile stage of NS reveals yellow lobed structures, bright yellow spots not associated with hair follicles. At this stage, it may be difficult to differentiate from aplasia cutis congenita.[4]

In childhood stage, there are yellowish globules seen in a cobblestone pattern, corresponding histopathologically to the hyperplastic sebaceous glands in the dermis. Crown vessels are seen occasionally due to vessels pushed to the periphery by the sebaceous glands.

In adult stage of NS, fissures and ridges arranged in cerebriform pattern, brown globules (**Fig. 4B**).[5]

Regular dermoscopic examination helps to detect benign and malignant neoplasms occurring on the adult NS. Arborizing telangiectasia, white structures and blue gray globules on tumorous growth are seen on dermoscopy of nodular basal cell carcinoma (BCC) arising within NS.[5]

Key Points

- Yellow lobed structures, bright yellow spots in infantile stage of NS
- Yellowish globules in cobblestone pattern in childhood stage of NS
- Brown globules, fissures and ridges in cerebriform pattern in adult stage of NS

Nevus Comedonicus

Clinical Features

Nevus comedonicus (NC) is a rare variant of epidermal nevus presenting as grouped dilated follicular openings with keratotic plugging arranged in unilateral, bilateral, linear, interrupted, segmental, or Blaschkoid pattern (**Fig. 5A**).[6]

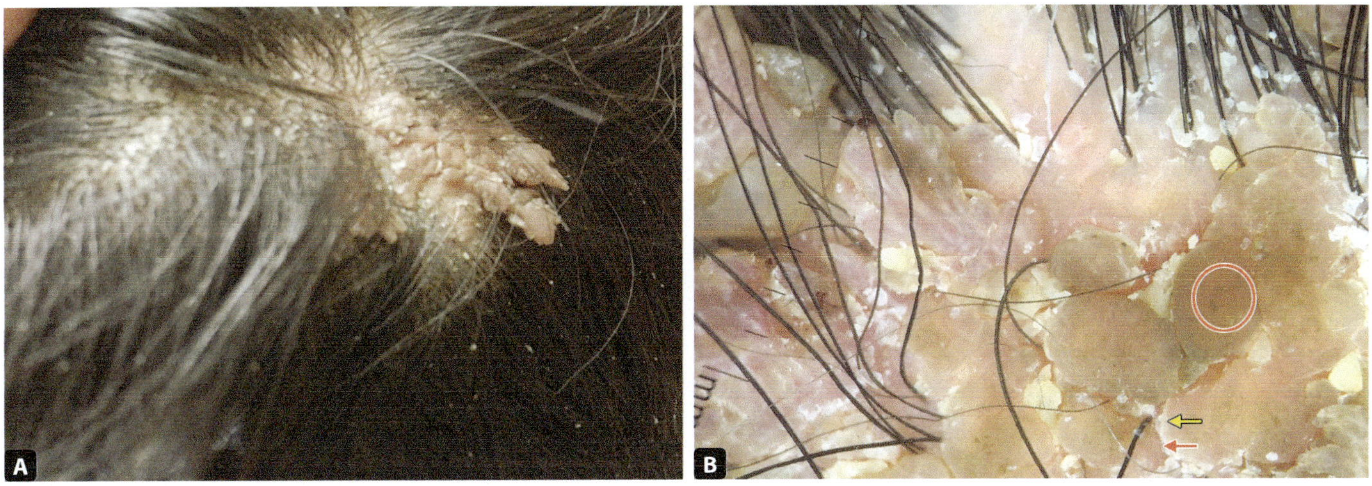

FIGS. 4A AND B: (A) Nevus sebaceous showing alopecic verrucous plaque over the scalp; (B) Dermoscopy showing yellowish globules, fissures (red arrow) and ridges (yellow arrow) arranged in cerebriform pattern, and brown globules (red circle) are seen (polarized, DermLite DL3N, 10×).

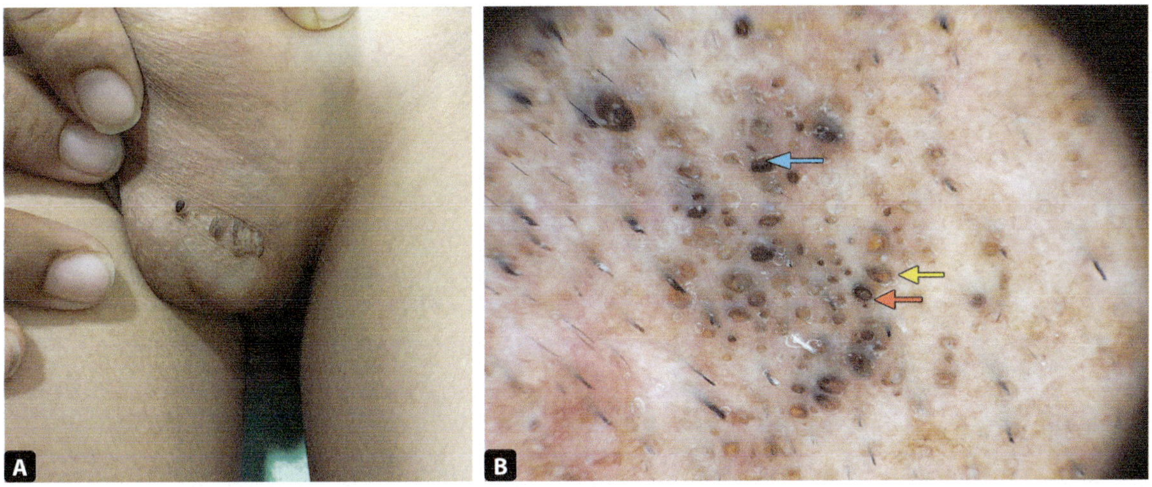

FIGS. 5A AND B: (A) Representative image of nevus comedonicus; (B) Dermoscopy of nevus comedonicus shows circular and barrel-shaped light (yellow arrow) and dark brownish (red arrow) structureless with keratinous plugs (blue arrow) (polarized, DermLite DL4, 10×).
Courtesy (Fig. A): Dr Swapnil Shah, Professor, Ashwini Rural Medical College, Solapur, Maharashtra, India.

Dermoscopic Features

It shows well-defined circular and barrel-shaped light and dark brownish structureless homogeneous areas with sharply demarcated keratinous plugs (**Fig. 5B**).[7,8]

Key Points

- Brownish structureless homogeneous areas with keratinous plugs

MELANOCYTIC NEVI

Congenital Melanocytic Nevi

Clinical Features

Congenital melanocytic nevi (CMN) are benign hamartomatous proliferations of melanocytes. They may be small-sized, medium-sized or large giant nevi (**Figs. 6A**, **7A**, and **8A**). They appear as pigmented nodules.

Dermoscopic Features

Large CMN show reticular-globular and cobblestone pattern. Other findings include atypical dots/globules, focal hypopigmentation, and perifollicular hypopigmentation. Medium-sized nevi show focal hypopigmentation, atypical dots, globules and milia-like cysts. Small-sized nevi show focal hypopigmentation, atypical dots, and globules (**Figs. 6B, 7B,** and **8B**). The presence of atypical dots/globules, asymmetry, and hypertrichosis correlates with the size of CMN.[9]

Key Points

- Globular, reticuloglobular, and cobblestone pattern.

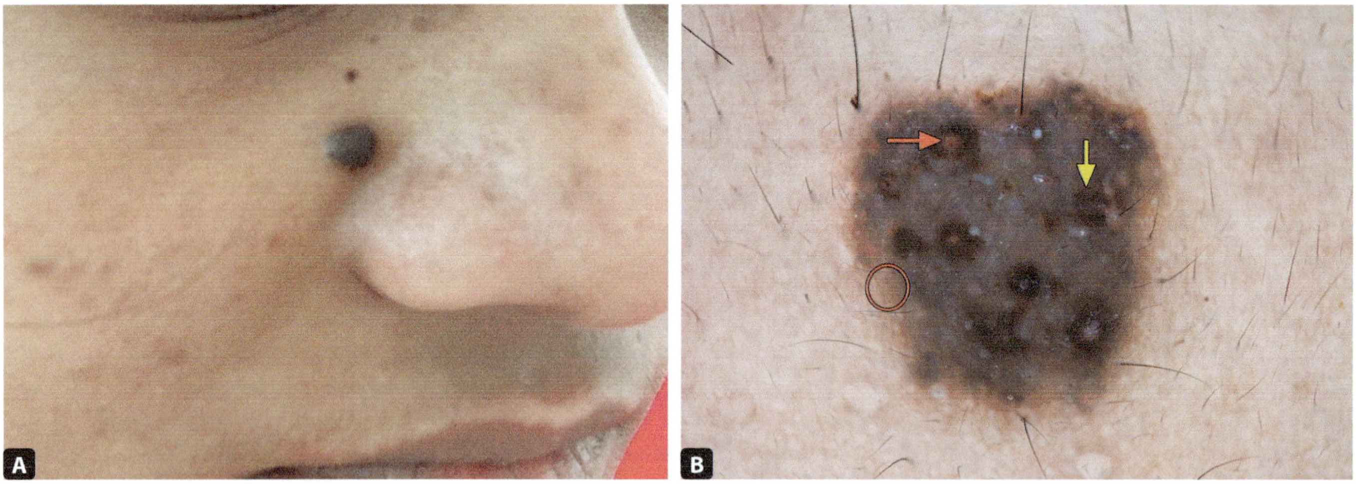

FIGS. 6A AND B: (A) Clinical image of congenital melanocytic nevus showing hyperpigmented papule on the nasolabial fold; (B) Dermoscopy of congenital melanocytic nevus shows pigment globules, focal hypopigmentation (red circle), perifollicular hypopigmentation (red arrow), and atypical globules (yellow arrow) (polarized, Illuco IDS, 10×).

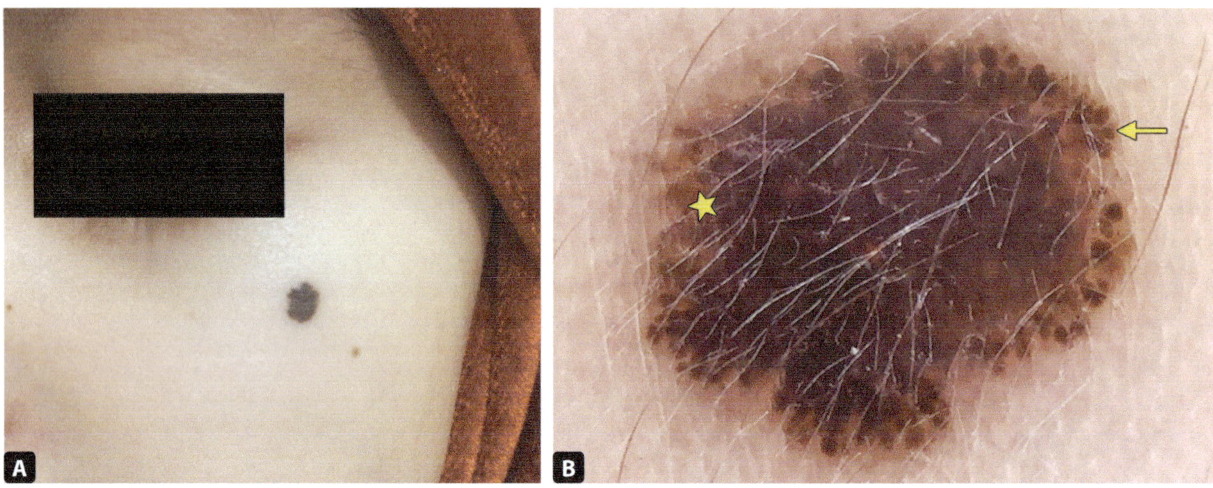

FIGS. 7A AND B: (A) Clinical image of congenital melanocytic nevus showing hyperpigmented papule on the cheek; (B) Dermoscopy of a small-sized nevus showing reticuloglobular pattern (star) and brown globules (arrow) arranged symmetrically at the periphery of the lesion (polarized, DermLite DL3N, 10×).

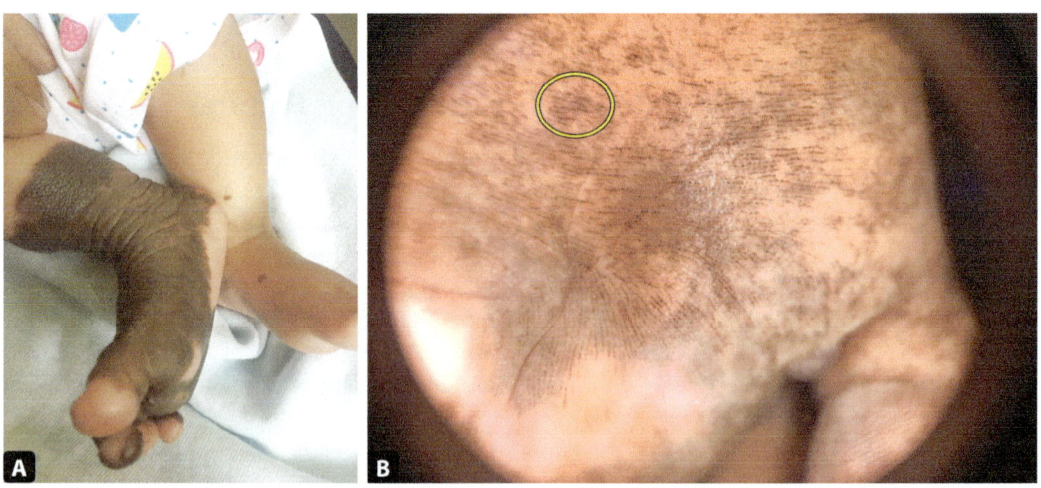

FIGS. 8A AND B: (A) Large giant congenital melanocytic nevus on the lower extremity of an infant; (B) Dermoscopy showing brown dots and globules arranged linearly in parallel fissure pattern (circle) (polarized, DermLite DL3N, 10×).

Acquired Melanocytic Nevi

Clinical Features

Acquired melanocytic nevi are benign melanocytic nevi and are classified as junctional (**Fig. 9A**), compound (**Fig. 10A**), and intradermal (**Fig. 11A**) nevi.

Dermoscopic Features

Junctional Nevus

It includes a light or dark brown honeycomb-like (network-like) pattern in a uniform distribution. The lines of the network are of uniform length and width; and the center is darker as compared to the periphery of the lesion (**Fig. 9B**). Small brown-black dots, globules, and heavy pigmentation may be present in the center and obscures the network at times. Reticular pattern is also commonly seen in junctional nevus.

Compound Nevus

Globular pattern characterized by homogeneous globules distributed uniformly throughout the lesion which corresponds to nests of pigmented melanocytes (**Fig. 10B**). Closely aggregated large regular globules form the cobblestone pattern. Homogeneous pattern may be seen.

Intradermal Nevus

Vascular structures like curvilinear streaks in mosaic arrangement around milia-like cysts are seen in intradermal nevi (**Fig. 11B**).[10]

Acral Nevus

It shows fissure pattern of pigment globules where in globules are mainly located in the fissures. The arrangement of globules can be lattice, branching or fibrillar pattern (**Figs. 12A** and **B**).

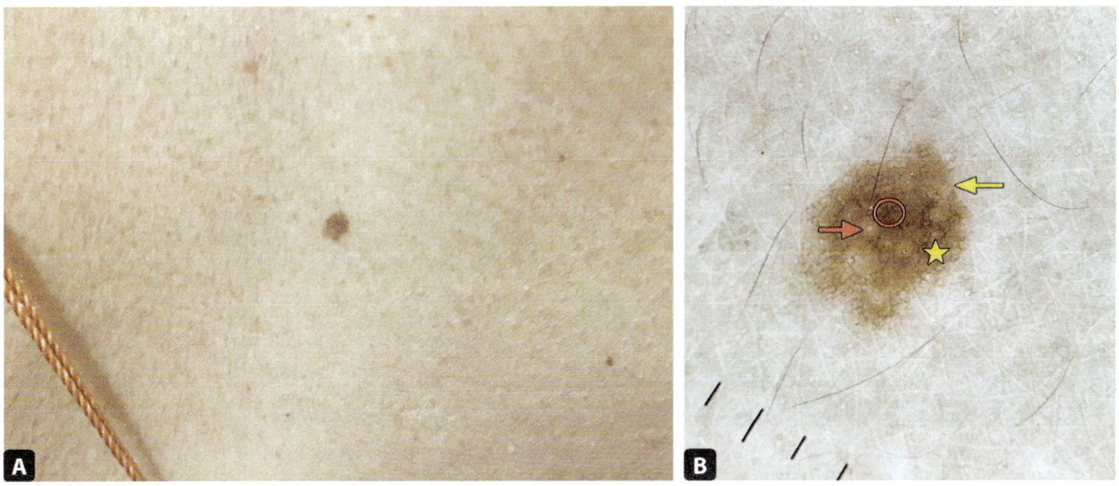

FIGS. 9A AND B: (A) Clinical image of junctional nevus showing ill-defined brown flat macule over the trunk; (B) Dermoscopy of junctional melanocytic nevus shows dark brown pigment network with uniform lines (yellow star), perifollicular hypopigmentation (red arrow), and central darker globules (red circle). Note the fading of borders in the normal skin (yellow arrow) (polarized, Illuco IDS, 10×).

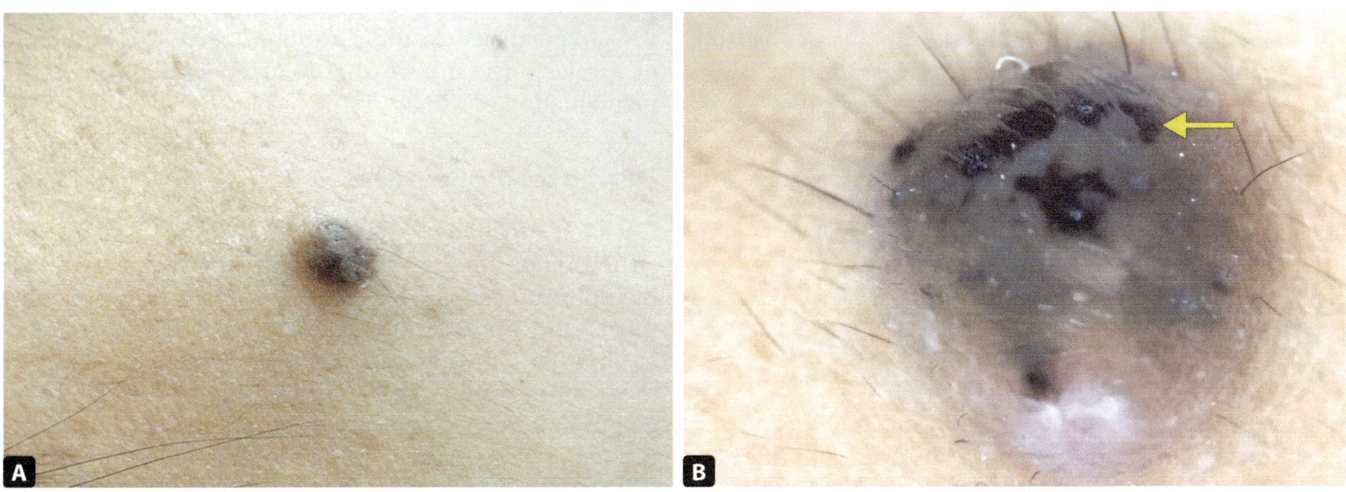

FIGS. 10A AND B: (A) Clinical image of compound melanocytic nevus shows pigmented nodule; (B) Dermoscopy of compound melanocytic nevus shows bluish-black pigment globules in a uniform distribution (yellow arrow) (polarized, DermLite DL4, 10×).
Courtesy: Dr Shashikumar BM, Associate Professor, Mandya Institute of Medical Sciences, Mandya, Karnataka, India.

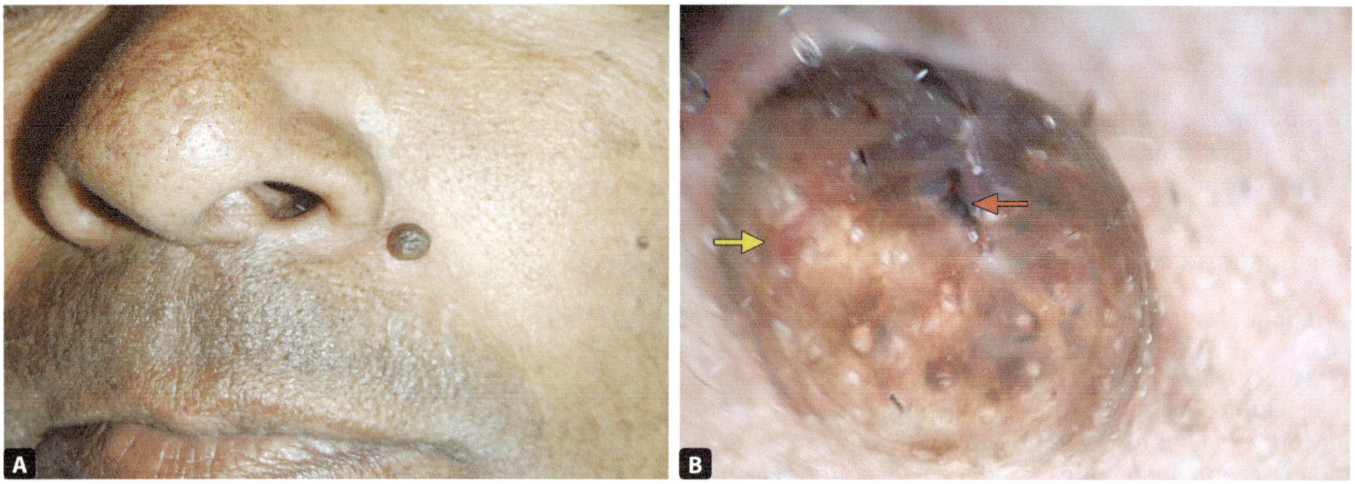

FIGS. 11A AND B: (A) Clinical image of intradermal melanocytic nevus shows nodule with less pigmentation; (B) Dermoscopy of intradermal melanocytic nevus shows curvilinear vessels (yellow arrow) with minimal pigment globules (red arrow) (polarized, Illuco IDS, 10×).

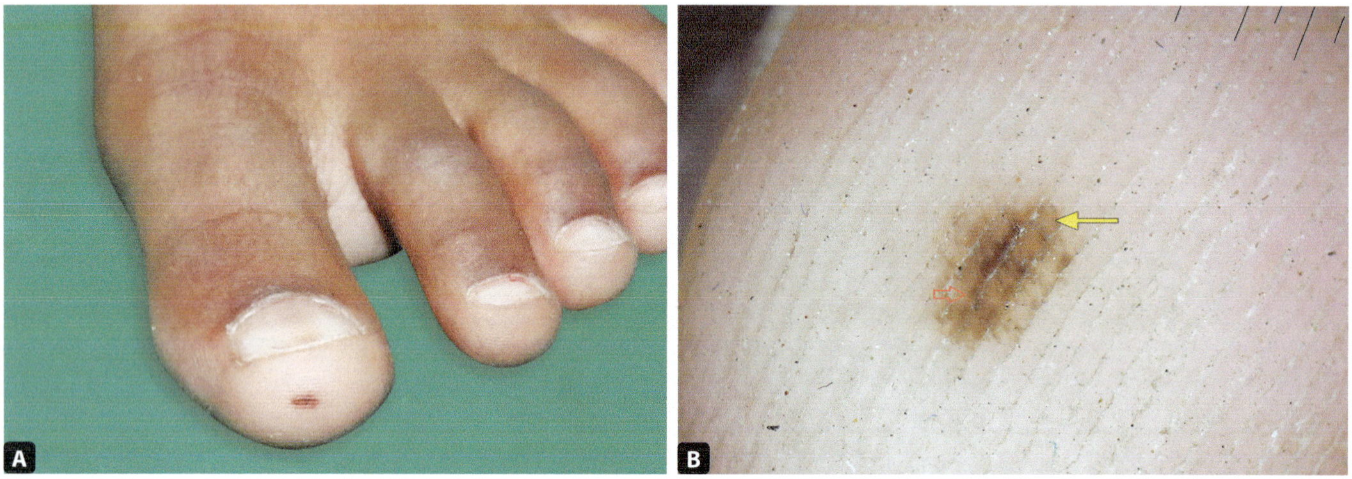

FIGS. 12A AND B: (A) Clinical image of acral melanocytic nevus shows pigmented lesion on the great toe; (B) Dermoscopy of acral melanocytic nevus shows fissure pattern of pigment globules (red arrow) with fibrillar pattern of pigmentation (yellow arrow) (polarized, DermLite Foto Pro II, 10×).

Unna Nevus

It shows globular pattern or cobblestone pattern consisting of large angulated globular structures (**Figs. 13A** and **B**).

Key Points

- Reticular pattern, globular pattern, and honeycomb-like pattern are seen in acquired melanocytic nevi.

Blue Nevus

Clinical Features

Blue nevus (BN) or dermal melanocytoma is characterized by solitary small, well-defined, round to oval shaped, flat to slightly-elevated papule with a predominant steel blue color seen on the extremities, face (**Fig. 14A**), and trunk. The clinical variants include common BN, cellular BN, malignant BN, large patch/plaque lesions, combined BN, atypical nevus, and eruptive BN.[11] The blue color of the lesion is due to the deeper location of melanin pigmentation.

Dermoscopic Features

Absence of pigment network with homogeneous and structureless blue pigmentation (other color variations include white-blue, steel blue-gray, blue-brown or blue-black, and multichromatic pattern). The pigmentation is confluent throughout the lesion and fades away at the periphery (**Fig. 14B**). Other findings include bluish globules, dots, network-like structures or peripheral out-of-focus streaks corresponding to pigmented projections of the nevus cells or melanophages within the deeper dermis.[12]

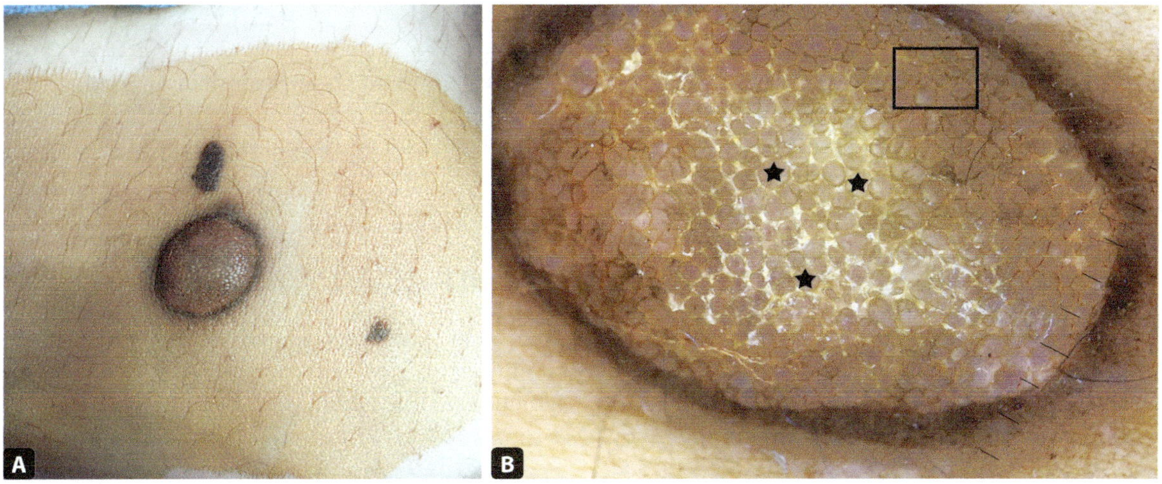

FIGS. 13A AND B: (A) Clinical image of Unna nevus showing soft, polypoid skin-colored nodule; (B) Dermoscopy showing numerous light brown globules (stars) distributed uniformly in a cobblestone pattern (box) (polarized, DermLite DL3N, 10×).

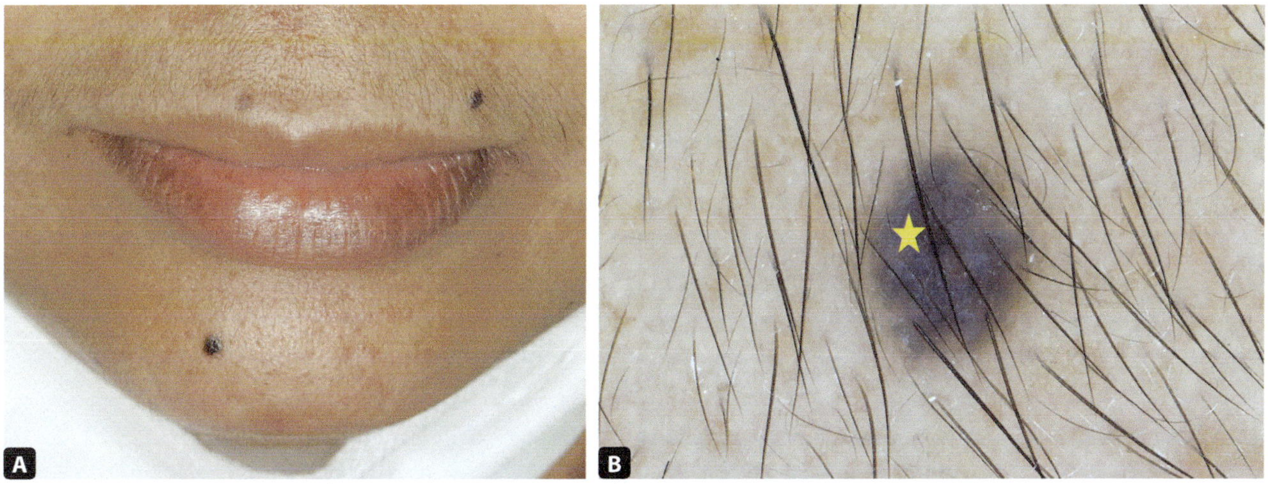

FIGS. 14A AND B: (A) Clinical image of blue nevus shows bluish papule over the chin; (B) Dermoscopy of blue nevus shows homogeneous steel blue (star) area covering the entire lesion (polarized, DermLite Foto Pro II, 10×).

Key Points

- Absence of pigment network, homogeneous structureless blue pigmentation, and multichromatic patterns.

Spitz Nevus

Clinical Features

Spitz nevi (SN) are benign melanocytic proliferations usually occurring in children and young adults, characterized as solitary, asymptomatic, round to oval, skin-colored or pinkish dome-shaped, papule or nodule on the head, neck or extremities (**Fig. 15A**). Two clinical subtypes include nonpigmented or pigmented (including Reed nevus).

Dermoscopic Features

Nonpigmented SN show a vascular pattern with monomorphic and uniformly distributed dotted vessels in a pink background. Occasionally, regularly distributed, symmetric red globules, and corkscrew or hairpin vessels may be seen. Other findings include reticular depigmentation, negative network, and chrysalis-like structures.[13]

Pigmented SN show gray-brown or blue globules distributed throughout the lesion mainly at the periphery (globular pattern) (**Fig. 15B**). Other patterns include starburst, reticular, atypical or homogeneous pattern dermoscopically.[14]

Key Points

- Nonpigmented SN show regularly distributed, symmetric red dots or globules on a pink background.
- Pigmented SN show globular, starburst, reticular, atypical or homogeneous pattern.

Atypical Melanocytic Nevi

Clinical Features

Clark's nevi (**Figs. 16A** and **17A**) or atypical melanocytic nevi (dysplastic nevi) are benign acquired melanocytic neoplasms that possess similar clinical morphology (asymmetry, border irregularity, color variability, diameter >6 mm, evolving) as melanoma.

Dermoscopic Features

The common dermoscopic patterns seen in Clark's nevus are reticular (pigment network with uniform thickness and color), reticular-homogeneous, and globular-homogeneous types of pigmentary patterns (**Figs. 16B**, and **17B** and **C**). These can be central, eccentric hyperpigmentation or central or eccentric hypopigmentation and multifocal hyper- or hypopigmentation.[15]

Key Points

- Clark's nevus shows reticular (pigment network with uniform thickness and color), reticular-homogeneous, and globular homogeneous types of pigmentary patterns.

Halo Nevus

Clinical Features

Halo nevi (HN), also known as Sutton's nevi, are benign melanocytic nevi surrounded by a depigmented area, which resemble a halo (**Fig. 18A**).

Dermoscopic Features

The most common dermoscopic findings are globular and/or homogeneous patterns (**Fig. 18B**). Regression of the

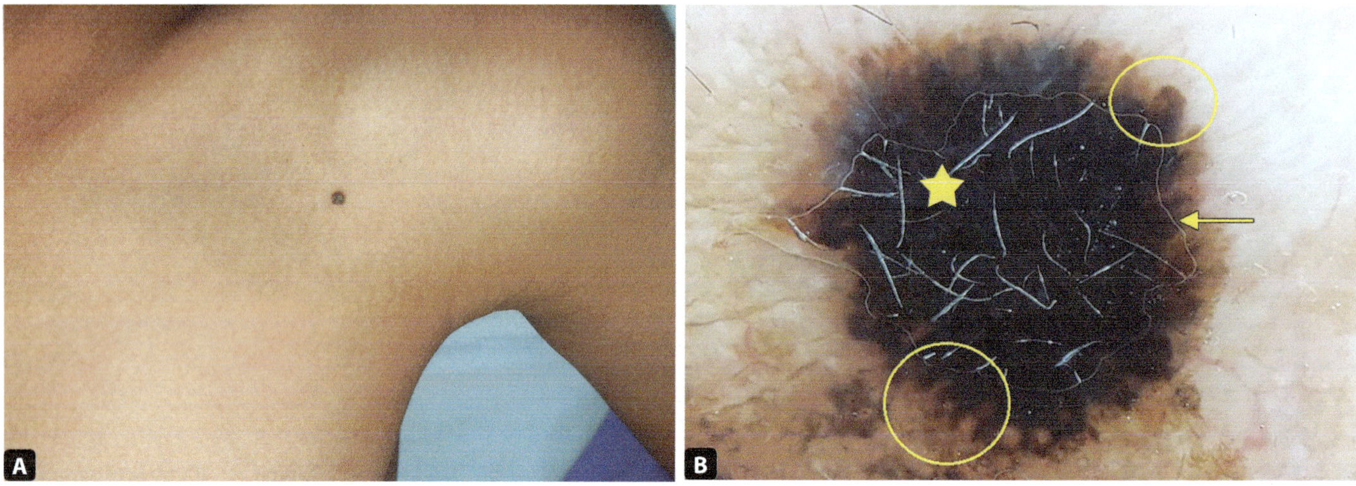

FIGS. 15A AND B: (A) Clinical image of Spitz nevus on the chest; (B) Dermoscopy of Spitz nevus shows dark brown pigment globules (arrow) at the periphery on a bluish background (star) with few pseudopods (circles).

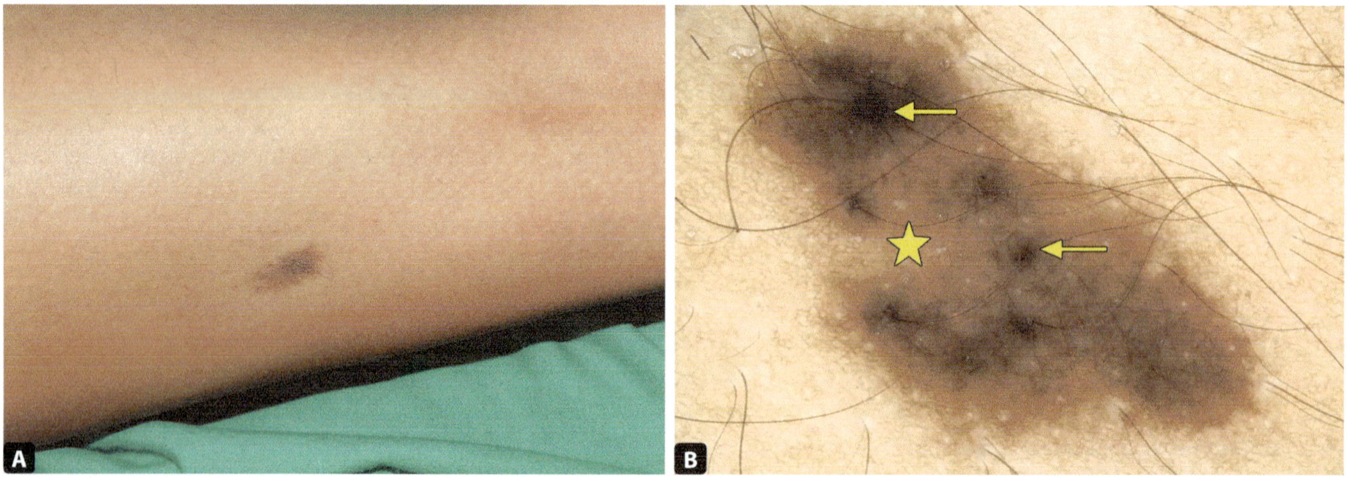

FIGS. 16A AND B: (A) Clinical image of Clark's nevus (atypical melanocytic) shows pigmented lesion on the leg; (B) Dermoscopy of Clark's nevus (atypical melanocytic) shows reticuloglobular pattern with accentuated pigment network (star) and few hyperpigmented areas (arrows) (polarized, DermLite DL4, 10×).

Courtesy (Fig. B): Dr Shweta P Bhadbhade, KVG Medical College, Sullia, Karnataka, India.

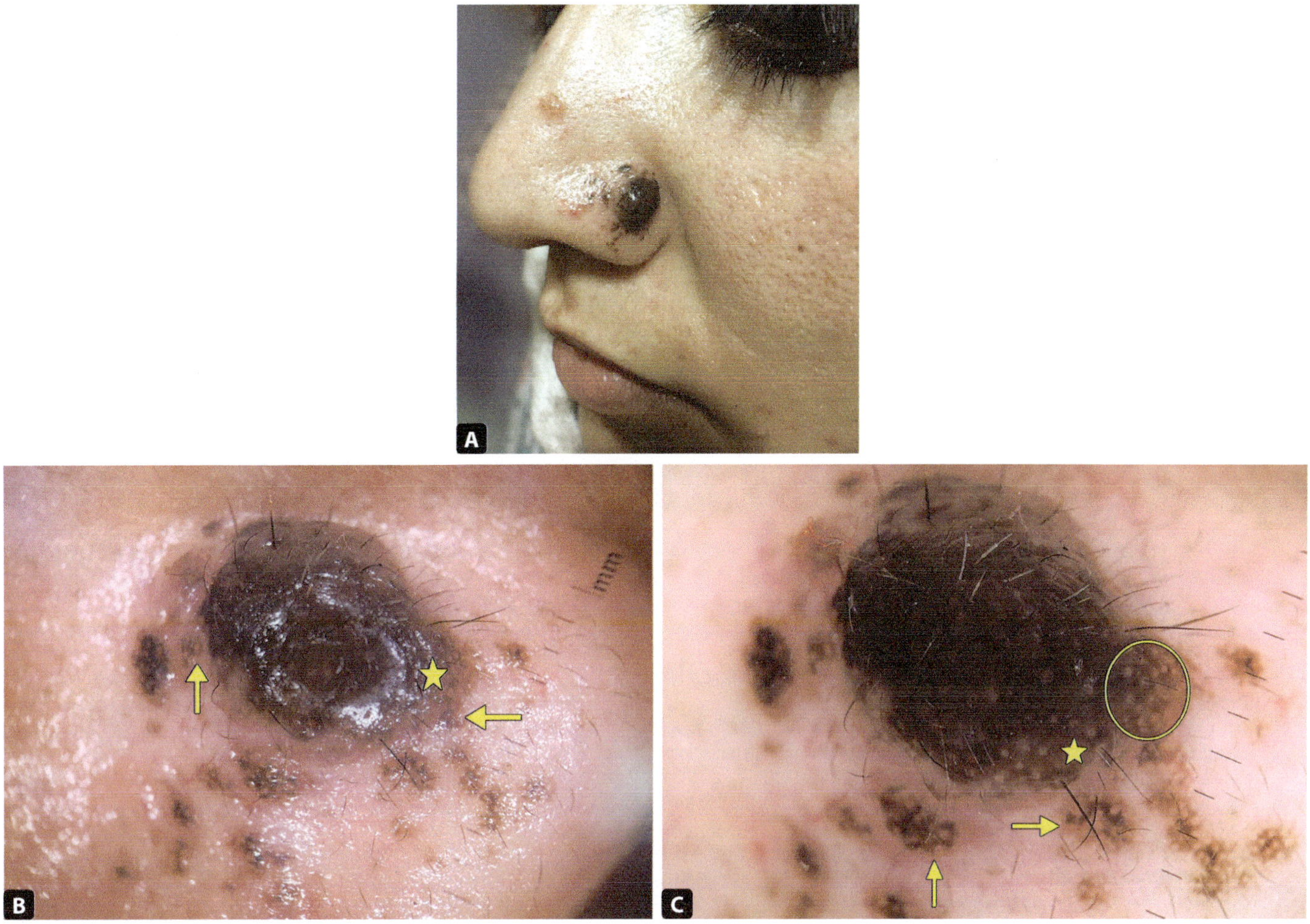

FIGS. 17A TO C: (A) Clinical image of Clark's nevus (atypical melanocytic) showing hyperpigmented papule over the nose; (B) Dermoscopy showing reticular-homogeneous pattern (star) and extension of pigment pattern to the periphery (arrows) (polarized, DermLite DL3N, 10×); (C) Dermoscopy showing reticular-homogeneous pattern of pigmentation (star) with multiple satellite nevi (arrows) and perifollicular hypopigmentation (circle) (polarized, DermLite DL3N, 10×).

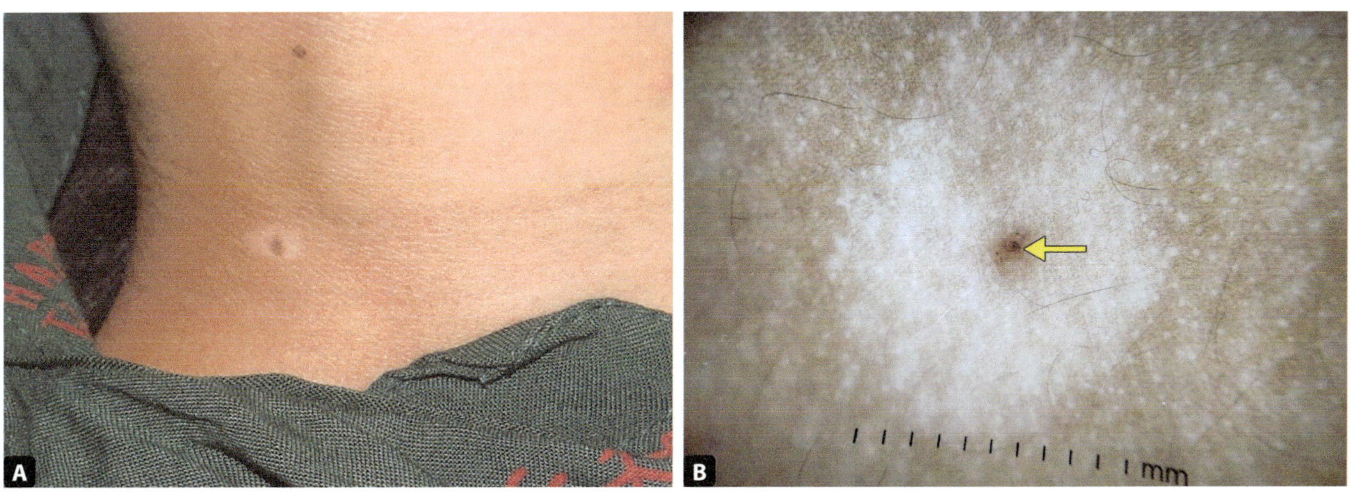

FIGS. 18A AND B: (A) Clinical image of halo nevus shows pigmented lesion with peripheral depigmented patch on the neck; (B) Dermoscopy of halo nevus shows globular pattern of pigment globules (arrow) in the pigmented area with peripheral white area (polarized, DermLite DL4, 10×).

Courtesy (Fig. B): Dr Savitha LB, Consultant Dermatologist, Bagalkot, Karnataka, India.

nevus component was characterized by light brown to pink central area with dotted vessels.[16]

Key Points

- Globular or homogeneous pattern of pigmentation is seen in HN.

KEY POINTS

- Dermoscopy of nevi and nevoid disorders demonstrate definitive features.
- A proper follow-up is possible for rapid growth or uncharacteristic patterns in a particular lesion.
- Early changes of malignant transformation are easily detected.

CONCLUSION

Frequently the differentiation between benign and malignant lesions only on clinical examination may be challenging for the physician. Dermoscopes are a valuable tool for the diagnosis of various benign and malignant keratinocytic and melanocytic nevi. They may be helpful in avoiding a biopsy in certain skin conditions.

REFERENCES

1. Elmas ÖF, Akdeniz N. Dermoscopic aspect of verrucous epidermal nevi: new findings. Turk J Med Sci. 2019;49:710-4.
2. Dickman J, Noparstak M, Nathoo R. Dermoscopy of inflammatory linear verrucous epidermal nevus: brown and red glomerular structures over a white background as an identifying feature. SKIN. 2019;3(5):341-3.
3. Sahu P, Lakra S, Dayal S. Nevus sebaceous on face: histopathological and dermoscopic correlation. Indian Dermatol Online J. 2020;11:878-80.
4. Neri I, Savoia F, Giacomini F, Raone B, Aprile S, Patrizi A. Usefulness of dermatoscopy for the early diagnosis of sebaceous naevus and differentiation from aplasia cutis congenita. Clin Exp Dermatol. 2009;34:e50-2.
5. Ankad BS, Beergouder SL, Domble V. Trichoscopy: the best auxiliary tool in the evaluation of nevus sebaceous. Int J Trichol. 2016;8:5-10.
6. Tchernev G, Ananiev J, Semkova K, Dourmishev LA, Schönlebe J, Wollina U. Nevus comedonicus: an updated review. Dermatol Ther (Heidelb). 2013;3:33-40.
7. Chauhan P, Meena D, Sharma S. Dermoscopy of nevus comedonicus: a case series. Indian J Paediatr Dermatol. 2020;21:232-4.
8. Vora RV, Kota RS, Sheth NK. Dermoscopy of nevus comedonicus. Indian Dermatol Online J. 2017;8(5):388-9.
9. Cengiz FP, Emiroglu N, Ozkaya DB, Su O, Onsun N. Dermoscopic features of small, medium, and large-sized congenital melanocytic nevi. Ann Dermatol. 2017;29:26-32.
10. Malladi NS, Chikhalkar SB, Khopkar U, Kharkar V. A descriptive observational study on clinical and dermoscopic features of benign melanocytic neoplasms. Indian J Dermatol Venereol Leprol. 2020;86:251-61.
11. Kesty K, Zargari O. Eruptive blue nevi. Indian J Dermatol Venereol Leprol. 2015;81:198-201.
12. Di Cesare A, Sera F, Gulia A, Coletti G, Micantonio T, Fargnoli MC, et al. The spectrum of dermatoscopic patterns in blue nevi. J Am Acad Dermatol. 2012;67:199-205.
13. Pedrosa AF, Lopes JM, Azevedo F, Mota A. Spitz/Reed nevi: a review of clinical-dermatoscopic and histological correlation. Dermatol Pract Concept. 2016;6:37-41.
14. Lallas A, Apalla Z, Ioannides D, Lazaridou E, Kyrgidis A, Broganelli P, et al. Update on dermoscopy of Spitz/Reed naevi and management guidelines by the International Dermoscopy Society. Br J Dermatol. 2017;177:645-55.
15. Hofmann-Wellenhof R, Blum A, Wolf IH, Piccolo D, Kerl H, Garbe C, et al. Dermoscopic classification of atypical melanocytic nevi (Clark nevi). Arch Dermatol. 2001;137:1575-80.
16. Kolm I, Di Stefani A, Hofmann-Wellenhof R, Fink-Puches R, Wolf IH, Richtig E, et al. Dermoscopy patterns of halo nevi. Arch Dermatol. 2006;142: 1627-32.

16 CHAPTER Trichoscopy

Part 1: Noncicatricial Alopecia

Rachita Dhurat, Samipa S Mukherjee, Harshit Ranpara

INTRODUCTION

Trichoscopy is a noninvasive technique of visualization of the skin of scalp and hair. It is an important tool to differentiate between scarring and nonscarring alopecia. It is also a valuable aid for the correct diagnosis and classification of the type of hair loss.

ANDROGENETIC ALOPECIA

Clinical Features

The clinical diagnosis of androgenetic alopecia (AGA) in men is straightforward. However, it is difficult to ascertain the diagnosis in women especially in early stages of AGA as Ludwig staging system (I–III) fails to detect early-stage female pattern hair loss (FPHL) as it relies mainly on assessing the visible hair thinning on the crown. Ludwig staging system is less useful for early diagnosis of FPHL.[1] Increase mid-scalp parting of hair is the clinical clue to diagnose FPHL. However, by the time women develop increased midscalp parting, there is substantial amount of hair loss.

Trichoscopic Features

Male AGA and female AGA share similar trichoscopic features. In 2001, De Lacharriere et al. considered hair follicle miniaturization as the key point of androgenic alopecia. Decrease in hair follicle size leading to progressive reduction in hair diameter (miniaturization) corresponds to transformation of terminal hair into thin/vellus hair. This hair shaft thickness heterogeneity is also named "hair diameter diversity" or "anisotrichosis."[1] Reduced hair shaft caliber ≥20% hair follicles has traditionally been deemed essential in diagnosing patterned hair loss; although a cutoff of 10% diversity may be more appropriate in females (**Fig. 1**).[2] Presence of >6 short thin hairs in the frontal scalp is diagnostic for early FPHL.[3] Other trichoscopy abnormalities include perifollicular discoloration (hyperpigmentation) (**Fig. 2**), and presence of variable number of yellow dots (**Fig. 3**) and "eraser"-like areas.[1]

Key Points

- Hair diameter diversity or "anisotrichosis" ≥10% for FPHL and ≥20% for AGA
- Presence of >6 short thin hairs in the frontal scalp
- Perifollicular discoloration
- Yellow dots
- Focal atrichia (eraser-like area)

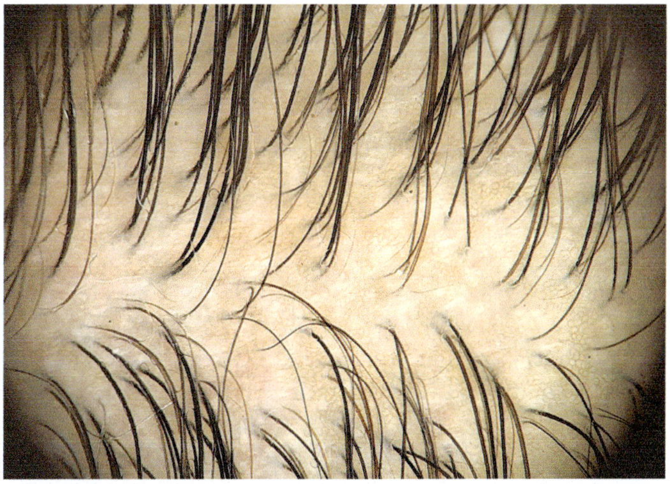

FIG. 1: Trichoscopy showing hair diameter diversity >30% in female pattern hair loss (polarized, FotoFinder, 20×).

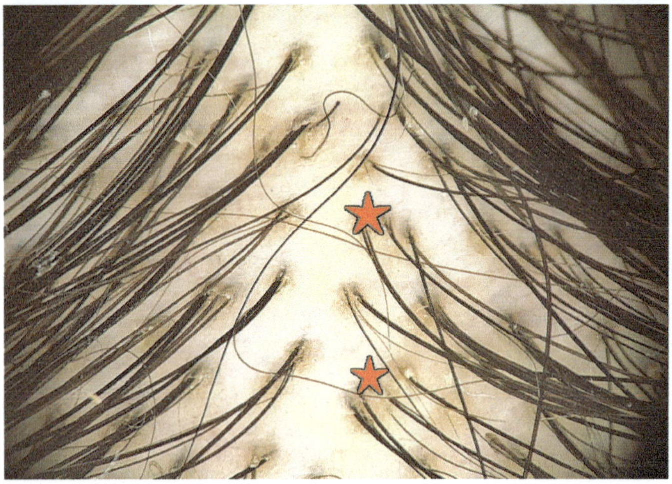

FIG. 2: Trichoscopy showing perifollicular hyperpigmentation (peripilar sign) (red stars) in a case of female pattern hair loss (polarized, FotoFinder, 20×).

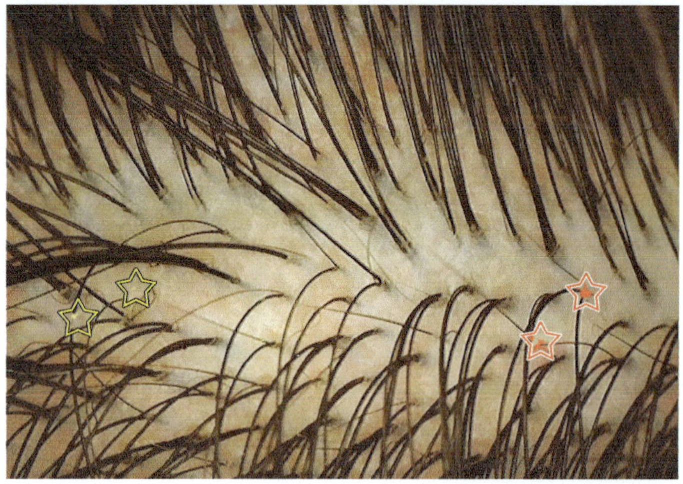

FIG. 4: Trichoscopy showing pigtail (yellow stars) and upright hair (red stars) in telogen effluvium (polarized, FotoFinder, 20×).

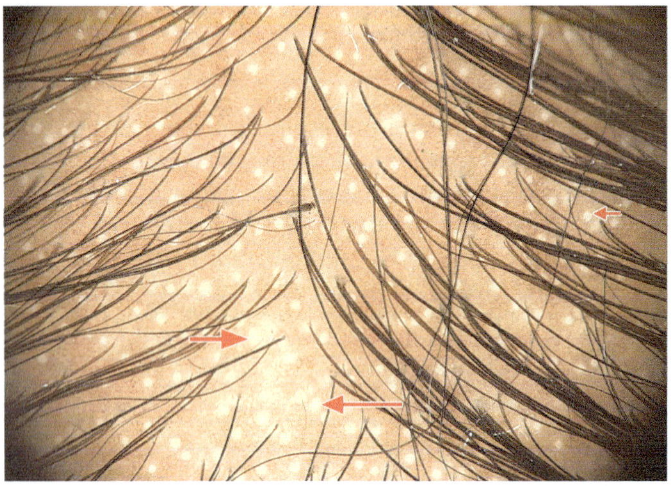

FIG. 3: Trichoscopy showing multiple yellow dots (red arrows) in a case of female pattern hair loss (polarized, FotoFinder, 20×).

TABLE 1: Differences between androgenetic alopecia and telogen effluvium.

Trichoscopic characteristics	Androgenetic alopecia	Telogen effluvium
Hair diameter diversity	Present	Absent
Vellus hair	Present	Absent
Focal atrichia	Present	Absent
Empty hair follicles with yellow dots	Present	Present
Peripilar sign	Present	Present
Regrowing hair	Present	Present
Honeycomb pigmentation	Present	Present/Absent
Predominance of abnormalities in frontal area	Present	Absent

TELOGEN EFFLUVIUM

Clinical Features

Telogen effluvium (TE) is characterized by persistent excessive hair shedding, yet the loss of hair is replaced as rapidly as it sheds, so patients never become bald unless hair loss is >50%. On scalp examination, the pull test is diffusely positive. The period of dramatic hair loss occurs diffusely from the scalp approximately 2–3 months after the triggering event.[4]

Trichoscopic Features

Although trichoscopic features of TE are not characteristic, upright short regrowing hairs have been described most commonly.[5,6]

Regrowing pigtail hairs are short, regularly twisted with tapered ends, lightly pigmented, and resemble a pig's tail (**Fig. 4**). They may be circular or oval. Regrowing pigtail hairs most probably result from rapid hair regrowth, before full recovery of the hair follicle. They have been described in alopecia areata (AA), trichotillomania (TTM), and even cicatricial alopecia. Other trichoscopic features include predominance of follicular units with only one hair, empty hair follicles/yellow dots, perifollicular discoloration (peripilar sign), and absence of hair diameter diversity. **Table 1** depicts the difference between AGA and TE.

Key Points

- Short, upright regrowing hairs and/or pigtail hair
- Single hair follicular units
- Peripilar sign
- No evidence of anisotrichosis

ALOPECIA AREATA

Clinical Features

It is one of the most common causes of patchy, nonscarring alopecia. It may involve any area of the scalp or can present

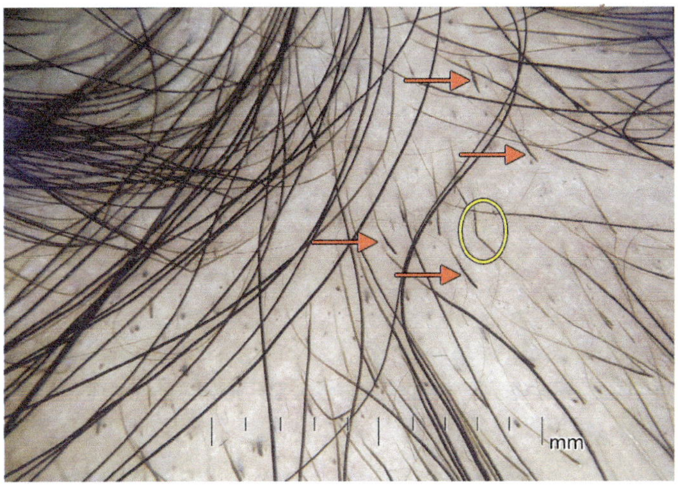

FIG. 5: Trichoscopy showing coudability hair (yellow circle) along with exclamation mark hair (red arrows) in alopecia areata (polarized, DermLite DL3N, 10×).

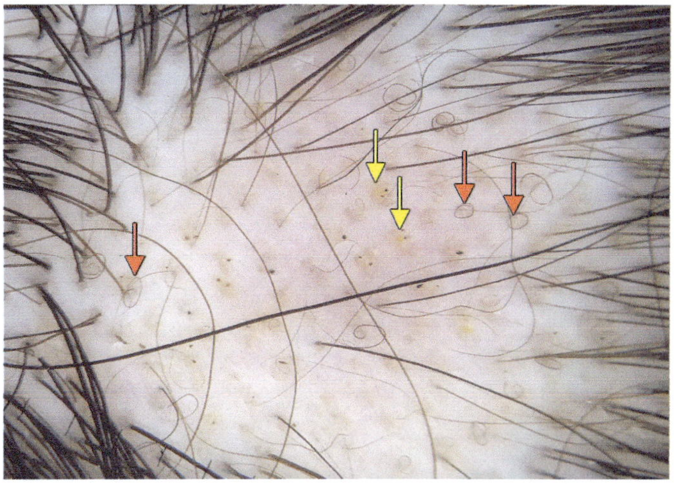

FIG. 6: Trichoscopy showing several circle hair (red arrows) and yellow dots (yellow arrows) in alopecia areata (polarized, DermLite DL3N, 10×).

with specific patterns such as the sisaphio or the ophiasis pattern. AA can also present with involvement of eyebrows and body hair.

Trichoscopic Features

Trichoscopy should be done from the periphery of the patch toward the central portion. It helps in not only establishing the diagnosis but also gauging the severity as well as monitoring the prognosis. Exclamation mark hairs are characterized by thinning of proximal portion, with uniform pigmentation along the distal two-thirds of the hair shaft and the proximal one-third is depigmented which are noted along the margin of the patch. When long exclamation mark hair is pushed inward toward scalp, the hair shaft kinks and is known as "coudability sign" and the hairs are "coudability hairs" (**Fig. 5**).[7] Short regrowing hair and pigtail hair or circle hair is trichoscopic indicators of hair regrowth.[5] Yellow dots which result due to accumulation of keratin and sebaceous material in the follicular openings are seen in all the stages of the disease and correlate with disease severity (**Fig. 6**).[8] Black dots are seen in both AA and TTM (**Fig. 7**).

Rakowska et al. observed that black dots tend to be uniform in size and shape in AA, whereas in TTM and tinea capitis are variable in diameter and round, oval, and irregular in shape.[9] The honeycomb reticular pigment network is unaltered. Recently "craters of the moon" has been described which signifies extensive yellow dots which resemble the craters on the moon.[10] Another type of hair described in AA are tulip hairs. Tulip hairs are short hairs with darker, tulip flower-shaped ends. These hairs have been attributed to the fracture of hair shafts diagonally. Traditionally described in TTM, they may also be seen in AA.

Key Points

- Black dots are sensitive indicators of disease activity and severity.

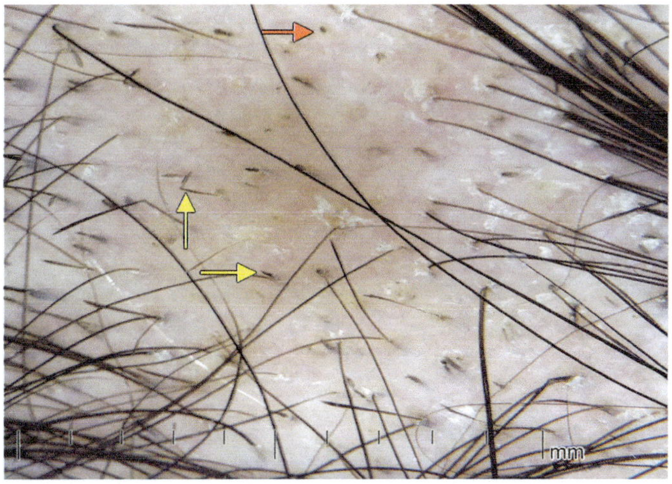

FIG. 7: Trichoscopy showing black dots (red arrow) and broken hair (yellow arrows) in alopecia areata (polarized, DermLite DL3N, 10×).

- Yellow dots correlate with disease severity
- Exclamation mark hair is seen at the periphery of the patch however is not specific for AA.
- Vascular changes may give a clue toward treatment with either topical or intralesional steroids.

ALOPECIA AREATA INCOGNITO

Clinical Features

It presents as diffuse thinning of hair without the classical patchy hair loss (**Fig. 8**). The disease mostly affects women who generally complain of acute diffuse thinning of hair and are often misdiagnosed as TE.

Trichoscopic Features

Trichoscopy shows the presence of numerous empty yellow dots, yellow dots with short vellus hairs, and short regrowing tip-shaped miniaturized hairs (**Fig. 9**).[11]

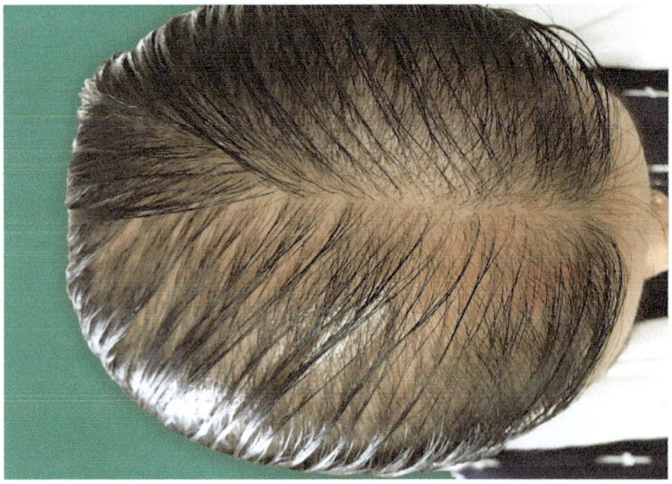

FIG. 8: Clinical image of alopecia areata incognito showing diffuse hair loss with extensive thinning.

Courtesy: Dr Chetan Rajput, SBH Government Medical College, Dhule, Maharashtra, India.

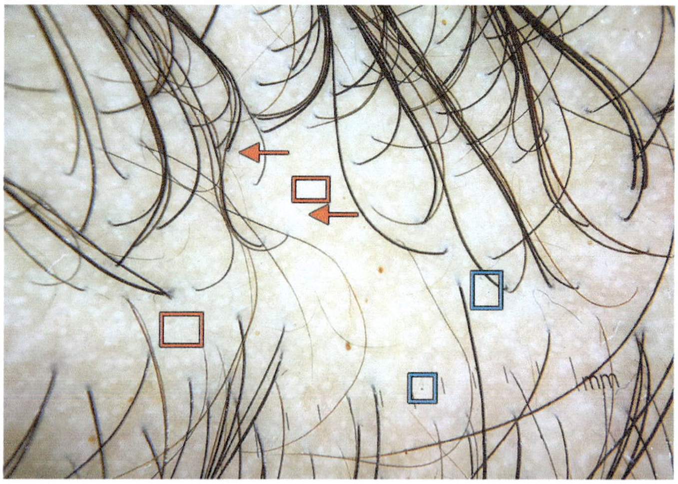

FIG. 9: Trichoscopy of alopecia areata incognito empty yellow dots (red boxes), yellow dots with vellus hair (blue boxes) and vellus hairs (red arrows) (polarized, DermLite DL4, 10×).

Courtesy: Dr Chetan Rajput, SBH Government Medical College, Dhule, Maharashtra, India.

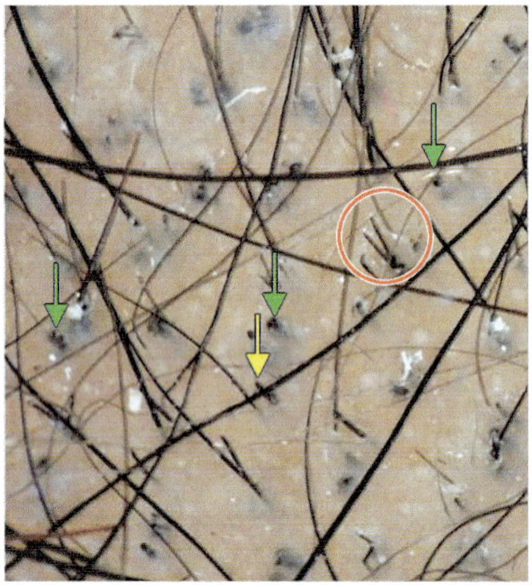

FIG. 10: Trichoscopy showing V-sign (red circle), broken hair (yellow arrow), and black dots (green arrows) in trichotillomania (TTM) (polarized, DermLite DL3N, 10×).

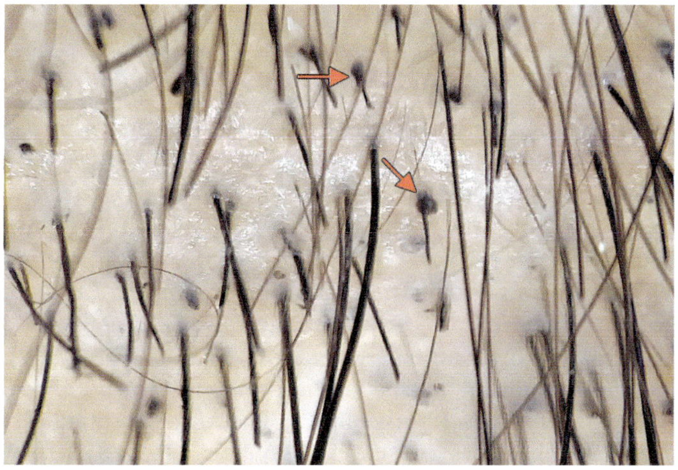

FIG. 11: Trichoscopy showing burnt matchstick sign (red arrows) (polarized, DermLite DL3N, 10×).

Key Points

- Diffuse hair thinning without patchy hair loss
- Abundant yellow dots with short miniaturized regrowing hairs

TRICHOTILLOMANIA

Clinical Features

Trichotillomania is characterized by a compulsive urge to pull the hair resulting in patches most commonly over scalp, eyebrows, or other hair-bearing areas. Of note is that the patches are formed on the easily accessible areas of the scalp and history may reveal an underlying stress.

Trichoscopic Features

"Flame hairs" are translucent, wavy hair with a broad base and a tapering jagged tip occurring due to the traction and external manipulation of the hair shaft. Tulip hair is short hair with the distal end being shaped like a tulip flower which is attributed to the diagonal fracture to the hair shaft,[11] whereas V-sign is referred to when two hairs emerging from a single follicular opening are broken at the same level (**Fig. 10**).[12] Recently "burnt match-stick sign" has been described, where the hair has a dark bulbar proximal tip with a linear uniformly pigmented stem of variable length (**Fig. 11**).[13] Another sign known as the "Mace sign" has been described which is defined as that is a broken terminal hair with uniform diameter and pigmentation with a bulge at

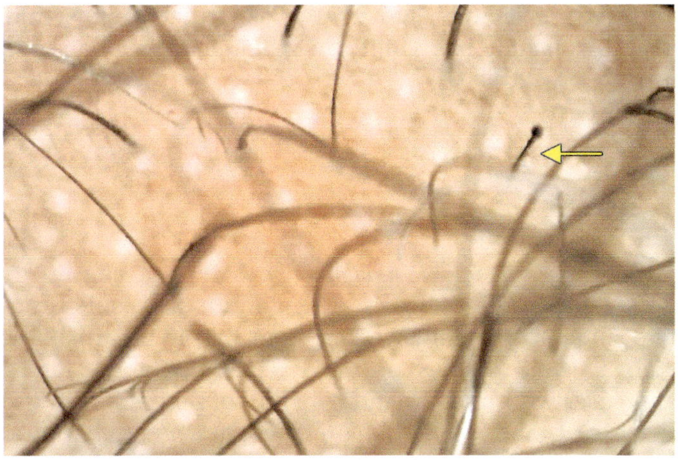

FIG. 12: Trichoscopy of trichotillomania shows mace hair (yellow arrow) with multiple broken hairs and white dots (polarized, DermLite DL3N, 10×).

Source: Reused with permission from Ankad BS, Mukherjee S, Smitha SV. Trichoscopy in hair disorders in darker skin: An approach to diagnosis. Clin Dermatol Rev. 2020;4:102-14.

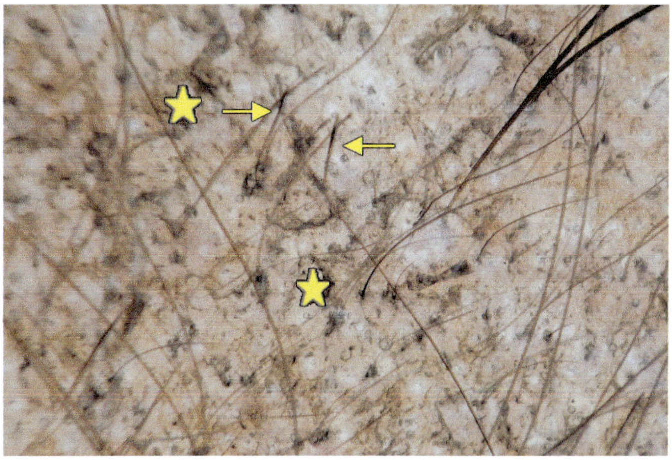

FIG. 13: Trichoscopy of trichotillomania shows tulip hairs (yellow arrows) and hair powder (yellow stars) in the interfollicular area (polarized, DermLite DL3N, 10×).

Source: Reused with permission from Ankad BS, Mukherjee S, Smitha SV. Trichoscopy in hair disorders in darker skin: An approach to diagnosis. Clin Dermatol Rev. 2020;4:102-14.

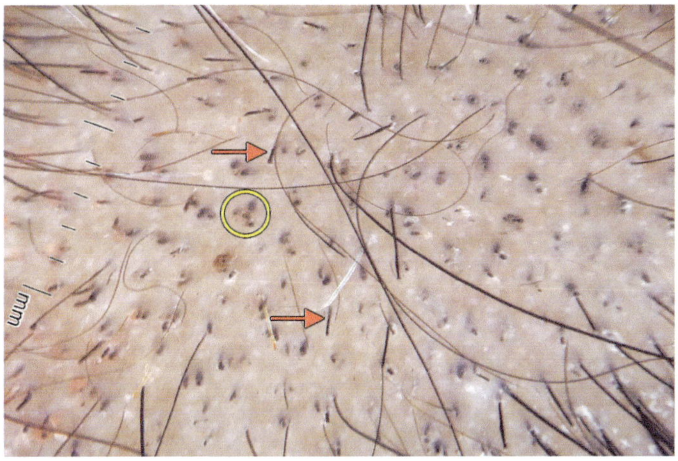

FIG. 14: Trichoscopy showing black dots (yellow circle) and broken hair (red arrows) in trichotillomania (polarized, DermLite DL3N, 10×).

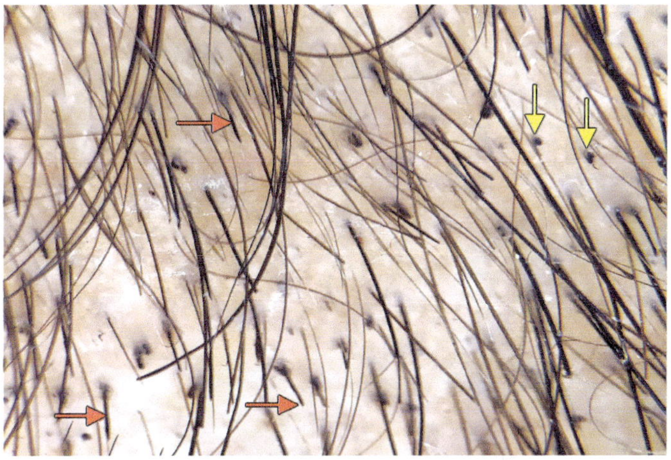

FIG. 15: Trichoscopy showing broken hair of variable length (red arrows) and coarse black dots (yellow arrows) are also noted in trichotillomania (polarized, DermLite DL3N, 10×).

distal end (**Fig. 12**).[14] Hair powder, residue of damaged hair, and keratin debris from the fractured shaft can be noticed as sprinklings in perifollicular area (**Fig. 13**).[9] Follicular patterns show black dots which are coarse and irregularly distributed (**Fig. 14**). Broken hair of variable length is noted (**Fig. 15**). Perifollicular hemorrhages which were once considered to be specific for TTM have now been associated with multiple pruritic conditions of the scalp. Trichoptilosis is also noted commonly due to longitudinal fracture of the hair shaft (**Fig. 16**). The trichoscopic key features of TTM are not exclusive. The diagnosis of TTM can conclusively be made by anamnesis, clinical, trichoscopic, and histopathologic examination.

Key Points

- Black dots are coarse and irregularly distributed.
- Multiple changes in the hair shaft patterns are noted due to the external traction, manipulation, and rubbing of the hair.

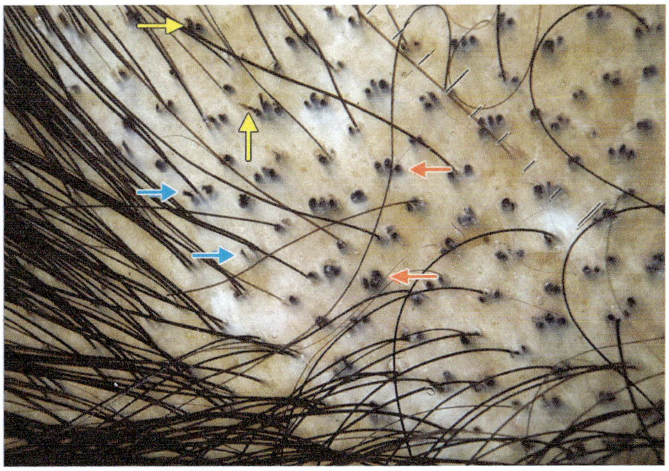

FIG. 16: Trichoscopy of trichotillomania shows trichoptilosis (blue arrows) with flame hairs (yellow arrows) and black dots (red arrows) (polarized, DermLite DL3N, 10×).

Source: Reused with permission from Ankad BS, Mukherjee S, Smitha SV. Trichoscopy in hair disorders in darker skin: An approach to diagnosis. Clin Dermatol Rev. 2020;4:102-14.

TINEA CAPITIS

Clinical Features

Tinea capitis presents as inflammatory and noninflammatory lesions of the scalp. Tinea capitis may present in several ways (**Fig. 17**).[15]

- Dry scaling-like dandruff but usually with moth-eaten hair loss
- Black dots—the hairs are broken off at the scalp surface, which is scaly
- Smooth areas of hair loss
- *Kerion*: A very inflamed mass, like an abscess
- *Favus*: Yellow crusts and matted hair

Trichoscopic Features

Comma hairs, corkscrew hairs, zigzag hairs, and Morse code-like hairs are found to be characteristic for tinea capitis (**Figs. 18** to **20**). However, corkscrew hairs are also observed in ectodermal dysplasias. Other trichoscopic features include bent hairs, block hairs, broken hair, and i-hairs (**Fig. 20**).[16]

TRACTION ALOPECIA

Clinical Features

Traction alopecia (TA) is hair loss that is caused by repeatedly pulling of hair. This commonly results from the sufferer frequently wearing their hair in a particularly tight ponytail, pigtails, or braids (**Fig. 21**). The risk for TA increases with traction and a history of relaxers. It is also seen occasionally in long-haired people who use barrettes to keep hair out of their faces.[17] It is clinically characterized by a fringe along the marginal hairline seen over the frontal and temporal scalp. It has also been reported over the submandibular area in Sikh males who tied their beard in a tight knot below the chin.[18,19]

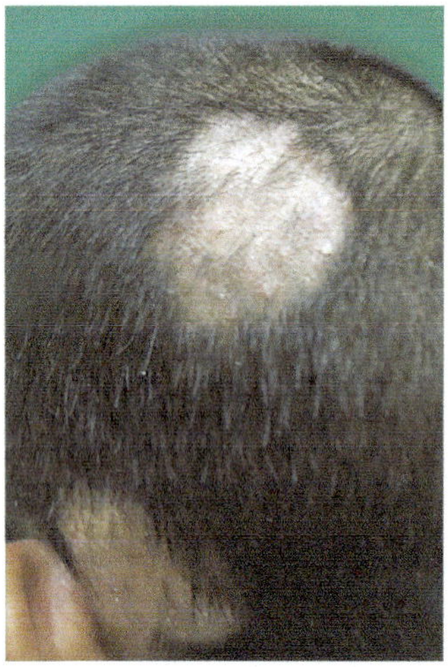

FIG. 17: Tinea capitis showing focal patches of hair loss over the scalp with scaling in a young boy.

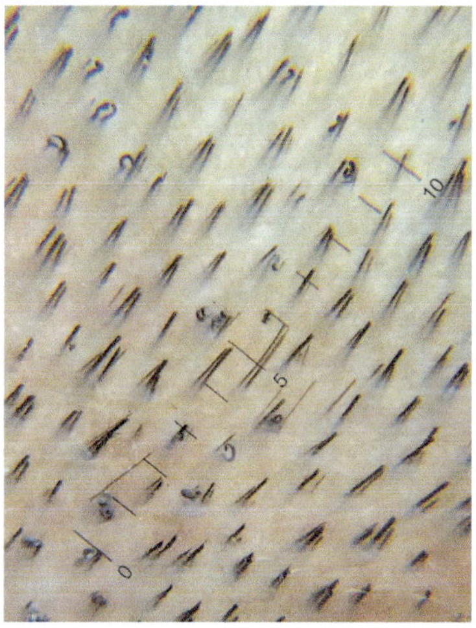

FIG. 18: Trichoscopy showing multiple comma hair in tinea capitis (polarized, FotoFinder, 20×).

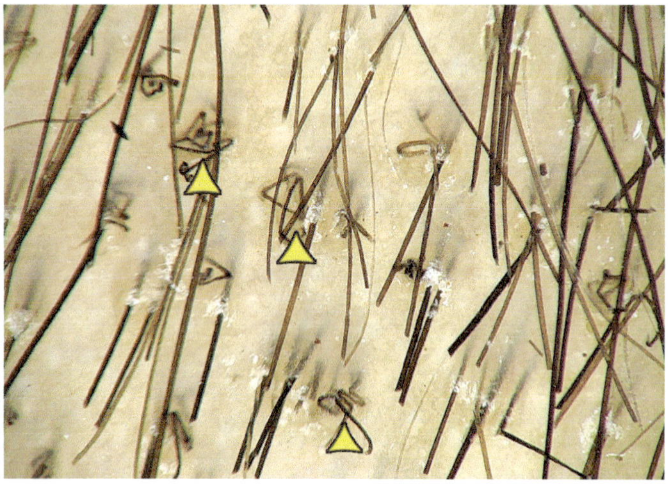

FIG. 19: Multiple zigzag hairs (arrowheads) in a case of tinea capitis (polarized, FotoFinder, 20×).

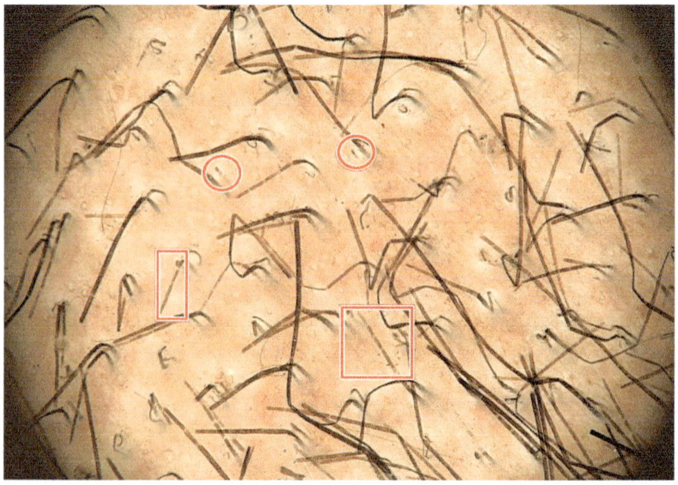

FIG. 20: Trichoscopy shows "i" hair (red circles) and Morse code-like hair (red boxes) in tinea capitis (polarized, FotoFinder, 20×).

Courtesy: Dr Swapnil Shah, Professor, Ashwini Rural Medical College, Solapur, Maharashtra, India.

Trichoscopic Features

Trichoscopy reveals multiple linear white tracks or hair casts at the base of the shaft of terminal hair in the direction of pull of hairs. These linear tracks in continuation with the shaft of hair at one end give the appearance of a flame or lit torch (**Fig. 22**).[20]

Key Points[21]

- Numerous hair casts, yellowish-white cylinders
- Reduced hair density with absence of follicular openings
- Presence of vellus hair
- Broken hair of different length in case of acute TA

TEMPORAL TRIANGULAR ALOPECIA

Clinical Features

Temporal triangular alopecia (TTA) can present as a triangular, oval, or lancet-shaped patch of alopecia (**Fig. 23**).

Trichoscopic Features

They are intact follicular openings, empty follicles, presence of vellus hairs in the bald patch and presence of terminal hairs surrounding the patch (**Fig. 24**).

Key Points

Inui et al. have proposed a criteria to diagnose TTA.[22]

- Triangular or lancet-shaped patch of alopecia involving frontotemporal scalp
- Trichoscopically normal follicular openings with vellus hairs surrounded by normal terminal hair area
- Trichoscopically no broken hairs, tapering hairs, black dots, yellow dots, and orifice loss
- Persistent without significant hair regrowth for 6 months after clinically or trichoscopically confirming the existence of vellus hairs

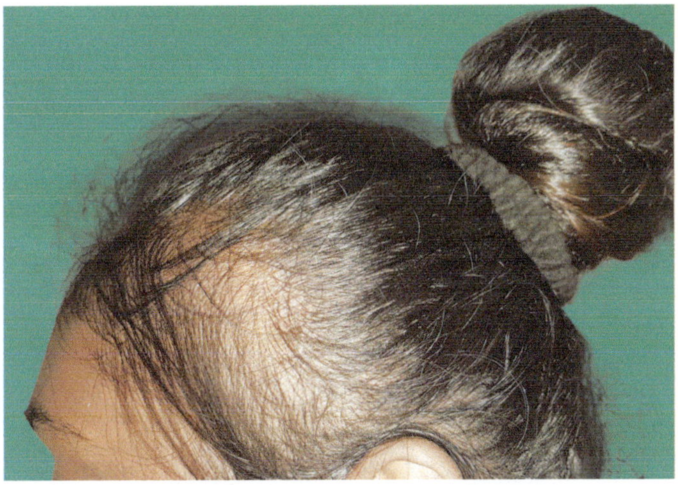

FIG. 21: Band of hair loss over the left temporal area with fringe sign in traction alopecia.

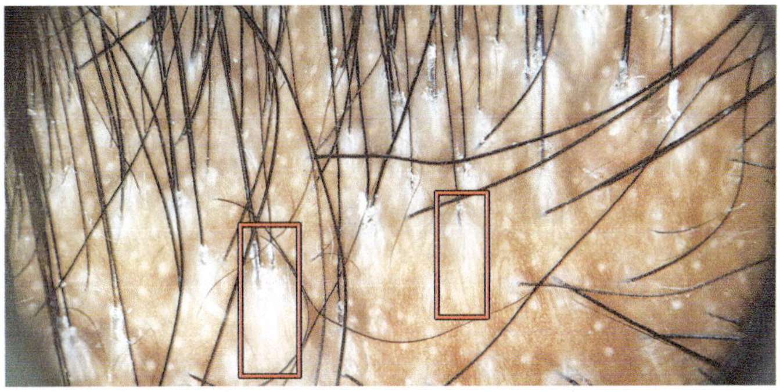

FIG. 22: Perifollicular scaling and linear white tracks over the scalp at the base of the shaft of terminal hair giving lit torch appearance (Flambeau sign) (red boxes) in traction alopecia (polarized, FotoFinder, 20×).

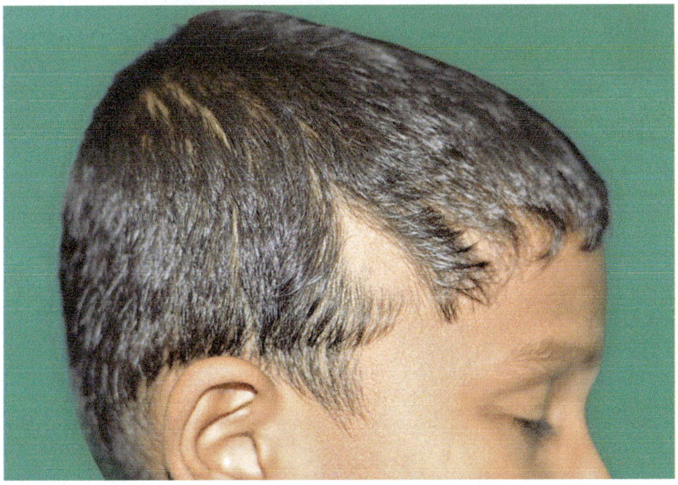

FIG. 23: Triangular patch of alopecia over the right frontotemporal area of scalp in case of triangular temporal alopecia.

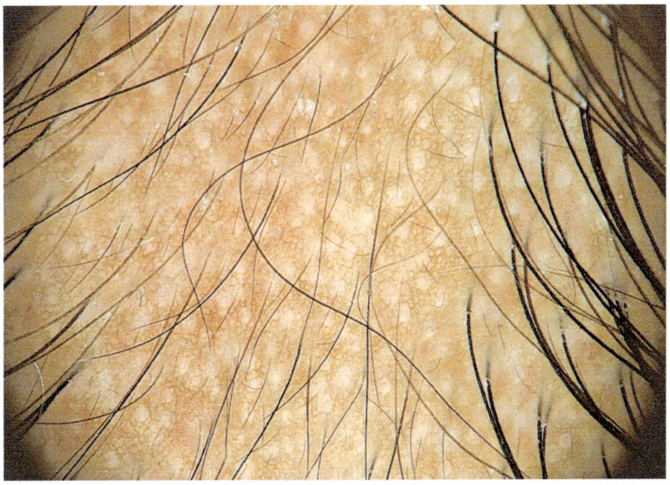

FIG. 24: Trichoscopy showing vellus hairs within the patch surrounded by terminal hairs at the periphery in temporal triangular alopecia (polarized, FotoFinder, 20×).

APLASIA CUTIS CONGENITA

Clinical Features

Aplasia cutis congenita, also known as congenital absence of skin, is a group of disorders characterized by the absence of a skin fragment at birth. The most common site involves the scalp; however, it may also be seen on the other areas of the body (**Fig. 25**).

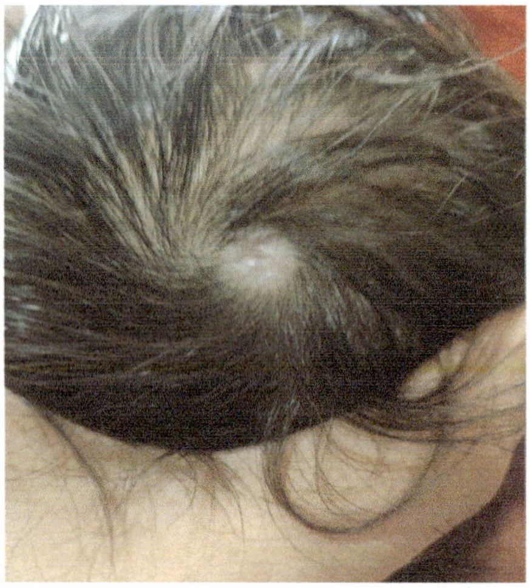

FIG. 25: Clinical image of aplasia cutis shows atrophic patch with loss of hair.

Courtesy: Dr Shailesh Malani, Consultant Dermatologist, Sailu, Maharashtra, India.

Trichoscopic Features

Rakowska et al. described a radial arrangement of hair shafts, visible elongated hair bulbs through the semitranslucent epidermis. There are presence of prominent vessels, skin atrophy, and no follicular openings at the center of the lesion (**Fig. 26**).[6] Trichoscopy helps in differentiating from other congenital disorders like a trauma or nevus sebaceous.

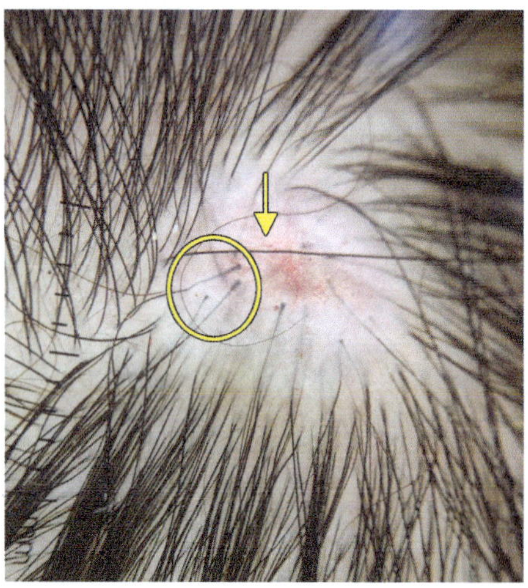

FIG. 26: Trichoscopic image of aplasia cutis shows numerous hair bulbs (yellow circle) that are visible through the transparent epidermis with vascular elements (yellow arrow) (polarized, DermLite DL4, 10×).

Courtesy: Dr Shailesh Malani, Consultant Dermatologist, Sailu, Maharashtra, India.

Key Points

- Translucent appearance of the skin with loss of appendages in the central portion and a radial arrangement of hair shafts in the hair margin gives a clue to diagnosis.
- Trichoscopy helps to differentiate between other congenital disorders.

MONILETHRIX

Clinical Features

Mostly presents in pediatric age group, however, may be present in adolescent age group as an acquired condition. It presents with short, brittle lusterless hair that do not grow in length. The eyebrows and side locks may be affected (**Fig. 27**).

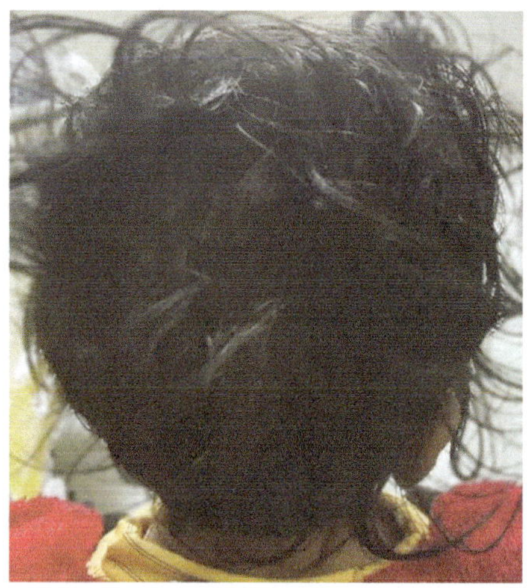

FIG. 27: Clinical of monilethrix with short and frizzy hairs.

Courtesy: Dr Savitha LB, Consultant Dermatologist, Bagalkot, Karnataka, India.

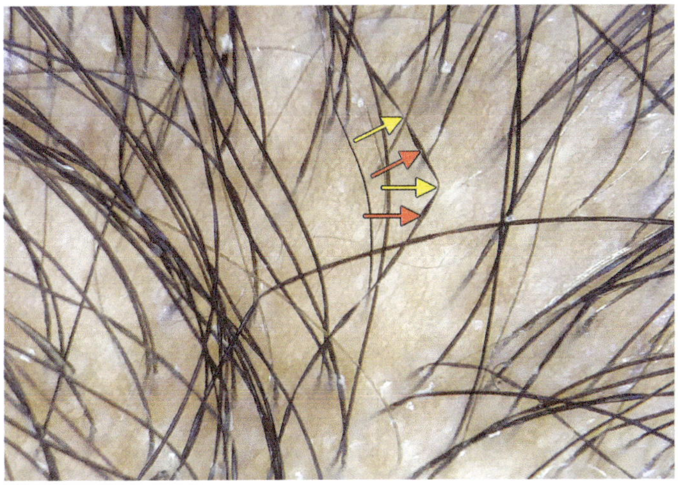

FIG. 28: Trichoscopy using showing equidistant nodes (red arrows) and internodes (yellow arrows) in monilethrix (polarized, DermLite DL3N, 10×).

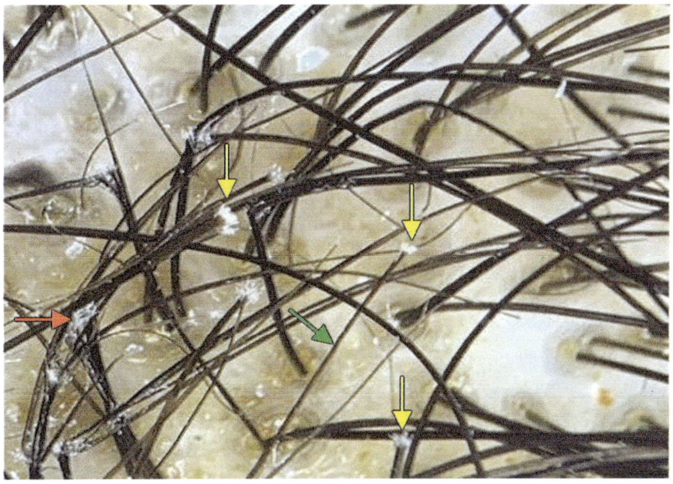

FIG. 29: Trichoscopy shows thrust paint brush appearance (red arrow), broken hair (green arrow) with trichoptilosis (yellow arrows) in trichorrhexis nodosa (polarized, DermLite DL3N, 10×).

Trichoscopic Features

Trichoscopy shows the presence of beaded hair with striking nodes and internodes which are placed in an equidistant fashion (**Fig. 28**).[23] There may also be presence of broken hair and black dots owing the breakage of the hair shaft.

Key Points

- Beaded hair
- Equidistant nodes and internodes
- Black dots and broken hair

TRICHORRHEXIS NODOSA

Clinical Features

It may be acquired or congenital. This condition presents as dry lusterless hair with easy breakability of the hair. Acquired cases can result from hair treatments such as styling, coloring, perming, harsh combing, or even due to friction. Examination of scalp and eyebrow hair yields maximum results.

Trichoscopic Features

The nodes appear as gray-white areas, and the classical paintbrush bristle appearance is seen on trichoscopy (**Fig. 29**). In acquired cases, these nodes are present distally as against in congenital cases where they are present in the proximal part of the shaft.[24]

Key Points

- Thrust paint brush appearance
- Gray white areas on the hair shaft
- Nodes are more distal in acquired cases, whereas they are proximal in congenital cases

WOOLLY HAIR

Clinical Features

It is a rare congenital disorder characterized by short tightly packed curly hair which is dry, brittle, and lusterless involving the entire scalp (**Fig. 30**).

Trichoscopic Features

Trichoscopy helps to distinguish between healthy curly hair and wooly hair syndrome. Woolly hair syndrome demonstrates hair shafts with a "crawling snake" appearance, with short wave cycles (**Fig. 31**).[25] Apart from that, the examination demonstrated broken hair shafts.

Key Points

- Useful for differentiating healthy curly hair and woolly hair syndrome

KEY POINTS

- Trichoscopic findings in hair shafts in the form of vellus, broken, exclamation, comma, tulip hairs, etc. are seen.
- Follicular findings in the form of black and yellow dots.

CONCLUSION

Trichoscopy is a noninvasive technique for the correct diagnosis and classification of the type of hair loss. It is an important tool to differentiate between scarring and nonscarring alopecia.

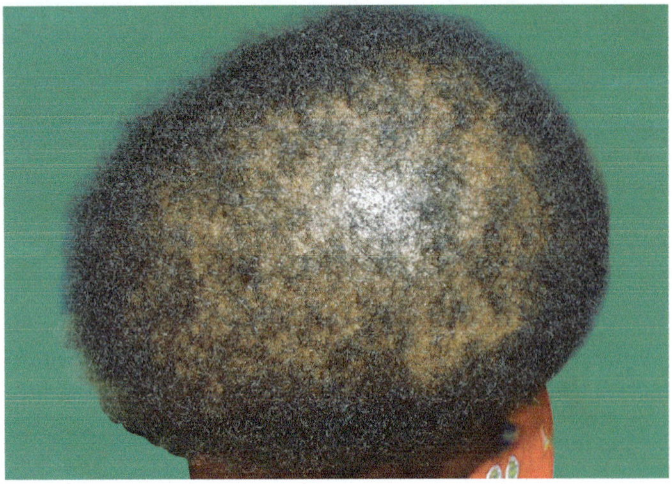

FIG. 30: Clinical image of woolly hair.

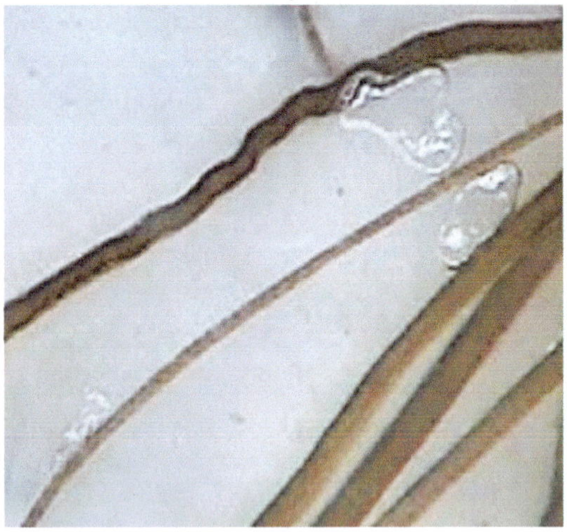

FIG. 31: Trichoscopy showing crawling snake appearance in woolly hair (polarized, FotoFinder, 120×).

REFERENCES

1. Harries M, Tosti A, Bergfeld W, Blume-Peytavi U, Shapiro J, Lutz G, et al. Towards a consensus on how to diagnose and quantify female pattern hair loss - The 'Female Pattern Hair Loss Severity Index (FPHL-SI). J Eur Acad Dermatol Venereol. 2016;30(4):667-76.
2. Hu R, Xu F, Han Y, Sheng Y, Qi S, Miao Y, et al. Trichoscopic findings of androgenetic alopecia and their association with disease severity. J Dermatol. 2015;42(6):602-7.
3. Herskovitz I, de Sousa IC, Tosti A. Vellus hairs in the frontal scalp in early female pattern hair loss. Int J Trichology. 2013;5(3):118-20.
4. Dhurat RS, Agrawal S, Sharma A, Ghate S. Pigtail hair in acute telogen effluvium - Lest we forget!. Indian Dermatol Online J. 2020;11(3):444-5.
5. Rudnicka L, Olszewska M, Rakowska A, Slowinska M. Trichoscopy update 2011. J Dermatol Case Rep. 2011;5(4):82-8.
6. Rudnicka L, Olszewska M, Rakowska A. Atlas of Trichoscopy: Dermoscopy in Hair and Scalp Disease. London: Springer; 2012. p. 191-202.
7. Pirmez R. Revisiting coudability hairs in alopecia areata: The story behind the name. Skin Appendage Disord. 2016;2(1-2):76-8.
8. Torres F, Tosti A. Trichoscopy: An update. G Ital Dermatol Venereol. 2014;149(1):83-91.
9. Rakowska A, Slowinska M, Olszewska M, Rudnicka L. New trichoscopy findings in trichotillomania: Flame hairs, V-sign, hook hairs, hair powder, tulip hairs. Acta Derm Venereol. 2014;94(3):303-6.
10. Malakar SS, Mehta PR, Malakar SS. Craters of the moon. A marker for disease severity in alopecia areata? Indian J Paediatr Dermatol. 2017;18(4):314-6.
11. Tosti A. Non scarring alopecias. In: Tosti A, (ed). Dermoscopy of the Hair and Nails, 2nd edition. Boca Raton: Springer; 2016. p. 40-1.
12. Rudnica L, Olszewska M, Rakowsa A, (eds). Trichotillomania and traction alopecia. In: Atlas of Trichoscopy. London: Springer; 2012. p. 263-7.
13. Malakar S, Mukherjee SS. Burnt matchstick sign – A new trichoscopic finding in trichotillomania. Int J Trichol. 2017;9(1):44-6.
14. Malakar S, Mukherjee SS. 'Mace sign'- A definitive sign of trichotillomania? Our Dermatol Online. 2017;8:491-2.
15. Higgins EM, Fuller LC, Smith CH. Guidelines for the management of tinea capitis. British Association of Dermatologists. Br J Dermatol. 2000;143(1):53-8.
16. Waśkiel-Burnat A, Rakowska A, Sikora M, Ciechanowicz P, Olszewska M, Rudnicka L. Trichoscopy of tinea capitis: A systematic review. Dermatol Ther (Heidelb). 2020;10(1):43-52.
17. Khumalo NP. (2012). "The 'fringe sign' for public education on traction alopecia". Dermatology Online Journal. 2012;18(9):16.
18. Kanwar AJ, Kaur S, Basak P, Sharma R. Traction alopecia in Sikh males. Arch Dermatol. 1989;125(11):1587.
19. Samrao A, Price VH, Zedek D, Mirmirani P. The "fringe sign" A useful clinical finding in traction alopecia of the marginal hair line. Dermatol Online J. 2011;17(11):1.
20. Agrawal S, Daruwalla SB, Dhurat RS. The flambeau sign - A new dermoscopy finding in a case of marginal traction alopecia. Australas J Dermatol. 2020;61(1):49-50.
21. Billero V, Miteva M. Traction alopecia: the root of the problem. Clin Cosmet Investig Dermatol. 2018;11():149-59.
22. Inui S, Nakajima T, Itami S. Temporal triangular alopecia: Trichoscopic diagnosis. J Dermatol. 2012;39:572-4.
23. Malakar S, Mehta PR, Mukherjee SS. Trichoscopy in pediatric age group. Indian J Paediatr Dermatol. 2018;19:93-101.
24. Mukherjee S, Malakar S. Paediatric hair disorders. In: Malakar S, Chandrashekhar BS, Mukherjee S, Mehta P, Pradhan P, (eds). Trichoscopy: A Text and Atlas. New Delhi: Jaypee; 2017. p. 316-8.
25. Rakowska A, Slowinska M, Kowalska-Oledzka E, Rudnicka L. Trichoscopy in genetic hair shaft abnormalities. J Dermatol Case Rep. 2008;2(2):14-20.

Part 2: Cicatricial Alopecias

Yasmeen J Bhat, Vrutika Hasmukh Shah

INTRODUCTION

Cicatricial alopecias are a group of heterogeneous disorders leading to irreversible destruction of hair follicles and subsequent scarring. Trichoscopy helps in diagnosis, guides in choosing the site of biopsy and monitoring disease activity. It should be done from periphery to center of the lesion.

LICHEN PLANOPILARIS

Clinical Features

Lichen planopilaris (LPP) is the most common cause of cicatricial alopecia. Clinically, LPP is characterized by keratotic follicular papules that coalesce to form plaques followed by multiple irregular cicatricial alopecic areas, perifollicular erythema, and absence of follicular openings with follicular plugging.[1,2]

Trichoscopy

Trichoscopy shows absence of follicular openings, peripilar cast, and blue-gray dots arranged in a "target" pattern. The "target" pattern corresponds to melanophages in papillary dermis and is a sign of pigmentary incontinence confined to the hair follicles (**Figs. 1A** to **G**).[1]

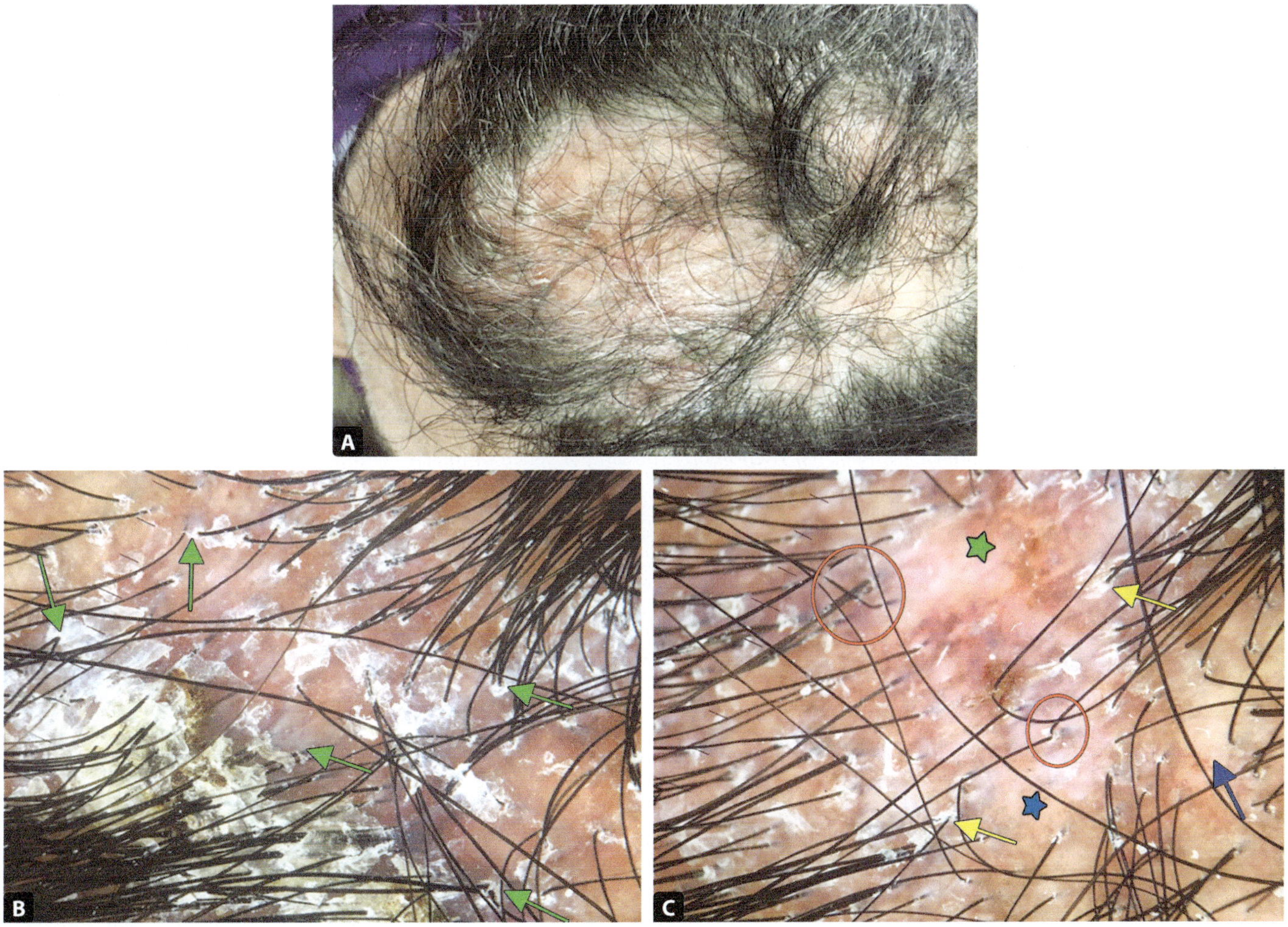

FIGS. 1A TO G: *(Continued)*

(*Continued*)

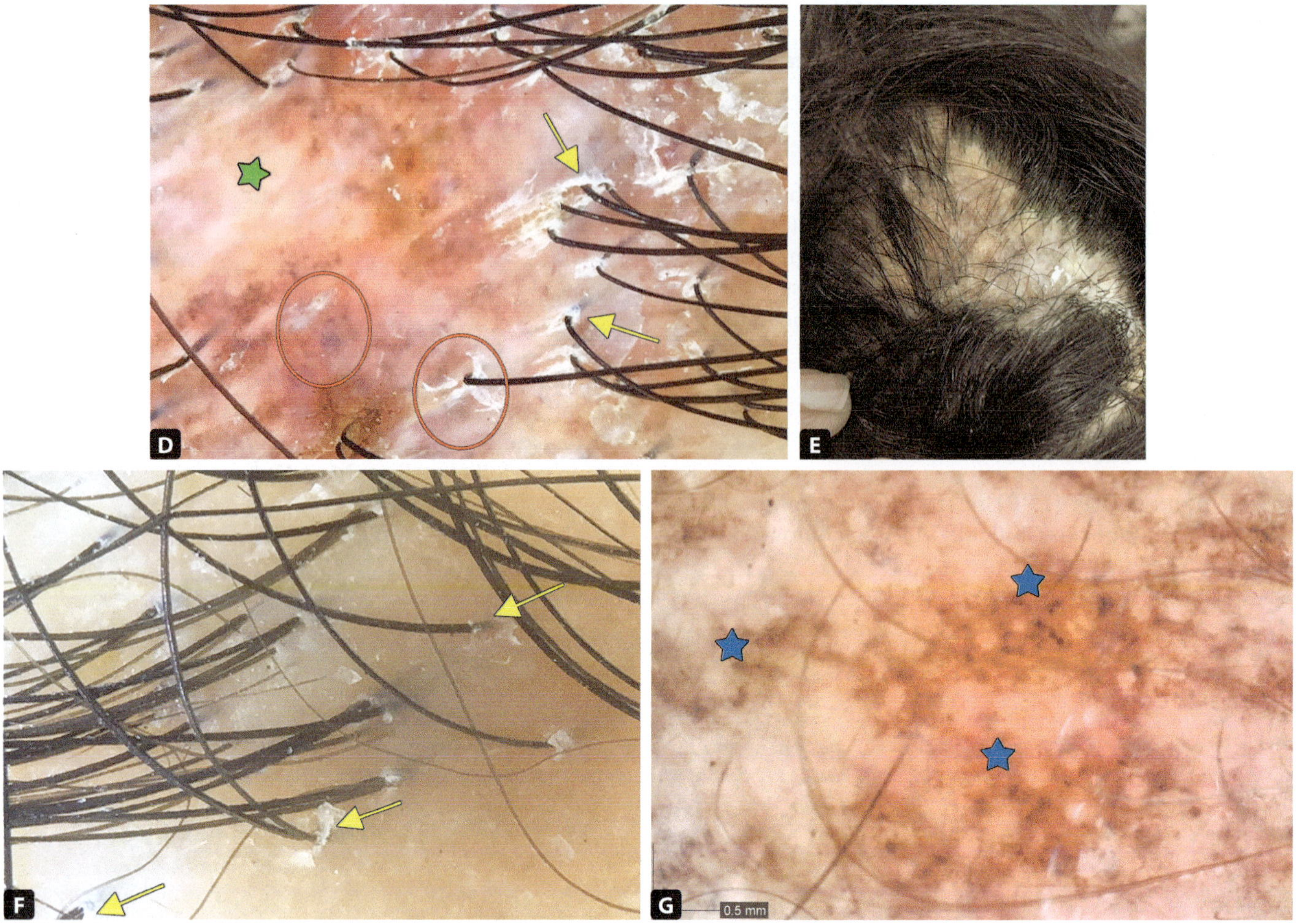

FIGS. 1A TO G: (A) Clinical image of early lichen planopilaris; (B) Trichoscopy shows peripilar scales in the form of white collar around the proximal hair (green arrows) (polarized, DermLite DL3N, 10×); (C) Trichoscopy shows peripilar scales (yellow arrows), peripilar bluish pigmentation (red circles), white areas (green star), absence of follicles with pigmentation (blue star), and linear vessels (blue arrow) (polarized, DermLite DL3N, 10×); (D) Trichoscopy shows peripilar scales (yellow arrows), peripilar bluish pigmentation (red circles), white areas (green star). (polarized, DermLite DL3N, 10×); (E) Clinical image of late lichen planopilaris; (F) Trichoscopy showing peripilar scales (yellow arrows) (polarized, DermLite DL3N, 10×); (G) Trichoscopy showing absence of follicles with pigmentation (blue stars) (polarized, Dino-Lite, 70×).

Key Points[2]

- Absence of follicular openings and vellus hair
- Peripilar cast
- Blue-gray dots in a target distribution around the hair follicles
- Fibrotic white patches
- *Pinpoint white dots in background of honeycomb-pigmented network*: Starry sky pattern

DISCOID LUPUS ERYTHEMATOSUS

Clinical Features

Cicatricial alopecia associated with single or multiple patches of alopecia with central atrophy, erythema, follicular plugging, and telangiectasia.[3]

Trichoscopy

Loss of follicular openings, white patches, peripilar casts, keratotic plugs, red dots, thick arborizing vessels, and blue-gray dots in a speckled pattern are seen on trichoscopy.[1] Red dots correspond to follicular openings surrounded by dilated vessels and if treated early, hair regrowth may be achieved.[4] Blue-gray dots in a "speckled" pattern correspond to interface dermatitis and melanophages in papillary dermis. Blue white veil is newly described trichoscopic feature seen secondary to melanin incontinence with overlying hyperkeratosis (**Figs. 2A** to **D**).[5]

Key Points[3,4]

- Loss of follicular openings
- Keratotic plugs

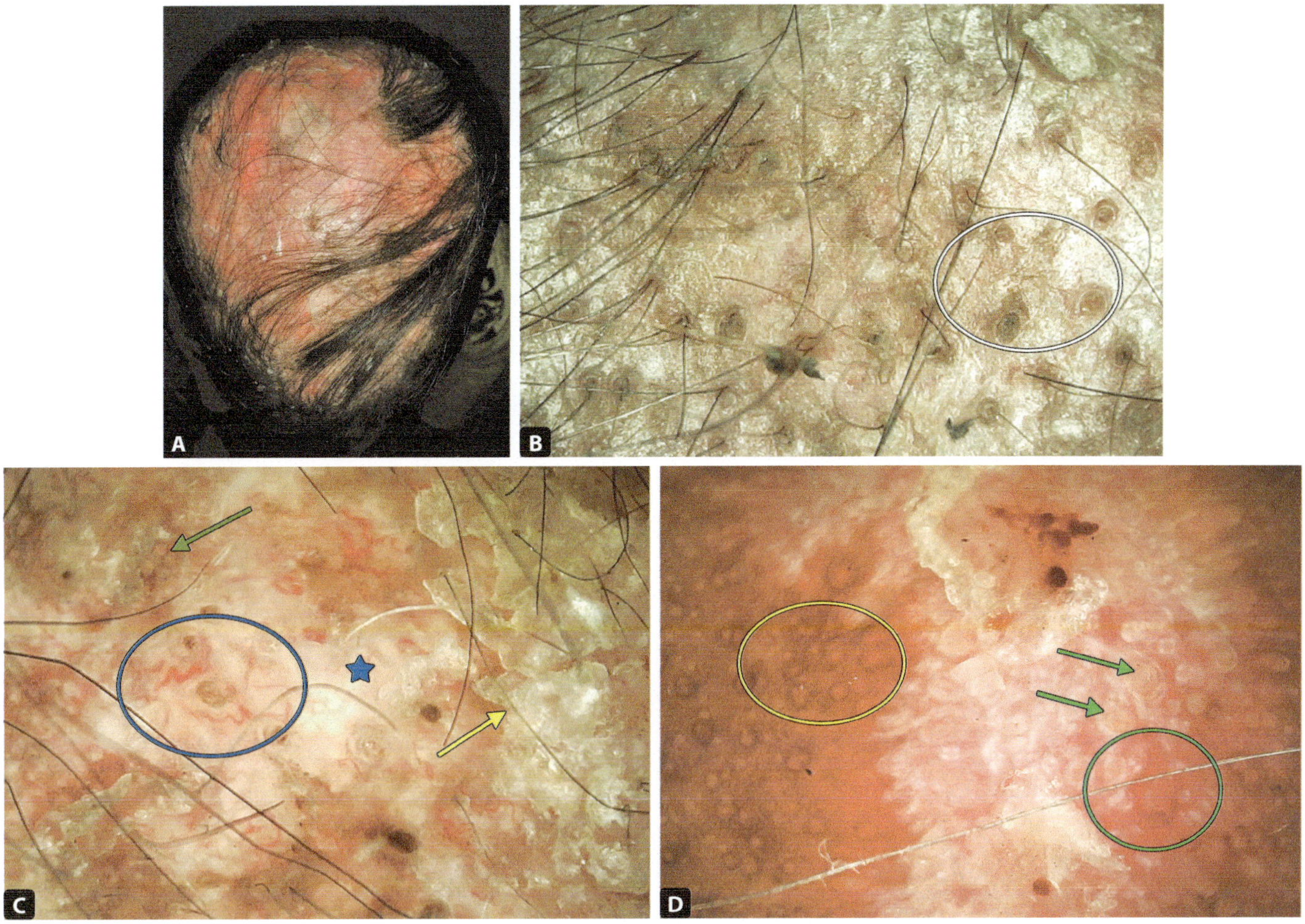

FIGS. 2A TO D: (A) Clinical image of discoid lupus erythematosus; (B) Trichoscopy showing follicular keratotic plugs (white circle) (nonpolarized, EScope Oitez, 20×); (C) Trichoscopy showing yellow dots (green arrow), arborizing vessels (blue circle), whitish interfollicular scale (yellow arrow), and white patches (blue star) (polarized, EScope Oitez, 20×); (D) Trichoscopy showing blue gray dots in a speckled pattern (yellow circle), follicular red dots (green circle), and perifollicular halo (green arrows) (polarized, EScope Oitez, 20×).

- Blue-gray dots in a speckled pattern
- Red dots
- Thick arborizing vessels

FRONTAL FIBROSING ALOPECIA

Clinical Features

Cicatricial alopecia is characterized by progressive symmetric recession of frontotemporal hairline along with patchy or total loss of eyebrows.[6,7]

Trichoscopy

On trichoscopy, absence of vellus hair, peripilar cast and erythema, broken hair, and black dots are seen (**Figs. 3A** to **D**).

Key Points[4]

- Absence of follicular openings and vellus hair
- Perifollicular erythema—characteristic
- Peripilar cast
- Lonely hair

FOLLICULITIS DECALVANS

Clinical Features

Folliculitis decalvans (FD) is a primary neutrophilic cicatricial alopecia characterized by recurrent papulo-pustular lesions with exudative crusted areas.[8]

Trichoscopy

Trichoscopy shows crusts and tufted hairs surrounded by thick concentric scales.[9] At the base of hair tufts, starburst sign is seen which is formed by a band of yellowish scales and white strands (due to perifollicular epidermal hyperplasia) (**Figs. 4A** to **E**).[10]

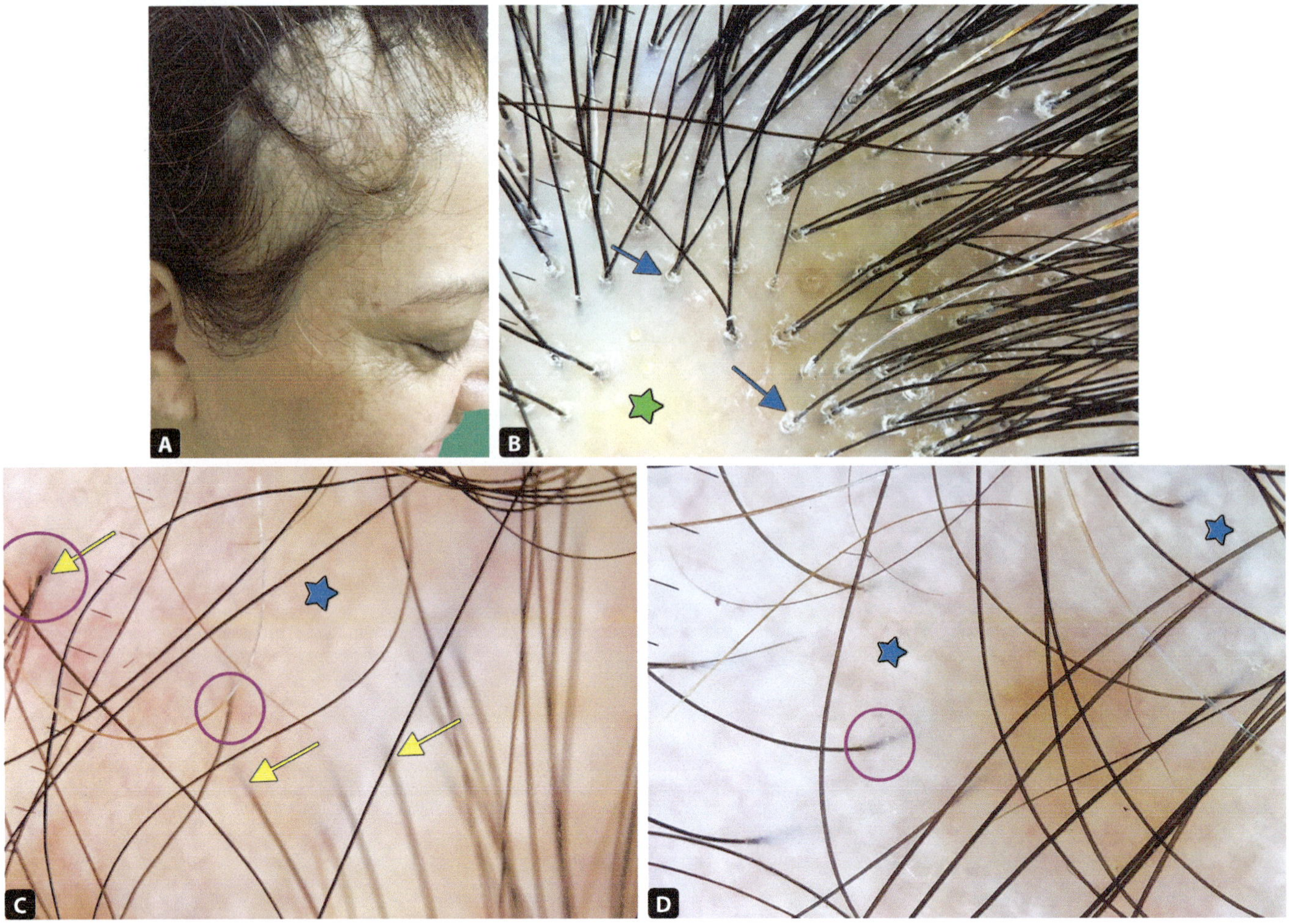

FIGS. 3A TO D: (A) Clinical image of frontal fibrosing alopecia; (B) Trichoscopy showing peripilar cast at the periphery (blue arrows) and absence of hair follicles (green star) (polarized, DermLite DL3N, 10×); (C) Trichoscopy showing peripilar lonely hairs (yellow arrows), white areas (blue star), and peripilar erythema (purple circles) (polarized, DermLite DL3N, 10×); (D) Trichoscopy showing white areas (blue stars) and peripilar erythema (purple circle) (polarized, DermLite DL3N, 10×).

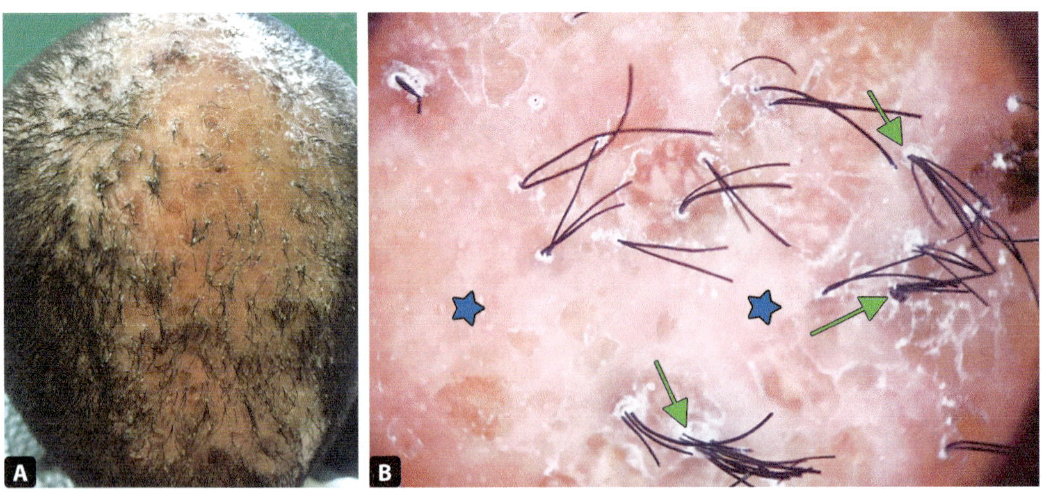

FIGS. 4A TO E: (*Continued*)

(*Continued*)

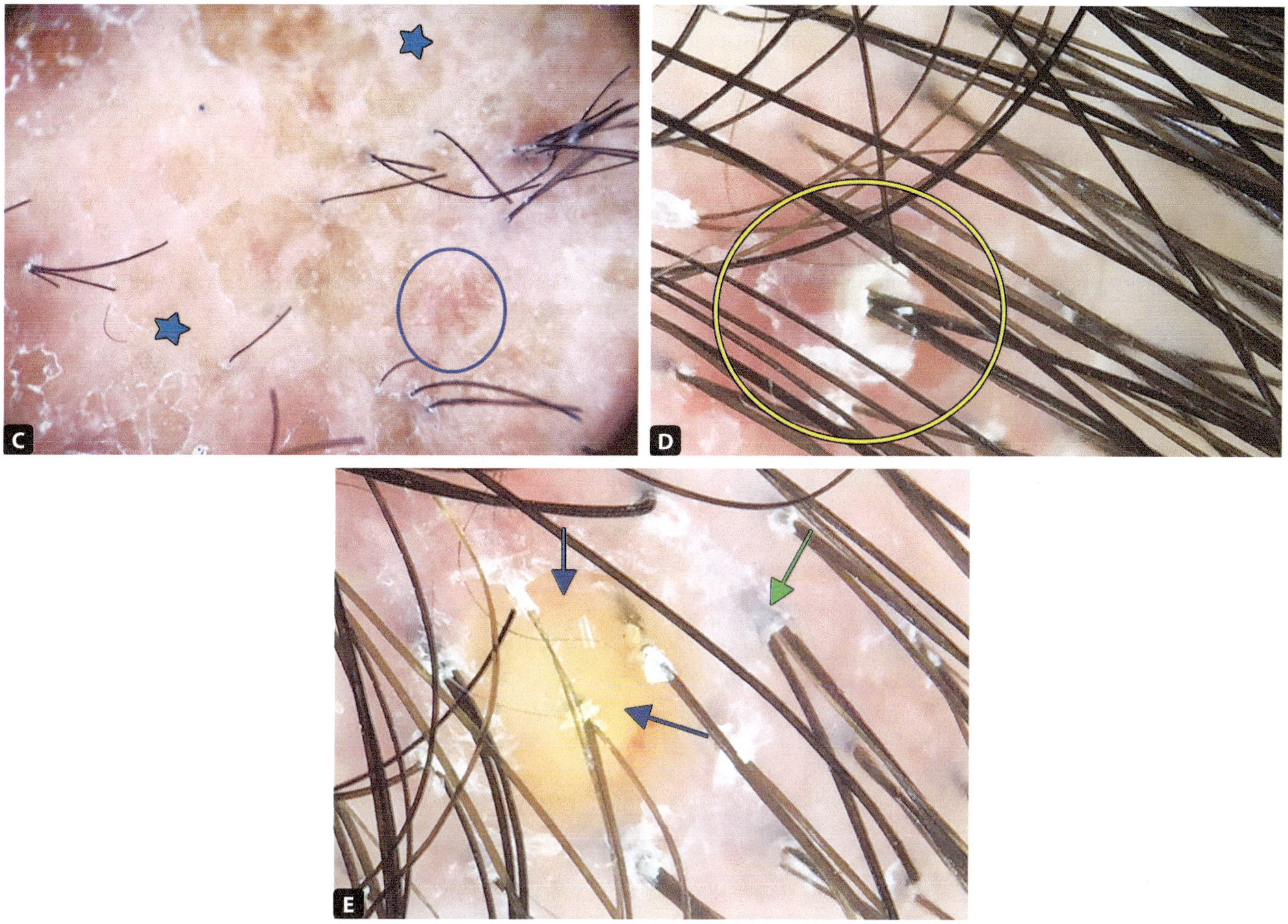

FIGS. 4A TO E: (A) Clinical image of folliculitis decalvans; (B) Trichoscopy showing tufts of hair with peripilar scales (green arrows) and absence of follicles (blue stars) (polarized, DermLite DL3N, 10×); (C) Trichoscopy showing absence of follicles (blue stars) and coiled dilated capillaries (blue circle) (polarized, DermLite DL3N, 10×); (D) Trichoscopy showing tufts of hair with perifollicular tubular scale (yellow circle) (polarized, DermLite DL3N, 10×); (E) Trichoscopy showing tufts of hair with peripilar scales (green arrow) and perifollicular pustule (blue arrows) (polarized, DermLite DL3N, 10×).

Key Points[9,10]

- Tufts of six or more hairs—diagnostic
- Perifollicular pustules and scaling
- Coiled dilated capillaries
- Peripilar casts—thicker than that of LPP
- Starburst sign

TUFTED FOLLICULITIS

Context

Tufted folliculitis (TF) is a variant of FD where circumscribed areas of scalp inflammation heal with scarring characterized by tufts of up to 30 hairs emerging from a single dilated follicular opening.[11]

Key Points[11]

- Doll hair—tuft of 5 to 30 hairs emerging from a single follicular orifice
- Yellowish tubular scaling
- Peripilar cast

DISSECTING CELLULITIS

Clinical Features

Dissecting cellulitis is a neutrophilic alopecia characterized by follicular occlusion and presents as painful nodules, boggy plaques, abscesses, and sinuses over the vertex or back of the scalp.[12] It is a part of follicular occlusion triad.

Trichoscopy

White fibrotic areas with loss of follicular ostia, large and few keratin plugs, broken hairs, pili torti, and yellow dot with three-dimensional (3D) structures are seen.[13] Yellow dot with 3D structures correspond to yellow dot imposed over dystrophic hair (**Figs. 5A** to **D**).[10]

Key Points[13]

- Accentuated plugged follicular openings
- Black dots
- Broken hairs
- Yellow dot with 3D structures

PSEUDOPELADE OF BROCQ

Clinical Features

Pseudopelade of Brocq is a lymphocytic cicatricial alopecia characterized by asymptomatic, noninflamed, white reticulate patches in the central scalp.[12]

Trichoscopy

Trichoscopy shows scarring areas devoid of inflammation (**Figs. 6A** to **C**).

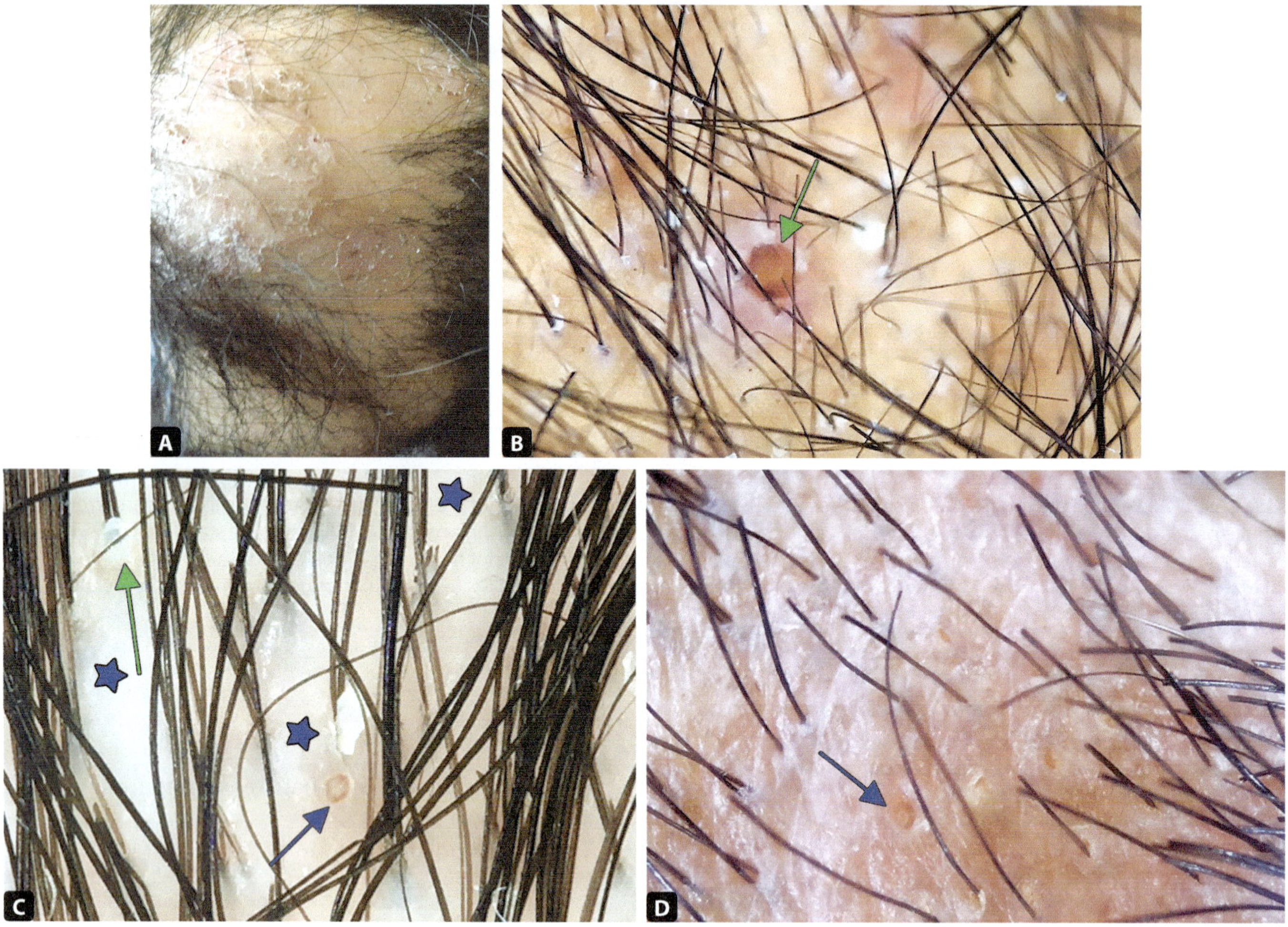

FIGS. 5A TO D: (A) Clinical image of dissecting folliculitis; (B) Trichoscopy showing perifollicular pustules (green arrow) (polarized, DermLite DL3N, 10×); (C) Trichoscopy showing perifollicular pustules (green arrow), absence of follicles (blue stars), and three-dimensional (3D) yellow dot (blue arrow) (polarized, DermLite DL3N, 10×); (D) Trichoscopy shows three-dimensional (3D) yellow dot (blue arrow) (nonpolarized, DermLite DL3N, 10×).

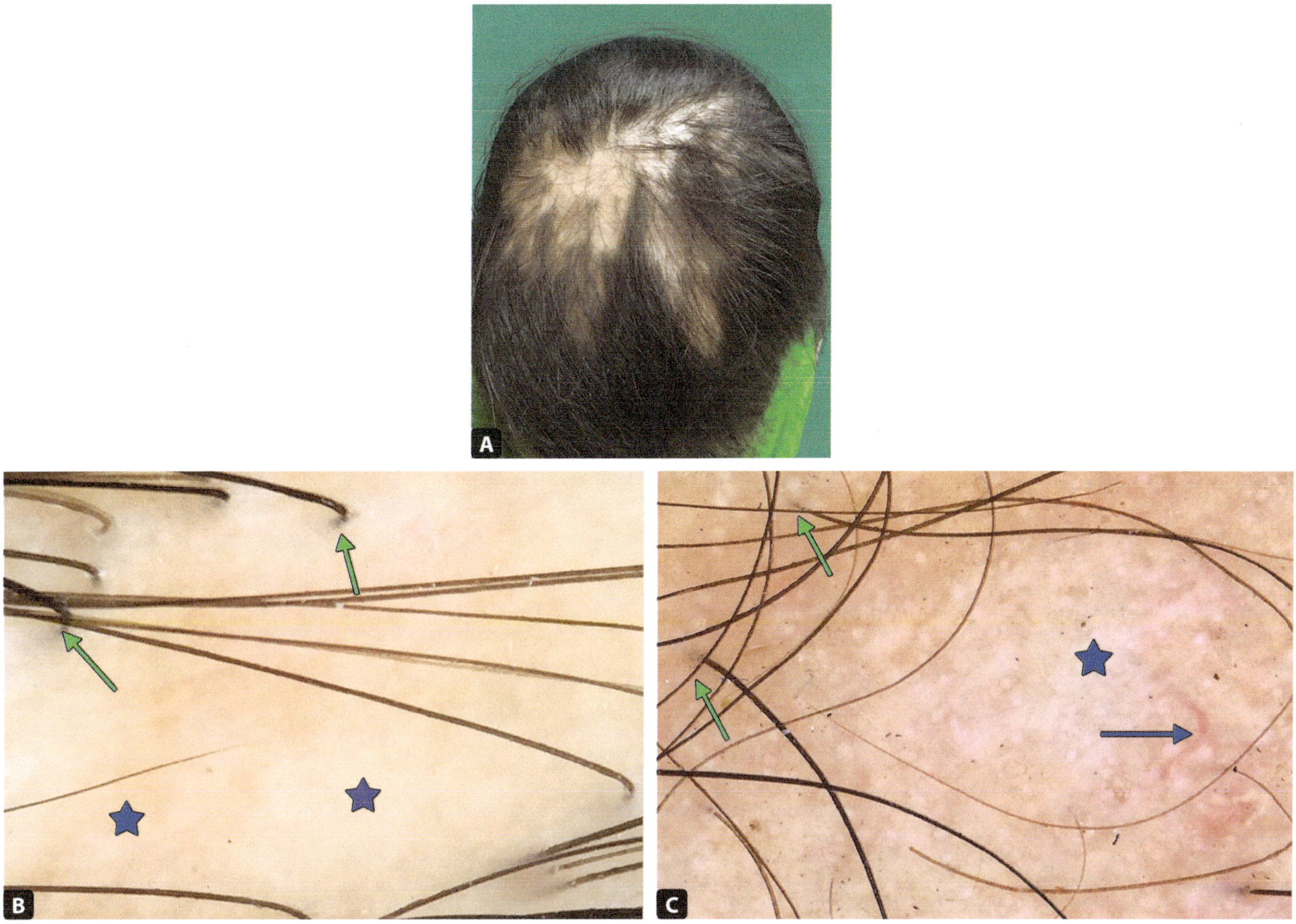

FIGS. 6A TO C: (A) Clinical image of pseudopelade of Brocq; (B) Trichoscopy showing single hairs at the periphery (green arrows) and absence of hair follicles (blue stars) (polarized, DermLite DL3N, 10×); (C) Trichoscopy showing single hairs at the periphery (green arrows), absence of hair follicles and white areas (blue star), and short linear vessels (blue arrow) (polarized, DermLite DL3N, 10×).

Key Points[14]

- Loss of follicular openings
- Lone dystrophic hairs at the margin
- Smooth white areas
- *Background*: Porcelain-white, gray, beige, and erythematous

CENTRAL CENTRIFUGAL CICATRCIAL ALOPECIA

Clinical Features

Central centrifugal cicatricial alopecia (CCCA) is cicatricial alopecia of central scalp that extends centrifugally, mostly secondary to hair care practices such as hot comb, relaxers, and tight extensions.[15]

Trichoscopy

Trichoscopy shows gray-white perifollicular halo, irregular white patches, absence of follicular ostia, irregularly distributed pinpoint white dots, asterisk-like brown macules, and broken hairs. Brown asterisk-like blotches correlate with postinflammatory hyperpigmentation and peripilar gray-white halo corresponds to lamellar fibrosis that destroys the normal melanization of outer root sheath (**Figs. 7A** and **B**).

Key Points[16]

- Preserved honeycomb pattern
- Irregularly distributed pinpoint white dots
- Irregular white patches
- *Peripilar white-gray halo*: Highly specific and sensitive
- Asterisk-like brown macules
- *Broken hairs*: Sign of occult CCCA

EROSIVE PUSTULAR DERMATOSIS OF THE SCALP

Clinical Features

Erosive pustular dermatosis of the scalp is rare and seen in elderly females, presenting as recurrent episodes of itchy and painful erosions and pustules on the scalp with adherent purulent crusts and beefy red color.

Trichoscopy

Nonspecific features such as erythema, brownish white crusts, hemorrhages, and reduced hair density (**Figs. 8A** and **B**). Histopathology shows epidermal atrophy, mixed inflammation, and reduced follicles.[12]

Key Points

- Beefy erythema
- Brownish white crusts
- Hemorrhages
- Reduced hair density

KEY POINTS

- Trichoscopy reveals mainly follicular findings and less hair shaft signs.
- Perifollicular scales and vascular findings are seen in early disease.
- White atrophic areas and pigmentation are seen in late cases of cicatricial alopecia.

CONCLUSION

The characteristic trichoscopic features that differentiate cicatricial from noncicatricial alopecia include—loss of white dots, white atrophic areas, vascular patterns, changes in pigmentary pattern, perifollicular scaling, and not much hair shaft changes.

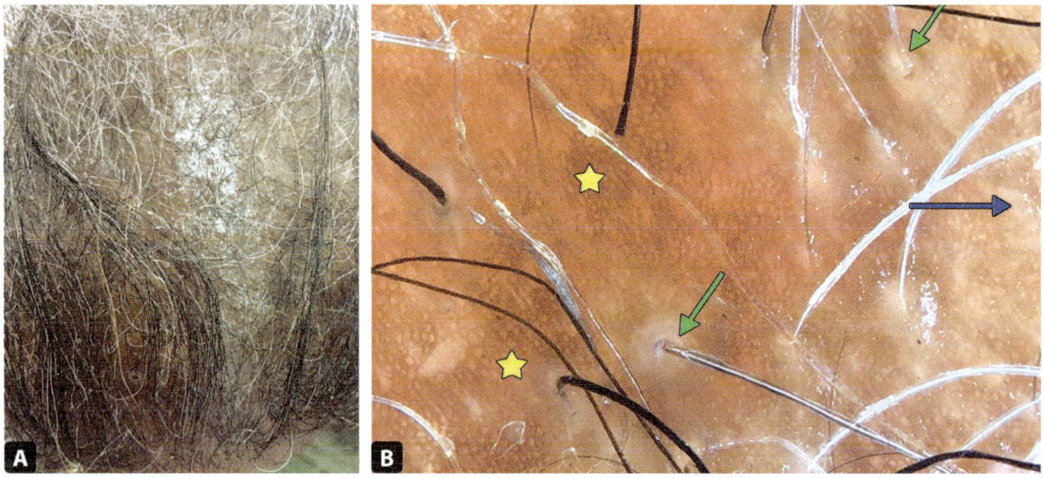

FIGS. 7A AND B: (A) Clinical image of central centrifugal cicatricial alopecia; (B) Trichoscopy showing preserved honeycomb pattern (yellow stars), gray-white perifollicular halo (green arrows), and irregular white patches (blue arrow) (polarized, DermLite DL3N, 20×).

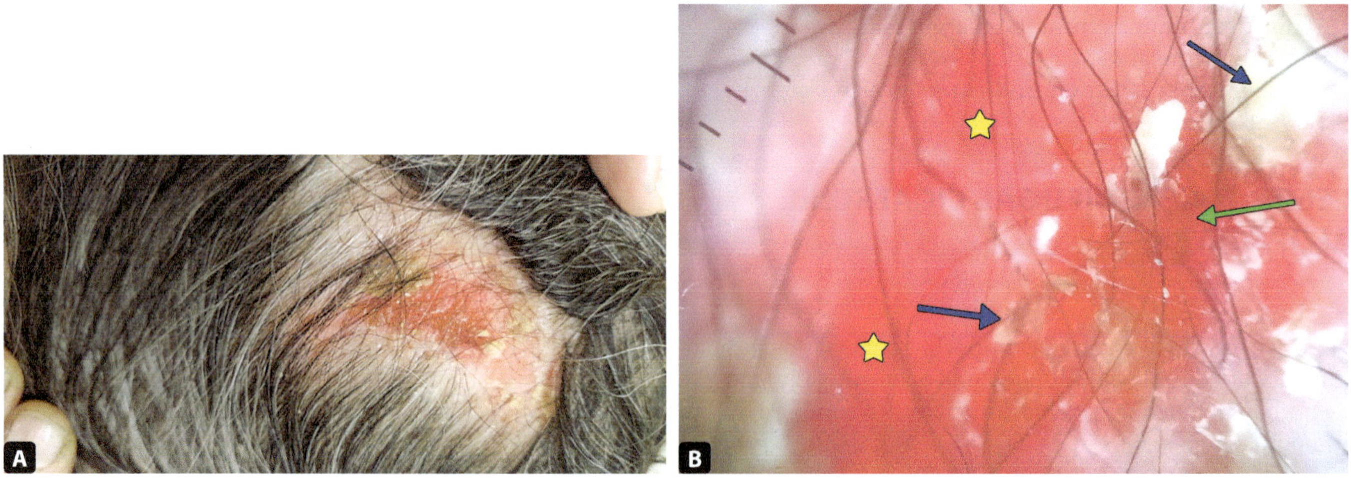

FIGS. 8A AND B: (A) Clinical image of erosive pustular dermatosis; (B) Trichoscopy showing background erythema (yellow stars), brownish white crusts (blue arrows), and hemorrhages (green arrow) with reduced hair density (polarized, DermLite DL4, 10×).

REFERENCES

1. Duque-Estrada B, Tamler C, Sodré CT, Barcaui CB, Pereira FB. Dermoscopy patterns of cicatricial alopecia resulting from discoid lupus erythematosus and lichen planopilaris. An Bras Dermatol. 2010;85(2):178-83.
2. Friedman P, Sabban EC, Marcucci C, Peralta R, Cabo H. Dermoscopic findings in different clinical variants of lichen planus. Is dermoscopy useful? Dermatol Pract Concept. 2015;5(5):51-5.
3. Tosti A. Primary scarring alopecias. In: Tosti A, (ed). Dermoscopy of the Hair and Nails, 2nd edition. Boca Raton: Springer; 2016. p.57.
4. Mathur M, Acharya P. Trichoscopy of primary cicatricial alopecias: an updated review. J Eur Acad Dermatol Venereol. 2020;34(3):473-84.
5. Cervantes J, Hafeez F, Miteva M. Blue-white veil as novel dermatoscopic feature in discoid lupus erythematosus in 2 African-American patients. Skin Appendage Disord. 2017;3(4):211-4.
6. Tosti A. Primary scarring alopecias. In: Tosti A, (ed). Dermoscopy of the Hair and Nails, 2nd edition. Boca Raton: Springer; 2016. p. 53.
7. Vañó-Galván S, Molina-Ruiz AM, Serrano-Falcón C, Arias-Santiago S, Rodrigues-Barata AR, Garnacho-Saucedo G, et al. Frontal fibrosing alopecia: a multicenter review of 355 patients. J Am Acad Dermatol. 2014;70(4):670-8.
8. Fernandez-Crehuet P, Va~no-Galvan S, Molina-Ruiz AM, Rodrigues-Barata AR, Serrano-Falcón C, Martorell-Calatayud A, et al. Trichoscopic features of folliculitis decalvans: results in 58 Patients. Int J Trichol. 2017;9(3):140-1.
9. Miteva M, Tosti A. Hair and scalp dermatoscopy. J Am Acad Dermatol. 2012;67(5):1040-8.
10. Rakowska A, Slowinska M, Kowalska-Oledzka E, Warszawik O, Czuwara J, Olszewska M, et al. Trichoscopy of cicatricial alopecia. J Drugs Dermatol. 2012;11(6):753-8.
11. Broshtilova V, Bardarov E, Kazandjieva J, Marina S. Tufted hair folliculitis: a case report and literature review. Acta Dermatovenerol Alp Pannonica Adriat. 2011;20(1):27-9.
12. Bolduc C, Sperling L, Shapiro J. Primary cicatricial alopecia: Other lymphocytic primary cicatricial alopecias and neutrophilic and mixed primary cicatricial alopecias. J Am Acad Dermatol. 2016;75(6):1101-17.
13. Verzi AE, Lacarrubba F, Micali G. Heterogeneity of trichoscopy findings in dissecting cellulitis of the scalp: correlation with disease activity and duration. Br J Dermatol. 2017;177(6):e331-2.
14. Nikam VV, Mehta HH. A nonrandomized study of trichoscopy patterns using nonpolarized (contact) and polarized (noncontact) dermatoscopy in hair and shaft disorders. Int J Trichol. 2014;6(2):54-62.
15. Summers P, Kyei A, Bergfeld W. Central centrifugal cicatricial alopecia - an approach to diagnosis and management. Int J Dermatol. 2011;50(12):1457-64.
16. Miteva M, Tosti A. Dermatoscopic features of central centrifugal cicatricial alopecia. J Am Acad Dermatol. 2014;71(3):443-9.

17 CHAPTER

Onychoscopy

Chander Grover, Dipali Rathod

INTRODUCTION

Although nail disorders constitute 10% of dermatological consultations, their clinical and dermoscopic evaluation remains a diagnostic challenge.[1] Onychoscopy (dermoscopy of nail unit) offers a noninvasive, cost-effective diagnostic tool enabling visualization of subtle changes,[2] providing insight into underlying systemic conditions, enabling visualization of subsurface changes, and vascular alterations.[3] It helps in differential diagnosis, choosing a biopsy site, and assessing therapeutic response.[4,5] There are essential differences between onychoscopy and dermoscopy (**Table 1**).

TABLE 1: Differences between onychoscopy and dermoscopy.

S. No.	Onychoscopy	Dermoscopy
1.	Technically difficult to perform and interpret	Technically easier procedure
2.	Taking pictures is more cumbersome due to the curvature and size of the nail unit	Taking pictures is easy
3.	The interface medium is needed in a larger quantity, especially if using ultrasound gel	Generally lesser quantity is needed
4.	Ultrasound gel is considered an ideal interface medium for contact dermoscopy	70% alcoholic solution is considered an ideal interface medium
5.	All parts of the nail unit cannot be focused as a whole in a single view	Depends upon the lesion to be examined

PROCEDURE OF ONYCHOSCOPY

- It is crucial to have a through knowledge of nail anatomy.
- Digit to be examined, and the pathological area should be identified.
- First examine under lower magnification (~10×) (global view) (**Fig. 1**), then shifted to higher magnification (~50–200×) (**Fig. 2**) for finer details.
- Surface abnormalities (nail plate changes) better evaluated by nonpolarized light source without fluid (dry mode) (**Fig. 2**).

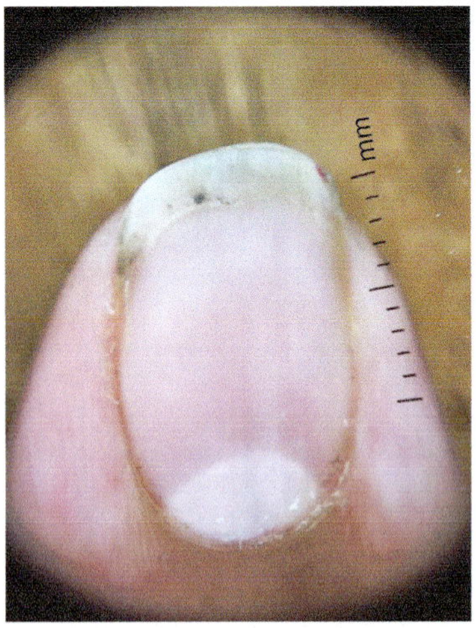

FIG. 1: Normal nail under low magnification. The proximal white semilunar structure is the lunula, and the pink zone distal to it represents the normal nail bed. The nail plate in this case is transparent except for the distal opaque free edge, with dirt trapped underneath. Hyperpigmented proximal nail fold and transparent cuticle overlying the nail plate can be seen (polarized, DermLite DL4, 10×).

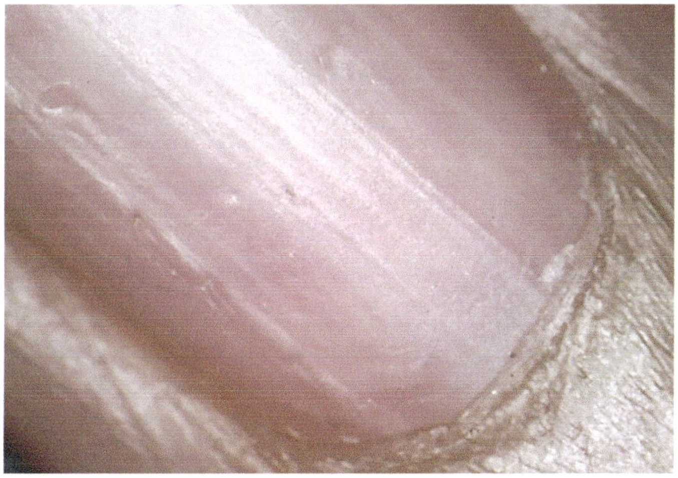

FIG. 2: Normal nail under higher magnification. Note the surface irregularities which are visible under the nonpolarized mode (nonpolarized, Dino-Lite AM7115MZT, 50×).

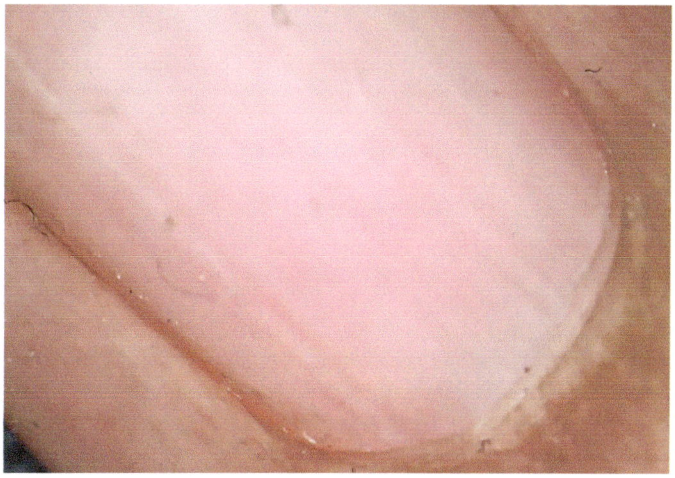

FIG. 3: Same nail plate under same magnification. However, polarization permits visualization of the pinkish nail bed (polarized, Dino-Lite AM7115MZT, 50×).

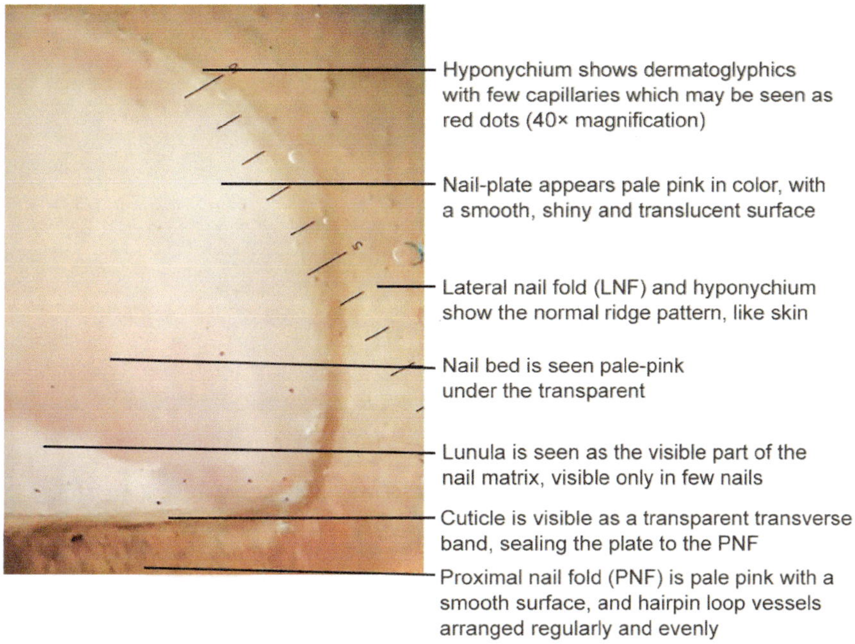

FIG. 4: Detailed onychoscopic features of a normal nail structure on onychoscopy. Prominent capillaries in the distal nail bed can be seen (polarized, Dino-Lite AM7115MZT, 50×).

- Subsurface abnormalities (nail bed, vascular and color changes) better evaluated by a polarized light source with fluid (wet mode) (**Fig. 3**).

The onychoscopic features of normal nail are depicted in **Figures 4** and **5**.

PIGMENTARY DISORDERS (CHROMONYCHIA)

Melanonychia

- Most extensively studied nail disorder.
- Onychoscopy helps differentiate benign causes from a malignant cause.
- Onychoscopic assessment of color and its intensity provides clues toward location of pigment source, ethnicity, and nail plate thickness.

Benign Longitudinal Melanonychia

- The causes of longitudinal melanonychia are either melanocyte activation (more common) or melanocyte proliferation (less common).
- *Regular pattern*—light-colored, parallel longitudinal lines, homogeneous in color, spacing, thickness, and orientation. However, a regular pattern may not be observed at times, especially in children.[6]

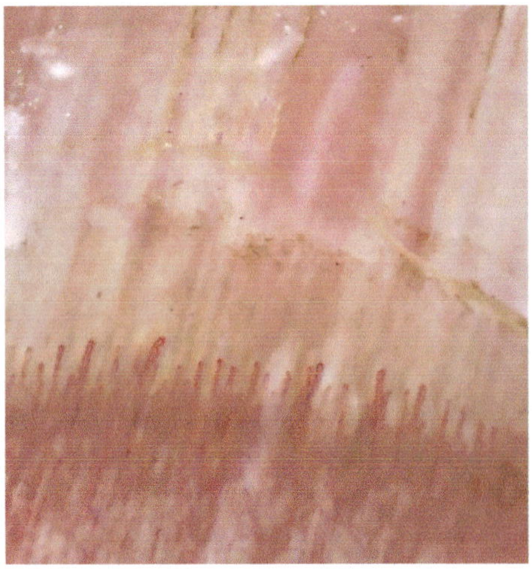

FIG. 5: Normal proximal nail fold with visible capillary loops (polarized, Dino-Lite AM7115MZT, 50×).

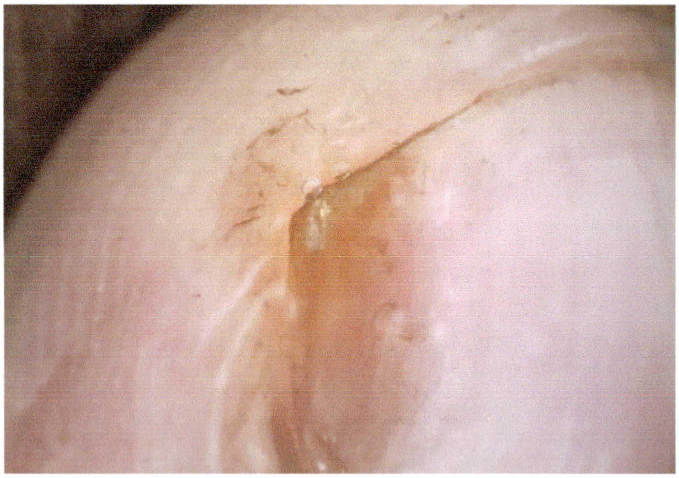

FIG. 6: Benign longitudinal melanonychia due to melanocyte activation seen in a toenail with frictional melanonychia (polarized, Dino-Lite AM7115MZT, 50×).

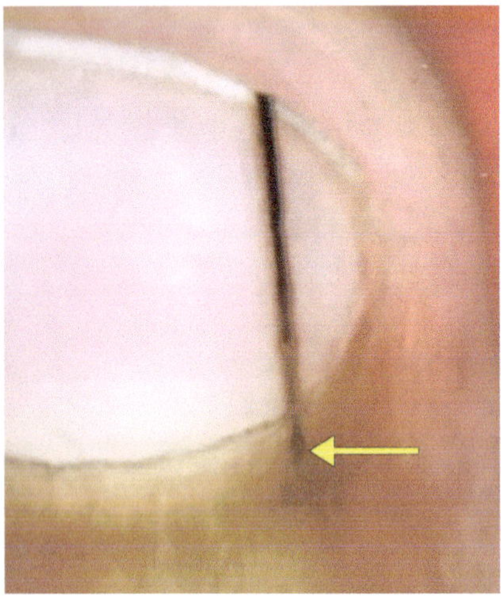

FIG. 7: Benign longitudinal melanonychia due to melanocyte proliferation. Uniform black band with parallel edges is noted. Pseudo-Hutchinson's sign (arrow) can be seen in the proximal nail fold (polarized, DermLite DL4, 10×).

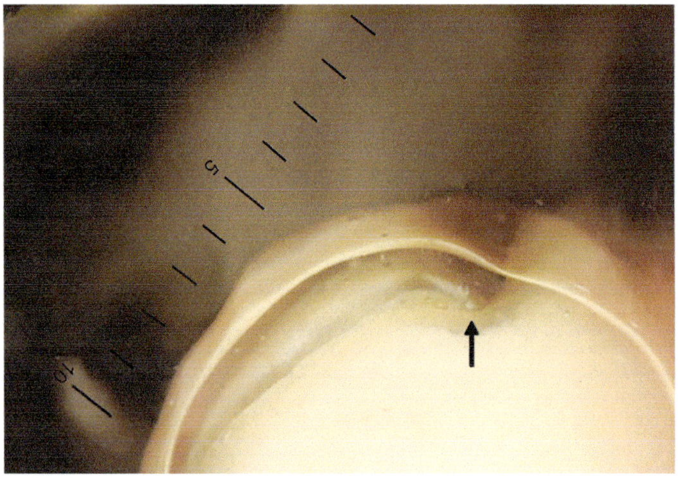

FIG. 8: Benign longitudinal melanonychia showing pigmentation of the lower half (arrow) of the nail plate when examined distally. This signifies a more distal matrix location of the pigment origin (polarized, Heine Delta 20T, 20×).

- Melanocyte activation (ethnic or drug-induced) shows a homogeneous gray-colored band with thin longitudinal gray lines (**Fig. 6**).
- Nevus (melanocyte proliferation) shows regular arrangement of parallel lines on a brown background (**Fig. 7**).
- Onychoscopic examination of free edge of nail plate helps determine origin of the pigment. Pigment present in lower half (ventrally) indicates a distal matrix origin, while that in upper half (dorsally) indicates origin in proximal matrix (**Fig. 8**). Pigmentation throughout the nail plate thickness indicates a wider origin.

Malignant Longitudinal Melanonychia

- *Irregular pattern*—longitudinal lines, irregular in color, spacing, thickness, and parallelism. There may also be a diffuse dark background with barely visible lines.
- Variability in hues of pigmentation favors malignancy.[7]
- *Hutchinson's sign*—a clinical sign which describes periungual extension of brown-black pigmentation onto the proximal and lateral nail folds indicating subungual melanoma.
- *Micro-Hutchinson's sign*—pigmentation seen only on onychoscopy of periungual tissue, not visible to the naked eye.
- *Pseudo-Hutchinson's sign*—nail bed and nail matrix hyperpigmentation observed through the transparent nail folds (**Fig. 7**).[8]

Leukonychia

- Whitish discoloration of nail plate
- Onychoscopy helps delineate true and pseudoleukonychia.

- Both may present as longitudinal and/or transverse white streaks.[9]
- Punctate leukonychia refers to small white cloud-like structures within the nail plate (**Fig. 9**).

Erythronychia

- Diffuse redness or longitudinal red-colored bands originating from the lunula
- The pattern can be seen in nail lichen planus (LP) while a single erythematous band (monodactylous erythronychia) is an indicator of tumors including onychopapilloma.
- Alternating red and white bands (candy-cane appearance) is seen in Darier's disease.

INFECTIONS OF NAIL

Onychomycosis

- Most common nail disorder, constituting approximately 50% of onychopathies[10]
- Most common clinical presentation is distal-lateral subungual onychomycosis (DLSO) having typical onychoscopic features as:
  - A "jagged edge with spikes" seen in the proximal border of onycholysis (**Fig. 10**)[11,12]
  - Subungual "ruin pattern"—distal pulverization with indented areas on the subungual keratosis (**Fig. 11**)
  - "Aurora borealis pattern"—a multitude of colors of longitudinal striae seen in the onycholytic nail plate (**Figs. 12** and **13**)

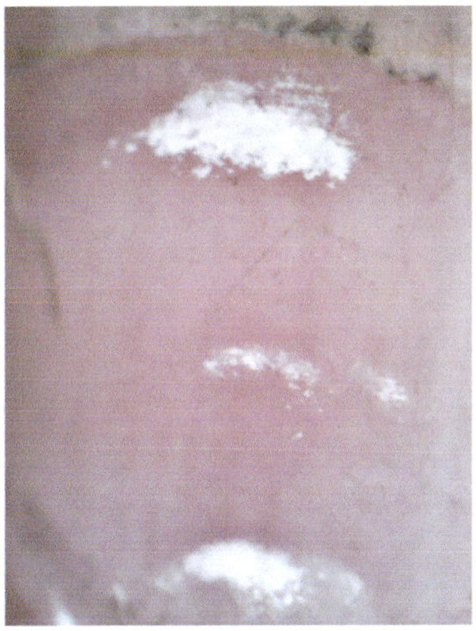

FIG. 9: Punctate leukonychia seen in a child (polarized, Dino-Lite AM7115, 50×).

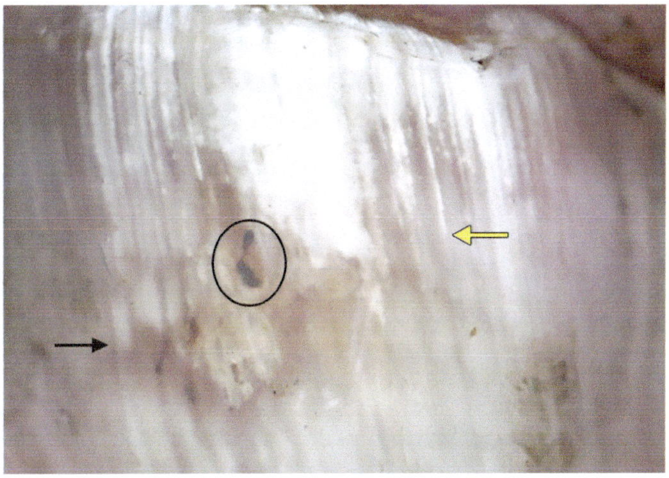

FIG. 10: Distal-lateral subungual onychomycosis with "spike pattern" (black arrow) and jagged edge (yellow arrow) of onycholysis. Few splinter hemorrhages (black circle) can also be seen which could be trauma induced (polarized, Dino-Lite AM7115, 50×).

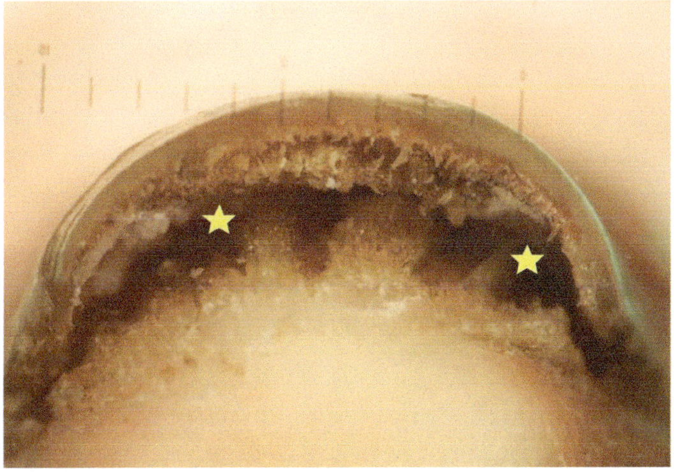

FIG. 11: Subungual hyperkeratosis in a patient with distal-lateral superficial onychomycosis. The friable debris with empty spaces (stars) is indicative of "ruinous pattern" which favors onychomycosis (polarized, Heine Delta 20T, 20×).

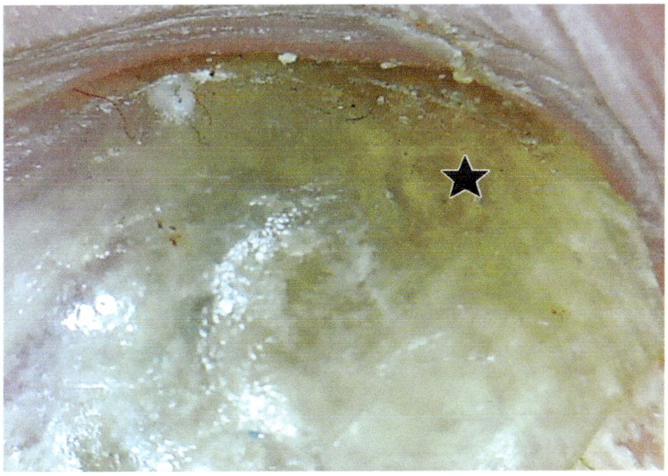

FIG. 12: "Aurora borealis" pattern of color changes seen in a nail with distal-lateral superficial onychomycosis. The gradation of color changes in the onycholysed nail plate, varying from white to yellow to green to brown (star), is highly suggestive of onychomycosis (nonpolarized, Dino-Lite AM7115, 50×).

- *Dermatophytoma* corresponds to yellowish-orange-colored patches in the nail plate connected to the distal nail plate by a narrow channel (**Fig. 14**).
- Proximal subungual onychomycosis (PSO) shows distal jagged edge and spikes corresponding to fungal invasion from proximal edge (**Fig. 15**).
- Endonyx onychomycosis shows a "dendritic pattern" at the periphery of the cloud-like patches of leukonychia (**Fig. 16**).[13]
- Superficial white onychomycosis (SWO) shows superficial white deposits on an irregular nail plate surface with a "grid pattern".[14]
- Other suggestive features include fungal melanonychia (black to brown-colored longitudinal or transverse pigment bands) and small splinter hemorrhages.[15]

Candida Infection

- Uncommonly causes onychomycosis in immunocompetent hosts or normal nails
- Associated with proximal nail fold (PNF) swelling, rounding, and disruption of the cuticle
- Total dystrophic changes may be seen in patients with chronic-mucocutaneous candidiasis.

Verrucae (Subungual and Periungual)

- Appear with a yellowish or whitish and rough-verrucous surface (hyperkeratotic surface) along with multiple reddish-black dots and/or streaks (corresponding to thrombosed dilated capillaries and small hemorrhages) (**Fig. 17**)[16,17]

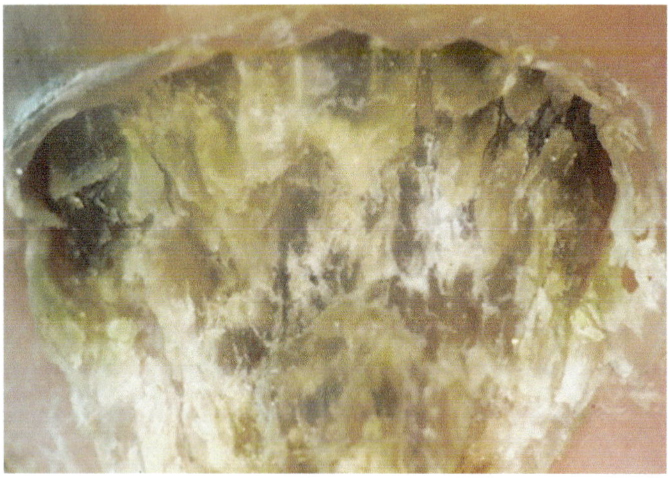

FIG. 13: Similar spectrum of color changes seen in a case with total dystrophic onychomycosis (polarized, Heine Delta 20T, 20×).

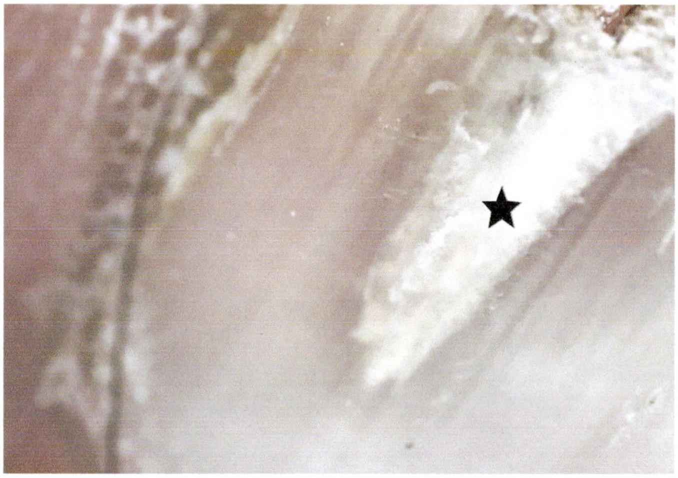

FIG. 14: A compact area of opacity and discoloration within the nail plate (star), connected distally by a narrow channel. This is suggestive of a dermatophytoma (polarized, Dino-Lite AM7115, 50×).

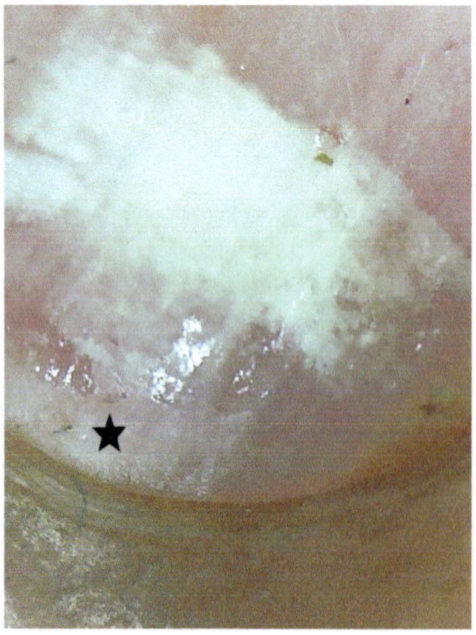

FIG. 15: Whitish discoloration arising under the proximal part of the nail plate (star) and extending distally, suggestive of proximal subungual onychomycosis (nonpolarized, Dino-Lite AM7115, 50×).

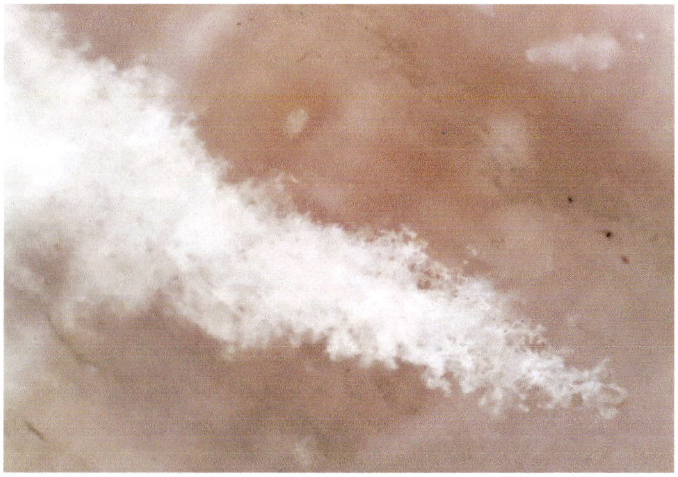

FIG. 16: Leukonychia involving a part of the nail plate with a dendritic pattern, suggestive of endonyx onychomycosis (nonpolarized, Dino-Lite AM7115, 70×).

- Lesions responding to treatment show a decreased capillary density.
- Onychoscopy can help to estimate the proximal extent of wart beneath the nail plate.[18]

Paronychia

- Acute paronychia shows yellowish-red crust, white lines, white scales with dotted vessels on pink background.
- Chronic paronychia is characterized by disrupted or ragged cuticle and transverse ridges over the nail plate. Occasional whitish structures are noted.

Pseudomonas Infections

- Chloronychia (green nails) shows greenish discoloration with a peripheral fading, typically arising near the nail folds (**Fig. 18**).

INFLAMMATORY NAIL DISORDERS

Nail Psoriasis

- Onychoscopic features of nail psoriasis depend on the part of nail unit affected.
- Nail pitting, splinter hemorrhages, and onycholysis have been reported as the most common onychoscopic findings.[19-21]
- *Nail matrix disease* manifests as:
  - Pits—irregular in size and shape, larger, coarse and deep depressions (**Figs. 19** to **21**)
  - Longitudinal and transverse ridging
  - Nail plate crumbling
  - Leukonychia (white irregular areas within the nail plate)[19,22]
  - "Red lunula" may be seen, signifying visible nail matrix inflammation (**Fig. 22**).

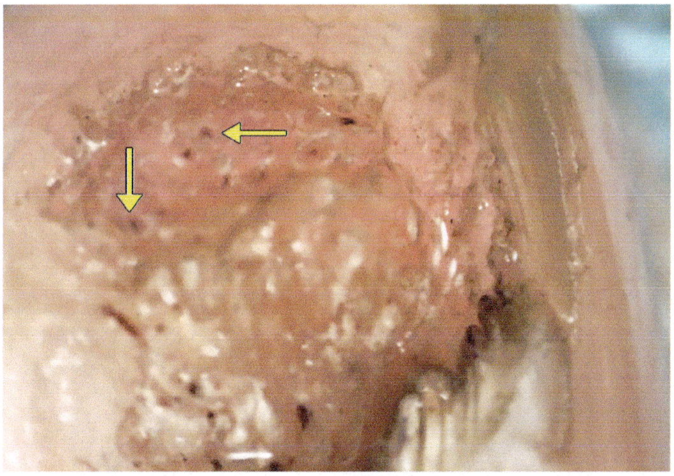

FIG. 17: Whitish, verrucous (hyperkeratotic) papule involving the distal nail fold and distal nail bed. Multiple reddish-black dots (arrows) surrounded by white scale are suggestive of subungual wart. The dots correspond to thrombosed and dilated capillaries (polarized, Dino-Lite AM7115, 70×).

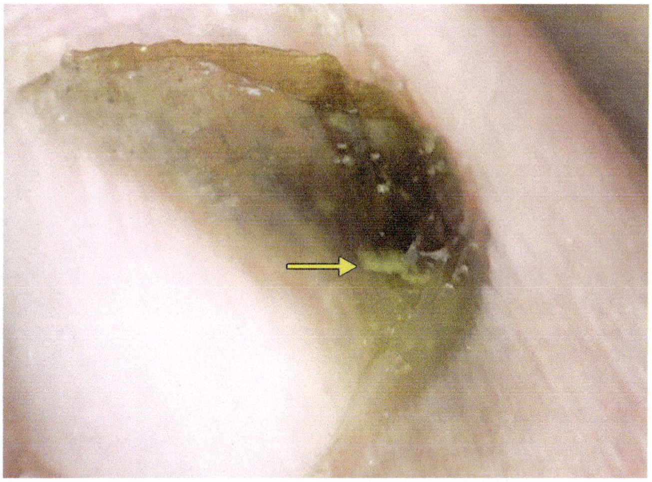

FIG. 18: Chloronychia seen in a lady with chronic paronychia. The greenish color (arrow) with peripheral fading is quite distinctive (polarized, Dino-Lite AM7115, 50×).

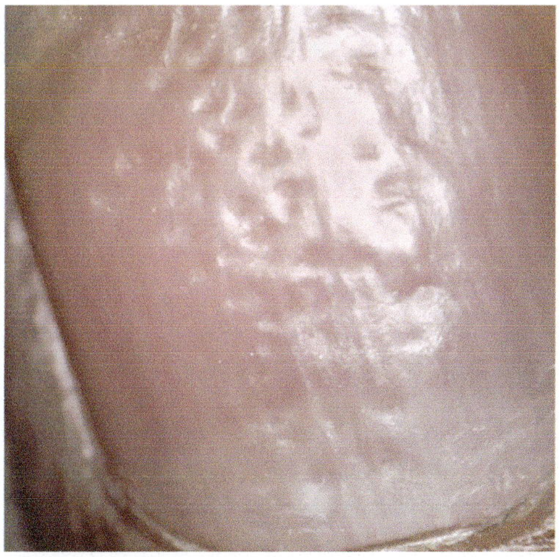

FIG. 19: Nail matrix changes seen as coarse and irregular pits in a patient with nail psoriasis. They are best visualized in a nonpolarized view (nonpolarized, Dino-Lite AM7115, 50×).

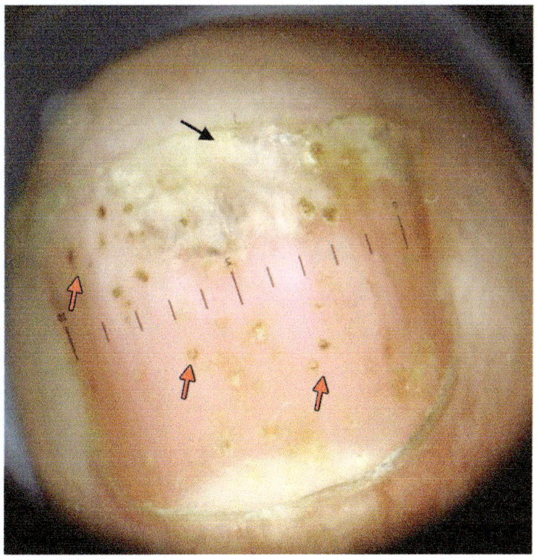

FIG. 20: Nail matrix changes seen as multiple pits (red arrows) surrounded by a keratotic scale, in a patient with nail psoriasis. Distal onycholysis with regular border (black arrow) is also seen (polarized, Heine Delta 20T, 20×).

- *Nail bed disease* manifests as:
  - Onycholysis usually surrounded by a proximal erythematous border (**Fig. 23**), composed of fusiform dilated vessels surrounded by a prominent halo[19,21]
  - Salmon patches or "oil drop" patches—seen as red to orange patches irregular in size and shape (**Figs. 24** and **25**)
  - Subungual hyperkeratosis which is compact when examined distally (**Fig. 26**).
  - Occasional yellowish-white structures (micropustules)
  - Vascular changes—seen as splinter hemorrhages (longitudinal fusiform streaks with color ranging from brown, black, or purple (**Fig. 25**); dilated tortuous capillaries in the hyponychium and PNF (**Fig. 27**) which correlate with disease activity;[23] reduced mean capillary density in PNF with architectural alterations including capillary dropouts and coiled capillaries.[24,25]

Lichen Planus

- Around 10% of cases with LP have nail involvement.[26,27]
- Onychoscopic features observed depend on the part of nail unit affected.
- *Nail matrix involvement* manifests as:
  - Dorsal pterygium, seen as variously colored pink bands with erythematous and whitish areas, converging toward the center (**Fig. 28**).
  - Pits seen as multiple small depressions giving rise to trachyonychia at times (**Fig. 29**).
  - Red lunula (**Fig. 30**), fissuring, longitudinal ridging, melanonychia, anonychia, whitish striations, nail fragmentation and atrophy (**Figs. 31** and **32**).[10,26,27]

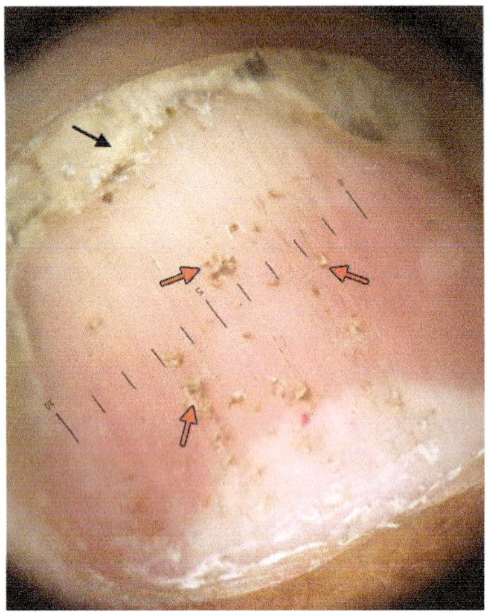

FIG. 21: Nail matrix changes seen as multiple smaller pits which are more whitish (red arrows). Many of these are overlying the lunula. Nail bed change in the form of distal onycholysis is less pronounced in this case (black arrow) (polarized, Heine Delta 20T, 20×).

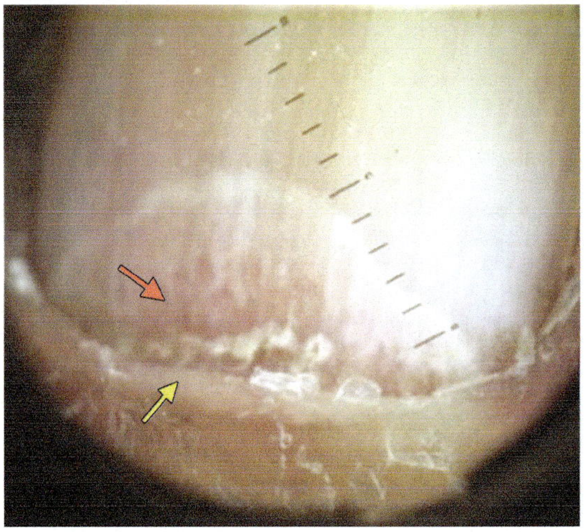

FIG. 22: Nail matrix changes seen as red lunula in a patient with nail psoriasis (red arrow). Ragged cuticle and swollen proximal nail fold (yellow arrow) (polarized, Heine Delta 20T, 20×).

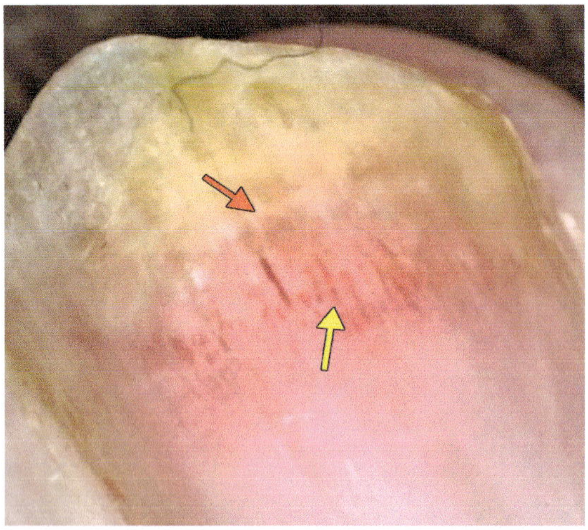

FIG. 23: Onycholysis with regular edge with a proximal erythematous border (red arrow). Prominent blood vessels with few splinter hemorrhages seen (yellow arrow) (polarized, Dino-Lite AM7115, 50×).

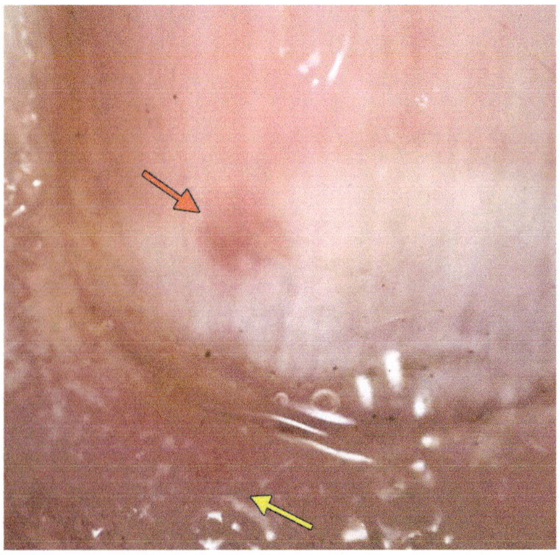

FIG. 24: "Salmon patch" seen in the nail bed (red arrow). Prominent dilated vessels seen as "red dots" in the proximal nail fold (yellow arrow) (polarized, Dino-Lite AM7115, 50×).

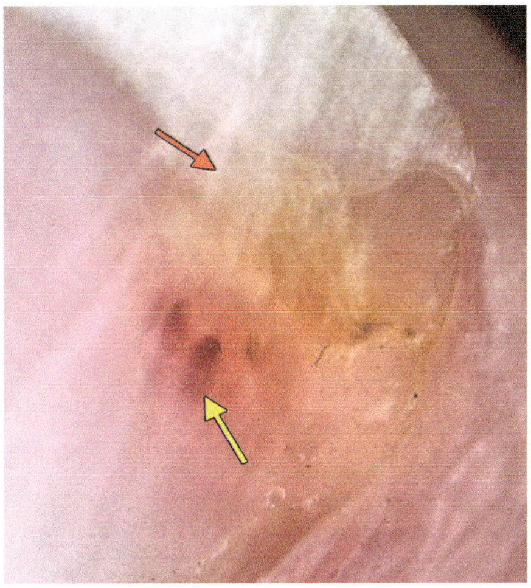

FIG. 25: Yellow structureless area suggestive of "oil drop" sign (red arrow) along with splinter hemorrhages (yellow arrow) in a case of nail psoriasis is seen (polarized, Dino-Lite AM7115, 50×).

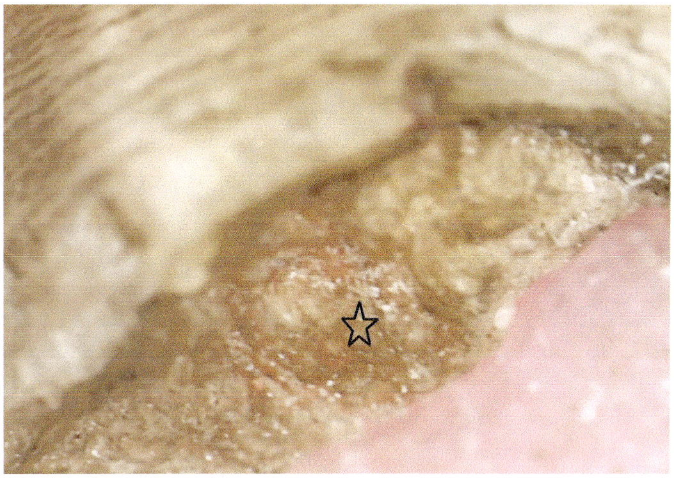

FIG. 26: Compact subungual hyperkeratosis (star) in a case of nail psoriasis (polarized, Dino-Lite AM7115, 50×).

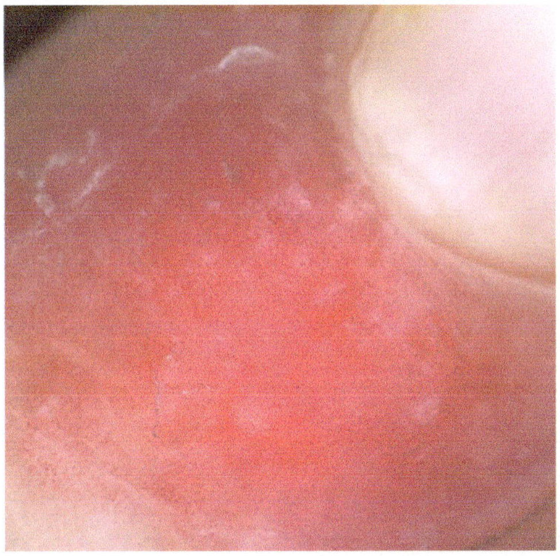

FIG. 27: Uniform red dots in psoriasis in the proximal nail fold (polarized, Dino-Lite AM7115, 35×).

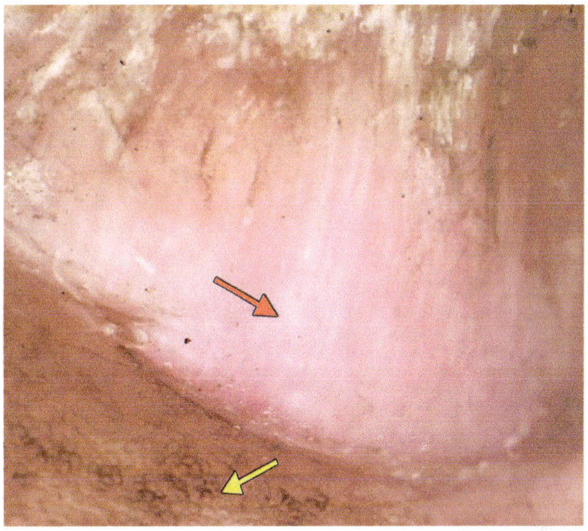

FIG. 28: Evolving pterygium in a case of nail lichen planus suggested by the prominent bulge in the nail matrix (red arrow). Proximal nail fold pigmentation (yellow arrow) and absent cuticle also seen (polarized, Dino-Lite AM7115, 70×).

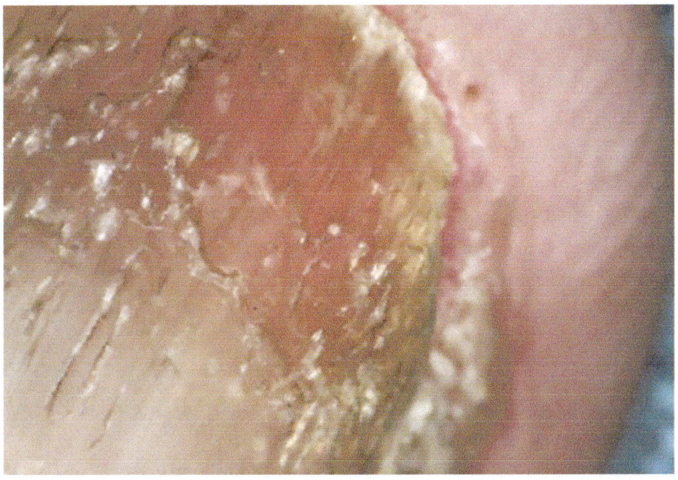

FIG. 29: Trachyonychia in a case of nail lichen planus (polarized, Dino-Lite AM7115, 50×).

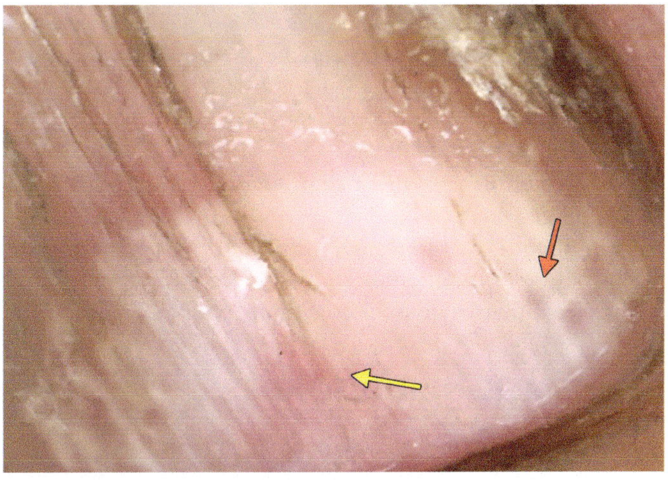

FIG. 30: Lunular changes in lichen planus. Erythematous lunula (yellow arrow) as well as spotted/dotted lunula (red arrow) is seen (polarized, Dino-Lite AM7115, 50×).

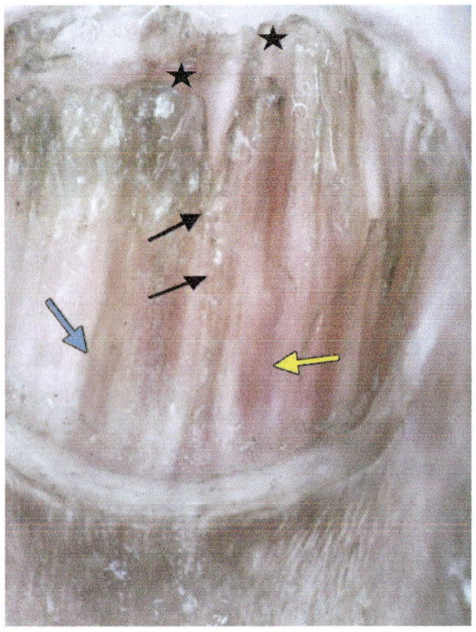

FIG. 31: Nail lichen planus with onychorrhexis or longitudinal splitting (black arrows), onychoschizia or lamellar splitting (black asterisks) and thinning of nail plate. Longitudinal melanonychia (blue arrow) as well as linear nail bed dyschromias (multicolored bands arising distal to lunula) (yellow arrow) can be seen (polarized, Dino-Lite AM7115, 50×).

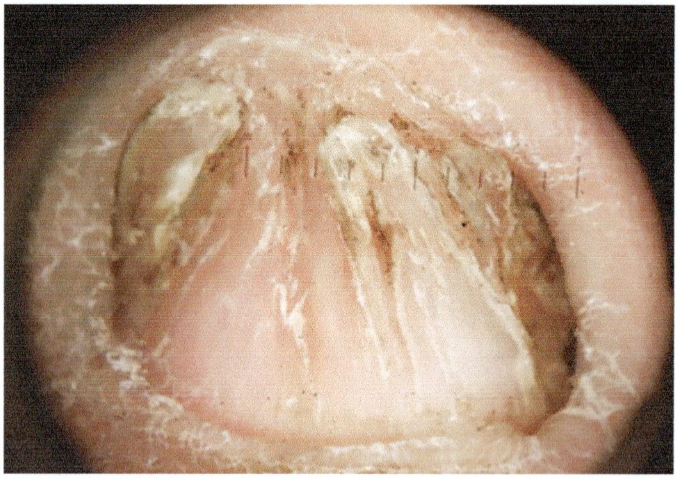

FIG. 32: Nail lichen planus with longitudinal grooves converging toward the center. This is a bad prognostic sign (polarized, Heine Delta 20T, 20×).

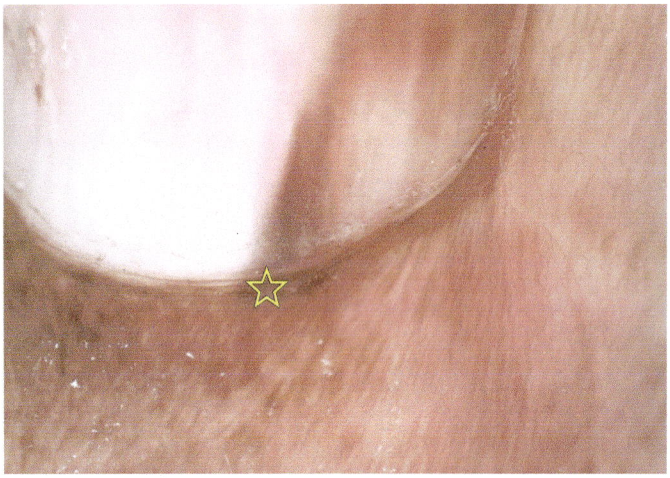

FIG. 33: Significant nail fold pigmentation (star) in a patient with nail lichen planus (polarized, Dino-Lite AM7115, 50×).

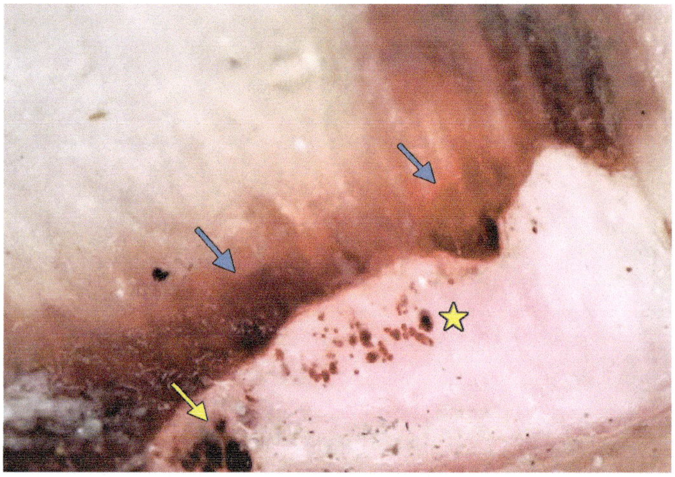

FIG. 34: Subungual hematoma seen as dots (yellow asterisk), streaks (yellow arrow) and larger collections with varying color changes (blue arrows) in a case with nail lichen planus on intramatricial injections (polarized, Dino-Lite AM7115, 35×).

- *Nail bed involvement* is seen as:
  - Chromonychia
  - Linear nail bed dyschromia (**Fig. 31**)[28]
  - Splinter hemorrhages
  - Onycholysis with a regular or irregular proximal edge
- Significant *nail fold changes* including pigmentation, swelling, and cuticular changes (**Fig. 33**), even though PNF capillaries do not show many changes.[27]

TRAUMATIC NAIL DISORDERS

Subungual Hemorrhage

- It is observed as globules of varying sizes, shapes, and colors, with or without distal streaks (**Figs. 34** and **35**).
- It may range from bright red, brown, or black depending on the duration of hemorrhage.
- Tend to move distally with time.
- It is important to remember that presence of blood does not rule out underlying melanin, especially when onychoscopy is being used for differentiating subungual hemorrhage (hematoma) from subungual melanoma.

Traumatic Onycholysis

- The line of detachment of nail plate from nail bed is linear, regular, and smooth (**Fig. 36**).
- It is surrounded by a normally pale pink bed, without subungual hyperkeratosis.

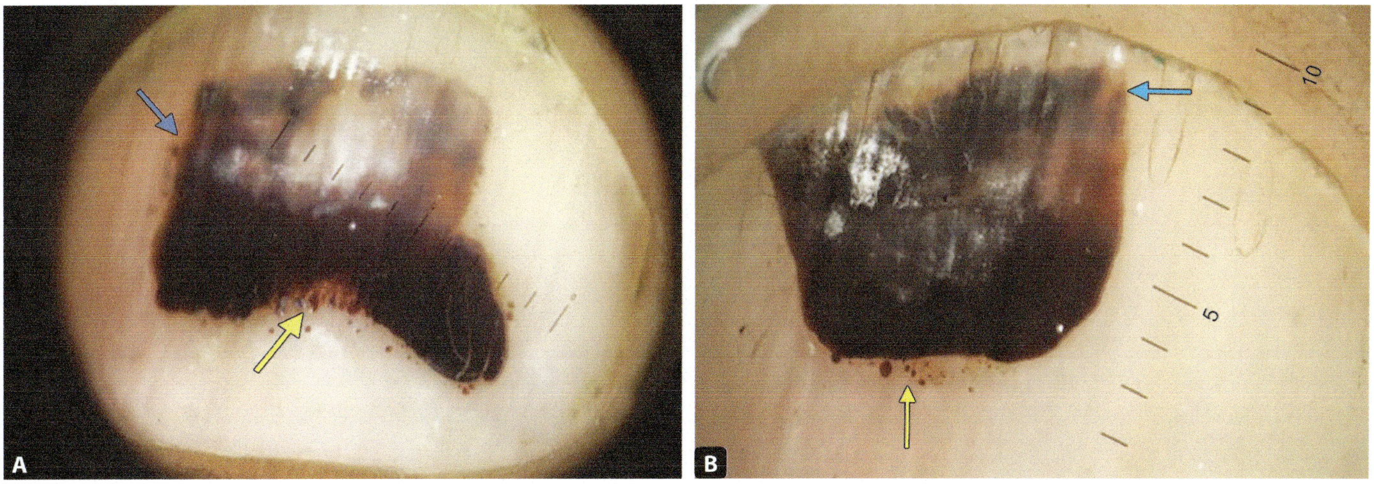

FIGS. 35A AND B: Subungual hematoma with dark red-purple color. Distal border shows longitudinal streaks (blue arrows) and proximally there are reddish brown spots and streaks (yellow arrows) (polarized, Heine Delta 20T, 20×).

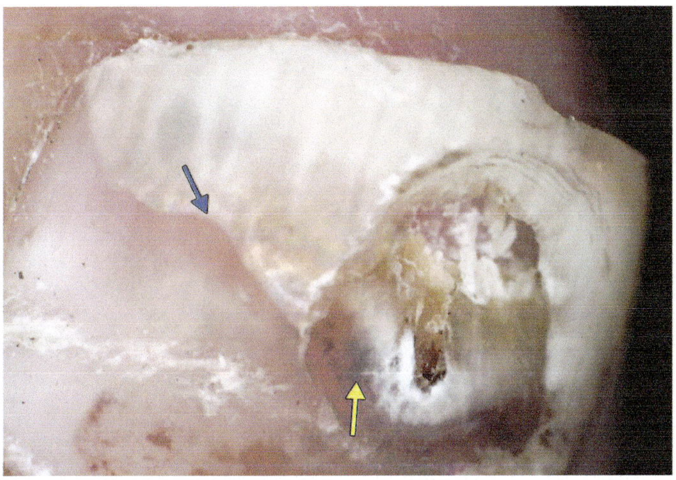

FIG. 36: Traumatic onycholysis with a regular border (blue arrow). Note the presence of subungual hemorrhages secondary to trauma (yellow arrow) (polarized, Dino-Lite AM7115, 35×).

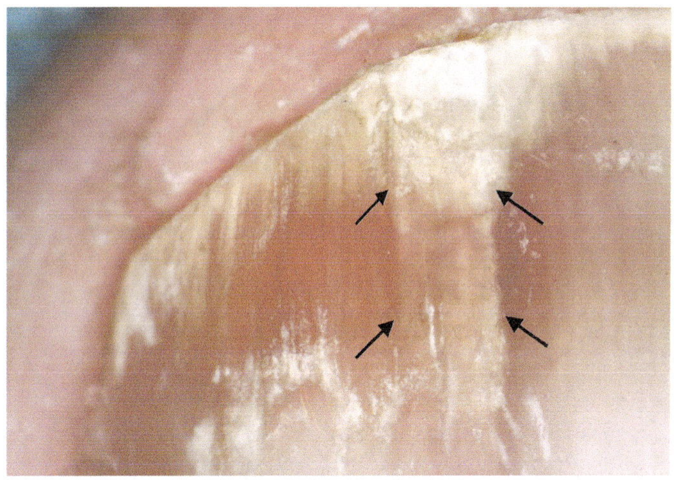

FIG. 37: Onychopapilloma showing a band of longitudinal leukonychia extending to distal edge of nail plate (black arrows) (polarized, Dino-Lite AM7115, 50×).

Onychotillomania

- Onychoscopic changes include presence of scales and crusts around the nail unit.[29]
- Partial absence of nail plate may be seen.
- Nail plate may show wavy lines and subungual hemorrhages.
- Nail bed may show pigmentation and speckled dots.
- Melanonychia is a common accompaniment.

NAIL TUMORS

Onychopapilloma

- Benign neoplasm of the distal matrix/proximal nail bed[30]
- Onychoscopy shows a band of longitudinal erythronychia, starting from the lunula (**Fig. 37**), extending to distal edge of nail plate, often associated with splinter hemorrhages.
- Characteristic keratotic subungual mass may be seen at the distal edge of nail plate (**Fig. 38**).[30]

Onychomatricoma

- An uncommon benign matrix tumor presenting with classical tetrad of ungual hyperkeratosis, splinter hemorrhages, xanthonychia, and overcurvature of nail plate, both transversely and longitudinally.
- Other features include parallel lateral edges, thickening of free edge, with "woodworm" appearance (**Fig. 39**), dark dots, splinter hemorrhages, and longitudinal parallel white lines.[31]

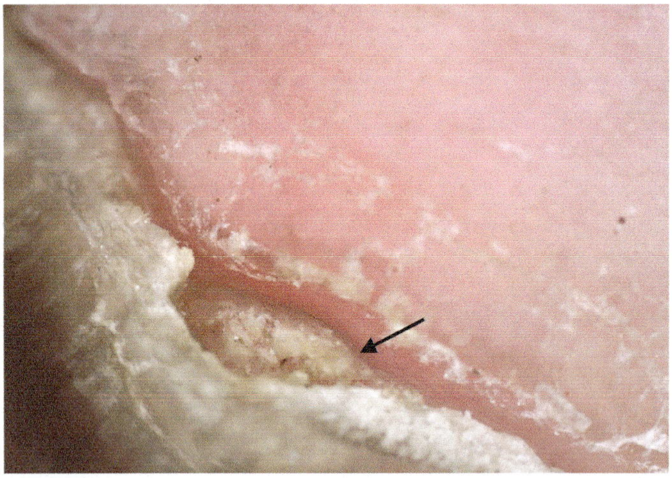

FIG. 38: Onychopapilloma showing a subungual keratotic mass (black arrow) underneath the distal edge of the nail plate (polarized, Dino-Lite AM7115, 50×).

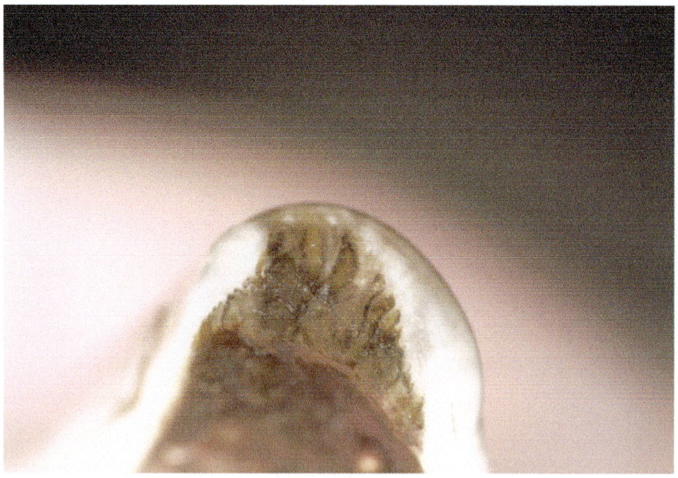

FIG. 39: Distal view of the nail plate edge showing "woodworm appearance" in a case with onychomatricoma (polarized, Dino-Lite AM7115, 50×).

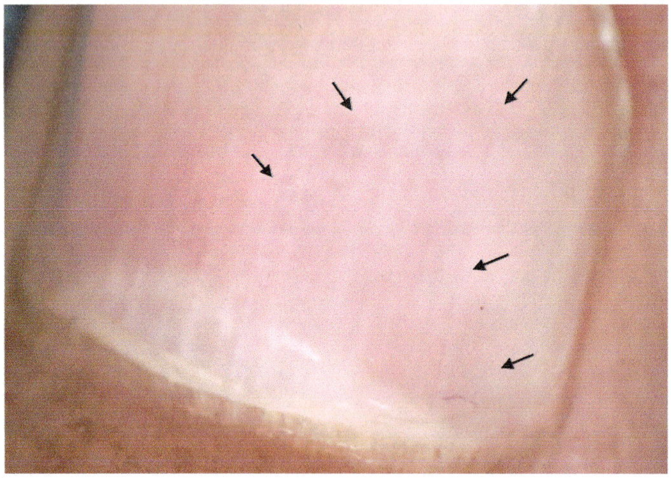

FIG. 40: Nail bed glomus tumor showing ill-defined area of erythema with indistinct borders (black arrows) (polarized, Dino-Lite AM7115, 35×).

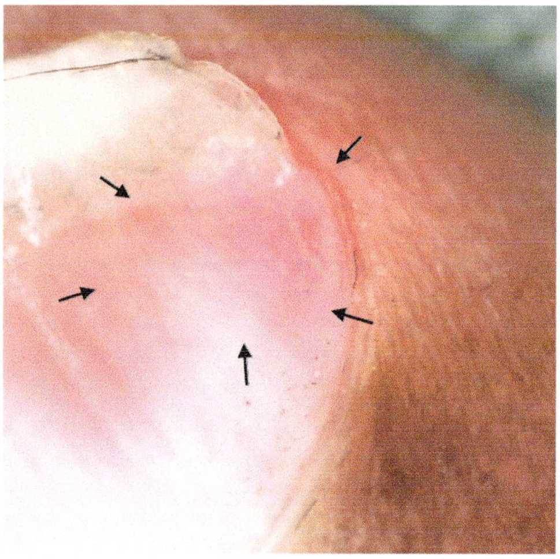

FIG. 41: A larger nail bed glomus tumor showing more marked erythema (black arrows) and overlying ramified capillaries (polarized, Dino-Lite AM7115, 35×).

Glomus Tumor

- A painful benign nail tumor arising from the glomus body[32,33] presenting with classic triad of symptoms including severe paroxysmal pain, cold sensitivity, and pinpoint tenderness.[34]
- Onychoscopy of nail bed glomus reveals an area with deep reddish-purple discoloration along with blurred borders and discrete linear vascular structures (**Figs. 40** and **41**).[32,33]
- Nail matrix glomus shows longitudinal erythronychia band or alternating red and white bands (**Fig. 42**).[34]
- Ultraviolet light dermoscopy may show a "pink glow" indicating the vascular nature of the tumor.[35]
- Intraoperative onychoscopy shows ramified capillaries over a blue background,[36] which disappear abruptly at the margins, helping determine the margins of tumor.[37]

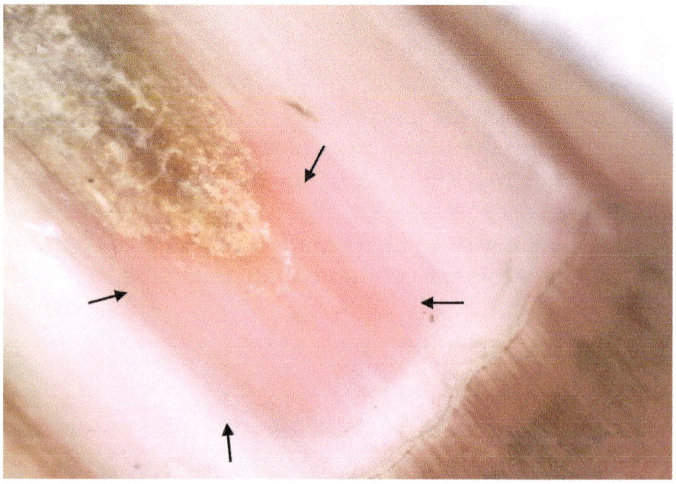

FIG. 42: Nail matrix glomus tumor showing longitudinal bands of red and white color (black arrows) (polarized, Dino-Lite AM7115, 35×).

NAIL FOLD CAPILLAROSCOPY

Dermoscopes can be useful in evaluating the horizontally placed nail fold capillaries (NFC) in the PNF.[38] The changes seen in this vascular bed are reflective of microangiopathy associated with many disorders such as connective tissue diseases.

Systemic sclerosis (SSc) is characterized by three different patterns of NFC changes:[39,40]

1. *Early pattern*: Few dilated and/or giant capillaries and a few hemorrhages. Capillary count and distribution are relatively preserved (**Fig. 43**).
2. *Active pattern*: Moderate loss of capillaries, large numbers of giant capillaries, hemorrhages, slight derangement and diffuse pericapillary edema (**Fig. 44**).
3. *Late pattern*: Severe loss of capillaries with extensive avascular areas, ramified and bushy capillaries, or more than one capillary loop in a dermal papilla (**Fig. 45**).

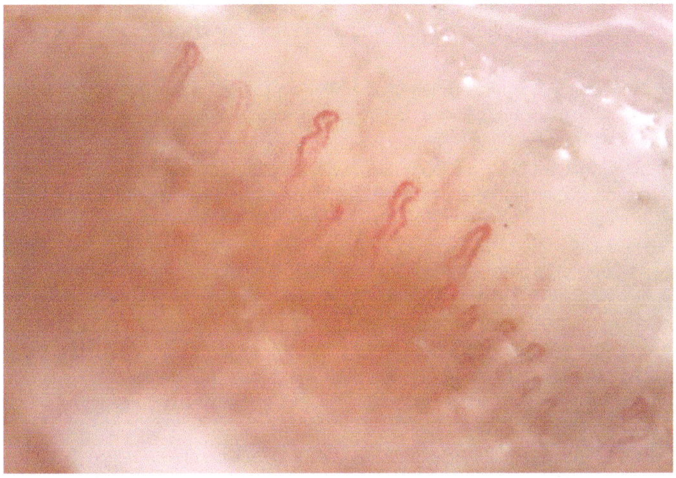

FIG. 43: Dilated and markedly tortuous capillaries in the proximal nail fold (polarized, Dino-Lite AM7115, 200×).

KEY POINTS

- Nail fold capillaroscopy shows dilated, tortuous and giant capillaries along with hemorrhages.
- Loss of capillaries, ramified and busy capillaries.
- Dermoscopic evaluation of nails (onychoscopy) is challenging due to anatomical constraints.
- At the same time, it is very rewarding as it overcomes limitations of other invasive diagnostic modalities in nail.
- Onychoscopy is a valuable, non-invasive, cost-effective diagnostic tool enabling visualization of subtle nail changes, changes in apparently uninvolved nails, subsurface changes (changes under the nail plate), as well as changes in nail fold capillaries which are associated with underlying systemic conditions.
- Onychoscopy is also useful in choosing a sampling site for direct microscopy, as well for biopsy, thus improving diagnostic outcomes.
- Onychoscopy also helps in treatment monitoring as it can pick up improvement or worsening early.

CONCLUSION

Onychoscopy is a noninvasive and rapid office-based technique applied for the better understanding of nail pathology. It is cost-effective and reproducible. It acts as a link between naked eye examination and histopathology. It also helps in locating the most proximal site for mycological sampling. It supports photographic documentation of changes seen, thus is useful for follow-up. However, it must be kept in mind that it cannot replace histopathology as the diagnostic benchmark.

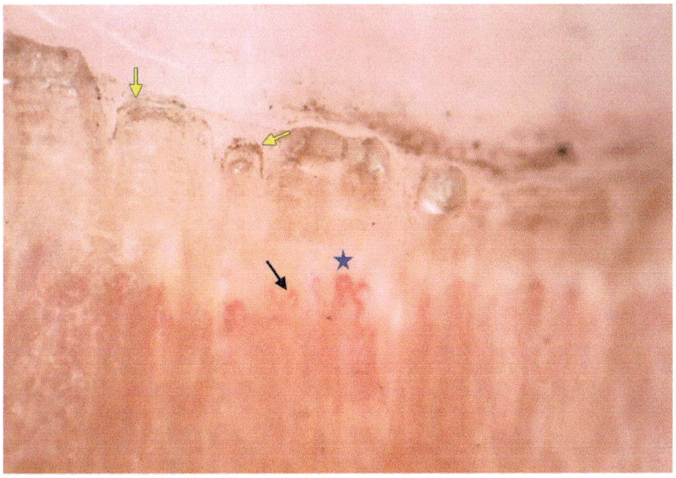

FIG. 44: Dilated (black arrow) and giant capillaries (blue asterisk) in the proximal nail fold. Ragged cuticle (yellow arrows) can also be seen (polarized, Dino-Lite AM7115, 150×).

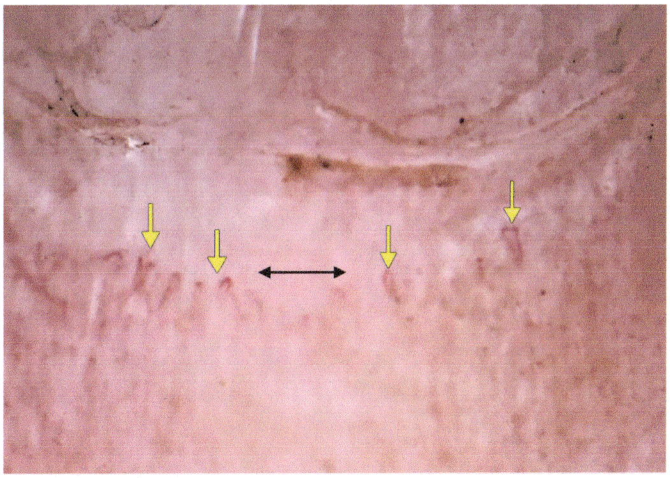

FIG. 45: Late pattern with avascular areas (black double arrow line) and dilated, distorted capillaries (yellow arrows) (polarized, Dino-Lite AM7115, 150×).

REFERENCES

1. Samman PD. The Nail in Disease, 2nd edition. London: Heinemann W; 1972. 1-176.
2. Campos-do-Carmo G, Ramos-e-Silva M. Dermoscopy: basic concepts. Int J Dermatol. 2008;47:712-9.
3. Grover C, Jakhar D. Onychoscopy: a practical guide. Indian J Dermatol Venereol Leprol. 2017;83:536-49.
4. Lencastre A, Lamas A, Sa D, Tosti A. Onychoscopy. Clin Dermatol. 2013;31:587-93.
5. Piraccini BM, Alessandrini A, Starace M. Onychoscopy: dermoscopy of the nails. Dermatol Clin. 2018;36:431-8.
6. Goettmann-Bonvallott S, André J, Belaich S. Longitudinal melanonychia in children: a clinical and histopathologic study of 40 cases. J Am Acad Dermatol. 1999;41:17-22.
7. Di Chiacchio ND, Farias DC, Piraccini BM, Hirata SH, Richert B, Zaiac M, et al. Consensus on melanonychia nail plate dermoscopy. An Bras Dermatol. 2013;88:309-13.
8. Tosti A, Piraccini BM, de Farias DC. Dealing with melanonychia. Semin Cutan Med Surg. 2009;28:49-54.
9. Piraccini BM, Bruni F, Starace M. Dermoscopy of non-skin cancer nail disorders. Dermatol Ther. 2012;25:594-602.
10. Nakamura RC, Costa MC. Dermatoscopic findings in the most frequent onychopathies: descriptive analysis of 500 cases. Int J Dermatol. 2012;51: 483-5.
11. De Crignis G, Valgas N, Rezende P, Leverone A, Nakamura R. Dermatoscopy of onychomycosis. Int J Dermatol. 2014;53:e97-9.
12. Piraccini BM, Balestri R, Starace M, Rech G. Nail digital dermoscopy (onychoscopy) in the diagnosis of onychomycosis. J Eur Acad Dermatol Venereol. 2013;27:509-13.
13. Jakhar D, Grover C, Kaur I. Dendritic pattern: unique onychoscopic feature in endonyx. J Am Acad Dermatol. 2019;81:e89-90.
14. Grover C, Jakhar D, Sharma S. The grid pattern of white superficial onychomycosis. Indian J Dermatol Venereol Leprol. 2020;86:568-70.
15. Starace M, Ambrogio F, Bruni F, Piraccini BM, Alessandrini A. Dermatophytic melanonychia: a case series of an increasing disease. Mycoses. 2021;64: 511-9.
16. Bae JM, Kang H, Kim HO, Park YM. Differential diagnosis of plantar wart from corn, callus and healed wart with the aid of dermoscopy. Br J Dermatol. 2009;160:220-2.
17. Lee DY, Park JH, Lee JH, Yang JM, Lee ES. The use of dermoscopy for the diagnosis of plantar wart. J Eur Acad Dermatol Venereol. 2009;23:726-7.
18. Haenssle HA, Blum A, Hofmann-Wellenhof R, Kreusch J, Stolz W, Argenziano G, et al. When all you have is a dermatoscope—start looking at the nails. Dermatol Pract Concept. 2014;4(2):11-20.
19. Yadav TA, Khopkar US. Dermoscopy to detect signs of sub-clinical nail involvement in chronic plaque psoriasis: a study of 68 patients. Indian J Dermatol. 2015;60(3):272-5.
20. Yorulmaz A, Artuz F. A study of dermoscopic features of nail psoriasis. Postepy Dermatol Alergol. 2017;34:28-35.
21. Chauhan A, Singal A, Grover C, Sharma S. Dermoscopic features of nail psoriasis: an observational, analytical study. Skin Appendage Disord. 2020;6: 207-15.
22. Grover C, Jakhar D. Diagnostic utility of onychoscopy: review of literature. Indian J Dermatopathol Diagn Dermatol. 2017;4:31-40.
23. Iorizzo M, Dahdah M, Vicenzi C, Tosti A. Videodermoscopy of the hyponychium in nail bed psoriasis. J Am Acad Dermatol. 2008;58:714-5.
24. Bhushan M, Moore T, Herrick AL, Griffiths CE. Nail-fold video capillaroscopy in psoriasis. Br J Dermatol. 2000;142:1171-6.
25. Ribeiro CF, Siqueira EB, Holler AP, Fabrício L, Skare TL. Periungual capillaroscopy in psoriasis. An Bras Dermatol. 2012;87:550-3.
26. Nakamura R, Broce AA, Palencia DP, Ortiz NI, Leverone A. Dermatoscopy of nail lichen planus. Int J Dermatol. 2013;52:684-7.
27. Kharghoria G, Grover C, Bhattacharya SN. Nail dermatoscopic (onychoscopic) features of nail lichen planus: a cross-sectional study. Australas J Dermatol. 2021;62:e79-82.
28. Grover C, Kharghoria G, Bhattacharya SN. Linear nail bed dyschromia: a distinctive dermoscopic feature of nail lichen planus. Clin Exp Dermatol. 2019;44:697-9.
29. Maddy AJ, Tosti A. Dermoscopic features of onychotillomania: a study of 36 cases. J Am Acad Dermatol. 2018;79:702-5.
30. Tosti A, Schneider SL, Ramirez-Quizon MN, Zaiac M, Miteva M. Clinical, dermoscopic, and pathologic features of onychopapilloma: a review of 47 cases. J Am Acad Dermatol. 2016;74:521-6.
31. Lesort C, Debarbieux S, Duru G, Dalle S, Poulhalon N, Thomas L. Dermoscopic features of onychomatricoma: a study of 34 cases. Dermatology. 2015;231:177-83.
32. Duarte AF, Correia O, Barreiros H, Haneke E. Giant subungual glomus tumor: clinical, dermoscopy, imagiologic and surgery details. Dermatol Online J. 2016;22:13030/qt66f7b8wt.
33. Grover C, Jayasree P, Kaliyadan F. Clinical and onychoscopic characteristics of subungual glomus tumor: a cross-sectional study. Int J Dermatol. 2021;60:693-702.
34. Kallis P, Miteva M, Patel T, Zaiac M, Tosti A. Onychomatricoma with concomitant subungual glomus tumor. Skin Appendage Disord. 2015;1:14-7.
35. Thatte SS, Chikhalkar SB, Khopkar US. "Pink glow": a new sign for the diagnosis of glomus tumor on ultraviolet light dermoscopy. Indian Dermatol Online J. 2015;6(Suppl 1):S21-3.
36. Maehara S, Ohe EM, Enokihara MY, Michalany NS, Yamada S, Hirata SH. Diagnosis of glomus tumor by nail bed and matrix dermoscopy. An Bras Dermatol. 2010;85(2):236-8.
37. Rai AK. Role of intraoperative dermoscopy in excision of nail unit glomus tumor. Indian Dermatol Online J. 2016;7:448-50.
38. Jakhar D, Grover C, Singal A. Nailfold capillaroscopy with USB dermatoscope: a cross-sectional study in healthy adults. Indian J Dermatol Venereol Leprol. 2020;86:33-8.
39. Cutolo M, Sulli A, Pizzorni C, Accardo S. Nail fold videocapillaroscopy assessment of microvascular damage in systemic sclerosis. J Rheumatol. 2000;27:155-60.
40. Jakhar D, Grover C, Singal A, Das GK. Nailfold capillaroscopy and retinal findings in patients with systemic sclerosis: is there an association? Indian Dermatol Online J. 2020;11:382-6.

18 CHAPTER

Miscellaneous Uses of Dermoscopy

Ishmeet Kaur, Faizan Younus Shah, Suman Patra

INTRODUCTION

Dermoscopy is perpetually being explored for its innovative utility at a great pace. It has received recognition in diagnosis of various pigmentary, inflammatory, infectious, granulomatous, hair, and nail disorders. However, It's recently described utility in prognosis, therapeutic assessment, understanding pathogenesis and depth of the pathology, newer modified techniques for increasing diagnostic yield of histopathology and other tests have unraveled many benefits in the field of dermatology. This chapter will highlight the innovative uses of dermoscopy that can aid in clinical practice beyond the purpose of diagnosis.

PROGNOSTIC AND THERAPEUTIC APPLICATIONS

Specific dermoscopic features have been described which can assess prognosis and therapeutic response. In case of non-neoplastic inflammatory diseases, it is now possible to differentiate active disease from inactive or burnout stage. This has been described in case of alopecia areata, lichen planus, discoid lupus erythematosus, and frontal fibrosing alopecia in **Table 1**.

In squamous cell carcinoma (SCC), dermoscopic evidence of branching and serpentine blood vessels indicates moderate to poorly differentiated SCCs as opposed to well-differentiated SCCs.[8] Black color and peripheral streaks pattern in dermoscopy indicate presence of mitoses in melanoma, while atypical pigment network and brown color indicate melanoma without mitoses.[9]

Dermoscopy has also been utilized to evaluate treatment response. Valuable clues can be picked up in serial dermoscopy of the lesions of hair disorders like alopecia areata (**Figs. 1A** and **B**) and pigmentary disorders like melasma and vitiligo (**Table 2**).

AESTHETIC APPLICATION

- *Dermoscopic photoaging scale (DPAS)*: The assessment of photoaging with dermoscopy provides a more

TABLE 1: Dermoscopic features defining the activity of disease.

Disease	Active stage	Inactive stage
Alopecia areata	Black dots, "exclamation mark" hairs, broken hairs, and clustered short vellus hairs[1]	White dots, yellow dots, atypical red vessels (may be secondary to treatment with topical steroid)[1]
Vitiligo	Altered pigment pattern, perifollicular pigment retention (PFP), and starburst appearance, diffuse white glow, comet-tail sign and "tapioca sago" appearance	Perifollicular depigmentation, sharply defined border, absent pigment network, reticulate pigment network, perifollicular pigmentation[2,3]
Frontal fibrosing alopecia	Presence of background erythema[4]	Cicatricial white areas[5]
Lichen planus	Wickham's striae (WS)	Absence of WS, only grayish brown dots and globules[6]
Discoid lupus erythematosus	Perifollicular whitish halos, lesional and perilesional scales, follicular keratotic plugging, thick arborizing vessels, follicular red dots and perifollicular scales	Variable patchy whitish hypopigmented areas, and the presence of white structureless areas, thin arborizing vessels[7]

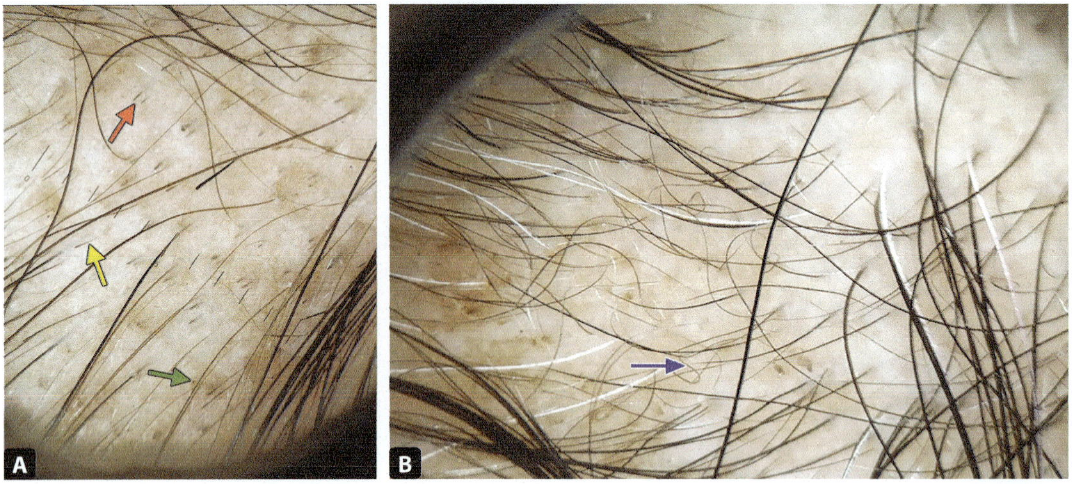

FIGS. 1A AND B: (A) Dermoscopic picture of active alopecia areata lesion showing multiple broken hairs (red arrow), black dots (green arrow) and exclamation mark hairs (yellow arrow); (B) Same lesion after treatment showing absence of black dots and broken hairs but presence of many regrowing coiled hairs (blue arrow) (polarized, Heine Delta 20T, 10×).

TABLE 2: Dermoscopic features indicating prognosis or successful treatment response.

Condition	Features for prognosis and post successful treatment
Alopecia areata	Black dots, tapered hair, broken hairs tend to decrease significantly, pig-tail, and upright regrowing hairs appear,[10] presence of "i" hairs[11]
Vitiligo	Perifollicular hyperpigmentation, marginal hyperpigmentation, ameboid or petaloid patterns, reticulate pigmentation, perilesional or intralesional erythema and telangiectasias[12]
Melasma	Significant reduction in globular pattern and perifollicular pigmentation was observed in treated patients[13]
Periorbital hyperpigmentation	Classification into pigmented, vascular or mixed type. Deciding therapeutic intervention and assess treatment response through decrease in number of vessels or decrease in grade of pigmentation
Laser hair reduction	Reduction in mean hair density (hairs/cm^2), terminal/vellus hair ratio, and hair thickness in trichoscopy can help to monitor treatment response[14]
Hair transplantation	Trichoscopy can be utilized to assess density, angle of exiting hairs, angle of the hairs in hairline and aesthetic appearance post-transplant[15]
Tinea capitis	Zigzag hairs, horseshoe hair and barcode hairs points to ectothrix infection *(Microsporum canis)* where griseofulvin can be chosen for treatment, comma hairs and corkscrew hairs without zigzag hairs and barcode hairs points to endothrix infection *(Trichophyton violaceum)*, and it is recommended to start treatment with terbinafine in usual dose[16,17]

objective and consistent valuation. DPAS is based on 11 criteria, with a maximal score of 44.[18] DPAS helps to detect photoaging before it becomes clinically evident.

- *Trichoscan*: Trichoscan is a technique which involves a combination of dermoscopy with automatic digital image analysis to assess biological parameters of human hair growth. This technique finds utility in evaluation of various alopecia particularly androgenetic alopecia and appraisal of treatment efficacy of newer modalities.[19]
- *Trichoscopy in laser hair reduction (LHR)*: Trichoscopic evaluation of area to be treated for hirsutism helps in deciding optimal laser parameters to provide maximum efficacy and minimizing adverse effects like post-laser burn and hyperpigmentation. The parameters can be fine-tuned based on the thickness of hair and can also be used to assess treatment response (**Figs. 2A** and **B**).[20]
- *Trichoscopy in hair transplant (HT)*: Trichoscopy is of great use in HT for selection of ideal candidate, assessment of donor and recipient areas, and evaluation of post-treatment results. It helps to differentiate cases of diffuse unpatterned alopecia (DUPA) from androgenetic alopecia which is important for the surgeon as HT in the former case would be a misadventure. Assessment of follicular density, number of hairs per follicular unit, post-follicular unit transplant (FUT) scar and residual hair density in donor area and evaluation of hair angle, post-transplant density and overall aesthetics in recipient area and early detection of complications are the other benefits offered.[15]

INTRAOPERATIVE APPLICATIONS

- *Dermoscopy in skin biopsy*: Dermoscopy helps in identification of the site most suitable for biopsy, thus increasing diagnostic yield. It can obviate the need for skin biopsy in certain cases and improve the malignant/

benign ratio in excised melanocytic lesions. Patients who need a biopsy but refuse it due to apprehensions regarding the procedure are more likely to consent following a demonstration of disease-specific features on dermoscopy.[21,22]

- *Excision of wart, nevi, and tumors*: Preoperative dermoscopy has been used for determination of appropriate minimal surgical margins in cases of lesions like wart, nevi, and tumors (**Figs. 3A** and **B**).[23,24] Real-time dermoscopy during procedures like surgical excision, electrocautery, radiofrequency, and cryotherapy can be a useful tool to preserve normal tissue and assure complete excision/removal. This allows for procedure to be conducted at a higher magnification with better precision at appropriate depth and has been popularly named as interventional dermoscopy.[25]
- *Nail unit tumors*: Onychoscopy, at certain times, may fail to completely assess the nail matrix and nail bed, necessitating a nail matrix biopsy; especially in cases of melanonychia with suspicious origin of melanocyte proliferation (**Fig. 4**). Intraoperative dermoscopy following removal of nail plate may allow better assessment of the nail matrix/bed and origin of pigment. This point has important cosmetic implications as biopsy from nail matrix may result in permanent nail dystrophy.[26]
- *Intraoperative dermoscopy*: It benefits in proper localization and margination of glomus tumor and onychomatricoma ensuring complete excision of tumor (already dealt with in chapter on onychoscopy). Margination of vague borders of glomus tumor becomes convenient with appreciation of ramified telangiectasia over a blue background with abrupt loss near the margin.[27,28] Intraoperative onychoscopy has also been successfully explored in understanding pathogenesis of nail presentations like red lunula.[29]
- *Foreign body removal*: Identification of retained foreign bodies and suture material, inconspicuous to the naked eye, is another benefit offered by dermoscopy (**Fig. 5**). The appreciation of a track and protruding tail-edge is a distinctive pointer toward an intracutaneous foreign body.[30]

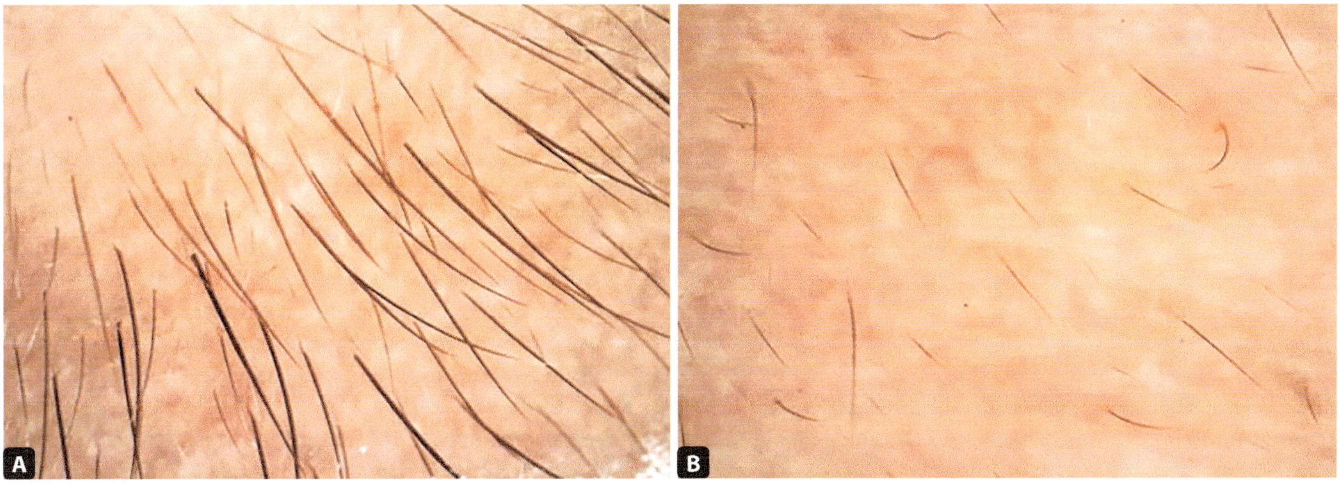

FIGS. 2A AND B: Monitoring treatment response of hirsutism at chin with dermoscopy that shows reduced density and hair diameter after 3 sessions of laser hair reduction with diode laser (polarized, Dino-Lite Edge 3.0 AM73915MZT, 50×).

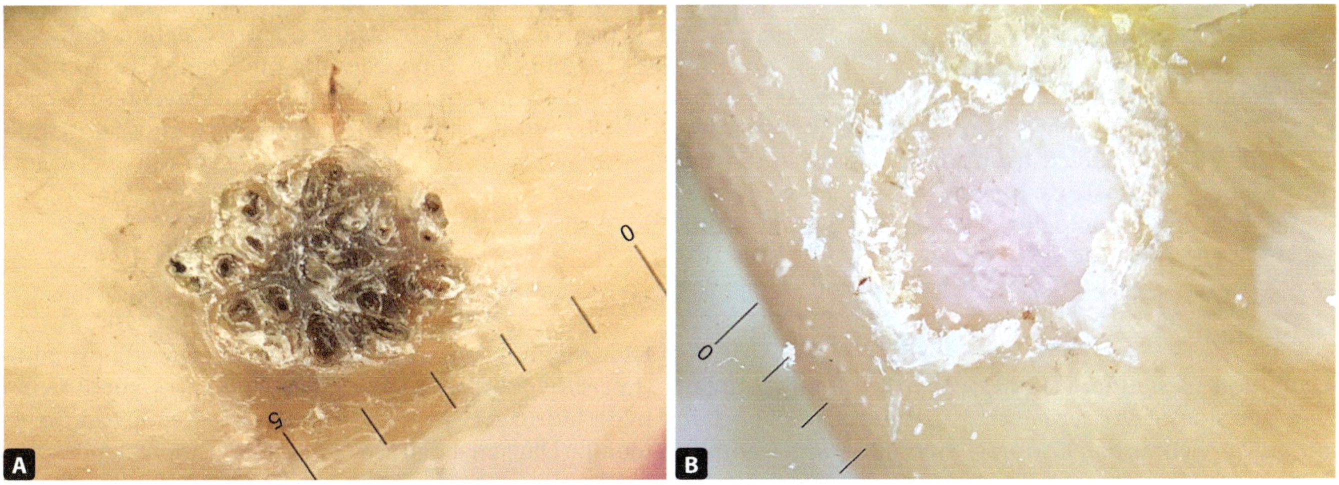

FIGS. 3A AND B: (A) Dermoscopic image of plantar wart showing thrombosed capillaries and verrucous surface; (B) Post-treatment picture of wart 2 weeks after single injection bleomycin showing disappearance of thrombosed vessels (polarized, Heine Delta 20T, 10×).

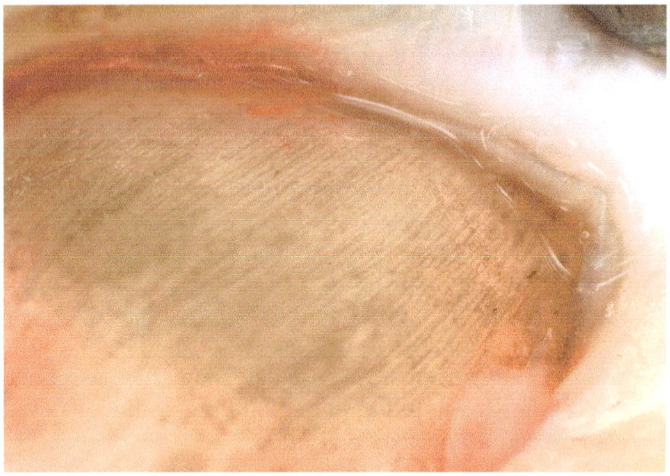

FIG. 4: Intraoperative onychoscopy of benign melanonychia showing fine light brown parallel lines restricted to proximal aspect of nail bed and nail matrix (polarized, Dino-Lite Edge 3.0 AM73915MZT, 150×).

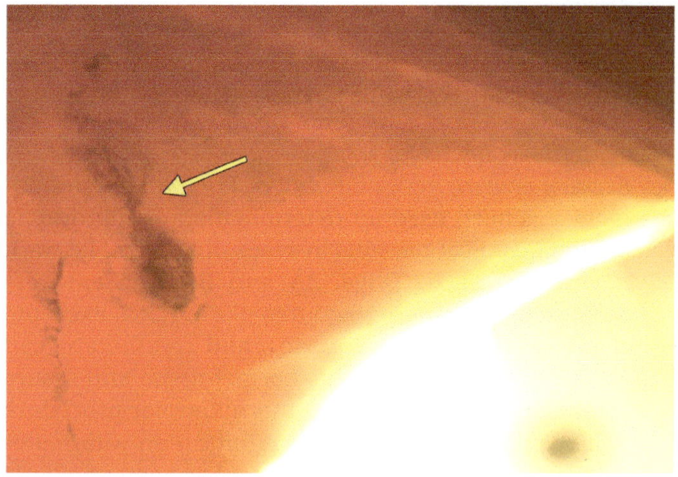

FIG. 6: Transillumination dermoscopy of finger web space showing black curvilinear structure against a red background indicating burrow (yellow arrow) (polarized, Dino-Lite Edge 3.0 AM73915MZT, 150×).

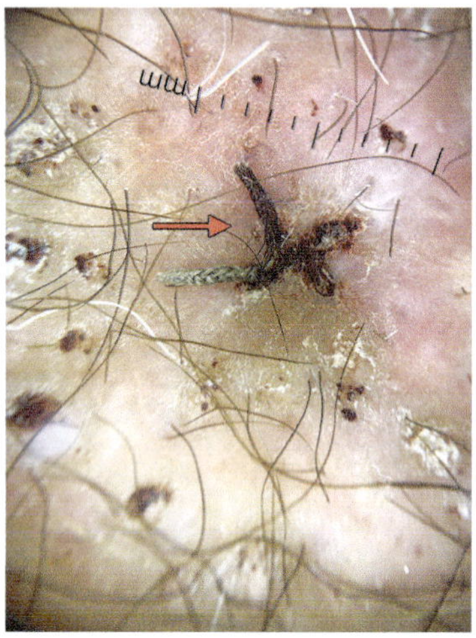

FIG. 5: Dermoscopy assisting in detection of occult retained suture (red arrow) (polarized, DermLite DL4, 10×).

MODIFIED TECHNIQUES

Transillumination Dermoscopy

As an adjuvant to dermoscopy, transillumination dermoscopy (TD) has only recently been described.[31-33] As most of the light gets reflected from the nail surface during conventional dermoscopy making it hard to study the deeper nail bed pathologies, TD can serve as a useful tool.[33-35]

Technique

In addition to standard dermoscopy of the target area, the other side of the target area (palmar aspect of nail unit, finger web or hair) is transilluminated with another light source (pen torch/cell phone torch) which should have a single, narrow, and strong beam. The light source of the dermatoscope can be further switched off to create a complete dark environment. The normal tissue gives a homogeneous reddish glow, while any obstruction/abnormality (wart/hematoma/etc.) or air entrapment (burrow) will appear black/dark.[33]

Uses

- *Nail bed*: The technique has been utilized to study nail bed pathology like nail psoriasis and subungual hematoma. In nail psoriasis, TD accentuates the nail bed features like splinter hemorrhages.[35] Similarly, the extent and course of evolution/resolution of subungual hematoma can be assessed in detail with this technique.[33,34]
- *Finger web space*: The technique has also been utilized to scope the finger web spaces to visualize burrows in scabies that appear black due to entrapment of air over a red background of normal tissue (**Fig. 6**).[33]
- *Hair*: It can be done with the classic TD method or with the help of a mirror (instead of the external light source) which reflects the polarized light coming from the dermatoscope from the other side. The technique utilizing mirror is called "cross-polarized dermoscopy". It has been used to better appreciate trichogram features of hair shaft abnormalities like "tiger tail appearance" seen in trichothiodystrophy, trichorrhexis nodosa, and the classic "floppy sock appearance."[36,37]

Hidroscopy

Hidroscopy can be utilized to appreciate abnormalities (hyper/hypohidrosis) as well as response to treatment of hyperhidrosis.[38] It has also been used as an adjunctive tool for Hansen's disease.[39] For better appreciation of the predominant areas involved, starch iodine test can be performed and visualized with dermatoscope. The sweat droplets are appreciated as blue-violet-colored drops coming out of gland opening.[40]

Oculoscopy

The USB dermatoscope has been utilized as oculoscope for visualization of Lisch nodule over iris[41] and can be utilized to better evaluate lesions over eyelid. Modification has been made to hold the dermatoscope at place using car holder.[42]

Tape Dermoscopy

Tape dermoscopy is a method used by Blum and Giacomel[43] which alleviate the need to use expensive dermatoscopic equipment for visualization of the lesion. The procedure involves putting an immersion fluid over the lesion and covering with a transparent tape. Photographs are captured at 25–30 cm distance.

Drop Dermoscopy

To facilitate patient initiated teledermoscopic consultation, a concept of "drop dermoscopy" has also been proposed.[44] A drop of alcohol-based sanitizer is applied over the lesion and picture is taken by any smartphone or digital camera through the fluid. The fluid reduces the reflection from the surface and helps to visualize subsurface structures.

Teledermoscopy

As an adjunctive tool in teledermatology, teledermoscopy has almost 90% concordance with histopathological diagnosis when both clinical and dermoscopic images are provided.[45,46] This is useful in pigmentary disorders, nevi, melanoma, and nonmelanoma skin cancers.[47,48] Total body dermoscopy[49] including total body photography (TBP) and sequential digital dermoscopic imaging (SDDI) is utilized to detect atypical nevi and screening of patients. Use of artificial intelligence to analyze teledermoscopic images further improves diagnostic accuracy.[50] "Mobile dermatoscopy"[45] by attaching smartphone with the dermoscope can further facilitate capturing and sharing of images.

OTHER USES

- *Ex vivo dermoscopy of tissue specimen*: Dermoscopic examination of tissue samples optimizes sectioning for histopathology by identifying concerned atypical features in melanocytic lesions.[51] This can be combined with derm dotting which is used to mark suspicious areas recognized on dermoscopy, thereby improving the diagnostic yield.[52]
- *Cosmetic wart mapping*: Cosmetic wart mapping refers to videodermoscopy of the affected areas which helps in identification and ablation of small warts which would otherwise be missed and lead to further dissemination.[19,53]
- *Patch test interpretation*: Correct interpretation of patch test is challenging, especially when differentiation between weak allergic and irritant reactions is not possible. Characteristic patterns on dermoscopy have helped in better interpretation of results (**Figs. 7A** and **B**). Vesicles and dotted vessels observed on dermoscopy are strong pointers in favor of allergic reaction.[54]
- *Pathergy test interpretation*: Use of dermoscope for evaluation of pathergy test result decreases the interobserver variation in interpretation and removes any subjective discrepancies.[55]
- *Dermoscopic self-examination by patients*: Patients with high risk of skin cancer are advised to perform self-examination to look for changes that may indicate melanoma. Dermoscopy can serve as a potential aid in such cases.[56]
- *Assessment of melanin distribution*: The depth of melanin deposition in skin can be crudely determined by dermoscope with built-in ultraviolet (UV) light. It offers a better alternative to Wood's lamp as the

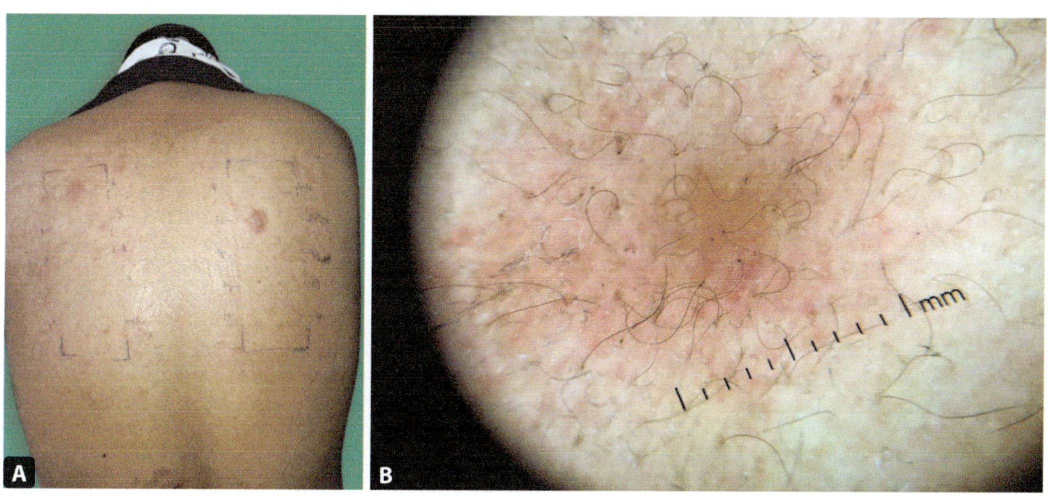

FIGS. 7A AND B: Patch test: (A) Clinical and (B) dermoscopic image showing absence of vesicle or dotted vessels make allergic contact dermatitis less likely (polarized, DermLite DL4, 10×).

requirement for eye protection and need for a dark room is obviated.[57]

KEY POINTS

- Dermoscopy has recently been explored for its utility in determining prognosis, therapeutic response, depth of pathology, and understanding pathogenesis.
- With appreciation of specific features, it can aid in assessment of activity and severity of various pigmentary and hair disorders.
- Besides diagnosis and response assessment, trichoscopy can also help in determining the optimal parameters for LHR and for hair transplantation.
- Intraoperative dermoscopy helps in marking most suitable site for biopsy, delineating margins of excision for benign lesions and foreign body and differentiating benign from malignant melanonychia.
- Certain modified forms of dermoscopy like TD, hidroscopy, oculoscopy, drop dermoscopy, tape dermoscopy can make the diagnostic process more convenient.
- Teledermoscopy is a relatively new aspect of dermoscopy that can enhance the diagnostic accuracy and screening process of suspicious lesions. It can also serve as a learning tool for beginners in dermoscopy.

CONCLUSION

The journey of exploring new gates of utility of dermoscopy is exciting and never-ending. It is imperative to stay aware of the newly explored utilities and advancements in this field. The future of intraoperative dermoscopy and utility of dermoscopy in understanding pathogenesis and mutational analysis holds concrete promise in the future.

REFERENCES

1. Kibar M, Aktan Ş, Lebe B, Bilgin M. Trichoscopic findings in alopecia areata and their relation to disease activity, severity and clinical subtype in Turkish patients. Australas J Dermatol. 2015;56(1):e1-6.
2. Jha AK, Sonthalia S, Lallas A. Dermoscopy as an evolving tool to assess vitiligo activity. J Am Acad Dermatol. 2018;78:1017-9.
3. Nirmal B, Antonisamy B, Peter CV, George L, George AA, Dinesh GM. Cross-sectional study of dermatoscopic findings in relation to activity in vitiligo: BPLeFoSK criteria for stability. J Cutan Aesthet Surg. 2019;12:36-41.
4. Sonthalia S, Jha AK, Tiwary PK. A dermoscopic diagnosis and activity evaluation of frontal fibrosing alopecia in an Indian lady. Indian Dermatol Online J. 2017;8:162-3.
5. Kose OK, Güleç AT. Evaluation of a handheld dermatoscope in clinical diagnosis of primary cicatricial alopecias. Dermatol Ther (Heidelb). 2019;9:525-35.
6. Baquero Sánchez E, Lorente-Lavirgen A, Domínguez Cruz J, Conejo-Mir J. Aportación de la dermatoscopia en el diagnóstico y pronóstico del liquen plano pigmentado lineal. Actas Dermosifiliogr. 2015;106:339-40.
7. Al-Refu K. The role of dermoscopy in assessment of the activity and scarring response in discoid lupus erythematosus. Open Dermatol J. 1918;12:99-111.
8. Pyne J, Sapkota D, Wong JC. Squamous cell carcinoma: variation in dermatoscopic vascular features between well and non-well differentiated tumors. Dermatol Pract Concept. 2012;2:204a05.
9. Ribero S, Argenziano G, Lallas A, Moscarella E, Benati E, Raucci M, et al. Dermoscopic features predicting the presence of mitoses in thin melanoma. J Dermatol Sci. 2017;86:158-61.
10. Ganjoo S, Thappa DM. Dermoscopic evaluation of therapeutic response to an intralesional corticosteroid in the treatment of alopecia areata. Indian J Dermatol Venereol Leprol. 2013;79:408-17.
11. Malakar S, Mehta PR. "i hair": a prognostic marker in alopecia areata and trichotillomania. Indian J Dermatol. 2017;62:658-60.
12. Chatterjee M, Neema S. Dermoscopy of pigmentary disorders in brown skin. Dermatol Clin. 2018;36:473-85.
13. Abdel Hay R, Mohammed FN, Sayed KS, Abd El Fattah NA, Ibrahim S. Dermoscopy as a useful tool for evaluating melasma and assessing the response to 1064-nm Q-switched Nd:YAG laser. Dermatol Ther. 2020;33: e13629.
14. Mohamed EE, Ahmed AM, Tawfik KM, Ibrahim SM. Trichoscopic changes in hair during treatment of hirsutism with 1064-nm neodymium:yttrium-aluminum-garnet laser. J Cosmet Dermatol. 2016;15:31-5.
15. Madura C, Ravipati N, Chandrashekhar BS. Clinical and trichoscopic correlation of scalp in patients who had undergone hair transplantation. Int J Dermoscopy. 2017;1:20-5.
16. Genedy RM, Sorour OA, Elokazy MA. Trichoscopic signs of tinea capitis: a guide for selection of appropriate antifungal. Int J Dermatol. 2021;60:471-81.
17. Kumar P, Pandhi D, Bhattacharya SN, Das S. Trichoscopy as a diagnostic tool for tinea capitis: a prospective, observational study. Int J Trichology. 2020;12:68-74.
18. Isik B, Gurel MS, Erdemir AT, Kesmezacar O. Development of skin aging scale by using dermoscopy. Skin Res Technol. 2013;19:69-74.
19. Hoffmann R. TrichoScan: a novel tool for the analysis of hair growth in vivo. J Investig Dermatol Symp Proc. 2003;8:109-15.
20. Sonthalia S, Pasquali P, Agrawal M, Sharma P, Jha AK, Errichetti E, et al. Dermoscopy update: review of its extradiagnostic and expanding indications and future prospects. Dermatol Pract Concept. 2019;9:253-64.
21. Carli P, De giorgi V, Crocetti E, Mannone F, Massi D, Chiarugi A, et al. Improvement of malignant/benign ratio in excised melanocytic lesions in the 'dermoscopy era': a retrospective study 1997-2001. Br J Dermatol. 2004; 150:687-92.
22. Sonthalia S, Errichetti E. Dermoscopy - not just for diagnosis and not just for dermatologists! Kathmandu Univ Med J (KUMJ). 2017;15:1-2.
23. Carducci M, Bozzetti M, Foscolo AM, Betti R. Margin detection using digital dermatoscopy improves the performance of traditional surgical excision of basal cell carcinomas of the head and neck. Dermatol Surg. 2011;37:280-5.
24. Piña RY, Piña RJ, Piña RJ, Castro MA, Darias DC. Dermoscopy for establishing the minimal surgical margins in basal cell carcinoma resection. Rev Méd Electrón. 2018;40:110-9.
25. Sonthalia S, Khurana R. Interventional dermoscopy. J Am Acad Dermatol. 2019;81:e129-30.
26. Kaur I, Chowdhry S, D'Souza P, Jakhar D, Yadav MK, Kaur O. Intra-operative dermoscopy in assessment of melanonychia and as a guide for biopsy. Indian Dermatol Online J. 2020;11:171-6.
27. Rai AK. Role of intraoperative dermoscopy in excision of nail unit glomus tumor. Indian Dermatol Online J. 2016;7:448-50.
28. Ginoux E, Perier muzet M, Poulalhon N, Debarbieux S, Dalle S, Thomas L. Intraoperative dermoscopic features of onychomatricoma: a review of 10 cases. Clin Exp Dermatol. 2017;42:395-9.
29. Kaur I, Jakhar D. Intraoperative onychoscopy and histopathological correlation of red lunula in nail lichen planus: a case series. Clin Exp Dermatol. 2020;45: 884-7.
30. Sonthalia S, Jha AK, Kaliyadan F. Dermoscopy for the detection and safe extraction of an intra-cutaneous foreign body. J Am Acad Dermatol. 2018;79:e19-20.
31. Goldman L. Transillumination of fingertip as aid in examination of nail changes. Arch Dermatol. 1962;85:644.
32. Ashique KT, Kaliyadan F. Transillumination: a simple tool to assess subungual extension in periungual warts. Indian Dermatol Online J. 2013;4:131-2.

33. Jakhar D, Kaur I. Transillumination dermoscopy for nail bed pathology. J Am Acad Dermatol. 2021;85(3):e137-8.
34. Kaliyadan F, Ashique KT. Nail transillumination combined with dermoscopy for enhancing diagnosis of subungual hematoma. Indian Dermatol Online J. 2018;9:105-6.
35. Kaur I, Jakhar D. Transillumination dermoscopy of finger web spaces for scabies. J Am Acad Dermatol. 2020;82:e87-8.
36. Yang YW, Yarbrough K, Mitkov M, Russi D, Price HN, Swanson DL. Polarized transilluminating dermoscopy: bedside trichoscopic diagnosis of trichothiodystrophy. Pediatr Dermatol. 2018;35:147-9.
37. Agrawal S, Dhurat R, Daruwalla S, Sharma A. A simple modification of a syringe barrel as an adaptor for dermoscopic guided biopsy. J Am Acad Dermatol. 2020;83:e5-6.
38. Jakhar D, Kaur I. Hidroscopy: in vivo videodermoscopy of the sweat glands. Skin Res Technol. 2019;25:410-1.
39. Kaur I, Jakhar D, Misri R. Hidroscopy as an adjunctive tool in the assessment of borderline tuberculoid Hansen's disease. Indian Dermatol Online J. 2020;11:1040-1.
40. Kaur I, Jakhar D. Starch-iodine test viewed through a dermoscope. J Am Acad Dermatol. 2020;83:e11-2.
41. Jakhar D, Grover C. Universal serial bus dermatoscope as an oculoscopy tool. J Am Acad Dermatol. 2018;78:e139-40.
42. Jakhar D, Grover C. Using a car phone holder for performing oculoscopy with a universal serial bus dermatoscope. J Am Acad Dermatol. 2019;80:e1-2.
43. Blum A, Giacomel J. Tape dermatoscopy: constructing a low-cost dermatoscope using a mobile phone, immersion fluid and transparent adhesive tape. Dermatol Pract Concept. 2015;5:87-93.
44. Kaliyadan F, Jayasree P, Ashique KT. Drop dermoscopy for teledermatology. J Am Acad Dermatol. 2021;84:e25-6.
45. Wu X, Oliveria SA, Yagerman S, Chen L, DeFazio J, Braun R, et al. Feasibility and efficacy of patient-initiated mobile teledermoscopy for short-term monitoring of clinically atypical nevi. JAMA Dermatol. 2015;151:489-96.
46. Vestergaard T, Prasad SC, Schuster A, Laurinaviciene R, Andersen MK, Bygum A. Diagnostic accuracy and interobserver concordance: teledermoscopy of 600 suspicious skin lesions in Southern Denmark. J Eur Acad Dermatol Venereol. 2020;34:1601-8.
47. Janda M, Horsham C, Vagenas D, Loescher LJ, Gillespie N, Koh U, et al. Accuracy of mobile digital teledermoscopy for skin self-examinations in adults at high risk of skin cancer: an open-label, randomized controlled trial. Lancet Digit Health. 2020;2:e129-37.
48. Barcaui CB, Lima PM. Application of teledermoscopy in the diagnosis of pigmented lesions. Int J Telemed Appl. 2018;2018:1624073.
49. Lee KJ, Soyer HP. Future developments in teledermoscopy and total body photography. Int J Dermatol Venereol. 2019;2:15-8.
50. Haenssle HA, Fink C, Schneiderbauer R, Toberer F, Buhl T, Blum A, et al. Man against machine: diagnostic performance of a deep learning convolutional neural network for dermoscopic melanoma recognition in comparison to 58 dermatologists. Ann Oncol. 2018;29:1836-42.
51. Merkel EA, Amin SM, Lee CY, Rademaker AW, Yazdan P, Martini MC, et al. The utility of dermoscopy-guided histologic sectioning for the diagnosis of melanocytic lesions: a case-control study. J Am Acad Dermatol. 2016;74:1107-13.
52. Moreno-Romero JA, Pérez-Muñoz N, Campoy-Sánchez A, Urbano-Carrillo M, Fernández-Figueras MT. Derm dotting: a new technique that improves diagnostic precision in the evaluation of skin lesions. Actas Dermosifiliogr. 2019;110:193-6.
53. Sonthalia S, Rahul A, Rashmi S. Cosmetic warts: pseudo-koebnerization of warts after cosmetic procedures for hair removal. J Clin Aesthet Dermatol. 2015;8:52-6.
54. Corazza M, Toni G, Scuderi V, Forconi R, Borghi A. Patch test reactions through the lens of dermoscopy: further insights, particularly on weak allergic reactions. Contact Derm. 2019;81:417-25.
55. Kecici AS, Kutlubay Z, Serdaroglu S, Tuzun Y. Pathergy testing: prospective comparison of dermatoscopic evaluation and naked eye examination. Intern Emerg Med. 2019;14:699-703.
56. Wu X, Marchetti MA, Marghoob AA. Dermoscopy: not just for dermatologists. Melanoma Manag. 2015;2:63-73.
57. Sano T, Minagawa A, Suzuki R, Koga H, Okuyama R. Dermoscopy with near-ultraviolet light highlights the demarcation of melanin distribution in cutaneous melanoma. J Am Acad Dermatol. 2021;84(1):e23-4.

19 CHAPTER

Oral Mucoscopy

Abhijeet Kumar Jha, Deepak Jakhar

INTRODUCTION

Mucoscopy is the dermoscopic examination of the mucosae (oral and genital mucosa) and its pathology.[1,2] The utility of dermoscope in examination of the mucosa is relatively new and indications of its use are expanding with time. The major challenge in mucoscopy is the standardization of the technique. Currently available instruments are less adapted for performing mucoscopy. The moist surface of mucosa, fear of contamination of instrument and cross-infection discourages many clinicians to use dermoscopes on the mucosal surfaces. Various modifications in the technique for performing mucoscopy have been suggested to overcome this challenge. The use of chalazion clamp in the oral mucosa has been suggested with contact dermoscopes (**Fig. 1**).[1] The ring part of the clamp faces the mucosal surface, following which the dermoscope can be used to scope the lesion. Similarly, for universal serial bus (USB) dermoscopes, polyethylene tube clinched between the teeth can serve as a portal for examining the oral mucosa.[2] With the ease of performing mucoscopy, the indications are expected to increase in near future. In this chapter, we have included the most commonly reported indications of mucoscopy.

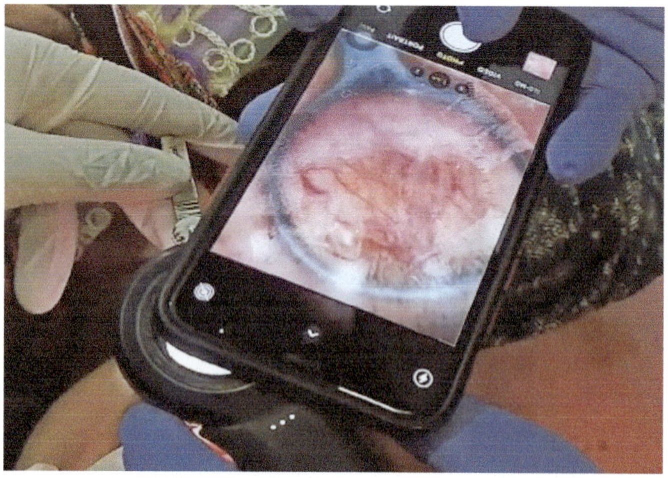

FIG. 1: Mucoscopy with a chalazion clamp. The rim of the clamp is shown in the mucoscopy image (polarized, DermLite DL4, 10×).

LICHEN PLANUS

Clinical Features

Oral lichen planus (LP) involves buccal mucosa, tongue, and gingiva and presents as reticular, papular, plaque-like, erosive, atrophic or bullous lesions.[3,4]

Dermoscopic Features

Lichen planus of the lips shows Wickham's striae (corresponding with compact orthokeratosis above zones of wedge-shaped hypergranulosis) over a pink or violaceous background and scaling (**Fig. 2**).[5,6]

Key Points

- Wickham's striae with pink or violaceous background and scales.

DISCOID LUPUS ERYTHEMATOSUS

Clinical Features

Erythematous plaque with crusting and oozing is characteristically seen on the lower lip.

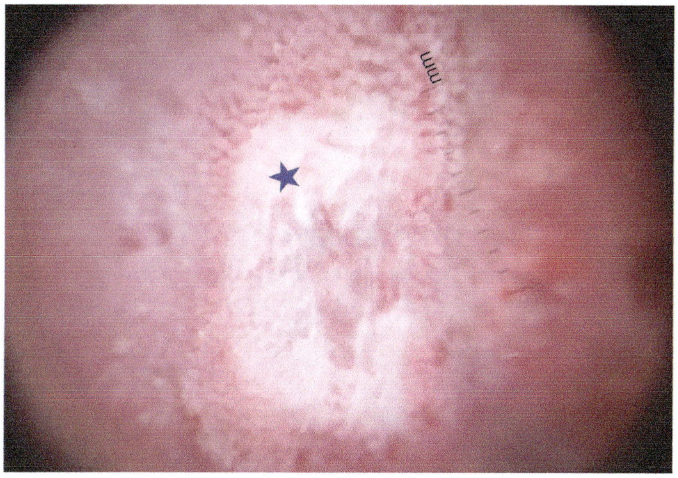

FIG. 2: Mucoscopy of lichen planus of the lip showing Wickham's striae (blue star) over a pink or violaceous background (polarized, DermLite DL4, 10×).

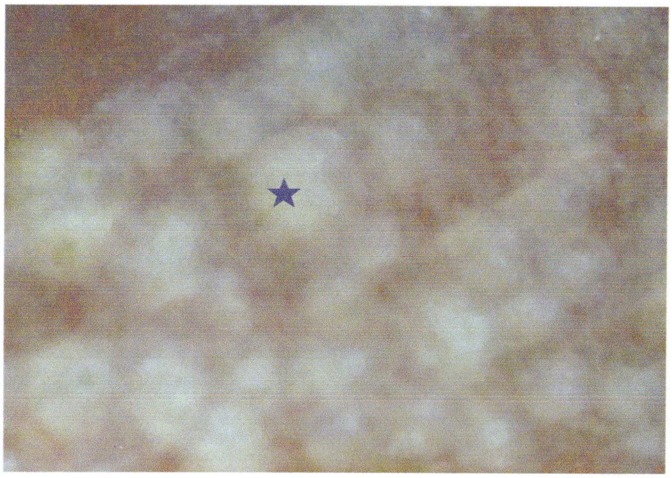

FIG. 3: Mucoscopy of Fordyce spot showing white to yellow-colored ovoid areas (blue star) (polarized, Dino-Lite AM4115ZT, 200×).

Dermoscopic Features

Hallmark of mucosal discoid lupus erythematosus (DLE) is telangiectasia, white structureless areas, and ulceration.[7] Labial DLE presents with telangiectasia, brown pigment spots, scales, white structureless areas, bleeding spots, and erosions.[8] Grayish-black to brown pigment dots observed on mucoscopy possibly represent pigment incontinence, whitish-yellow scales correlate with hyperparakeratosis, white structureless areas with irregular hyperplasia, and finally pink background and dilated vessels represent the prominent inflammatory infiltrate.

Key Points

- Telangiectasia, brown pigment spots, scales, white structureless areas, bleeding spots, and erosions are definitive features.

FORDYCE SPOTS

Clinical Features

Fordyce spots (FSs) are ectopic sebaceous glands commonly reported on lips, buccal mucosa, and genital mucosa.

Dermoscopic Features

Mucoscopy of FS shows whitish to yellowish discrete ovoid structures surrounded by linear and branching vessels (**Fig. 3**). Each FS shows opacity in the center indicating the opening of the sebaceous gland onto the epithelial surface.[9]

Key Points

- Mucoscopy of FS shows whitish to yellowish discrete ovoid structures surrounded by linear and branching vessels.

VASCULAR LESIONS

Venous Lake

Clinical Features

Venous lake (VL) most commonly appears as a dark blue or red, soft nodule/plaque on the lower lip (**Fig. 4**).

Dermoscopic Features

It shows either structureless pattern or globules of purple, red or bluish color which correspond to the spaces filled with erythrocytes, sometimes with thrombi.[10-12] On polarized mucoscopy, shiny white lines or shiny white structureless areas may be observed (**Fig. 5**).

Key Points

- Purple or blue or red globules with white shiny streaks are noted.

Pyogenic Granuloma

Clinical Features

Pyogenic granuloma (PG) is an acquired, benign vascular proliferation affecting skin and mucosa.

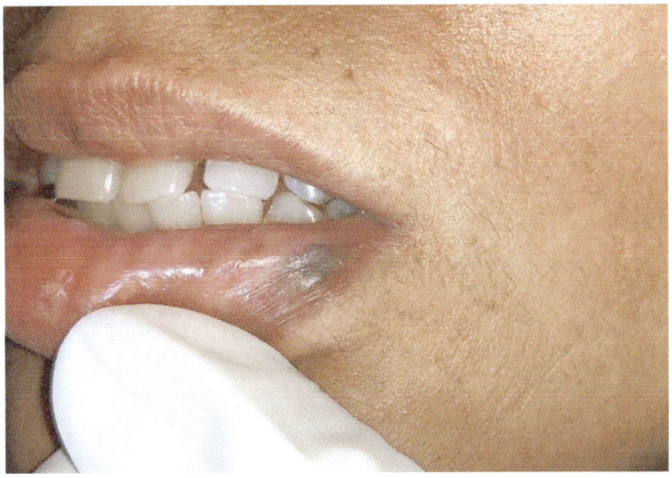

FIG. 4: Clinical image of venous lake shows bluish plaque on the lower lip.
Courtesy: Dr Sneha Gandhi, Consultant Dermatologist, Karnal, Haryana, India.

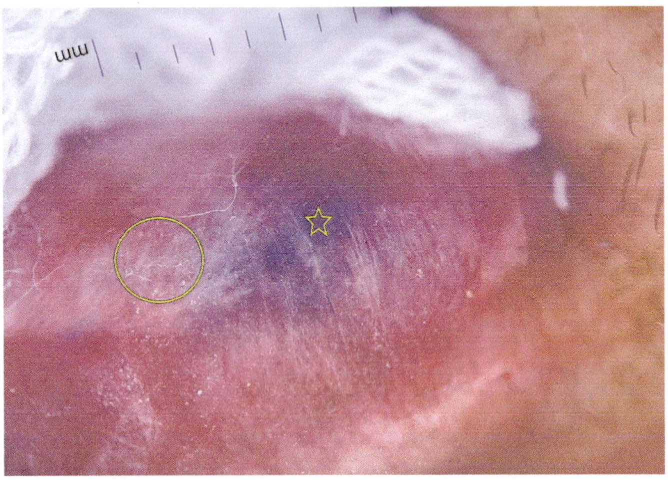

FIG. 5: Mucoscopy of venous lake shows bluish globules (star) with white shiny streaks (circle) (polarized, DermLite DL4, 10×).
Courtesy: Dr Sneha Gandhi, Consultant Dermatologist, Karnal, Haryana, India.

Dermoscopic Features

Mucoscopy shows reddish homogeneous areas (corresponding with proliferating vessels), white collarette (hyperplastic adnexal epithelium that embraces the lesion at the periphery) as well as white lines corresponding to a fibrous septa intersecting the lobules (**Fig. 6**).[13,14]

Key Points

- Reddish homogeneous areas, white collarette as well as white lines.

Angiokeratoma

Clinical Features

It presents with small red to purplish papule with slight scaling.

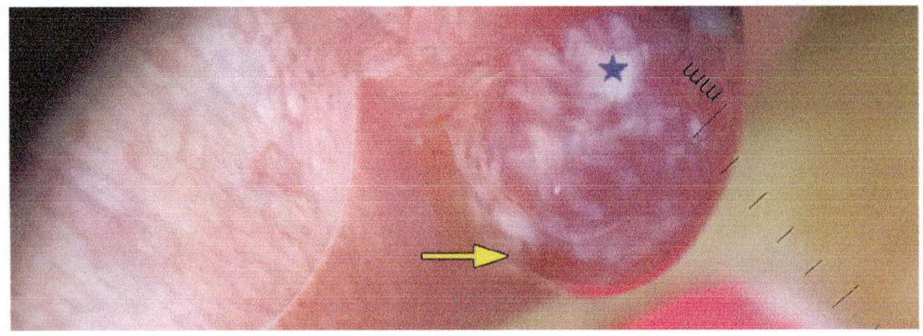

FIG. 6: Mucoscopy of pyogenic granuloma showing reddish homogeneous areas (yellow arrow), white-to-yellow collarette as well as white lines (blue star) corresponding to fibrous septa intersecting the lobules (polarized, DermLite DL4, 10×).

Dermoscopic Features

Only one dermoscopic report concerning oral localization of angiokeratoma (AK), namely angiokeratoma circumscriptum of the tongue, has been reported. The lesion showed multiple red-bluish lacunae, whitish veil, and milky-red areas corresponding with dilated and congested vessels underlying hyperplastic squamous epithelium.[15]

Key Points

- Multiple red-bluish lacunae, whitish veil, and milky-red areas.

Mucocele

Clinical Features

Extravasation mucocele (EM) is associated with extravasation of salivary gland secretions from the salivary gland duct into surrounding tissues. In contrast, obstruction of the salivary gland duct leads to retention mucocele (RM) formation.

Dermoscopic Features

Mucoscopy features reported include shiny surface with extensive vascular network (linear and branched vessels) and white structureless areas (corresponding to the hyperplastic epithelium) (**Fig. 7**).[16,17]

Key Points

- Shiny surface with extensive vascular network and white structureless areas are characteristics.

Fixed Drug Eruption

Clinical Features

Fixed drug eruption (FDE) is one of the most prevalent cutaneous drug-induced reactions with wide clinical spectrum.

Dermoscopic Features

In a patient with FDE involving the lower lip area, dermoscopy revealed the presence of brownish-black, gray, and steel blue dots (**Fig. 8**).[18,19]

Key Points

- Brownish-black, gray, and steel blue dots.

Mucosal Wart

Clinical Features

It appears as soft, pink or white papule on the gingival mucosa.

Dermoscopic Features

Mucoscopy shows finger-like projection with hairpin-like/glomerular vessel within the projection (**Fig. 9**).

Key Points

- Finger-like projection with hairpin-like/glomerular vessel.

Leukoplakia

Clinical Features

Asymptomatic white patch on the labial mucosa, which cannot be rubbed off, is characteristic.

Dermoscopic Features

Mucoscopy of leukoplakia shows white structureless areas, surface corrugations, intervening pink lines and dotted vessels in irregular distribution (**Fig. 10**).[20]

Key Points

- White structureless areas with surface corrugations and intervening pink lines.

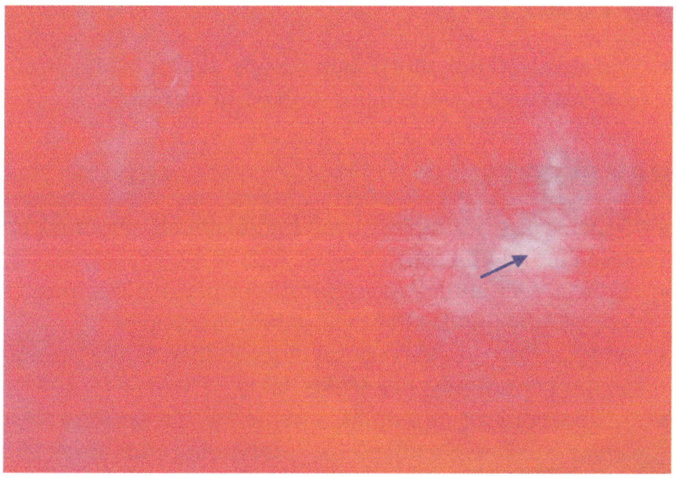

FIG. 7: Mucoscopy of mucocele showing shiny surface with extensive vascular network (linear and branched vessels) and white structureless areas (blue arrow) (polarized, Dino-Lite AM4115ZT, 200×).

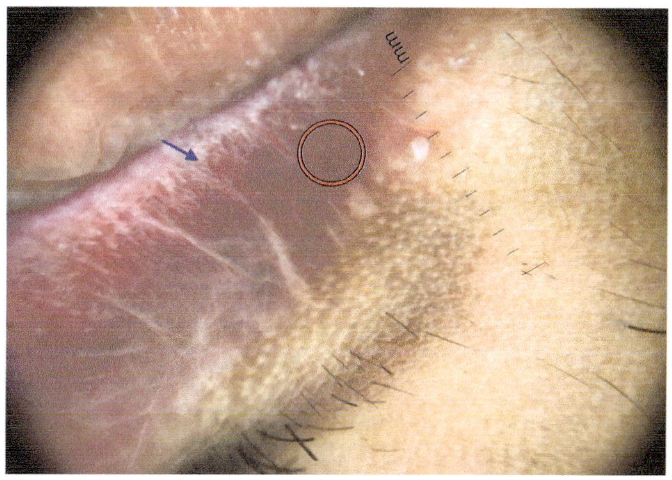

FIG. 8: Mucoscopy of fixed drug eruption on lower lip showing brownish-black, gray, and steel blue-colored areas (red circle) and dots (blue arrow) (polarized, DermLite DL4, 10×).

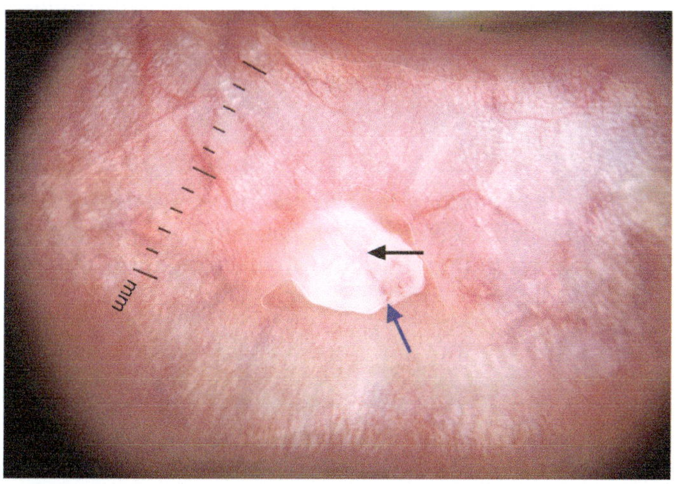

FIG. 9: Mucoscopy of wart showing finger-like projection with hairpin-like (black arrow) and glomerular (blue arrow) vessel within the projection (polarized, Dino-Lite AM4115ZT, 50×).

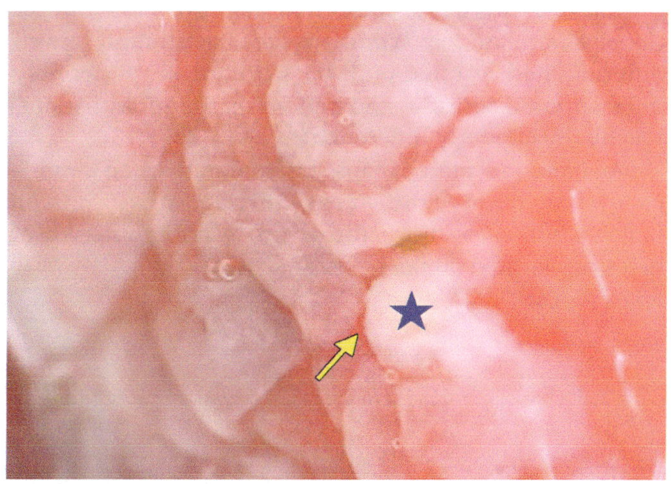

FIG. 10: Mucoscopy of leukoplakia showing white structureless areas (blue star), surface corrugations and intervening pink lines (yellow arrow) (polarized, Dino-Lite AM4115ZT, 50×).

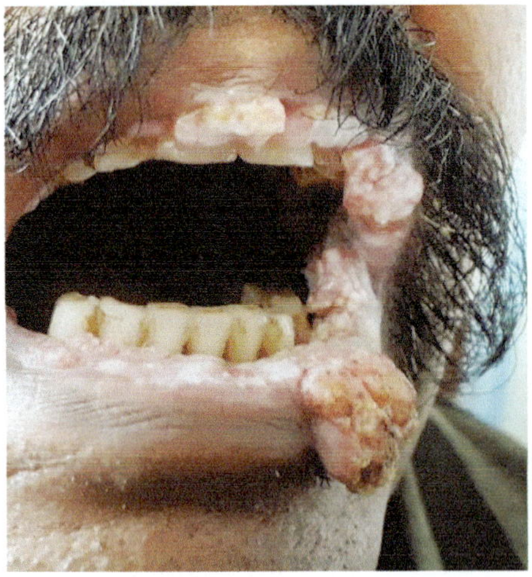

FIG. 11: Clinical image of squamous cell carcinoma shows fungating cauliflower-like growth on the firm nodules.

Courtesy: Dr Nagesh TS, Sapthagiri Medical College, Bengaluru, Karnataka, India.

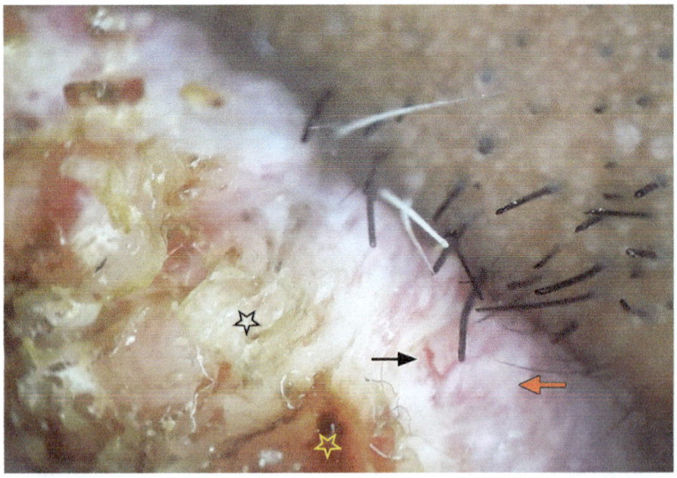

FIG. 12: Mucoscopy of squamous cell carcinoma shows white areas (red arrow), atypical vessels (black arrow), and white-crusted areas (black star). Note the blood spots (yellow star) (polarized, DermLite DL4, 10×).

Courtesy: Dr Nagesh TS, Sapthagiri Medical College, Bengaluru, Karnataka, India.

Squamous Cell Carcinoma

Clinical Features

It presents as firm nodule with scaling, crusting, and oozing (**Fig. 11**).

Dermoscopic Features

Mucoscopy of lip squamous cell carcinoma (SCC) is characterized by the presence of small nonfocused polymorphous vessels, scales, white structureless areas, white halos, and white circles (**Fig. 12**). White circles, on mucoscopy, are useful clues for diagnosing lip SCCs, and differentiating it from actinic cheilitis. White circles are seen predominantly in SCCs (59%) as compared to actinic cheilitis (13%).[21]

Presence of white color in various mucoscopy structures is related to well- or moderately-differentiated variants of SCC. Dark phototypes may also show brown-to-gray dots/globules. Background coloration also provides clue for tumor differentiation: Whitish-yellow background in well-differentiated lesions, pink background in moderately-differentiated lesions, and red background with dense vascularity in poorly-differentiated lesions.[22]

An incisional punch biopsy is mandatory when dermoscopy reveals one or more of these criteria such as ulceration, scales, white-colored structures, and polymorphous vessels in lesions located on the lower lip.

Key Points

- Nonfocused polymorphous vessels, scales, white structureless areas, white halos, and white circles.

KEY POINTS

- Mucoscopy is a rapidly evolving diagnostic tool for oral and genital mucosae.
- Special techniques are required for performing mucoscopy using handheld or videodermatoscopes.
- Mucoscopy provides useful clues in identifying premalignant conditions like leukoplakia.
- Mucoscopy of leukoplakia shows white structureless areas, surface corrugations, intervening pink lines and dotted vessels.
- Mucoscopy of DLE shows telangiectasia, white structureless areas, and ulceration.
- White circles on mucoscopy give a clue toward SCC.
- Biopsy is indicated if mucoscopy shows—ulceration, scales, white-colored structures, and polymorphous vessels in lesions.

CONCLUSION

The rapidly expanding field of mucoscopy gives valuable clues to aid in the diagnosis of various mucosal pathologies. Initial reports in literature are encouraging to propose its use in daily clinical practice.

REFERENCES

1. Jha AK, Pathak J. Using a chalazion clamp to enhance dermoscopy of oral mucosal lesions. J Am Acad Dermatol. 2017;76(3):e91-2.
2. Jakhar D, Grover C. Innovative modification of the USB dermatoscope for mucoscopy. J Am Acad Dermatol. 2018;78(1):e3-4.
3. Lavanya N, Jayanthi P, Rao UK, Ranganathan K. Oral lichen planus: an update on pathogenesis and treatment. J Oral Maxillofac Pathol. 2011;15(2): 127-32.
4. Martinez JK, Guevara BE, Visitacion LR. Atypical cutaneous and mucosal lichen planus in a 53-year-old Filipino male: case report. SPMC J Health Care Serv. 2017;3(1):1.
5. Mathur M, Acharya P, Karki A, Kc N, Shah J, Jha A. Isolated lichen planus of lip: diagnosis and treatment monitoring using dermoscopy. Clin Case Rep. 2018;7(1):146-8.
6. Sonthalia S, Varma S, Jha AK, Jakhar D, Kaliyadan F. Case report: dermoscopic features of oral lichen planus - the evolution of mucoscopy. F1000Res. 2018;7:284.
7. Chandela M, Misri R, Jakhar D. Mucoscopy of discoid lupus erythematosus on lower lip. Indian Dermatol Online J. 2020;11:296-7.
8. Salah E. Clinical and dermoscopic spectrum of discoid lupus erythematosus: novel observations from lips and oral mucosa. Int J Dermatol. 2018;57(7): 830-6.
9. Jakhar D, Kaur I. Mucoscopy of Fordyce's spots on lips. Indian Dermatol Online J. 2019;10(4):498-9.
10. Jha AK, Pathak J. Mucoscopy of a venous lake. Dermatol Pract Concept. 2019;9(1):20-1.
11. Jha AK, Zeeshan MD, Jha Amar AK. Mucoscopy in lingual varicosities. Dermatol Pract Concept. 2018;8(1):54-5.
12. Lee JS, Mun JH. Dermoscopy of venous lake on the lips: a comparative study with labial melanotic macule. PLoS One. 2018;13(10):e0206768.
13. Oiso N, Kawada A. Dermoscopy of pyogenic granuloma on the lip: the differing appearances of vascular structures with and without pressure. Eur J Dermatol. 2011;21(3):441.
14. Kissou A, Hassam BE. Dermoscopy of pyogenic granuloma. Pan Afr Med J. 2017;27:110.
15. Eskiizmir G, Gencoglan G, Temiz P, Ermertcan AT. Angiokeratoma circumscriptum of the tongue. Cutan Ocul Toxicol. 2011;30(3):231-3.
16. Ayhan E, Toprak SF, Kaya Ş, Akkaynak Ş. Dermoscopy of oral mucocele: three types of extravasation mucoceles. Turk J Med Sci. 2020;50(1):96-102.
17. Kaur I, Jakhar D, Anand P. Mucoscopy of mucocele. Indian Dermatol Online J. 2019;10(3):358-9.
18. Sławińska M, Barańska-Rybak W, Wilkowska A, Nowicki R. Bullous fixed drug eruption due to fluconazole, imitating herpes simplex. Clin Exp Dermatol. 2017;42(5):544-5.
19. Kumar Jha A, Vinay K, Sławińska M, Sonthalia S, Sobjanek M, Kami⊠ska-Winciorek G, et al. Application of mucous membrane dermoscopy (mucoscopy) in diagnostics of benign oral lesions - literature review and preliminary observations from International Dermoscopy Society study. Dermatol Ther. 2021;34(1):e14478.
20. Okamoto T, Tanaka M, Kaibuchi N, Kuwazawa T, Ando T. Correlation between dermoscopic and histopathological findings of leucoplakia of the tongue: a case report. Br J Oral Maxillofac Surg. 2018;56(8):758-60.
21. Benati E, Persechino F, Piana S, Argenziano G, Lallas A, Moscarella E, et al. Dermoscopic features of squamous cell carcinoma on the lips. Br J Dermatol. 2017;177:e41-3.
22. Jha AK, Sonthalia S, Sławińska M, Lallas A, Vinay K, Sobjanek M, et al. Mucoscopy of lip squamous cell carcinoma and correlation with skin phototype and histological differentiation: a multicentric retrospective observational study by the International Dermoscopy Society. Int J Dermatol. 2021;60(4):489-96.

R

S

T

U

V

W

X

Y